S0-AFE-800

Broadribb's *Introductory Pediatric Nursing*

Fourth Edition

Broadribb's *Introductory Pediatric Nursing*

Fourth Edition

Margaret G. Marks, RN, BSNE

Instructor
Juniata-Mifflin Area Vocational Technical School
Lewistown, Pennsylvania

J. B. Lippincott Company
Philadelphia

Sponsoring Editor: Jennifer E. Brogan
Project Editor: Jim Slade
Indexer: Ellen Murray
Design Coordinator: Melissa Olson
Interior Designer: Anne O'Donnell
Cover Designer: William T. Donnelly
Production Manager: Helen Ewan
Production Coordinator: Nannette Winski
Compositor: Circle Graphics
Printer/Binder: Courier Book Company/Kendallville
Cover Printer: Lehigh Press

Fourth Edition

Copyright © 1994, by J. B. Lippincott Company.

Copyright © 1983, 1973, 1967 by J. B. Lippincott Company. All rights reserved. No part of this book may be used or reproduced in any manner whatsoever without written permission except for brief quotations embodied in critical articles and reviews. Printed in the United States of America. For information write J. B. Lippincott Company, 227 East Washington Square, Philadelphia, PA 19106.

Cover photograph of jigsaw puzzle "Child's Play" used with permission by Ceaco, Inc. © 1988.

1 3 5 6 4 2

Library of Congress Cataloging-in-Publication Data

Marks, Margaret G.
    Broadribb's introductory pediatric nursing.—4th ed. / Margaret
G. Marks.
        p. cm.
    Rev. ed of: Introductory pediatric nursing / Violet Broadribb. 3rd
ed. c1983.
    Includes bibliographical references and index.
    ISBN 0-397-54946-6
    1. Pediatric nursing.   I. Broadribb, Violet.   Introductory
pediatric nursing.   II. Title.   III. Title: Introductory pediatric
nursing.
    [DNLM: 1. Pediatric Nursing.   WY 159 M3455b   1994]
RJ245.B764   1994
610.73'62—dc20
DNLM/DLC
for Library of Congress   93-34321
                                                                CIP

Any procedure or practice described in this book should be applied by the health care practitioner under appropriate supervision in accordance with professional standards of care used with regard to the unique circumstances that apply in each practice situation. Care has been taken to confirm the accuracy of information presented and to describe generally accepted practices. However, the authors, editors, and publisher cannot accept any responsibility for errors or omissions or for any consequences from application of the information in this book and make no warranty, express or implied, with respect to the contents of the book.

Every effort has been made to ensure drug selections and dosages are in accordance with current recommendations and practice. Because of ongoing research, changes in government regulations, and the constant flow of information on drug therapy, reactions, and interactions, the reader is cautioned to check the package insert for each drug for indications, dosages, warnings, and precautions, particularly if the drug is new or infrequently used.

To April, Eddie, Shane, and Chelsea—
the lights of my life—
with much love from their Honey,
and to their parents,
Jeff and Anita and Tracey and Randy,
my wonderful, supporting children.

Reviewers

Deborah Cooper Connelly, RNC, MSN, CDE
Coordinator Level IV
Department of Practical Nursing
Bishop State Community College, Southwest Campus
Mobile, Alabama

Sherry G. Fader, RNC, BSN, MSN
Chair, Practical Nursing
Quincy College
Quincy, Massachusetts

Sheila F. Guidry, RN, DSN
Director Practical Nursing Program and
    Nursing Assistant/Home Health Aide Program
Wallace Community College
Selma, Alabama

Margrit E. (Betsy) Hayes, BSN, RN
Instructor
Otsego Area School of Practical Nursing
Milford, New York

Marion E. Monahan, RN, BSE, MAEd
Coordinator of Practical Nursing
Jeff Tech Practical Nursing Program
Reynoldsville, Pennsylvania

Bennita W. Vaughans, RN, MSN
Instructor
Trenholm State Technical College
Montgomery, Alabama

Preface

*I*n the last decade social changes have occurred that have deeply affected the lives of children and their families. In addition, health care delivery has changed and will continue to change throughout the remainder of this century, primarily due to the demands for health care cost containment. We have used previous editions of Broadribb's *Introductory Pediatric Nursing* with pleasure and believed it had an important role to fulfill in educating basic nurses in the care of children and their families. We believed that the obvious love and caring for children that was evident in past editions was fundamental to the flavor of the text. However, because of the social, cultural, and technological changes since the last edition, a revision was greatly needed. With this in mind, we undertook a major revision.

In revising this text we recognized that some of the underlying suppositions of the previous edition were no longer relevant. The child is no longer referred to as "he," but, throughout the text, is referred to in nongender specific terms or, when needed for clarity, is referred to as "he or she." Likewise, terminology was changed to family caregivers rather than parents because a large number of children no longer live in two-parent family homes. Nurses also are referred to in nongender specific terms in recognition that there are many excellent nurses, both male and female, who provide nursing care to children in a variety of settings. The cultural views of the text also have been broadened to represent the current cultural blend in the United States.

As health care has changed, more of the responsibility for caring for ill children has fallen on the family caregivers. With this in mind, increased emphasis has been placed on the responsibilities of the nurse in teaching the child and family. The nursing process has been used as the foundation for presenting nursing care. Although planning and implementation are individual steps in the nursing process, they are combined in this text in order to provide a structure for a narrative presentation. In this way, possible interventions are discussed on the basis from which planning and implementation can be put into action.

A concentrated effort was made to keep the readability of the text to a level with which the new student can be comfortable. In recognition of the limited time that the student has and the frustration that can result from having to turn to a dictionary or glossary for words that are unfamiliar, we have attempted to identify all possible unfamiliar terms and define them within the text. This increases the reading ease for the student, decreasing the time necessary to complete the assigned reading and enhancing the understanding of the information.

Features

In an effort to provide the instructor and student with a text that is informative, exciting, and easy to use, we have incorporated a number of features throughout the text, many of which are included in each chapter. The principal features include:

Chapter Outline—Each chapter opens with an outline providing the reader with an overall view of the chapter's main topics and organization.

Key Terms—A list of terms that may be unfamiliar to students and that are considered essential to the chapter's understanding appears at the beginning of each chapter. The first appearance in the chapter of each of these terms is in boldface type, with the definition included in the text. All key terms also are included in a glossary at the end of the text.

Student Objectives—Behavioral objectives also are included at the beginning of each chapter. These help to guide the student in recognizing the focus of the chapter.

Nursing Process—The nursing process serves as an organizing structure for the discussion of nursing care for many of the health problems covered in the text. These provide the student with a foundation from which individualized care plans can be developed. Each nursing process section includes nursing assessment, relevant nursing diagnoses, planning and implementation, and evaluation criteria for each of the proposed diagnoses. Emphasis is placed on the importance of involving the child and the family caregivers in the assessment process. We have selected nursing diagnoses to represent appropriate concerns for a particular condition, but we do not attempt to include all diagnoses that could be identified. Evaluation criteria provide guidelines for specific observations that encourage identification of measurable results.

Nursing Care Plans—Throughout the text nursing care plans are presented to provide the student with a model to follow in using the information from the nursing process to develop specific nursing care plans.

Parent Teaching Boxes—Information that the student can use in teaching family caregivers and children is presented in highlighted boxes ready for use.

Tables, Drawings, and Photographs—These important aspects of the text have been updated and clarified with the addition of new material throughout.

Chapter Summaries—Summaries are brief but serve to give the student and the instructor a review of the important aspects of information in the chapter.

Review Questions—Review questions at the end of each chapter encourage the student to think about the chapter content in practical terms. Many situational questions require the student to incorporate the knowledge gained from the chapter and apply it to real life problems. The review questions also can serve the instructor as a tool for stimulating class discussion.

Bibliography—Each bibliography contains updated references that the student can readily turn to for additional information on conditions discussed in the chapter.

Organization

The text is divided into five units to provide for an orderly approach to the content. The basic approach to the study of health problems of children is organized within a framework of growth and development. Growth and development is presented for an age group, and the specific health problems that commonly affect that age group are discussed in the following chapter. This approach has been well received by nursing students and continues to provide a user-friendly approach to the study of nursing care of children.

Unit I, The Child, the Family, and Health Care, introduces the student in Chapter 1 to a brief history of pediatrics and pediatric nursing and a glimpse at the change that has taken place in the nursing care of children. Following this is a discussion of the family, its structure, and the family factors that influence the growth and development of children. Concepts of child development are presented to provide a foundation for discussion in later chapters on growth and development. Chapter 2, The Child in the Hospital, covers admission of the child to the hospital, an introduction to the nursing process, and special aspects

of pediatric nursing, emphasizing the importance of safety in pediatric nursing. Chapter 3 presents basic nursing procedures, infection control in the pediatric setting, and general preoperative and postoperative care of the child undergoing surgery. This unit serves as an introduction to pediatric nursing so that the student can function in a pediatric unit while completing the remainder of the course of study.

Unit II, A Child is Born, presents prenatal and newborn nursing care. Chapter 4 covers prenatal growth and development including the influence of heredity and environment and parenthood education. Chapter 5 covers the normal newborn, daily care, and family interaction. Chapter 6 addresses the health problems of the high-risk newborn, including the premature infant. Chapter 7 covers the newborn with special needs and includes congenital anomalies, inborn errors of metabolism, and other congenital problems.

Unit III, A Child Grows, is organized by developmental stages, from infancy through adolescence. The even-numbered chapters cover growth and development of the designated age group and the odd-numbered chapters follow with health problems common to that age. Although many conditions are not limited to a specific age, they are included in the age group in which they most often occur. The nursing process and nursing care plans are integrated through this unit.

Unit IV, A Child in a Troubled Society, focuses on several societal problems and their effect on children. Chapter 18 discusses the impact that substance abuse has on the child, related health problems, and nursing care of the child and the family. Chapter 19 explores the problems of the child in a stressed family, including the issues of child abuse, runaway children, latchkey children, children of divorces, and homeless children and families.

Unit V, A Child Faces Chronic or Terminal Illness, examines in Chapter 20 the concerns that face the family of a child with a chronic illness. The impact on the family of caring for a child with a chronic illness and the nurse's role in assisting and supporting these families is discussed. Chapter 21 concludes with the dying child. Included in this chapter is a teaching aid to help the nurse perform a self-examination of personal attitudes about death and dying as well as concrete guidelines to use when interacting with a grieving child or adult.

Throughout the text family-centered care is stressed. Developmental enrichment and stimulation are stressed in the sections on nursing process. The basic premise of each child's self worth is fundamental in all of the nursing care presented.

Acknowledgments

When the thought of revising Broadribb's *Introductory Pediatric Nursing* was first introduced to me, I was more than a little overwhelmed. However, with the encouragement and support of my family, friends, and colleagues it has slowly become a reality. The process has turned into one that was much more encompassing than I had ever imagined, and it has been a very exciting experience.

I wish to thank Sylvia Swineford, our nursing program coordinator, for her early and continuous support, especially when I became frustrated and depressed over my own lack of progress at times. She helped make time available to me within the constraints of my teaching responsibilities and always acknowledged the magnitude of the undertaking.

Special thanks to Ann West, who has helped in countless ways and was always there for me when I needed support or someone to "go to bat" for me. She performed so many of the mundane jobs for me that were essential to the successful completion of the text. Ann's expertise is evident in much of the finished chapters.

The reviewers, who remained anonymous to me, made significant contributions. The enthusiasm that was conveyed in their responses was deeply appreciated.

I especially wish to thank Ruth Anne Sieber for sharing so generously with me her materials on children, death, and dying. Ruth Anne's experience as a pediatric nurse and a hospice nurse gave her the outstanding credentials to supply me with just what I needed to make the last chapter of the text a sensitive and warm treatment of a difficult subject.

My appreciation for everyone at Lippincott who had a part in seeing this edition through to the final production stage. My editor, Jennifer Brogan, was very supportive and always had a positive and kind word for me. Special thanks to Melissa Olson for the wonderful cover and design. Jim Slade, Project Editor, Helen Ewan, Production Manager, and many other people unknown to me personally have been instrumental in its completion, for which I am very grateful.

Contents

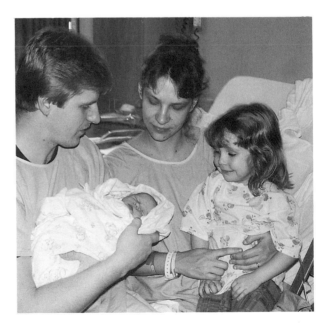

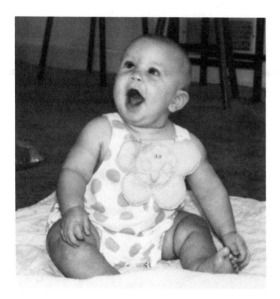

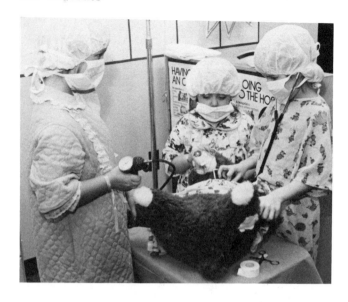

Broadribb's *Introductory Pediatric Nursing*

Fourth Edition

The Child, the Family, and Health Care

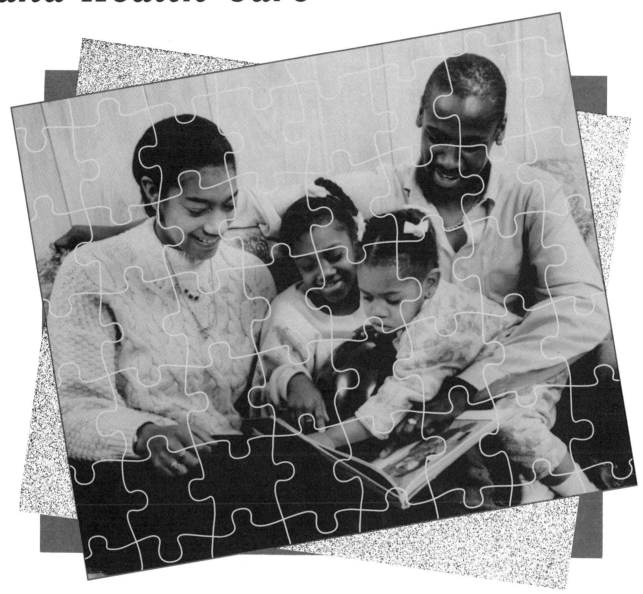

Unit I

Health Care, the Child, and the Family

Student Objectives

Upon completion of this chapter, the student will be able to:

1. State where the infant mortality rate in the United States ranks when compared with the infant mortality rate of other developed countries.
2. State two causes of the high rate of infant mortality in the United States.
3. Describe the post-World War I atmosphere in the care of children and its effect on those children.
4. Identify the principles on which family-centered nursing is based.
5. Identify the primary purpose of the family in society.
6. List the functions of the family in relation to children.
7. Describe the process of socialization.
8. Describe how parents influence the psychological and emotional health of a child.
9. Name and discuss the two traditional kinds of family structure.
10. List four factors that have contributed to the growing number of single-parent families.
11. Describe three types of nontraditional families.
12. Describe how children are affected by the following: a) Family size; b) Sibling order.
13. Explain how family relationships and communications are affected by the following: a) Working parents; b) Other parental behaviors.
14. State three factors that influence the way that children react to divorce.
15. List and discuss the six stages of psychosexual development according to Sigmund Freud.
16. Describe Erikson's theory of psychosocial development.
17. Name the eight stages of Erikson's psychosocial development, and list developmental tasks in each.
18. Identify and describe the four stages of Piaget's theory of cognitive development.

Marks MG: BROADRIBB'S INTRODUCTORY PEDIATRIC NURSING, 4th ed. © 1994 J.B. Lippincott Company.

Key Terms

archetypes	id
blended family	libido
cognitive development	nuclear family
communal family	pediatric nurse
development	practitioner (PNP)
developmental task	primary nursing
ego	single-parent family
egocentric	socialization
extended family	stepfamily
growth	sublimation
health maintenance organizations (HMOs)	superego

*T*he nurse preparing to care for today's and tomorrow's children and families faces vastly different responsibilities and challenges than did the pediatric nurse of three or four decades ago. Nurses and other health professionals are becoming increasingly concerned with much more than the care of sick children. Health teaching, prevention of illness, and promotion of optimal (most desirable or satisfactory) physical, developmental, and emotional health are all part of contemporary nursing (Table 1-1).

Scientific and technologic advances have reduced the incidence of communicable disease and have helped to control metabolic disorders such as diabetes. Much of health care takes place outside the hospital, either at home or in clinics or physicians' offices. Prenatal diagnosis of birth defects, transfusions, and other treatments for the unborn fetus as well as improved life-support systems for premature infants are but a few examples of the remarkable progress in child care.

Controversy rages about choices in family planning. In January 1973, a Supreme Court decision declared abortion legal anywhere in the United States. In 1981, efforts were made to convince Congress that legislation should be passed to make all abortions illegal on the alleged

grounds that the fetus is a person and therefore has the right to life. In the 1990s, bitter debate between pro-life and pro-choice groups is still raging and seems likely to continue for some years.

Tremendous sociologic changes have affected attitudes toward, and concepts in, child health. American society is largely suburban, with a population of highly mobile people and families. The women's movement has focused new attention on the needs of families in which the mother works outside the home. Escalation in divorce rates, changes in attitudes toward sexual roles, and general acceptance of unmarried mothers have increased the number of single-parent families. Many people have come to regard health care as a right, not a privilege, and expect fair value received for their investment.

The reduction in communicable and infectious diseases has made it possible to devote more attention to such critical problems as child abuse, learning and behavior disorders, developmental disabilities, and chronic illness. Research in these areas continues, and as these findings become available, nurses will be among the practitioners who will help translate this research into improved health care for children and families.

The ability of nurses to translate the relevant medical research into practice, however, is based on their understanding of the predictable but variable phases of a child's growth and development and their understanding of and sensitivity to the importance of family interactions.

Changing Concepts in Child Health Care

Child health care has evolved from a sideline of internal medicine to a specialty that focuses on the child and the child's family in health and illness, through all phases of development. Technologic advances account for many of the changes seen in the last 100 years, but sociologic changes, in particular, society's view of the child and the child's needs, have been just as important.

Infant Mortality

Despite remarkable advances in many areas of maternal and child health, the maternal and infant mortality statistics are still grim. Infant mortality declined steadily in the 1960s and 1970s, but the 1980s saw a stall in that decline.

Table 1-1. United States Goals for the Year 2000

Categories	Targeted for Reduction
Physical activity and fitness	Overweight among adolescents
Nutrition	Growth retardation among low-income children 5 years of age and younger
Tobacco	Start of cigarette smoking by children and youth Smoking during pregnancy Exposure of children ≤6 years of age to smoking in the home Smokeless tobacco use by adolescent and young adult males
Alcohol and other drugs	Alcohol-related accidents causing death Drug-related deaths Hospital visits resulting from drug abuse
Family planning	Number of pregnancies in females ≤17 years of age Number of unplanned pregnancies Number of infertile couples
Mental health and mental disorders	Suicides among 15–19 year olds Suicide attempts among 14–17 year olds Mental disorders in children and adolescents
Violent and abusive behavior	Homicides in 15–35 year olds Violent deaths related to weapons Physical, sexual, and emotional abuse and neglect in children Spousal abuse against women Assault injuries in those older than 12 years of age Rape and attempted rape of women 12–34 years of age
Unintentional injuries	Drownings in children ≤4 years of age Death in home fires in children ≤4 years of age Poisonings in children ≤4 years of age
Environmental health	Asthma in children ≤14 years of age Mental retardation in school-age children Blood lead levels over 15μg/dL in children ≤5 years of age
Oral health	Dental caries in children of all ages
Maternal and infant health	Infant mortality by 1/3 Fetal death rate by 1/3 Maternal death rate by 1/2 Incidence of fetal alcohol syndrome
HIV infection	HIV infection in women giving birth to live-born infants

Sexually transmitted diseases	Incidence of:
	   Gonorrhea in adolescents 15–19 years of age
	   Chlamydia trachomatis infections
	   Primary and secondary syphilis
	   Congenital syphilis
	   Genital herpes and genital warts
	   Pelvic inflammatory disease
	   Sexually transmitted hepatitis B

Immunization and infectious diseases	Diarrhea in children in child care centers Acute otitis media in children ≤4 years of age
Age-related objectives	Death rate for children and adolescents

Adapted from U.S. Department of Health and Human Services. Healthy People, 2000. Washington, DC: Public Health Service, 1990.

In 1990, the United States ranked 21st in the rate of infant deaths among developed countries (Figure 1-1).

Both infant and maternal mortality rates are much higher among nonwhite populations, a fact that studies repeatedly attribute to lack of adequate prenatal care and an increased birth rate among women 15 to 19 years of age, a high-risk group (Figure 1-2). Of even greater concern is the fact that cities such as Washington, DC, Philadelphia, and Detroit have twice the national infant mortality rate, making them infant mortality "disaster areas."[1]

National Commission to Prevent Infant Mortality

In 1986, Congress established the National Commission to Prevent Infant Mortality and charged it with the responsibility of creating a national strategic plan to reduce infant mortality and morbidity rates in the United States. The Commission's first report, in 1988, *Death Before Life: The Tragedy of Infant Mortality*, set out recommendations on which the Commission vowed to concentrate listing two primary objectives: to make the health of mothers and babies a national priority and to provide universal access to care for all pregnant women and children. The Commission concluded that educating the nation about the health needs of mothers and babies will cause national response to the problem. Women must be empowered with information and motivation to reduce infant mortality and morbidity rates. The Commission also has stated that barriers of finances, geography, education, social position, behavior, and program administration problems must be eliminated to provide universal access to health care. In various reports published by the Commission, ample evidence indicated that low birth weight and late or nonexistent prenatal care were main factors in our country's poor rank in infant mortality. In February 1990, the Commission published *Troubling Trends: The Health of the Next Generation*, which concluded that early prenatal care, along with smoking cessation, pregnancy planning, and nutrition counseling with food supplementation, will result in heavier and healthier infants. In the statistics that the Commission gathered and published, clear evidence showed that low birth weight and infant mortality were closely linked.

Institutional Care

Pediatrics is a relatively new medical specialty, developing only in the mid-1800s. The first children's hospital opened in Philadelphia in 1855. Until that point in Western civilization, children were not considered important except as contributors to family income. Children had been cared for in hospitals as adults were, often in the same bed.

Unfortunately, early institutions for children were notorious for their unsanitary conditions, neglect, and lack of proper infant nutrition. Well into the 19th century, mortality rates were commonly 50% to 100% among institutionalized children, whether in asylums or hospitals.

During the early 1900s, a primary cause of death in children's institutions was the intractable diarrhea most of these children developed. Initiation of the simple prac-

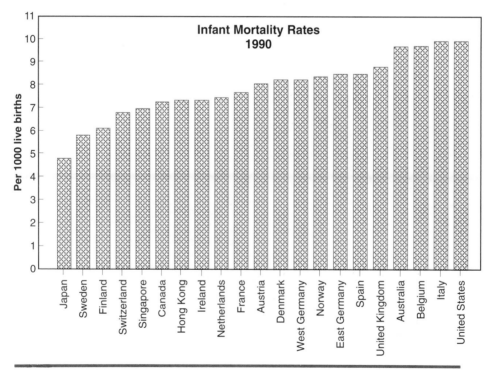

Figure 1-1. Infant mortality rates ranking of the developed countries, 1990. (Adapted from United Nations Statistical Office. Infant Mortality. Geneva: Author 1990.)

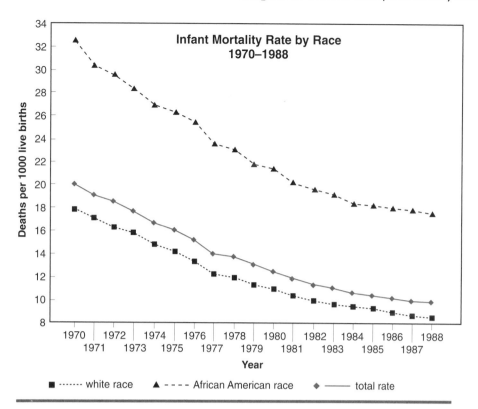

Figure 1-2. Infant mortality statistics by race, 1970–1988. (From National Center for Health Statistics, Hyattsville, MD, 1990.)

tice of boiling milk and isolating children with septic conditions lowered the incidence of diarrhea.

Following World War I, a period of strict asepsis began. Babies were placed in individual cubicles, and the nurses were strictly forbidden to pick up the children except when absolutely necessary. Crib sides were draped with clean sheets, leaving infants with nothing to do but stare at the ceiling. The importance of toys in a child's environment appears not to have been recognized; besides, it was thought that such objects could transmit infection. Parents were allowed to visit for half an hour or perhaps 1 hour each week. They were forbidden to pick up their children under penalty of having their visiting privileges taken away entirely.

Despite these precautions, the high infant mortality rates continued. One of the first people to suspect the cause was Joseph Brennaman, a physician of Children's Memorial Hospital, Chicago. In 1932, he suggested that the infants suffered from a lack of stimulation; other concerned child specialists became interested. In the 1940s, René Spitz published the results of studies that supported his contention that deprivation of maternal care caused a state of dazed stupor in an infant. He believed this condition could become irreversible if the child were not returned to the mother promptly. He termed this state anaclitic depression. He also coined the term hospitalism, which he defined as "a vitiated condition of the body due

to long confinement in the hospital [*vitiated* means feeble or weak]." Later, the term came to be used almost entirely to denote the harmful effects of institutional care on infants. Another physician, Bakwin, found that infants hospitalized for a long time actually developed physical symptoms, which he attributed to a lack of emotional stimulation and a lack of feeding satisfaction.

John Bowlby of London explored the subject of maternal deprivation thoroughly, working under the auspices of the World Health Organization (WHO). His 1951 study, which received worldwide attention, revealed the negative results of the separation of child and mother owing to hospitalization. Bowlby's work, together with that of John Robertson, his associate, led to a reevaluation and liberalization of hospital-visiting policies for children.

Marshall Klaus and John Kennell, physicians at Rainbow Babies and Children's Hospital, Cleveland, carried out important studies in the 1970s and 1980s on the effect of the separation of newborns and parents. They established that this early separation may have long-term effects on family relationships and that offering the new family an opportunity to be together at birth, and for a significant period after birth, may provide benefits that last well into early childhood (Figure 1-3). These findings also have helped to modify hospital policies.

Hospital regulations changed slowly, but gradually

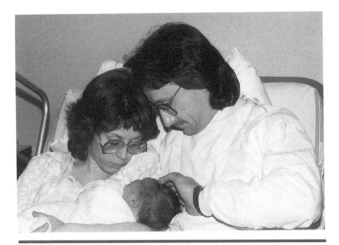

Figure 1-3. The mother, father, and infant son soon after birth. (From Castiglia PT, Harbin RE. Child Health Care: Process and Practice. Philadelphia: JB Lippincott, 1992, p. 185.)

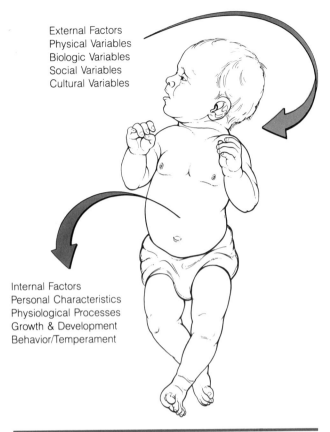

External Factors
Physical Variables
Biologic Variables
Social Variables
Cultural Variables

Internal Factors
Personal Characteristics
Physiological Processes
Growth & Development
Behavior/Temperament

Figure 1-4. Internal and external factors that influence the health and illness patterns of the child.

they began to reflect the needs of children and their families. Isolation practices have been relaxed for children who do not have infectious diseases; children are encouraged to ambulate as early as possible and to visit the playroom, where they can be with other children. Nurses at all levels who work with children are prepared to understand, value, and use play as a therapeutic tool in the daily care of children.

Family-Centered Care

Family-centered nursing is a new and broadened concept in the health care institutions of the United States. No longer are pediatric patients treated as clinical cases with attention given exclusively to their medical problems. Instead, health caregivers recognize that children belong to a family, a community, and a particular way of life or culture, and their health is influenced by these and other factors (Figure 1-4). Separating children from their background means that their needs are met only in a superficial manner, if at all. Even if nursing takes place entirely inside hospital walls, family-centered care pays attention to each child's unique emotional, developmental, social, and scholastic needs as well as physical ones.

Regionalized Care

During the past several decades there has been a definite trend toward centralization and regionalization of pediatric services. Providing high-quality medical care in pediatrics necessitated moving the pediatric patient to medical teaching centers with the best resources for diagnosis and treatment.

To avoid duplication of services and equipment, the most intricate and expensive services and the most highly specialized personnel were made available in the central-

ized location: pediatric neurologists, adolescent allergy specialists, pediatric oncologists, nurse play therapists, child psychiatrists, pediatric nurse practitioners, and clinical nurse specialists. Here are found geneticists, neonatal intensive care units, computed tomography scanners, and burn care units.

Regionalized care often takes the pediatric patient far from home. It is a longer distance for the family caregivers to travel to visit than it would be for them to travel to the local suburban hospital. Family-centered care becomes even more important under these circumstances. Measures are always taken to keep the child's hospitalization as brief as possible, the child as ambulatory as possible, and the family as close as possible. For the child to be separated from the family is traumatic and may actually retard recovery. Many of these regionalized centers (tertiary care hospitals) have accommodations in which families may stay while their child is hospitalized.

Other Innovative Child Health Care Programs

Many pediatric hospitals have home care programs for children with chronic illness, such as leukemia, hemophilia, and cystic fibrosis. Between hospitalizations, the child's condition is monitored at home by the hospital's nurses, offering continuity of care.

Some pediatric hospitals have **primary nursing**, a system whereby one nurse plans the total care for a child and directs the efforts of nurses on the other two shifts. The primary nurse is responsible for the child's care at all times and often makes home visits to the child after discharge and before readmission. In those hospitals in which primary nursing is not practiced, a good procedure is to assign the same nurse to a child to provide stability in the child's care.

Many children are now being cared for in **health maintenance organizations (*HMOs*)**. HMOs are professional groups of physicians, laboratory service personnel, nurse practitioners, nurses, and consultants who care for the health of a family on a continuing basis and are geared to health care and disease prevention. The family pays a set fee for total care; any necessary hospitalization is covered by that fee. The emphasis is on health and prevention in contrast with the acute care, cure-oriented pediatric medical center.

In some private practices and in many clinic settings, the child is cared for by a **pediatric nurse practitioner (*PNP*)**, a professional nurse prepared at the postbaccalaureate level, to give primary health care to children and families. PNPs use pediatricians or family physicians as consultants but offer day-to-day assessment and care.

The Nurse's Changing Role in Child Health Care

The image of nursing has changed in the last 20 years, and the horizons and responsibilities have broadened tremendously. Child care now involves surveillance of growth and development, anticipatory guidance about maturational and common health problems, and teaching and follow-up about immunization and health teaching in addition to the treatment of disease and physical problems.

Nurses at all levels are legally accountable for their actions, assuming new responsibilities and accountability with every advance in education. Nurses practicing in any pediatric setting and at all levels must keep up-to-date with education and information on how to help their young patients and where to direct families for help when other resources are needed. When the nurse functions as a teacher, advisor, and resource person, it is important that the information and advice provided be correct, pertinent, and useful to the person in need.

Community Resources

There are multiple sources of help for families in need of guidance or physical care. Specialized centers and clinics, usually functioning through government grants and private contributions, are able to give free or inexpensive help. The United States Department of Health and Human Ser-

vices has provided grants to large numbers of community-health projects in the cities and rural areas of all states. Among these are children and youth projects, neighborhood health centers, maternal and infant care, programs for disabled children, and migrant health projects.

The Family as a Social Unit

The birth of a baby alters forever the relationship of the parents and establishes a new social unit—a family—in which all members influence and are influenced by each other. Each subsequent child born into that family continues the process of reshaping the individual members and the family unit. In addition, family members are individually and collectively affected by the larger community around them.

Nursing care of children demands a solid understanding of normal patterns of growth and development—physical, psychological, social, and intellectual (cognitive)—and an awareness of the many factors that influence those patterns. It also demands an appreciation for the uniqueness of each child and each family. To be complete and therefore as effective as possible, a child must be considered as a member of a family and a larger community.

Today's American child enters a family that may resemble only faintly the traditional nuclear family of 30 or 40 years ago, in which the father worked outside the home and the mother cared for the children. Family structure is changing in response to turbulent social and economic conditions. For instance, it is estimated that in 60% to 70% of families of school-age children only one parent lives at home. More than 50% of American women with a child younger than 1 year of age now work outside the home. Changes such as these create bigger demands on parents and have contributed to the growing demands on public institutions to fill in the gaps. "Blended" or stepfamilies have created other major changes in family structure and interactions within the family. Divorce, abandonment, and delays in childbearing are all contributing factors.

Family Function

The family is civilization's oldest and most basic social unit. The family's primary purpose is to ensure survival of the unit and individual members and to continue the society and its knowledge, customs, values, and beliefs. It establishes a primary connection with a group responsible for a person until that person becomes independent. Although family structure varies among different cultures, its functions related to children are similar: providing physical care, educating and training children, and protecting children's psychological and emotional health.

Physical Care

The family is responsible for meeting each child's basic needs for food, clothing, shelter, and protection from harm, including illness. The work necessary to meet these needs was once clearly divided between mother and father, with the mother providing total care for the child and the father providing the resources that made it possible. These attitudes have changed, so that in a two-parent family, each parent has an opportunity to share in the joys and trials of child care and other aspects of family living. In the single-parent family, all these responsibilities must be assumed by one person.

Education and Training
Within the family unit, a child learns the rules of the society and the culture in which the family lives: its language, values, ethics, and acceptable behaviors. This process is called **socialization** and is accomplished by training and education. The family teaches children acceptable ways of meeting physical needs, such as eating and elimination, and certain skills, such as dressing oneself. The family educates children about relationships to other people within and outside the family. Children learn what is permitted and approved within their society and what is forbidden.

Psychological and Emotional Health
Research studies continue to support the importance of early parent–child relationships to emotional adjustment in later life. Even a few hours may constitute a critical period in the emotional bond between parents and child. Although the results of these studies are controversial, it is generally agreed that young children are highly sensitive to psychological influences, and those influences may have long-range effects, either positive or negative.

Within the family, children learn who they are and how their behavior affects other family members. Children observe and imitate the behavior of family members, learning quickly which behaviors are rewarded and which are punished. Participation in a family is a child's only rehearsal for parenthood. How parents treat the child has a powerful influence on how the child will treat future children. Studies have shown that, often, parents who abuse their children had been abused by their parents as children.

Family Structure

There are a variety of traditional and nontraditional family structures in place. The traditional structures that occur in many cultures are the nuclear family and the extended family. Nontraditional variations include the single-parent family, the communal family, the stepfamily, and the gay or lesbian family.

Nuclear Family
The **nuclear family** is composed of a man, a woman, and their children (either biologic or adopted) who share a common household (Figure 1-5). This was once the typical American family structure; now fewer than one third of

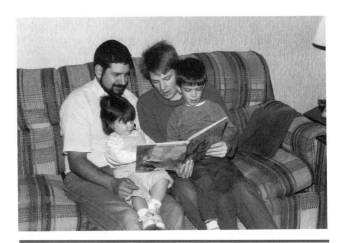

Figure 1-5. The nuclear family: mother, father, and children. (From Jackson DB, Saunders RB. Child Health Nursing. Philadelphia: JB Lippincott, 1993, p. 36.)

families in the United States fit this pattern. The nuclear family is a more mobile and independent unit than is an extended family but is often part of a network of related nuclear families within close geographic proximity.

Extended Family
Typical of agricultural societies, the **extended family** consists of one or more nuclear families plus other relatives, often crossing generations to include grandparents, aunts, uncles, and cousins. The needs of individual members are subordinate to the needs of the group, and children are considered an economic asset. Grandparents aid in childrearing, and children learn respect for their elders by observing their parents' behavior toward the older generation.

Nontraditional Family Structures
Rising divorce rates, the women's movement, increasing acceptance of children born out of wedlock, and changes in adoption laws reflecting a more liberal attitude toward adoption have combined to produce a growing number of **single-parent families**. Approximately 23% of households in the United States are included in this category, and most are headed by women.[2] Although this family situation places a heavy burden on the parent, no conclusive evidence is available to show its effects on children. At some time in their lives, more than 50% of children in the United States may be part of a single-parent family.

During the early 1960s, increasing numbers of young adults began to challenge the values and traditions of the American social system. One of the results of that challenge was the establishing of communal groups and collectives, or **communal families**. This alternative structure occurs in many settings and may favor either a primitive or a modern lifestyle. Members of a communal family share responsibility for homemaking and childrearing; all children are the collective responsibility of adult members. Not actually a new family structure, the communal family is a variation of the extended family.

In the gay or lesbian family, two people of the same sex live together, bound by formal or informal commitment, with or without children. Children may be the result of a prior heterosexual mating or a product of the foster-child system, adoption, artificial insemination, or surrogacy. Although these families often face some complex issues, including discrimination, studies of children in such families show that they are not negatively influenced by membership in this type of family.

The **stepfamily** is made up of the custodial parent and children and a new spouse. As the divorce rate has climbed, the number of stepfamilies has increased. If both partners in the marriage bring children from a previous marriage into the household, the family is usually termed a **blended family**. The stress that remarriage of the custodial parent places on a child seems to depend in part on the child's age. Initially, there is an increase in the number of problems in children of all ages. However, younger children apparently are able to form an attachment to the new parent and accept that person in the parenting role better than do adolescents. Adolescents, already engaged in searching for identity and exploring their own sexuality, may view the presence of a non-

biologic parent as an intrusion. When children from each partner's former marriage are brought into the family, the incidence of problems increases. Second marriages often produce children of that union, which contributes to adjustment problems of the family members. However, remarriage may provide the stability of a two-parent family that may offer additional resources for the child. Each family is unique and has its own set of problems.

Family Factors that Influence Children

Family Size

The number of children in the family has a significant impact on family interactions. The smaller the family, the more time there is for individual attention to each child. Children in small families, particularly "only" children, often spend more time with adults and therefore relate better with them than with their peers. Only children tend to be more advanced in language development and intellectual achievement.

A large family understandably emphasizes the group more than the child. There is greater interdependence among these children and less dependence on the parents (Figure 1-6). Less time is available for parental attention to each child.

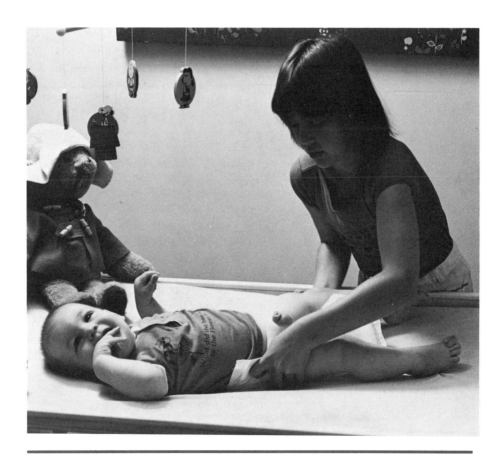

Figure 1-6. Children from larger families learn to care for each other and are not as dependent on parents as "only" children. (Photo by Bruce Grindle.)

Sibling Order and Sex

Whether a child is the firstborn, the middle child, or the youngest also makes a difference in the child's relationships and behavior. Firstborn children command a great deal of attention from parents and grandparents and also are affected by their parents' inexperience, anxieties, and uncertainties. Often the parents' expectations for the oldest child are greater than for subsequent children. Generally, firstborn children are greater achievers than their siblings.

With second and subsequent children, parents tend to be more relaxed and permissive. These children are likely to be more relaxed and are slower to develop language skills. They often identify more with peers than with parents.

Sexual identity in relation to siblings also affects a child's development. Girls raised with older brothers tend to have more masculine characteristics than girls raised with older sisters. Boys raised with older brothers tend to be more aggressive than boys who have older sisters.[3]

Parental Behavior

Many factors have contributed to the change in the traditional mother-at-home, father-at-work image of the American family (Figure 1-7). Sixty-five percent of American mothers of children younger than 18 years of age work outside the home, some because they are the family's only source of income, others because the family's economic goals demand a second income.[1] This fact means that more than half of all children between the ages of 3 and 5 years spend part of their day being cared for by someone other than their parent.

Many factors contribute to families spending less

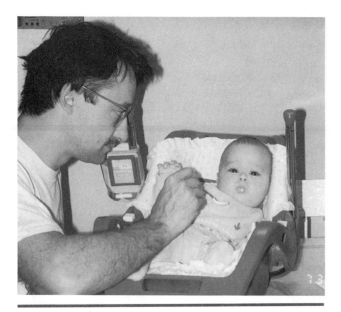

Figure 1-7. Father feeding an infant. (From Castiglia PT, Harbin RE. Child Health Care: Process and Practice. Philadelphia: JB Lippincott, 1992, p. 244.)

time together. Separate jobs for mother and father, school activities for children, absorption in television rather than family conversation at mealtime, more fast food or individual meals without sitting down together as a family, and an emphasis on the acquisition of material goods rather than the development of relationships all contribute to a breakdown in family communication, which is typical of many families and unmeasured in its impact on today's children, the parents of tomorrow.

Divorce

From 1970 to 1980, the number of divorces granted increased every year. Although there has been a slight decrease in this number in recent years, more than 1 million children younger than 18 years of age have been involved in a divorce. This fact holds nothing good for the children involved, but it is difficult to determine the exact extent of the damage. Children whose lives were seriously disrupted before a divorce may feel relieved when the situation is resolved. Others who felt that their lives were happy may feel frightened and abandoned. All these emotions depend on the people involved, their ages, and the kind of care and relationships they experience with their parents after the divorce.

Concepts of Child Development

Growth and development refers to the total growth of the child from birth toward maturity. **Growth** is the physical increase in size and appearance of the body caused by increasing numbers of new cells. **Development** is the progressive change in the child's maturation. **Developmental tasks** are basic achievements associated with each stage of development. These tasks must be mastered to successfully move on to the next developmental stage. Developmental tasks must be completed successfully at each stage for a person to achieve maturity. How a helpless infant grows and develops into a fully functioning independent adult has fascinated scientists for years. Three pioneering researchers in this area whose theories are widely accepted are Sigmund Freud, Erik Erikson, and Jean Piaget (Table 1-2). Their theories present human development as a series of overlapping stages that occur in predictable patterns in a person's life. These stages are only approximations of what is likely to happen at various ages in a child's life, and each child's development may differ from these stages in varying degrees.

Sigmund Freud

Most modern psychologists base their understanding of children at least partly on the work of Sigmund Freud. His theories are concerned primarily with the **libido** (sexual drive or development). Although Freud did not study chil-

Table 1-2. Comparative Summary of Freud, Erikson, and Piaget Theories

Age (years)	Stage	Erikson (Psychosocial Development)	Freud (Psychosexual Development)	Piaget (Intellectual Development)
1	Infancy	Trust vs mistrust	Oral stage	Sensorimotor phase
2–3	Toddlerhood	Autonomy vs shame	Anal stage	
4–6	Preschool age (early childhood)	Initiative vs guilt	Phallic (infant genital) stage Oedipal stage	Preoperational phase
7–12	School age (middle childhood)	Industry vs inferiority	Latency stage	Concrete operational phase
13–18	Adolescence	Identity vs identity confusion	Genital stage (puberty)	Formal operational phase

dren, his work focused on childhood development as a cause of later conflict. Freud believed that a child who did not adequately resolve a particular stage of development would have a fixation (compulsion) that correlated with that stage. Freud described three levels of consciousness: the **id**, which controls physical need and instincts of the body; the **ego**, the conscious self, which controls the pleasure principle of the id by delaying the instincts until an appropriate time; and the **superego**, the conscience or parental value system. These consciousness levels interact to check behavior and balance each other. The psychosexual stages in Freud's theory are the oral, the anal, the phallic, the latency, and the genital stages of development.

Oral Stage (Ages 0 to 2 Years)

The newborn first relates almost entirely to the mother (or someone taking a motherly role), and the first experiences with body satisfaction come through the mouth. This is true not only of sucking but also of making noises, crying, and often, breathing. It is through the mouth that the baby expresses needs and finds satisfaction and thus begins to make sense of the world. Fixations that Freud believed applied to the oral stage are obsessive eating, bathing, or smoking; alcoholism; unrealistic self-confidence; and depression. The id is in control throughout this stage, but the ego is beginning to develop and it functions well by the end of the stage.

Anal Stage (Ages 2 to 3 Years)

This stage is the child's first encounter with the serious need to learn self-control and to take responsibility. Toilet training looms large in the minds of many people as an important phase in childhood. Because elimination is one of the child's first experiences of creativity, it represents the beginnings of the desire to mold and control the environment—the "mudpie period" in a person's life.

The child has pride in the product created. Cleanliness and this natural pride do not always go together, so it may be necessary to help direct this pride and interest

into more acceptable behaviors. This achievement is an important part of learning to take part in society. Playing with such materials as modeling clay, crayons, and dough helps put the child's natural interests to good use, a process called **sublimation**. Fixations of the anal stage are obstinacy, compulsiveness, autocratic dogmatism (tyrannical beliefs), extravagance, passive resistance, and aggression.

Phallic (Infant Genital) Stage (Ages 3 to 6 Years)

It is only natural that interest moves to the genital area as a source of pride and curiosity. To the child's mind, this area constitutes the difference between boys and girls, a difference that the child is beginning to be aware of socially. The superego begins to develop during this stage, and by 10 years of age (the end of the latency stage), it is well established.

Until this time, girls and boys enjoy the same toys and games and generally are treated alike. Then, the boy begins to take pride in being a male and the girl in being a female. In many families, a new brother or sister arrives at about this time, arousing the child's natural interest in human origins. A hospital setting may prompt questions that might be delayed or avoided at home and also may provide answers the child might not get at home.

This stage is when the child begins to understand what it means to be a boy or a girl. Parents' reaction to the child's genital exploration may determine whether the child learns to feel satisfied with himself or herself as a sexual being or is laden with feelings of guilt and dissatisfaction throughout his or her life.

Freud hypothesized that this awareness of genital differences leads to a time of conflict in the child's emotional relationships with parents. The conflict occurs between attachment to and imitation of the parent of the same sex and the appeal of the other parent. The boy who for years has depended on his mother for all his emotional and physical needs is now confronted by his desire to be a man (Oedipus complex). The girl, who has imitated her mother, now finds her father a real attraction (Electra complex). This is not only social but sexual; it is through contact with parents that the child learns to relate to the opposite sex. This is not just a physical interest but a need to learn the interests, attitudes, concerns, and wishes of the opposite sex.

A child usually feels ambivalent at this age, sometimes wanting the comfort and support of others of the same sex, at other times disdaining it. It is also the time when embarrassment begins, when a boy may be acutely embarrassed by undressing in front of a female nurse but less uncomfortable undressing in front of a male nurse.

For most children of this age, boys as well as girls, playing with dolls is a way of working out family relationships and expressing feelings that naturally build up without fear of punishment. Fixations of the phallic stage are narcissism, arrogance, flamboyance, and chauvinism.

Latency Stage (Ages 6 to 10 Years)
The latency stage is the time of primary schooling, when the child is preparing for adult life but must await maturity to exercise initiative in adult living. It is the time when the child's sense of moral responsibility (the superego) is built, based on what has been taught through the parents' words and actions.

When placed in an unfamiliar setting, children in this stage may become confused because they do not know what is expected of them. They need the sense of security that comes from approval and praise and usually respond favorably to a brief explanation of "how we do things here."

Genital Stage (Ages 11 to 13 Years)
Physical puberty continues to occur at an increasingly early age, and social puberty occurs even earlier, owing largely to the influence of sexual frankness on television and in movies and the print media. At puberty, all the child's earlier learning is concentrated on the powerful biologic drive, finding and relating to a mate. In earlier societies, mating and forming a family took place at a young age. Our society delays mating for many years after puberty, creating a time of confusion and turmoil during which biologic readiness must take second place to educational and economic goals. This is a sensitive period when privacy is important, and great uncertainty exists about relating to any members of the opposite sex.

Erik Erikson

Building on Freud's theories, Erikson described human psychosocial development as a series of tasks or crises. This development depends on a self-healing process within the person that helps counterbalance the stresses created by natural and accidental crises. The self-healing process is delayed by any major crisis, such as hospitalization, which interrupts normal development. Interruptions may cause regression to an earlier stage, such as the

older child who begins to wet the bed when hospitalized. Erikson commented that "children 'fall apart' repeatedly, and unlike Humpty Dumpty, grow together again," if they are given time and sympathy and are not interfered with.[4]

Erikson formulated a series of eight developmental tasks or crises, the first five of which pertain to children and youth. In each, the person must master the central problem before moving on to the next one. Each holds positive and negative counterparts, and each of the first five implies new developmental tasks for parents (Table 1-3).

Trust Versus Mistrust (Ages 0 to 1 Year)
The infant has no way to control the world other than crying for help and hoping for rescue. During the first year, the child learns whether the world can be trusted to give love and concern or only frustration, fear, and despair. The infant who is fed on demand learns to trust that cries communicating need will be answered. The baby fed according to the schedule of the hospital or mother does not understand the importance of routine but only that these cries may go unanswered.

Autonomy Versus Doubt and Shame (Ages 1 to 3 Years)
Even the smallest child wants to feel in control and needs to learn to perform tasks independently, even when this takes a long time or makes a mess. The toddler gains reassurance from self-feeding, from crawling or walking alone where it is safe, and from being free to handle materials and learn about things in the environment.

A toddler exploring the environment begins to explore and learn about his or her body, too. If caregivers react appropriately to this normal behavior, the child will gain self-respect and pride. If, however, they shame the child for responding to this natural curiosity, the belief that somehow the body is "dirty, nasty, and bad" may develop and remain.

Initiative Versus Guilt (Ages 3 to 6 Years)
During this period, the child engages in active, assertive play. Steadily improving physical coordination and expanding social skills encourage "showing off" to gain adult attention, and the child hopes, approval. The preschool child, still self-centered, plays alone, although in the company of other children. Interaction comes later. These children want to know what the rules are and enjoy "being good" and the adult approval that action gains. During this time, the child develops a conscience and accepts punishment for doing wrong because it relieves feelings of guilt.

Children in this phase of development generally do not have a concept of time and the changes it imposes on nursing shifts. Explaining that it is time for a nurse to go home to the nurse's own family may help an unhappy child realize that the nurse is not leaving because of any

Table 1-3. Child and Parent Development

Developmental Level	Basic Task	Stage of Parental Development	Parental Task
Infant	Trust	Learning to recognize and interpret infant's cues	To interpret cues and respond positively to the infant's needs; hold, cuddle, and talk to infant
Toddler	Autonomy	Learning to accept child's need for self-mastery	To accept child's growing need for freedom while setting consistent, realistic limits; offer support and understanding when separation anxiety occurs
Preschooler	Initiative	Learning to allow child to explore surrounding environment	To allow independent development while modeling necessary standards; generously praise child's endeavors to build child's self-esteem
School-age	Industry	Learning to accept rejection without deserting	To accept child's successes and defeats, assuring child of acceptance; to be there when needed without intruding unnecessarily
Adolescent	Identity	Learning to build a new life, supporting the emergence of the adolescent as an individual	To be available when adolescent feels need; provide examples of positive moral values; keep communication channels open; adjust to changing family roles and relationships during and after the adolescent's struggle to establish an identity

negative behavior of the child's. The child needs a familiar frame of reference to understand when something is going to happen. For example, the parent or caregiver may say, "I will be back when your lunch tray comes" or "I will be back when the cartoons come on (television)."

Industry Versus Inferiority (Ages 6 to 12 Years)
Children begin to seek achievement in this phase. They learn to interact with others and, sometimes, to compete with them. They like activities they can follow through to completion and tangible results.

Competition is healthy as long as the standards are not so high that the child feels there is no chance of winning. Praise, not criticism, helps the child to build self-esteem and avoid feelings of inferiority. It is important to emphasize that everyone is a unique person and deserves to be appreciated for his or her own special qualities.

Identity Versus Identity Confusion (Ages 12 to 18 Years)
Adolescents are confronted by marked physical and emotional changes and the knowledge that soon they will be responsible for their own lives. The adolescent develops a sense of being an independent person with unique ideals and goals and may feel that parents, caregivers, and other adults refuse to grant that independence. Adolescents may break rules just to prove that they can. Stress, anxiety, and mood swings are typical of this phase. Relationships with peers are more important than ever.

Intimacy Versus Isolation (Early Adulthood)
This is the period during which the person tries to establish intimate personal relationships with friends and an intimate love relationship with one person. Difficulty in establishing intimacy results in feelings of isolation.

Generativity Versus Self-Absorption (Young and Middle Adulthood)
For many people, this phase means marriage and family, but for others it may mean fulfillment in some other way—a professional or business career or a religious vocation. The person who does not find this fulfillment becomes self-absorbed and ceases to develop socially.

Ego Integrity Versus Despair (Old Age)
This final phase is the least understood of all, for it means finding satisfaction with oneself, one's achievements, and present condition, without regret for the past or fear for the future.

Jean Piaget

Freud and Erikson studied psychosexual and psychosocial development; Piaget brought new insight into **cognitive** (intellectual) **development**—how a child learns and develops that quality called intelligence. He described intellectual development as a sequence of four principal stages, each made up of several substages.[5] All children move through these stages in the same order, but each moves at his or her own pace.

Sensorimotor Phase (Ages 0 to 2 Years)
The newborn behaves at a sensorimotor level linked entirely to desires for physical satisfaction. The newborn feels, hears, sees, tastes, and smells countless new things and moves in an apparently random way. Purposeful ac-

tivities are controlled by reflexive responses to the environment. For example, while nursing, the newborn gazes intently at mother's face, grasps her finger, smells the nipple, and tastes the milk, thus involving all senses.

As the infant grows, an understanding of cause and effect develops. When random arm motions strike the string of bells stretched across the crib, the newborn hears the sound that is made and eventually is able to manipulate the arms to deliberately make the bells ring.

In the same way, newborns cannot understand words or even the tone of voice, but only through hearing conversation directed to them can they pick out sounds and begin to understand. As the infant produces verbal noises, the response of those nearby are encouraging and eventually help the infant learn to talk.

Preoperational Phase (Ages 2 to 7 Years)

The child in this phase of development is **egocentric**; that is, the child cannot look at something from another's point of view. The child's interpretation of the world is from a self-centered point of view and in terms of what is seen, heard, or otherwise experienced directly.

This child has no concept of quantity; if it looks like more, it *is* more. Four ounces of juice poured into two glasses looks like more than four ounces in one glass. A sense of time is not yet developed, and thus the preschooler or early school-age child cannot always tell whether something happened a day ago, a week ago, or a year ago.

Concrete Operations (Ages 7 to 11 Years)

During this stage, children develop the ability to begin problem solving in a concrete, systematic way. They can classify and organize information about their environment, and they begin to understand that volume or weight may remain the same even though the appearance changes, unlike in the preoperational stage. These children can consider another's point of view and can deal simultaneously with more than one aspect of a situation.

Formal Operations (Ages 12 to 15 Years)

The adolescent is capable of dealing with ideas, abstract concepts described only in words or symbols. The person of this age begins to understand jokes based on double meanings and enjoys reading and discussing theories and philosophies. Adolescents can observe and then draw logical conclusions from their observations.

Other Theorists

Freud, Erikson, and Piaget are only three of the many researchers who have studied the development of children and families. During the 1940s and 1950s, Arnold Gesell studied many infants and talked with their parents concerning children's behavior. From his studies emerged a series of developmental landmarks that are

still considered valid and the observation that children progress through a series of "easy" and "difficult" phases as they develop. For example, he labeled one period the "terrible twos," the time when a toddler begins to assert new mobility and coordination to gain parental attention, even if the attention is unfavorable. Knowing that these cycles are normal makes it easier for parents to cope.

Carl Jung's contribution to the study of child growth and development focused on the inner sequence of events that shape the personality. He emphasized that human development follows predetermined patterns called **archetypes**. These archetypes replace the instinctive behavior present in other animal life. Interaction of the archetypes with the outside environment is evident throughout human life. For example, a normal child learns to suck, crawl, walk, and talk without any instruction, but the details of how the child does these things come from observation and imitation of others.

Jung believed that the first 3 years of a child's life are spent in coordinating experiences and learning to make a conscious personality, a distinct person who is separate from the rest of the environment. In the following years, the child learns to make sense of the environment by associating new discoveries to a general approach to the world. Dreams and nightmares help express developments of the personality that for some reason do not find a conscious outlet.

Jung points out that what happens to a child is not so critical to the child's development as the responses to these happenings. A hospital experience may permanently scar a child's personality if the child's natural feeling of terror is overlooked. It may be accepted and even become a point of pride, however, if carried out in an atmosphere of assurance and support of the child's emotional concern and the need for love and acceptance.

The interaction between inner development and the environment is particularly clear in studies of young children who have been deprived in some way. Bowlby's studies of children who were not held or loved and Bettelheim's studies of children given good physical care but little or no emotional satisfaction indicate how vital psychological interaction is.

Summary

Many changes have taken place in the care of children in this century. Until the early part of the 20th century, children were treated as miniature adults and were expected to behave that way. Sociologic changes and scientific advances have contributed to a much healthier environment for children, but the United States continues to lag behind many developed nations in improving the rate of infant mortality. Although progress has been made recently on a national level to develop agencies that are charged with working to improve the health of infants and children, much more needs to be done.

The current attitude of caring for the child as a member of a family is sensitive and sensible. Progress in medical science has advanced so rapidly and become so sophisticated that many children with chronic or serious conditions are taken care of in regionalized centers, creating a need for caring for the family in a "home away from home" atmosphere.

Throughout all of these changes, the nurses' role has changed also, and the nurse now has the responsibilities of teacher, advisor, and resource person as well as caretaker. Pediatric nursing consists of preventive care of the well child as much or more than care of the ill child.

The family unit has changed, too. Many children no longer have two parents, one of whom stays home. Many social changes have influenced these differences. Research begun by Freud and followed by Erikson, Piaget, and others continues to explore how children and parents develop together and what specific skills and abilities children acquire at various ages. It is now recognized that infants respond to parents from birth, and parents, in turn, respond to infants' behavior. Nurses and other health professionals must understand those patterns of response to contribute to the healthy growth and development of children and families.

Review Questions

1. What sociologic changes have affected child health concepts and attitudes?
2. Name the country that has the lowest infant mortality rate (least number of infant deaths per 1000).
3. Discuss how children were cared for in institutions in the 19th and early 20th centuries.
4. Describe the hospital care of infants and children in the period immediately following World War I.
5. While working, you overhear an older nurse complain about family caregivers "being underfoot so much and interfering with patient care." How would you defend open visiting for family caregivers to this person?
6. Explain why it is important for the nurse to know the community resources available for children.
7. Describe changes in family structure that have occurred since the middle of the 20th century.
8. Discuss in detail the influence the family has on a child and what the child learns from the family.
9. Why does the firstborn child usually have the "roughest road" in a family?
10. Freud's latency stage, Erikson's industry stage, and Piaget's concrete operational stage all involve the early elementary years. Compare the three psychologists' interpretations of these stages, pointing out similarities.
11. The developmental task identified by Erikson for the first stage of life is trust. Discuss why successful accomplishment of this task is essential to the person's future happiness and adjustment.

References

1. Chiles L. Troubling Trends: The Health of America's Next Generation. Washington, DC: National Commission to Prevent Infant Mortality, 1990.
2. United States Bureau of Census. Statistical Abstract of the United States: 1990, 110th ed. Washington, DC: Superintendent of Documents, 1990.
3. Craig G. Human Development, 6th ed. Englewood Cliffs, NJ: Prentice-Hall, 1992.
4. Erikson EH, Senn MJE. Symposium on the Healthy Personality. New York: Macy Foundation, 1958.
5. Piaget J. The Language and Thought of the Child. Cleveland: World Publishing, 1967.

Bibliography

Bowlby J. Attachment. New York: Basic Books, 1969.

Erikson EH. Childhood and Society, 2nd ed. New York: Norton, 1963.

Kalman N, Waughfield CG. Mental Health Concepts, 2nd ed. Albany: Delmar, 1987.

Schuster C, Ashburn S. The Process of Human Development, 3rd ed. Philadelphia: JB Lippincott, 1992.

Wadsworth BJ. Piaget's Theory of Cognitive and Affective Development. New York: Longman, 1984.

The Child Enters the Hospital

Chapter 2

Student Objectives

Upon completion of this chapter, the student will be able to:

1. List nine possible influences on the family's response to a child's illness.
2. Describe how a preadmission visit differs from an open house program.
3. Explain the family caregivers' role in preparing a child for hospitalization.
4. State how the caregiver may be involved in the child's admission physical.
5. Discuss the need for written discharge instructions for the caregiver.
6. State how family members should react to the postdischarge child during this period of adjustment.
7. List the five steps of the nursing process.
8. State who is involved in setting goals of nursing care for the child.
9. Compare observations indicating health or illness of an infant or young child.
10. Describe three additional useful observations of the older child.
11. Name one of the most important aspects of communication.
12. State the purpose of reflective statements when communicating with a caregiver or child.
13. List four categories of cultural attitudes that influence planning of care for the child.
14. Identify and differentiate the three stages of response to separation seen in the young child.
15. Describe the benefits of rooming-in.
16. Describe therapeutic use for puppets.
17. State how stress affects the frequency of accidents.
18. List safety measures to consider when using restraints.

Marks MG: BROADRIBB'S INTRODUCTORY PEDIATRIC NURSING, 4th ed. © 1994 J.B. Lippincott Company.

Key Terms

actual nursing diagnoses	interdependent nursing actions
child-life program	mummy restraint
clove hitch restraint	nursing process
dependent nursing actions	objective data
	papoose board
elbow restraint	play therapy
high-risk nursing diagnoses	rooming-in
	subjective data
independent nursing actions	therapeutic play
	wellness nursing diagnoses

*H*ospitalization may cause anxiety and stress at any age. Fear of the unknown is always threatening. The child who faces hospitalization is no exception. Children are often too young to understand what is happening or are afraid to ask questions. Short hospital stays are becoming more frequent, but even during a short stay the child may be apprehensive. In addition, the child may pick up on the fears of family caregivers. These negative emotions may have a negative effect on the child's progress.

The child's family suffers stress for a number of reasons. The cause of the illness, its treatment, guilt about the illness, past experiences of illness and hospitalization, disruption in family life, the threat to the child's long-term state of health, cultural or religious influences, coping methods within the family, and financial impact of the hospitalization all may affect how the family responds to the child's illness. Although these are concerns of the family and not specifically the child, they nevertheless influence how the child feels. Children are "tuned in" to the feelings and emotions of their caregivers.

The child's developmental level also plays an important role in determining how that child handles the stress of illness and hospitalization. The nurse who understands the developmental needs of the child may significantly improve the child's hospital stay and overall recovery. Many hospitals have a **child-life program** to make hospitalization less threatening for children and their parents. These programs are usually under the direction of a child-life specialist whose background is in psychology and early childhood development. This person works with nurses, physicians, and other health team members to help them meet the developmental, emotional, and intellectual needs of hospitalized children. The child-life specialist also works with students interested in child health care to help further their education. Sometimes, however, the best way to ease the stress of hospitalization is to make sure the child has been well prepared for the hospital experience.

The Pediatric Hospital Setting

Early Childhood Education About Hospitals

Hospitals are part of the child's community just as police and fire departments are. When the child is capable of understanding the basic functions of these community resources and the people who staff them, it is time for an explanation. Some hospitals have open house programs for well children on a monthly or biweekly basis. Children may attend with parents or caregivers or in an organized community or school group. A room is set aside where children can handle equipment (Figure 2-1), try out call bells, try on masks and gowns, have their blood pressure taken to feel the "squeeze" of the blood pressure cuff, and see a hospital pediatric bed and compare it with their bed at home. Hospital staff members explain simple procedures and answer children's questions. A tour of the pediatric department, including the playroom, may be offered. Some hospitals have puppet shows, show slides, or videos about admission and care. Child-life specialists, nurses, and volunteers help with these orientation programs.

Families are encouraged to help children develop a positive attitude about hospitals, beginning at an early age. Care should be taken within the family to avoid negative attitudes about hospitals. Young children need to know that the hospital is more than a place where "mommies go to get babies." But it is also important to

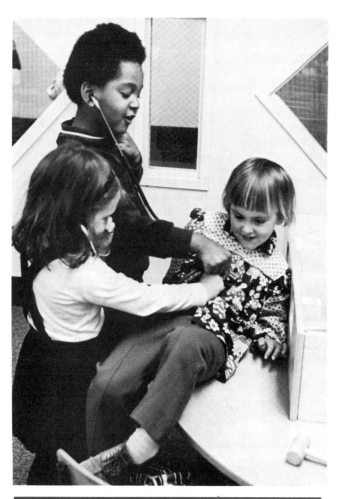

Figure 2-1. Listening to each other's heart beat shows children how the stethoscope works.

avoid fostering the view of the hospital as a place where people go to die. This is a particular concern if the child knows someone who died in the hospital. A careful explanation of the person's illness and simple, honest answers to questions about the death are necessary.

The Pediatric Unit Atmosphere

An effort by pediatric units and hospitals to create friendly, warm surroundings for children has produced many attractive, colorful pediatric settings. Walls are colorful, often decorated with murals, wallpaper, photos, and paintings specifically designed for children. Furniture is attractive, appropriate in size, and designed with safety in mind. Curtains and drapes are often coordinated with wall coverings in colors or designs that are appealing.

The staff members of the pediatric unit often wear colored smocks, colorful sweatshirts, or printed "scrub" suits. Research has shown that children react with greatest anxiety toward the traditional white uniform. Children often are encouraged to wear their own clothing during

the day. Colorful printed pajamas are provided for children who need to wear hospital clothing.

Treatments are not performed in the child's room but in a treatment room. Using a separate room where procedures are performed promotes the concept that the child's bed is a "safe" place. All treatments, with no exceptions, should be performed in the treatment room to reassure the child.

Play is the work of children, and a playroom, or area, is a vital part of all pediatric units. The playroom should be a place that is safe from any kind of procedures. Some hospitals provide a person trained in therapeutic play to coordinate and direct the play activities.

Most pediatric settings provide **rooming-in** facilities and encourage parents or family caregivers to visit as frequently as possible. This approach helps minimize the separation anxiety of the young child, in particular. Caregivers are involved in much of the young child's care, providing comfort and reassurance to the child. Families also are encouraged to bring a few favorite toys to the hospital for the child. Many pediatric units use **primary nursing** assignments so that the same nurse will be with a child as much as is possible. This approach gives the nurse the opportunity to establish a trusting relationship with the child.

Planning meals that include the child's favorite food selections within the limitations of any special dietary restrictions may perk up a flagging appetite. In addition, when space permits, several children may eat together at a small table. Younger children should be seated in high chairs or other suitable seats. Mealtimes should be planned to be served out of bed, if possible, and in a pleasant atmosphere. Some pediatric units use the playroom to serve meals to those children who are ambulatory.

Planned Admissions

Preadmission preparation may make the experience less threatening and the adjustment to admission as smooth as possible. Children who are candidates for admission to the hospital may attend open house programs or other special programs that are more detailed and specifically related to their upcoming experience. It is important for family caregivers and siblings to attend the preadmission tour along with the future patient to reduce anxiety in all family members.

During the preadmission visit, children may be given surgical masks, caps, and shoe covers and the opportunity to "operate" on a doll or other stuffed toy specifically designed for teaching purposes (Figure 2-2). Many hospitals have developed special coloring books to help prepare children for tonsillectomy, cardiac, or other specific surgical procedures. These books are given to children during the preadmission visit or sent to children at home before admission. Questions may be answered and anxieties explored during the visit. Children and their

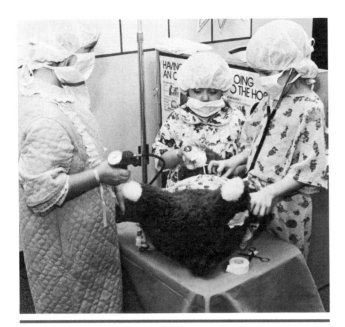

Figure 2-2. Children who are going to have surgery may act out the procedures on toys and thereby reduce some of their fear. (From Castiglia PT, Harbin RE: Child Health Care: Process and Practice. Philadelphia: JB Lippincott, 1992, p. 374.)

families often may be hesitant to ask questions or express feelings, thus the staff must be sensitive to this problem and discuss common questions and feelings. Children are told that some things will hurt but that doctors and nurses will do everything they can to make the hurt go away. Honesty must be a keynote to any program of this kind. The preadmission orientation staff also must be sensitive to cultural and language differences and make adjustments whenever appropriate.

Emergency Admissions

Emergencies leave little time for explanation. The emergency itself is frightening to the child and the family, and the need for treatment is urgent. Even though a caregiver tries to act calm and composed, the child often may sense the anxiety. If the hospital is still a great unknown, it only will add to the child's fear and panic. If the child has even a basic understanding about hospitals and what happens there, the emergency may seem a little less frightening.

In an emergency, physical needs assume priority over emotional needs. The presence, when possible, of a family caregiver who can conceal his or her own fear often is comforting to the child; however, the child may be angry that the caregiver does not prevent invasive procedures from being performed. Sometimes, however, it is not possible for the caregiver to stay with the child. A staff member may use this time to collect information about the child from the family member. This helps the family member to feel involved in the child's care.

Emergency department (ED) nurses need to be sensitive to the child and the family's needs. Recognizing the cognitive level of the child and how that affects the child's reactions is important. In addition, the ED staff must give explanations for procedures and conduct themselves in a caring, calm manner to provide reassurance to both the child and the family.

Pediatric Intensive Care Units

A child's admission to a pediatric intensive care unit (PICU) may be overwhelming for both the child and the family, especially if the admission is unexpected. Highly technical equipment, bright lights, and the crisis atmosphere may be frightening. Visiting may be restricted. Many stressors are present to cause an added effect on the child and the family. Great care should be taken by PICU nurses to prepare the family for how the child will look when they first visit. The family should be provided with a schedule of visiting hours so that they may plan to visit when permitted. The family should be encouraged to bring in a special doll or toy of the child's to provide comfort and security. The child's developmental level must be assessed so that appropriate explanations and reassurances may be provided before and during procedures. Positive reinforcements, such as stickers and small badges, may provide a symbol of courage. The nurse also needs to interpret technical information for family members. The nurse should promote the relationship between the family caregiver and the child as much as possible. The caregiver should be encouraged to touch and talk to the child. The caregiver may hold and rock the child, if possible, but if not, he or she can comfort the child by caressing and stroking. Visiting hours should be flexible enough to accommodate the best interests of the child.

Admission and Discharge Planning

Although admission may be a frightening experience, the child feels in much better control of the situation if the person taking the child to the hospital has explained where they are going and why and has answered questions truthfully. When the caregiver and the child arrive on the nursing unit, they should be greeted in a warm, friendly manner and taken to the child's room or to a room set aside specifically for the admission procedure. The caregiver and the child need to be oriented to the child's room, the nursing unit, and regulations (Box 2-1).

The Admission Interview

An admission interview is conducted as soon as possible after the child has been admitted. A quiet, private place

Box 2-1

Guidelines to Orient Child to Pediatric Unit

1. Introduce the primary nurse
2. Orient to the child's room:
   a. Demonstrate bed, bed controls, side rails
   b. Demonstrate call light
   c. Demonstrate television, include cost, if any
   d. Show bathroom facilities
   e. Explain telephone and rules that apply
3. Introduce to roommate(s); include families
4. Give directions to or show "special" rooms
   a. Playroom—rules that apply, hours available, toys or equipment that may be taken to child's room
   b. Treatment room—explain purpose
   c. Unit kitchen—rules that apply
   d. Other special rooms
5. Explain pediatric rules—give written rules, if available
   a. Visiting hours; who may visit
   b. Mealtimes; rules about bringing in food
   c. Bedtimes; naptimes or quiet time
   d. Rooming-in arrangements
6. Guidelines of daily routines
   a. Vital signs routine
   b. Bath routine
   c. Other routines
7. Guidelines for involvement of family caregiver

is desirable, where interruptions and noise are kept to a minimum. The caregiver and the nurse should be comfortably seated, and the child should be included. The nurse should be introduced to the caregiver and the child and should address each of them by name. The admission questionnaire should ask for the child's nickname, feeding habits, food likes and dislikes, sleeping schedule, toilet-training status, and any special words the child uses or understands to indicate needs or desires, such as words used for urinating and bowel movements. Figure 2-3 provides an example of an assessment form that may be used during this interview.

Rather than simply asking the caregiver to fill out a form, the nurse may ask the questions and write down the answers, gaining the opportunity to observe the reactions of the child and the caregiver as they interact with each other and answer the questions. In addition, this eases the problem of the caregiver who is not able to read or write. The nurse must be nonjudgmental, being careful not to indicate disapproval by verbal or nonverbal responses. The child's comments should be listened to attentively, and the child should be made to feel important in the interview.

The reason for the child's admission is the primary concern of the caregiver. While gathering information about the child's physical condition, the nurse also must allow the caregiver to express concerns and anxieties. The caregiver needs to answer the nurse's questions about the problem, including the child's symptoms, how long the symptoms have been present, a description of the symptoms and their intensity and frequency, and treatments up to this time. The nurse should ask the questions in a way that encourages the caregiver to be specific. The nurse also should ask the caregiver about any other concerns regarding the child.

Questions concerning the child's social and family history are important. The nurse should preface these questions with an explanation that the answers will help in caring for the child. Useful information includes the following:

- The child's primary caregiver
- Other adults in the home
- Siblings in the family, including names the child calls them
- Type of housing the child lives in
- If this is a child of separation or divorce, who has custody of the child and whether this affects who may visit the child
- Whether the child sleeps alone or with others
- Pets in the household
- Favorite toys and types of play
- If all adults work outside of the home, what the child care arrangements are

Through careful questioning, the interviewer tries to determine what the family's previous experience with hospitals and health care providers has been. It is also important to ascertain how much the caregiver and the child understand about the child's condition and their expectations of this hospitalization, what support systems are available when the child returns home, and any disturbing or threatening concerns on the part of the caregiver or the child. These findings, in addition to a careful history and physical assessment, form the basis for the patient's total plan of care while hospitalized.

During the interview, an identification bracelet is placed on the child's wrist. It is important that the child be prepared for even this simple procedure with an explanation of why it is necessary.

The nurse who receives the child on the pediatric unit should be friendly and casual, remembering that even a well-informed child may be shy and suspicious of excessive friendliness. The child who reacts with fear to well-meaning advances and clings to the caregiver is telling the nurse to go more slowly with the acquaintance process. Children who know that the caregiver may stay with them are more quickly put at ease.

The Admission Physical Assessment

After the child has been oriented to the new surroundings, perhaps clinging to the family caregiver's hand or carrying a favorite toy or blanket, the caregiver may undress the child for the physical examination. This procedure may be familiar from previous health care visits. If comfortable with helping, the caregiver may take a young child's temperature and help obtain the urine specimen. Arrangements should be made so that the caregiver also may be present, if possible, for tests or examinations that need to be performed. The nurse completes a baseline assessment of height, weight, blood pressure, temperature, pulse, and respiration. Included in this initial assessment is an inspection of the child's body. All observations are recorded. The nurse carefully documents any finding that is not within normal limits.

The nurse conducts or assists in conducting a complete physical assessment with special attention to any symptoms that the caregiver has identified. The nurse's primary role in this complete assessment may be to support the child. All the information gathered is used to plan the care of the child.

Discharge Planning

Planning for discharge and care of the child at home begins early in the hospital experience. Nurses and other health team members need to assess the level of understanding of the child and family and their ability to learn about the child's condition and about the care that will be necessary after the child goes home. Giving medications, using special equipment, and enforcing necessary restrictions must be discussed with the person who will be the primary caregiver and with one other person, if possible. It is necessary to provide specific, written instructions for reference at home; the anxiety and strangeness of hospitalization often limit the amount of information retained from teaching sessions.

If the treatment necessary at home appears too complex for the caregiver to manage, it may be helpful to arrange for a visiting nurse to assist for a period after the child is sent home.

Shortly before the child is discharged from the hospital, a conference may be arranged to review information and procedures with which the family caregivers need to become familiar. This conference may or may not include the child, depending on age and cognitive level. Questions and concerns need to be dealt with honestly, and a resource should be offered for questions that arise after discharge.

The return home may be a difficult period of adjustment for the entire family. The preschool child may be aloof at first, followed by a period of clinging, demanding behavior. Other behaviors such as regression, temper tantrums, excessive attachment to a toy or blanket, night waking, and nightmares may demonstrate fear of another separation. The older child may demonstrate anger or jealousy of siblings. The family may be advised to encourage positive behavior and avoid making the child the center of attention because of the illness. Discipline should be firm, loving, and consistent. The child may express feelings verbally or in play activities. The family may be reassured that this is not unusual.

The Nurse's Role in Caring for the Hospitalized Child

Implications for hospital care of children specific to each developmental stage are discussed in the respective chapters on growth and development. Certain elements are fairly constant through different stages of development, however. Reaction to hospitalization varies from child to child, but at all age levels a positive reaction varies in direct proportion to the amount of prehospitalization preparation the child received. Any child who arrives unexpectedly in a situation that may be frightening, and even threatening, reacts in a negative fashion. The nursing staff is immediately called on to use all of their expertise to help diffuse the child's anger and begin to turn the reaction toward a positive solution. This situation is just one example of how the pediatric nurse assesses and identifies problems, plans and undertakes actions, and then evaluates the results, that is, performs the nursing process, to meet the child's health care needs.

The Nursing Process

The **nursing process** is a proven form of problem solving based on the scientific method. The nursing process consists of five components:

- Assessment
- Nursing diagnosis
- Planning
- Implementation
- Evaluation

Based on the data collected during the assessment, nursing diagnoses are determined, nursing care is planned and implemented, and the results are evaluated. The process does not end here but continues through reassessment, establishment of new diagnoses, additional plans, implementation, and evaluation until all of the child's nursing problems are identified and dealt with (Figure 2-4).

Assessment

Nursing assessment is a skill that must be practiced and perfected through study and experience. The nurse must

(text continued on page 26)

PEDIATRIC NURSING ASSESSMENT FORM

1. Name _____ Date/Time of Admission _____ Via _____

2. Birth Date _____ Information obtained from:_____ Relationship to child _____

3. Child's legal guardian: _____ Child's Nickname: _____

VITAL SIGNS	Temp	Apical Pulse	Radial Pulse	Respirations	BP	Height	Weight	Head Circum

CURRENT CHIEF COMPLAINT/DIAGNOSIS:
Symptoms and Duration

Child's/Caregivers' Understanding of Condition:

PREVIOUS ILLNESS/INJURIES/DIAGNOSIS:
Illness, Symptoms, and Duration

Injuries or Surgery:

Anesthesia Complications?

Allergies and Reactions:	Immunizations	Dates:	Exposure to Infectious Disease Date
	DPT (DT)		(chicken pox, measles, etc.)
	Oral Polio		
	Hepatitis B		
	Hib (type)		
	MMR (measles, mumps, rubella)		
	TB skin test Result		

Medications: Name:	Dose	Frequency	Time of Last Dose

Child's reaction to previous hospitalizations: _____

Special fears of child about hospitalization? _____

Family History: (Check all that apply—indicate relationship to child)

_____ Cancer _____   _____ Seizures _____   _____ TB _____
_____ Heart disease _____   _____ Asthma _____   _____ Anesthesia complications _____
_____ Allergy _____   _____ Smoking _____   _____ Other (specify) _____
_____ Diabetes _____   _____ Hypertension _____

Living Facilities (check)

_____ House _____ Apartment _____ Trailer _____ Steps to travel?_____

Who does child live with? _____

Names, ages, of siblings in home_____

Names, ages of other children in home _____

Other persons in home _____

Special interests, toys, games, hobbies: _____

_____

Security object:_____ Was it brought to hospital? _____

Bowel/Bladder Habits:

Toilet Training(if applicable)

Started	_____ Yes	_____ No
Completed	_____ Yes	_____ No

Diapers:

Day	_____ Yes	_____ No
Night	_____ Yes	_____ No

Potty Chair:	_____ Yes	_____ No
Toilet:	_____ Yes	_____ No
Bedwetter:	_____ Yes	_____ No

Terms Used for:

Bowel Movement _____ Urination _____

Frequency of BM _____ Color _____ Consistency _____

Does child have problems with diarrhea or constipation?_____

_____

Does child have urinary frequency, burning, discomfort: _____ Yes _____ No

If yes, please explain:_____

_____

_____

Patterns of:

Sleep/rest:

Bedtime_____ Wakeup _____

Nap ____ Yes ____ No — When? _____

Activity:

Does infant roll over? _____

Does child stand/walk? _____

Does child climb? _____

Does child dress self? _____

Does child go up and down stairs? _____

Does child talk in formed sentences? _____

Eating Habits:

Does child: Feed self _____ Yes _____ No

Does child need help to eat? _____

Food and beverage:

Likes:_____

_____

Dislikes: _____

_____

Usual appetite? _____

Appetite now? _____

Last time child had food or beverage: _____

Items brought to hospital:

Glasses	_____ Yes	_____ No
Contacts	_____ Yes	_____ No
Hearing Aid	_____ Yes	_____ No
Dentures	_____ Yes	_____ No
Braces	_____ Yes	_____ No
Retainer	_____ Yes	_____ No
Special bottle	_____ Yes	_____ No
Own pacifier	_____ Yes	_____ No

Does child smoke or drink alcoholic beverages? _____ Yes _____ No

If yes, please give details _____

_____

Does child use street drugs? _____ Yes _____ No

If yes, please give details_____

_____

Other behavior habits of the child (Please check)

Thumbsucking _____ ; Nailbiting _____ ; Headbanging _____

Rituals (Explain) _____

_____

Disposition (Describe)_____

_____

Skin Assessment:

_____ Jaundice _____ Cyanosis _____ Pallor _____ Redness

_____ Cool _____ Warm _____ Clammy _____ Dry

_____ Normal appearance

Describe: (Location and character)

Rash _____

Abrasions _____

Lacerations _____

Contusions _____

Respiratory Assessment:

_____ Clear _____ Stridor _____ Rales (___moist, ___ dry) _____ Wheezing

_____ Rhonchi _____ Retractions (type) _____

_____ Coughing, Sneezing _____ Nasal Discharge (describe) _____

Child/Caregiver oriented to unit? _____ Yes _____ No; understanding verbalized by child _____, caregiver _____

Reviewed safety measures with child _____, caregiver _____; understanding verbalized by child _____, caregiver _____

Additional information nursing staff should know:

Figure 2-3. A sample pediatric nursing assessment form.

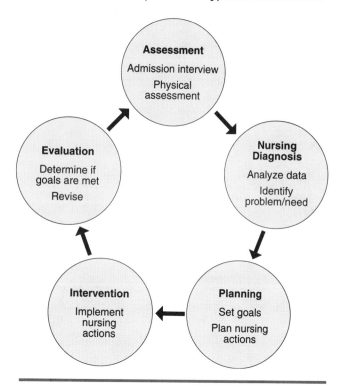

Figure 2-4. Diagram of the nursing process.

be skilled in understanding the concepts of communication, both verbal and nonverbal; concepts of growth and development; anatomy, physiology, and pathophysiology; and the influence of cultural heritage and family social structure. The data collected during the assessment of the child and family form the basis of all nursing care of the child.

Assessment begins with the admission interview and physical assessment. During this phase, a relationship of trust begins to build between the nurse, the child, and the family caregivers. This relationship forms more quickly when the nurse is sensitive to the cultural background of the family. Careful listening and recording of **subjective data** (data spoken by the child or family) and care observation and recording of **objective data** (observable by the nurse) are essential to obtain a complete picture.

Nursing Diagnosis

The process of determining a nursing diagnosis begins with the analysis of information (data) gathered during the assessment. A nursing diagnosis then may be made, based on actual or potential health problems that fall within the range of nursing practice. These diagnoses are not medical diagnoses but are based on the individual's response to a disease process, condition, or situation. Nursing diagnoses change as the patient's responses change, therefore they are in a continual state of reevaluation and modification. Nursing diagnoses are subdivided into three types: actual, high-risk, and wellness diagnoses.

Actual nursing diagnoses identify existing health problems. For example, a child who has asthma may have an actual diagnosis stated as *Ineffective airway clearance related to increased mucus production as evidenced by dyspnea and wheezing*. This statement identifies a health problem the child actually has (ineffective airway clearance), the factor that contributes to its cause (increased mucus production), and the signs and symptoms. Because of the presence of signs and symptoms of the child's inability to effectively clear the airway, this is an actual nursing diagnosis.

High-risk nursing diagnoses, a category that became effective in 1992, identify those health problems to which the patient is especially vulnerable. These identify those patients at high risk for a particular problem. For example: *High risk for injury related to uncontrolled muscular activity secondary to seizure*.

Wellness nursing diagnoses are those that identify the potential of an individual, family, or community to move from one level of wellness to a higher level. For example, a wellness diagnosis for a family adapting well to the birth of a second child might be *Potential for enhanced parenting*.

An approved list of nursing diagnoses were first published by the North American Nursing Diagnosis Association (NANDA) in 1973. NANDA has revised and added to these periodically since then. Currently, there are approximately 100 approved diagnoses.

Planning and Implementation

Planning nursing care for the child requires that data have been collected (assessment) and analyzed (nursing diagnosis) and goals have been set in cooperation with the child and family caregiver. These goals should be stated in measurable terms, with a specified time frame. For example, a short-term goal for a child with asthma could be "Child demonstrates use of metered dose inhaler within 2 days." After mutual goal setting has been accomplished, nursing actions are proposed. Although a number of possible diagnoses may be identified, the nurse must review them, rank by urgency, and select those that require the most immediate attention.

On completing the selection of the nursing goals to be accomplished first, the nurse must propose nursing interventions to achieve these goals. These nursing interventions may be based on clinical experience, knowledge of the health problem, standards of care, standard care plans, or other resources. The interventions should be discussed with the child and family caregiver to determine if they are practical and workable. Proposed interventions are modified to fit the individual child. If standardized care plans are used, they must be individualized to reflect the child's age and developmental level, cognitive level, and family, economic, and cultural influences.

Implementation is putting the nursing care plan into action. These actions may be independent, dependent, or interdependent. **Independent nursing actions** are those actions that may be performed based on the nurse's own clinical judgment, for example, initiating protective skin care for an area that might break down. **Dependent nursing actions** are those actions that the nurse performs as a result of a physician's orders, such as administering analgesics for pain. **Interdependent nursing actions** are those actions that the nurse must work with other health team members to accomplish, such as meal planning with the dietary therapist and teaching breathing exercises with the respiratory therapist.

Evaluation

Evaluation is a vital part of the nursing process—it measures the success or failure of the nursing care plan. Like assessment, evaluation is an ongoing process. Evaluation is achieved by determining if the goals have been met. The criteria of the nursing goals determine if the interventions were effective. If the goals have not been met in the specified time, or if implementation is not successful, a particular intervention may need to be reassessed and revised. Possibly the goal is unrealistic and needs to be discarded or adjusted. The child and the family must be assessed to adequately determine progress. Both objective data, which can be measured, and subjective data (responses from the child and family) are used in the evaluation.

Observation and Recording

As noted earlier, one of the most important parts of nursing care is continuous, careful observation of the patient's behavior and recording those observations in clear, specific terms. Nurses' notes often provide vital clues to a child's condition that health team members depend on for further diagnosis and treatment.

Observation of behavior should include the factors that influenced the behavior and how often the behavior is repeated. Physical behavior as well as emotional and intellectual responses should be noted, considering the child's age and developmental level, the abnormal environment of the hospital, and whether the child has been hospitalized previously or otherwise separated from family caregivers. It is important to note whether the behavior is consistent or unpredictable and any apparent reasons for changed behavior.

The Infant

Characteristic behaviors of the healthy infant compared with behaviors that may indicate signs of illness are shown in Table 2-1. The nurse must be cautious when using the type of information shown in such a table. Occasional evidence of one or more of the behaviors may not be significant. Any instance of behavior indicating illness needs to be documented and further evaluated in light of

frequency of the behavior as well as the usual behavior of the infant. If the caregiver has indicated in the assessment interview or on further questioning that this behavior is not out of the ordinary for the infant, it may not be indicative of a problem.

The Older Child

Most of the observations in Table 2-1 are valid for the older child as well. In addition, there are a few different or more mature reactions that may indicate an unhealthy state.

Covering Up for Pain or Discomfort. Few children get any enjoyment from illness or hospitalization. Going home is usually the child's burning desire, and the child often goes to great lengths to cover up any discomfort. Observing when the child is unaware of being watched helps the nurse determine if the child is showing any signs of pain, such as limping, holding one side of the abdomen, and grimacing. Then note what happens when the child realizes you are watching. Does the child straighten up and say, "I was just kidding around."? This is behavior that should be reported.

Extremes of Aggression or Passivity. How does this child behave? Is the child aggressive, resisting any and all advances, and striking out against playmates or adults? Or is the child passive, accepting everything? Even more important, is this a change in behavior? To know the answers, you must be consistently observant and record the child's behavior.

Reaction with Family Caregivers. Get a feeling of the interaction between the child and family caregivers—how they interact may be a reflection of their feelings toward each other. It also may reflect the caregivers' attitude to the situation of illness and hospitalization or to the care that the child is receiving.

Communication

Although most people think of communication as an oral or written exchange of words, communication also includes the body language, facial expression, voice intonations, and emotions behind the words that are exchanged between two or more people. One of the most important aspects of communication is listening to the other person. Listening is more than hearing. It includes "tuning in" to the other person, being sensitive to feelings, and concentrating on what the other person is trying to express. The nurse must be aware of underlying emotions and recognize the effect they have on the communication process. It is also important to clarify statements and feelings expressed by the child or caregiver. A reflective statement may indicate what the nurse believed was expressed. For instance, the nurse might say, "You are worried about Maria's loss of appetite." In this way the speaker may confirm or deny that the nurse has inter-

Table 2-1. Comparison of Observations of an Infant's Physical and Emotional Behavior

Observation	Healthy Activity	Behavior Indicating Illness*
Activity	Constantly active; some infants are more intense and curious than others	Lies quietly; little or no interest in surroundings; may stay in the same position
State of muscular tension	Muscular state is tense; grasp tight, head raised when prone, kicks are vigorous When supine, there is a space between the mattress and the infant's back	Lies relaxed with arms and legs straight and lax; makes no attempt to turn or raise head if placed in prone position; does not move about in crib
Constancy of reaction	Shows a constancy in reaction, does not regress in development; peppy and vigorous; interested in food; responds to caregiver's presence or voice	Not as peppy as previously; responds to discomfort and pain in apathetic manner; turns away from food that had once interested; turns head and cries instead of usual response
Behavior indicating pain	Appreciates being picked up Activity is not restlessness Shows activity in every part of body	Cries or protests when handled, seems to want to be left alone. May cry when picked up, but settles down after being held for a time, indicating something hurts when moved Turns head fretfully from side to side; pulls ear or rubs head; turns and rolls constantly, seemingly to try to get away from pain
Cry	Strong, vigorous cry	Weak, feeble cry, or whimper High-pitched cry, shrill cry may indicate increased intracranial pressure
Skin color	Healthy tint to skin; nailbeds and oral mucosa, conjunctivae, and tongue reddish-pink	Light-skinned babies may show unusual pallor or blueness around the eyes and nose. All babies may have dark or cyanotic nailbeds; pale oral mucosa, conjunctivae, and tongue
Appetite or feeding pattern	Exhibits an eagerness and impatience to satisfy hunger	May show indifference toward formula; sucking half-heartedly; vomits feeding; habitually regurgitates. May exhibit discomfort after feeding
Bizarre behavior		Any behavior that differs from expected for level of development; unusually good, or passive, when in strange surroundings; responds with rejection to every overture, friendly or otherwise; extremely clinging, never satisfied with amount of attention received

* Any *one* manifestation in itself may not be significant. The important thing is whether this behavior is consistent with this particular child or is a change from previous behavior. The significance depends greatly on the constancy of the behavior.

preted correctly. The pediatric nurse must be especially skilled in listening to communicate successfully with children and caregivers.

Communication with Children
The nurse is constantly communicating with patients, even though they may not be able to understand the words or respond. Infants evaluate actions, not realizing that nurses who handle them abruptly and hurriedly may be rushed or insecure; these small patients feel only that these nurses are frightening and unloving.

The child who is old enough to distinguish between people (generally some time after 6 months of age) tends to be frightened of strangers. Sudden, abrupt, or noisy approaches are almost certain to signal danger to the child. The child needs time to make an evaluation of the situation while still secure in the familiar arms of the caregiver. The nurse should not rush the situation but allow time for the child to initiate the relationship. Often the conversation may be started through a doll or stuffed animal the child brings to the hospital setting. Ask the toy's name, and address the toy, or just call it "Dolly," "Teddy," "Puppy," or "Kitty" if the child will not reveal the name. Ask the toy how it feels, referring to the part of the body that is the child's problem. For example, "Are you having trouble breathing today, Dolly?"

Distrust of strangers may last through the first 3 or 4 years of life. A casual approach with reluctant children is usually more effective. Those children who show rejecting or aggressive behavior are putting up a defense against their own fears, and the behavior should be ignored unless it threatens the child's own well-being or that of someone else.

Some nurses have difficulty in accepting their own feelings while working with children. Each nurse brings personal feelings, fears, and conflicts to a new situation. Many nurses feel inadequate when beginning relationships with children. Nurses need to be willing to accept the fact that they are also human. A good nurse is self-accepting and self-confident but does not necessarily begin that way; this comes with maturity and insight.

When speaking with small or young children, the nurse should not stand over them and talk down to them but should get down on eye level with them. The best plan is to speak in a slow, clear, positive voice, using simple words. Sentences should be short, and statements or questions should be expressed positively. Choices should be simple and only offered if a choice actually exists. Do not say, "Do you want to take your medicine now?" if there is no other option. Listen to the child's fears and worries; be honest in your answers. In addition, the perceptions of young children are literal. For instance, if the nurse says, "This will only be a little bee sting," children actually visualize being stung by a bee and that may be traumatic. As a result of this characteristic, the nurse must be careful to use positive explanations in terms that are familiar and nonthreatening to the child.

The school-age child is interested in knowing what and why. Explanations that help them understand how equipment works are important to them. The child does not need a complex or detailed explanation. A simple response is best. The child of this age will ask more questions if his or her curiosity was not satisfied.

It may be challenging to communicate with adolescents. Young teenagers frequently waver between thinking like a child and thinking like an adult. Sometimes the adolescent does not want to reveal much if a parent is present. Teens may need to relate information that they do not wish others to know. A discussion about confidentiality may set the adolescent's concerns at ease. The adolescent needs to know that the nurse will listen attentively, in an open-minded, nonjudgmental way.

The adolescent and the family may not view a problem in the same way. If this is the case, the problem may need to be defined more clearly so that an agreement may be reached, if possible. The nurse may be instrumental in assisting with the resolution of disagreements between the family and the adolescent.

Cultural Factors in Communication. Each child is the product of a family, a culture, and a community. The culture determines not only the language but the health

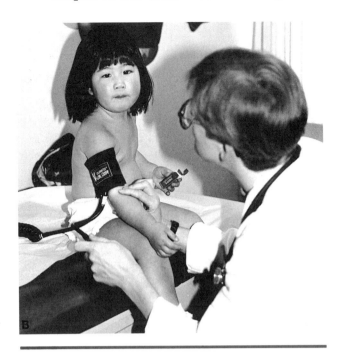

Figure 2-5. Children whose cultural heritage is different from that of the hospital staff have special problems in adjustment. (From Jackson DB, Saunders RB. Child Health Nursing. Philadelphia: JB Lippincott, 1993, p. 996.)

beliefs and practices of the family. Nurses who care for children need an understanding of the health practices and lifestyle of families from various cultures to plan culturally appropriate and acceptable care (Figure 2-5).

In some cultures, family life is gentle, permissive, and loving; in others, unquestioning obedience is demanded and pain and hardship are to be stoically endured. The child may be from a cultural group that places a high value on children, giving them lots of attention from many relatives and friends, or the child may be from a group that has taught the child that from early childhood one must fend for oneself.

Cultural attitudes toward food, cleanliness, respect, and freedom are all important in planning care for the child while in the hospital and after returning home. The behavior and cooperation of child and family are essential to achieving restoration of good health.

Children from families who are new to this country or whose social contacts have been primarily with their own cultural group are likely to feel bewildered or antagonistic. Hospitals may be strange to children raised in middle-class America. Is it any wonder that a Navaho Native American child reacts negatively to an atmosphere where food, language, people, and surroundings are totally alien?

Respect for a child's cultural heritage and individuality is an essential part of nursing care. The objective is to restore health so that the child may once again be a functioning part of the family and the community, whatever the cultural background.

Communication with Family Caregivers

Routine conferences among the nursing staff, physicians, child-life workers, physical therapists, and other personnel concerned with children in the hospital are helpful in gaining an understanding of child patients. A clearer picture of the child is obtained, his or her behavior is better understood, and an opportunity is presented to consider differing types of treatment and relationships. These outcomes may be rewarding to both the patient and the staff. When appropriate, the family caregivers may be invited to attend, and they may gain valuable insights and understanding.

Some hospitals prefer to hold parent group sessions. In either instance, it is most important that family caregivers are kept well informed about what is going on and what is being planned for their sick child (Figure 2-6).

Much may be done to make the caregivers feel welcome and important. When a procedure is planned, the caregiver may be told what is going to happen and invited to help, if practical. However, no caregiver who is reluctant to help with or observe a procedure should be urged to stay or made to feel it is a duty that should be fulfilled. Some caregivers are so anxious and apprehensive that they communicate their concern to the child rather than provide support. Attitudes from the caregiver may easily be conveyed to the child, sometimes causing negative reactions from the child. The nurse must be alert for any negative attitudes. Giving the caregiver time to discuss anxieties and concerns, exploring these problems with the caregiver, and demonstrating genuine caring and concern help ease these feelings. The nurse must remember that part of the nursing role is to be an ambassador of good will to the child and the family.

An older child may feel self-sufficient and may view the family caregiver's presence as being treated like a baby. However, it is normal to regress during illness, and most children of any age appreciate the presence of an assuring, self-controlled person during trying, uncomfortable times. The child needs to be able to trust the environment. If, as often happens, the child regresses in handling the overwhelming distress, the presence of a family caregiver may offer support.

Importance of Caregiver Participation

Research findings have clearly shown that separating young children from their family caregivers, especially during times of stress, may have damaging effects. Young children have no concept of time, so separation from their primary caregivers is especially difficult for them to understand. Three characteristic stages of response to the separation have been identified: protest, despair, and denial. Protest is the first stage. During this time the young child cries, often refusing to be comforted by others and constantly seeking the primary caregiver in every sight and sound. When the caregiver does not appear, the child enters the second stage—despair—and becomes apathetic and listless. Health care personnel often interpret this as a sign that the child is accepting the situation, but this is not the case; the child has given up.

In the third stage—denial—the child begins taking interest in the surroundings and appears to accept the situation. However, the damage is revealed when the caregivers do visit: the child often turns away from them, showing distrust and rejection. It may take a long time before the child accepts them again, and even then, remnants of the damage linger. The child may always have a memory of being abandoned at the hospital. Childhood impressions have a deep effect, regardless of how mistaken they may be.

A large number of hospitals provide for family caregivers to "room-in," which helps remove the hurt and depressions of the young hospitalized child. Although it is generally considered that separation from primary caregivers causes the greatest upset in children younger than 5 years of age, all years of childhood should be considered when setting up a rooming-in system.

One advantage of rooming-in is the measure of security the child feels as a result of the caregiver's care and attention. The primary caregiver may participate in bathing, dressing, and feeding; preparing the child for bed; and providing recreational activities. However, this system should not be used to relieve staff shortage. If treatments are to be continued at home, rooming-in creates an excel-

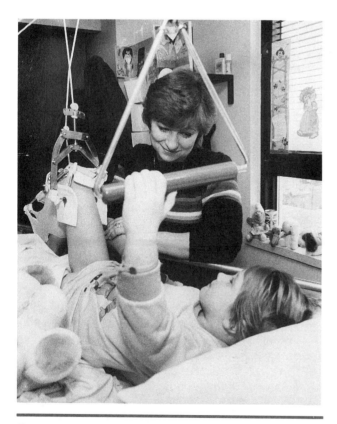

Figure 2-6. The close proximity of a parent is reassuring to the ill child.

lent opportunity for the caregiver to observe and practice before leaving the hospital.

Rules should be clearly understood before admission, and facilities for caregivers should be clearly explained. The hospital may provide a folding cot or reclining chair in the child's room. Provision for meals should be explained to the caregiver.

The nursing staff should be careful to avoid creating a situation in which they appear to be expecting the primary caregivers to perform as health care technicians. The basic role of the primary caregiver is to provide security and stability to the child.

Many pediatric units also have recognized the importance of allowing siblings to visit the hospitalized child. This policy provides benefits to both the hospitalized child and the sibling. The sibling at home may be imagining a much more serious illness than is actually the case. Visiting policies usually require that a family adult accompanies and is responsible for the child and that the visiting period is not too long. There also should be a policy requiring that the visiting sibling does not have a cold or other contagious illness and is up to date in immunizations.

The nursing staff also should be aware of the caregiver's needs. The caregiver needs to be encouraged to leave for meals or a break or to go home, if possible, for a shower and rest. The child may be given a possession of the caregiver's to help reassure that the caregiver will return.

The Hospital Play Program

Play is the business of children and a principal way in which they learn, grow, develop, and act out feelings and problems. Playing is a normal activity, and the more it can be part of hospital care, the more normal and more comfortable this environment becomes.

Play helps children come to terms with the hurts, anxieties, and separation that hospitalization brings. In the hospital playroom children may express frustrations, hostilities, and aggressions through play without the fear of being scolded by the nursing staff. Children who keep these negative emotions bottled up suffer much greater damage than those who are allowed to let them out where they may be handled constructively. Children must feel secure enough in the situation to express negative emotions without fear of disapproval.

Children must not be allowed to harm themselves or others, however. Although it is important to express feelings, acceptable or not, unlimited permissiveness is as harmful as excessive strictness. Children rely on adults to guide them and set limits for behavior because this means the adults care about them. When disapproval is necessary, it is important to make it clear that the child's action is being disapproved, not the child.

The Hospital Play Environment

Although a well-equipped playroom is of major importance in any pediatric department, children may play out their fantasies and emotions in their own crib or bed if for some reason they cannot be brought to the playroom. Materials for their particular use may be brought to them, and someone, a nurse or student volunteer, should be available to give the necessary support and attention needed.

An organized and well-planned play area is of considerable importance in the overall care of the hospitalized child (Figure 2-7). The play area should be large enough to accommodate cribs, wheelchairs, intravenous poles, and children in casts. It should provide a variety of play materials suitable for the ages and needs of all children. The child chooses the toy and the kind of play needed or desired; thus, the selection and kind of play may usually be left unstructured. This rule does not, however, mean that the child should be ignored by the play leaders or that nonparticipation is acceptable.

Adolescents should have a separate recreation room or area, if at all possible. Ideally, this is an area in which adolescents may gather to talk, play pool or table tennis, and have access to soft drinks (if permitted) and snacks. Tables and chairs should be provided to encourage interaction among the adolescents. Television with a videocassette tape player, computer games, and shuffle board are also desirable. These activities should be in an area away from young children. Rules may be clearly spelled out and posted.

Therapeutic Play

The nurse should understand the difference between play therapy and therapeutic play. **Play therapy** is a technique of psychoanalysis that psychiatrists or psychiatric nurse clinicians use to uncover a disturbed child's underlying thoughts, feelings, and motivations to help understand them better. **Therapeutic play** is a play technique that may be used by play therapists, nurses, child-life specialists, or trained volunteers.

The play leader should be alert to the needs of the child who is afraid to act independently as a result of strict home discipline. Even normally sociable children may carry their fears of the hospital environment into the playroom. It could be some time before timid, fearful, or nonassertive children are able to feel free enough to take advantage of the play opportunities. Too much enthusiasm on the part of the play leader in trying to get the child to participate may defeat the play leader's purpose and make the child withdraw. The leader must decide carefully whether to initiate an activity for a child or let the child advance at a self-set pace.

Often, other children provide the best incentive by doing something interesting so the timid child forgets apprehensions and tries it, or a child says, "Come and help me with this," and soon the other child becomes

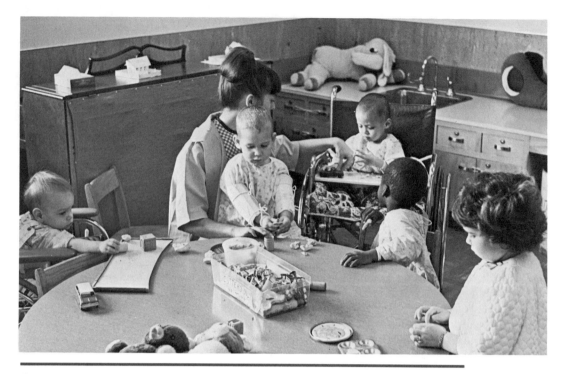

Figure 2-7. Children in a hospital playroom.

involved. A fearful child trusts a peer before trusting an adult who represents authority. Naturally, this fact does not mean the child's presence should be ignored. The leader shows the child around the playroom, indicating that the children are free to play with whatever they wish and that the leader is there to answer questions and to help when a child wishes or desires help.

When group play is initiated, the leader may invite the timid child to participate but should not insist. The leader must give the child time to adjust and gain confidence.

Play Material

All play material should be chosen with safety in mind: no sharp edges and no small parts that can be swallowed or aspirated. Toys and equipment should be inspected regularly for broken parts or sharp edges. Constant supervision of children while they are playing is necessary to provide for safety.

One important function of a playroom is the provision of opportunities for the child to dramatize hospital experiences. One section of the playroom containing hospital equipment, miniature or real, gives the child opportunity to play out feelings concerning the hospital environment and treatments. Stethoscopes, simulated thermometers, stretchers, wheelchairs, examining tables, instruments, bandages, and other medical and hospital equipment are useful for this purpose.

Dolls or puppets dressed to represent the people with whom the child comes in contact daily—boy, girl, and infant, as well as adult family members, nurses, physicians, therapists, and other personnel—should be available. Hospital scrub suits, scrub caps, isolation-type gowns, masks, or other types of uniforms may be provided for children to use in acting out their hospital experiences. These simulated hospitals also serve an educational purpose; the child who is to have surgery, tests, or special treatments may be helped to better understand the projected procedures and why they are done.

Other useful materials for the child's play (these are only a few samples of the many possibilities) are listed as follows:

- Ingredients for homemade play dough. Allowing and helping a child to make play dough gives the child greater satisfaction in using it than if the finished material is simply provided.

- Finger paints, water colors, crayons, and colored pencils; easels and drawing paper to use for the child's creations.

- Cut-out books, scissors, paste; pictures to paste on paper, perhaps to make the child's own scrapbook.

- Games, blocks, jigsaw puzzles, and building sets.

- For children who can be more physically active: tricycles, small sliding boards, and seesaws.

- Miniature stores with scales, counters, play models of store products.

Table 2-2. Games and Activities Using Materials
Available on a Nursing Unit

Age	Activity
Infant	Make a mobile from roller gauze and tongue blades to hang over a crib Ask the pharmacy or central supply for different size boxes to use for put-in, take-out toys (Do not use round vials from pharmacy; if accidentally aspirated, these can completely occlude the airway) Blow up a glove as a balloon; draw a smiling face on it with a marker Play "Patty Cake," "So Big," "Peek-a-Boo"
Toddler	Ask central supply for boxes to use as blocks for stacking Tie roller gauze to a glove box for a pull toy Sing or recite familiar nursery rhymes such as "Peter, Peter, Pumpkin Eater"
Preschool	Play "Simon Says" or "Mother, May I?" Draw a picture of a dog; ask child to close eyes; add an additional feature to the dog; ask the child to guess the added part, and repeat until a full picture is drawn Make a puppet from a lunch bag or draw a face on your hand with a marker Cut out a picture from a nursing journal (or draw a picture); cut it into large puzzle pieces Pour breakfast cereal into a basin; furnish boxes to pour and spoons to dig Furnish chart paper and a Magic Marker for coloring Make modeling clay from 1 cup salt, ½ cup flour, ½ cup water from diet kitchen Play "Ring-Around-the-Rosey" or "London Bridge"
School-age	Play "I Spy" or charades Make a deck of cards to play "Go Fish" or "Old Maid"; invent cards such as Nicholas Nurse, Doctor Dolittle, Irene Intern, Polly Patient Play "Hangman" Furnish scale or table paper and a Magic Marker for a huge drawing or sign Hide an object in the child's room and have the child look for it (have the child name places for you to look if the child cannot be out of bed)
Adolescent	Color squares on a chart form to make a checkerboard Have adolescent make a deck of cards to use for "Hearts" or "Rummy" Compete to see how many words the adolescent can make from the letters in the child's name Compete to guess whether the next person to enter room will be a man or woman, next car to go by window will be red or black, and so forth Compete to see who can name the most episodes of the television shows "Star Trek" or reruns of "The Brady Bunch"

From Pillitteri A. Maternal and Child Health. Philadelphia: JB Lippincott, 1992, p 1051.

Sometimes, only a little imagination is needed to be used to initiate an interesting play time. Table 2-2 suggests some activities at various age levels, most of which may be played in the child's room. These are especially useful for the child who is not able to go to the playroom.

Books for all age groups are also important. Puppets play an important part in the children's department. The use of hand puppets does much to orient or assure a hospitalized child. The doctor or nurse puppet on the play leader's hand answers questions (and discusses feelings) that the puppet on the child's hand has asked. A child often finds it easier to express feelings, fears, and questions through a puppet than to verbalize them directly. A ready sense of magic can let the child make believe that the puppet is really expressing things that one hesitates to ask oneself (Figure 2-8).

Ambulatory Play Facilities
The pediatric ambulatory departments are busy places. Growing knowledge of childhood diseases and their

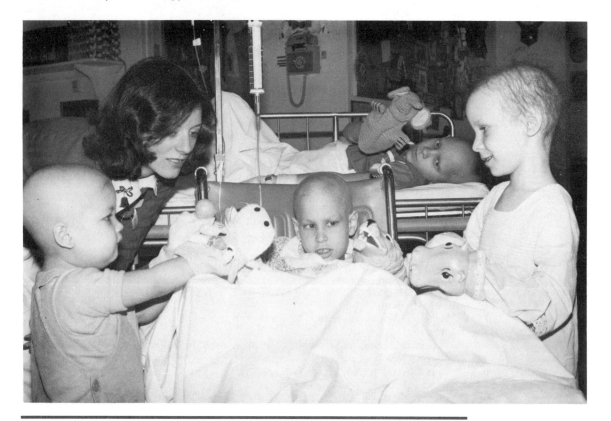

Figure 2-8. A puppet play group led by a pediatric nurse oncologist allows children to talk about what it's like to be in the hospital. Group sessions inform children that others have similar feelings.

treatment has made possible the treatment of more children as outpatients, allowing them to live at home. Because they must also be treated as children, a properly equipped and adequately staffed playroom is needed in a pediatric ambulatory setting.

Many children with serious but chronic diseases become frequent visitors to the ambulatory department. The provision of a playroom is not only enjoyable but helpful to children who are to undergo medical procedures, which may be frightening to the unprepared child. Play workers have an excellent opportunity to help an anxious child work through fears. Toys should be durable and easily cleaned. They should not require a specific time commitment so that children may leave when called for examination. They should also allow for both individual and group play. A play house, for instance, allows children to use their imaginations and incorporate one another in and out of the play as they arrive and leave for their appointments.

Some children who have become engrossed in a play project may resent having to leave it when called for examination. The child may be assured that the project may be finished after the treatment if the family caregiver is willing or able to take the time. If for any reason a child must be left in the playroom without the caregiver, name bands or name tags should be available, particularly for a new child or one unfamiliar to the staff.

Safety

Safety is an essential aspect of pediatric nursing care. It is a fact that accidents occur more often when people are in stressful situations. Infants, children, and their caregivers experience additional stress when a child is hospitalized. They are removed from a familiar home environment, faced with anxieties and fear, and have to adjust to an unfamiliar schedule. The pediatric nurse must have safety in mind at all times, consciously assessing every situation for accident potential.

The environment should meet all of the safety standards appropriate for other areas of the hospital, including good lighting, dry floors with no obstacles that may cause falls, electrical equipment checked for hazards, safe bath and shower facilities, and beds in low position for ambulatory patients.

The age and developmental level of the child must be considered. Toddlers are explorers whose developmental task is to develop autonomy. Toddlers love to put small objects into equally small openings, whether the opening is in their body, the oxygen tent, or elsewhere in the pediatric unit. Careful observation may prevent the toddler from having access to small objects, eliminating some of the dangers. Toddlers are also often climbers and must be protected from climbing and falling. Toddlers and preschoolers need special watching to protect them

Box 2-2

Safety Precautions for Pediatric Units

1. Cover electrical outlets.
2. Keep floor dry and free of clutter.
3. Use tape or Velcro closures when possible.
4. Always close safety pins when not in use.
5. Inspect toys (child's or hospital's) for loose or small parts, sharp edges, dangerous cords, or other hazards.
6. Do not permit friction toys where oxygen is in use.
7. Do not leave child unattended in high chair.
8. Keep crib sides up the full way, except when caring for child.
9. If the crib side is down, keep hand firmly on infant at all times.
10. Use crib with top if child stands or climbs.
11. Always check temperature of bath water to prevent burns.
12. Never leave infant or child unattended in bath water.
13. Keep beds of ambulatory children locked in low position.
14. Turn off motor of electric bed if young children might have access to controls.
15. Always use safety belts or straps for children in infant seats, feeding chairs, strollers, wheelchairs, or stretchers.
16. Use restraints only when necessary.
17. When restraints are used, remove and check for skin integrity, circulation, and correct application at least every hour or two.
18. Never tie a restraint to the crib side; tie to bed frame only.
19. Keep medications securely locked in designated area; children should never be permitted in this area.
20. Set limits and enforce them consistently; do not let children get out of control.
21. Place needles and syringes in sharps containers; make sure children have no access to these containers.
22. Always pick up any equipment after a procedure.
23. Never leave scissors or other sharp instruments within child's reach.

from danger. Nurses also must encourage family members to keep the crib sides up when they are not directly caring for the infant in the crib. One unguarded moment may mean a fall out of a crib for an infant. Box 2-2 presents a summary of pediatric safety precautions.

Restraints

Restraints often are needed to protect a child from injury during a procedure or an examination or to ensure the infant or child's safety and comfort. Restraints should never be used as a form of punishment. When possible, restraining by hand is the best method. However, for securing a child during intravenous infusions, to protect a surgical site from injury, such as cleft lip and cleft palate, or other times when restraint by hand is not practical, mechanical restraints must be used. Various types of restraints may be used.

A **mummy restraint** is used for an infant or small child during a procedure. (Figure 2-9). This device is a snug wrap that is effective when performing a scalp venipuncture, inserting a nasogastric tube, or performing other procedures that involve only the head or neck. A **papoose board** is commercially available for use with toddlers or preschool-age children.

Clove hitch restraints are used to secure an arm or leg, most often when a child is receiving an intravenous infusion. The restraint is made of soft cloth formed in a figure eight. Padding under the restraint is desirable if the child puts any pull on it. The site should be checked and loosened at least every 2 hours. Commercial restraints also are available to use for this purpose. **Elbow restraints** often are made of muslin that has two layers. Pockets wide enough to fit tongue depressors are placed vertically the width of the fabric. The top flap folds over to close the pockets. The restraint is wrapped around the child's arm and tied securely, preventing the child from bending the elbow. Care must be taken that the elbow restraints fit the child properly. They should not be too high under the axillae. They may be pinned to the child's shirt to keep them from slipping.

Jacket restraints are used to secure the child from climbing out of bed or a chair or to keep the child in a horizontal position. The restraint must be the correct size for the child. A child in a jacket restraint should be checked frequently to prevent the child from slipping and choking on the neck of the jacket. Ties must be secure to the bed frame, not the sides, so that the jacket is not pulled when the sides are put up and down. Whatever the type of restraint, caution is essential. Close and conscientious observation is a necessary part of nursing care. The nurse also must be alert to concerns of the family when the child is in restraints. Explanations about the need for restraints help the family understand and be cooperative. The caregiver may wish to physically restrain the child to prevent use of restraints, and this action is often possible. Each situation must be judged on its own merits.

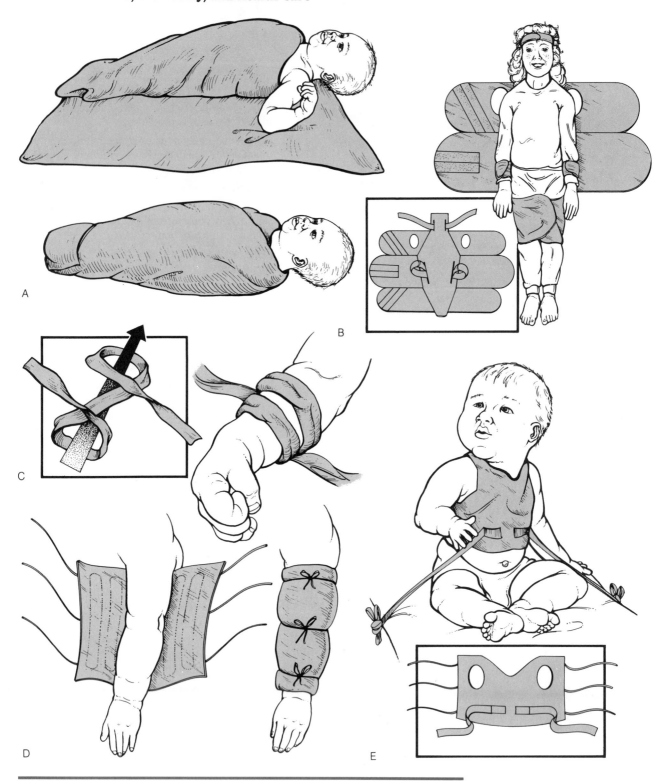

Figure 2-9. **A**, Mummy restraint. **B**, Papoose board. **C**, Clove hitch restraint. **D**, Elbow restraint. **E**, Jacket restraint.

Summary

Hospitalization places great stress on the child and the family. Many factors affect the way the family reacts to hospitalization of the child. Pediatric units are designed to present a warm, friendly, nonthreatening atmosphere for the child. Preadmission education also may help prepare the child for the event. Nevertheless, many anxieties persist. Emergency admissions and admissions to the PICUs may be especially traumatic. The nurse must be prepared to help the family and the child adjust. Liberal visiting policies, encouraging family caregivers to stay with young children, and sibling visiting contribute to decreasing the stress of hospitalization.

The admission interview sets the stage for the hospitalization, providing information that assists the health care team to provide the best possible care for the child and assist in the child's adjustment to the hospitalization. Using the nursing process, the nurse gathers, analyzes, plans, implements, and evaluates the care of the child. The nurse must be familiar with the characteristics of growth and development of each age level to accurately observe and record the child's progress.

Communication with child and family is a skill that the nurse must practice to perfect. Good communication skills are necessary to successfully care for children and their families.

Play is fundamental to the care of children. Therapeutic play offers the child the opportunity to express anger and fear in a safe environment. Expressing these emotions is beneficial to the child. Adolescents need a special area in which they may enjoy activities suited to their age.

Safety is an essential aspect of pediatric care. Children must be protected from any hazards that can cause harm to them. Understanding the growth and development levels of each age group helps the nurse be alert to possible dangers for each child. When restraints are necessary, care must be taken to protect the child from injury from the restraints by regular, careful observation.

Review Questions

1. Your neighbor's little girl, 3-year-old Angel, is going to be admitted to the pediatric unit for tests and possible surgery. How can you help her mother prepare her for this event?

2. Miguel, a 4-year-old child of migrant workers, is hurt in a farming accident. You are working in the ED when he is brought in for treatment. His grandmother, who speaks little English, is with him. How are you going to help this grandmother and child? What do you need to consider?

3. Shantel is an 8-month-old infant admitted to the pediatric unit. Her mother is unsure of whether she should stay because of other children at home. She asks for your advice. What will you say to her?

4. On a playground, you hear a child's caregiver say, "If you don't stop that you're going to hurt yourself and end up in the hospital!" How do you feel about this? Would you make any response?

5. Why is a treatment room necessary on the pediatric unit?

6. Would you do a fingerstick for a blood glucose determination in the playroom? Defend your answer.

7. Plan an orientation visit for a group of preschoolers from a nursery school. Check and use what is available in the pediatric unit where you have your clinical experience.

8. Develop a questionnaire to use in an admission interview (or redesign one currently in use where you have your clinical experience).

9. How would you prepare 2½-year-old Jason for a spinal tap? Would you let Martha, his primary caregiver, accompany him? Defend your answer.

10. How can rooming-in be considered helpful in discharge planning?

11. A nurse, Jim, complains that he feels that 5-year-old Kara's father is spoiling her with all the attention he is showering on her. How would you respond to Jim?

12. You are caring for 8-year-old Luiz who is scheduled for surgery. He has been quiet and sullen. What can you to do establish communication with him? Explore several options.

13. Shy 7-year-old Josette is sitting by herself in the playroom. How will you attempt to involve her?

14. Design and plan the ideal "teen" activity room. List all furniture and equipment you would have, and state the use(s) for each.

Bibliography

Austin JK. Assessment of coping mechanisms used by parents and children with chronic illness. MCN 15:98–102, 1990.

Brazelton TB. To Listen to a Child. New York: Addison-Wesley, 1984.

Carpenito LJ. Handbook of Nursing Diagnosis, 4th ed. Philadelphia: JB Lippincott, 1991.

Castiglia PT, Harbin RE. Child Health Care: Process and Practice. Philadelphia: JB Lippincott, 1992.

Greenberg LA. Teaching children who are learning disabled about illness and hospitalization. MCN 16:260–263, 1991.

Meyer D. Children's responses to nursing attire. Pediatr Nurs 18:157–160, 1992.

Nugent KE. Routine care: Promoting development in hospitalized infants. MCN 14:318–321, 1989.

Pillitteri A. Maternal and Child Health Nursing. Philadelphia: JB Lippincott, 1992.

Pizzi M. Occupational therapy: Creating possibilities for children with HIV infection, ARC, and AIDS. AIDS Patient Care 3:31–36, 1989.

Ramsey AM, Siroky AS. (1988). The use of puppets to teach school-age children with asthma. Pediatr Nurs 14:187–190, 1988.

Schuster CS, Ashburn SS. The Process of Human Development, 3rd ed. Boston: Little, Brown, 1992.

Summers KH. Providing for play in the care of children. Pediatr Nurs 18:266–267, 1992.

Swanwick M. Development and chronic illness. Nurs (Lond) 4:24–27, 1990.

Vessey JA, Farley JA, Risom LR. Iatrogenic developmental effects of pediatric intensive care. Pediatr Nurs 18:229–232, 1992.

Whaley L, Wong D. Nursing Care of Infants and Children, 4th ed. St. Louis: Mosby-Year Book, 1991.

Care of the Hospitalized Child

Chapter 3

Student Objectives

Upon completion of this chapter, the student will be able to:

1. List the types of patients on whom a rectal temperature should not be taken.
2. Identify the five types of respiratory retractions and the location of each.
3. Name four methods of obtaining blood pressure.
4. State the purpose of pulse oximetry.
5. Identify the purpose of using the Glasgow coma scale for neurologic assessment.
6. List four methods of reducing fever in a child.
7. Identify four ways that pathogens are transmitted, and give an example of each.
8. Identify the role that handwashing plays in infection control.
9. Identify the five "rights" of medication administration.
10. Identify the muscle preferred for intramuscular injections in the infant.
11. State the reason that a pediatric intravenous set-up has a burette chamber in the line.
12. Name some of the fears that children have about surgery, and state how the nurse can help to relieve them.
13. Identify behavioral characteristics that may indicate that an infant or a young child is having pain.

Marks MG: BROADRIBB'S INTRODUCTORY PEDIATRIC
NURSING, 4th ed. © 1994 J.B. Lippincott Company.

Key Terms

acid–base balance

anuria

azotemia

body surface area (BSA) method

electrolytes

extracellular fluid

extravasation

gastrostomy tube

gavage feeding

homeostasis

hyperalimentation

induration

interstitial fluid

intracellular fluid

intravascular fluid

patient-controlled analgesia (PCA)

total parenteral nutrition (TPN)

tympanic membrane sensor

West nomogram

*C*aring for children in a pediatric setting varies greatly from caring for adults. The nurse must know the growth and development characteristics of each age level, understand the relationship of children and their caregivers, and know the modifications of nursing procedures that are necessary in caring for children. Most important, the nurse must remember that children should never be viewed as "miniature adults." Every procedure, including assessment of temperature and pulse, fever reduction, medication administration, and preparation for surgery, requires a keen awareness of the specific needs of the child undergoing the procedure.

Physical Care of the Hospitalized Child

Physical care of the hospitalized child requires a wide variety of nursing skills and includes ongoing and continuous assessment of vital signs and specific system functioning, regulation of body temperature, therapeutic application of heat and cold, and assistance in medical procedures and diagnostic tests. Understanding and respecting a child's developmental age and stage, as de-

scribed in Chapter 2, is an essential component of all of these skills. Using this information, the nurse is able to tailor procedures and teaching to best meet the needs of these young patients and their families.

Assessment of Vital Signs and Growth

Assessment of the child's vital signs is an essential part of the admission procedure. The results of the initial assessment serve as a baseline for determining the progress of the child's condition.

Temperature

The method of measuring a child's temperature commonly is set by the policy of the pediatric unit. The temperature can be measured by oral, rectal, axillary, or tympanic method. Temperatures are recorded in Celsius or Fahrenheit according to the policy of the hospital. Any deviation from the normal range of temperature should be reported. Temperatures vary with the method by which they are taken, thus it is important to record the route of temperature measurement along with the measured temperature.

Mercury or electronic thermometers may be used to measure temperature by the oral, rectal, and axillary routes. Electronic thermometers have oral and rectal probes. The nurse should be careful to select the correct probe when using the thermometer. In pediatrics, oral temperatures usually are taken only on children older than 4 to 6 years of age who are conscious and cooperative. Oral thermometers should be placed in the side of the child's mouth. The child should not be left unattended while any temperature is being taken (Figure 3-1).

Rectal temperatures commonly are measured in infants and children younger than 4 to 6 years of age. They are not desirable in the newborn because of the danger of irritation to the rectal mucosa. When a rectal temperature is taken, the bulb end should be lubricated with a water-soluble lubricant. The infant is placed in a prone position, the buttocks are gently separated with one hand, and the thermometer is inserted gently approximately $1/4$ to $1/2$ inch into the rectum (Figure 3-2**A** and **B**). If any resistance is felt, the nurse should remove the thermometer immediately and take the temperature by some other method. The nurse must keep one hand on the child's buttocks and

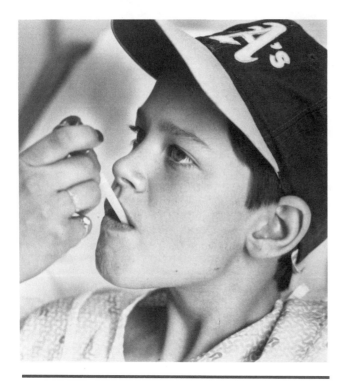

Figure 3-1. Placement of thermometer for oral temperature. (Courtesy of Nursing Department, Thomason Hospital, El Paso, TX.) (From Castiglia PT, Harbin RE. Child Health Care: Process and Practice. Philadelphia: JB Lippincott, 1992, p. 96.)

the other on the thermometer during the entire time the rectal thermometer is in place. A mercury thermometer is left in place for 3 or 4 minutes. An electronic thermometer is removed as soon as it signals that the temperature has been recorded.

Axillary temperatures are taken on newborns, infants and children with diarrhea, or when a rectal temperature is contraindicated. When taking an axillary temperature on an infant or child, the nurse must be certain to place the bulb of the thermometer well into the armpit, bringing the child's arm down close to the body. The nurse must check to see that there is skin-to-skin contact and that no clothing is in the way. The thermometer is left in place for 10 minutes or until the electronic thermometer signals (Figure 3-3).

Tympanic membrane sensors have been adopted by an increasing number of facilities. The tympanic thermometer offers the advantage of recording the temperature rapidly with little disturbance to the child. Tympanic thermometers are used according to the manufacturer's directions and hospital policy. A disposable speculum is used for each child. These thermometers are quick (registering in approximately 2 seconds) and noninvasive. A temperature often can be obtained without awakening a sleeping infant or child.

Pulse

Counting an apical rate is the preferred method to determine the pulse in an infant or young child. The nurse should try to accomplish this while the child is quiet. Approaching the child in a soothing, calm, quiet manner is helpful. The apical pulse should be counted before the child is disturbed for other procedures. A child can be held on the caregiver's lap for security for the full minute that the pulse is counted. The stethoscope is placed between the child's left nipple and sternum. A radial pulse may be taken on an older child. This pulse may be counted for 30 seconds and multiplied by 2. If the pulse is unusual in quality, rate, or rhythm, it should be counted for 1 full minute. Any rate that deviates from the normal rate should be reported. Pulse rates vary with age, from the 100 to 180 beats per minute for a neonate (birth to

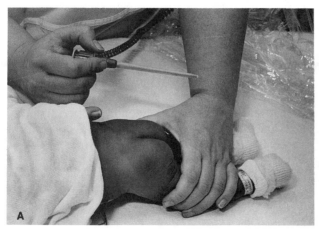
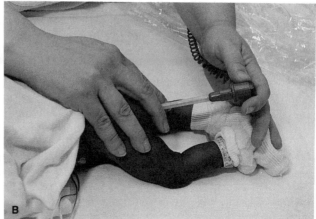

Figure 3-2. Taking rectal temperature of infant. **A**, Placing infant in prone position. **B**, Holding probe until signal sounds. (From Skale N. Manual of Pediatric Procedures. Philadelphia: JB Lippincott, 1992, p. 31.)

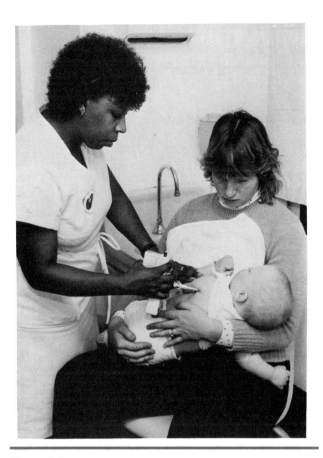

Figure 3-3. Taking an axillary temperature on an infant. (From Pillitteri A. Maternal and Child Health Nursing. Philadelphia: JB Lippincott, 1992, p. 1085.)

Table 3-1. Normal Pulse Ranges in Children

Age	Normal Range	Average
0–24 hours	70–170 bpm	120 bpm
1–7 days	100–180 bpm	140 bpm
1 month	110–188 bpm	160 bpm
1 month–1 year	80–180 bpm	120–130 bpm
2 years	80–140 bpm	110 bpm
4 years	80–120 bpm	100 bpm
6 years	70–115 bpm	100 bpm
10 years	70–110 bpm	90 bpm
12–14 years	60–110 bpm	85–90 bpm
14–18 years	50–95 bpm	70–75 bpm

bpm, beats per minute.
From Skale N. Manual of Pediatric Nursing Procedures. Philadelphia: JB Lippincott, 1992, p. 35.

should have an admission blood pressure taken. Obtaining a blood pressure measurement in an infant or small child is difficult, but equipment of the proper size helps ease the problem. The cuff should cover approximately two thirds of the arm. The blood pressure can be taken by the auscultation, palpation, Doppler, or flush method (Box 3-1). The Doppler method is used with increasing frequency to monitor pediatric blood pressure; however, the cuff still must be the correct size. Normal blood pressure values gradually increase from infancy through adolescence (Table 3-2).

30 days old) to 50 to 95 beats per minute for the 14- to 18-year-old adolescent (Table 3-1).

Respirations
Respirations of an infant or young child also must be counted during a quiet time. The child can be observed while he or she is lying or sitting quietly. Infants are abdominal breathers, therefore the rise and fall of the infant's abdomen are observed to count respirations; the older child's chest can be observed much as an adult's would be. The infant's respirations must be counted for 1 full minute because of normal irregularity. The chest of the infant or young child must be observed for retractions that indicate respiratory distress (Figure 3-4). Retractions are noted as substernal (below the sternum), subcostal (below the ribs), intercostal (between the ribs), suprasternal (above the sternum), or supraclavicular (above the clavicle).

Blood Pressure
For children 3 years of age and older, blood pressure monitoring is part of a routine physical assessment. All children of any age who are admitted to the hospital

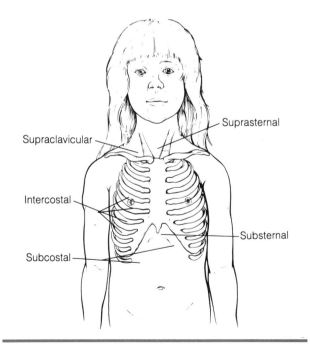

Figure 3-4. Sites of respiratory retraction.

Box 3-1

Methods for Measuring Pediatric Blood Pressures

For any method of measuring blood pressure, allow the child to handle the equipment. Use terminology appropriate to child's age. A preschool or young school-age child may want to use equipment to take the "blood pressure" of a doll or stuffed animal.

Auscultation

1. Place the correct size of cuff on the infant's or child's bare arm.
2. Locate the artery by palpating the antecubital fossa.
3. Inflate the cuff until radial pulse disappears or about 30 mm Hg above expected systolic reading.
4. Place stethoscope lightly over artery and slowly release air until pulse is heard.
5. Record readings as in adults.

Palpation

1. Follow steps 1 and 2 above.
2. Keep the palpating finger over the artery and inflate the cuff as above.
3. The point at which the pulse is felt is recorded as the systolic pressure.

Doppler

1. Obtain the monitor, dual air hose, and proper cuff size.
2. If monitor is not on a mobile stand be certain that it is placed on a firm surface.
3. Plug in monitor (unless battery operated) and attach dual hose, if necessary.
4. Attach appropriate size blood pressure cuff and wrap around child's limb.
5. Turn power switch ON. Record the reading.

Flush

(Used for newborns or small infants)

1. Apply cuff to distal limb (if arm outer edge is at wrist, if leg outer edge at ankle).
2. Wrap extremity distal to cuff with elastic bandage.
3. Inflate cuff to 150–200 mm Hg and remove elastic bandage.
4. Lower cuff pressure 5 mm Hg, leave at that level 3–4 seconds. Repeat until flush appears in blanched limb.
5. Repeat at least twice to confirm reading. This is recorded as the mean arterial pressure.

From Skale N. Manual of Pediatric Procedures. Philadelphia: JB Lippincott, 1992.

Table 3-2. Normal Blood Pressure Ranges

Age	Systolic (mm Hg)	Diastolic (mm Hg)
Newborn—12 hr (less than 1000 g)	39–59	16–36
Newborn—12 hr (3000 g)	50–70	24–45
Newborn—96 hr (3000 g)	60–90	20–60
Infant	74–100	50–70
Toddler	80–112	50–80
Preschooler	82–110	50–78
School-age	84–120	54–80
Adolescent	94–140	62–88

From Skale N. Manual of Pediatric Nursing Procedures. Philadelphia: JB Lippincott, 1992 p. 46.

Weight and Height

The weight and the height of the child are helpful indicators of the child's growth and development. Weight and height should be measured and recorded each time the child has a routine physical examination and at other health care visits. These measurements must be charted and compared with norms for the child's age. This process gives a good picture of how the child is progressing; however, the size of family members, the child's illnesses, general nutritional status, and developmental milestones also must be considered.

The infant or child should be weighed at the same time each day, on the same scales, wearing the same amount of clothing. An infant is weighed naked, with no shirt or diaper. The nurse must keep a hand within 1 inch of the infant at all times to be ready to prevent the infant from injury. The scale is covered with a fresh paper towel or clean sheet of paper as a means of infection control. An older infant may sit up on the scale, but the nurse must keep a hand ready to protect the infant from injury. A child who can stand alone steadily is weighed on platform-type scales. The child should be weighed without shoes, and if weighed daily in the hospital, must be weighed at the same time and in the same clothing. Bed scales may be used if the child cannot get out of bed. Weights are recorded in grams and kilograms (metric) or pounds and ounces.

The child who can stand is usually measured for height at the same time. The standing scales have an adjustable measuring device that may be used. An infant is measured while lying on a flat surface. Usually, examining tables have a measuring device mounted along the side of the table. The infant is measured flat with knees held flat to the table. Height is recorded in centimeters or inches according to the practice of the health care facility. The nurse needs to be aware of which measuring system is being used.

Assessment of Cardiovascular and Respiratory Status

A variety of monitors are used with infants and children to measure cardiovascular and respiratory status. Noninvasive methods are preferred when possible. The following are several of the noninvasive monitors that may be used.

Pulse Oximetry

Pulse oximetry measures the oxygen saturation of arterial hemoglobin. The probe can be taped to the toe or finger or clipped on the child's earlobe (Figure 3-5) and changed at least every 4 hours to prevent skin irritation. In an infant, the foot may be used. The probe is connected to the oximetry unit. The site should be checked every 2 hours to make certain that the probe is secure and tissue perfusion is adequate. Alarms can be set to sound when oxygen saturation decreases lower than a predetermined limit.

Apnea Monitor

An apnea monitor detects the infant's respiratory movement. Electrodes or a belt are placed on the chest of the infant where the greatest amount of respiratory movement is detected and are attached to the monitor by a cable. An alarm is set to sound when the infant does not breathe for a predetermined number of seconds. These monitors can be used in a hospital setting and often are used in the home for an infant who is at risk for apnea or who has a tracheostomy. Family caregivers are taught to stimulate the infant when the monitor sounds and to perform cardiopulmonary resuscitation if the infant does not begin breathing.

Cardiopulmonary Monitor

Cardiac monitors assess cardiac and respiratory function. Many of these monitors have a visual display of the

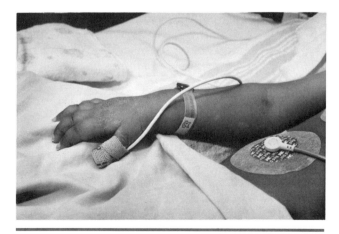

Figure 3-5. Pulse oximetry sensor taped to infant's thumb. (From Skale N. Manual of Pediatric Procedures. Philadelphia: JB Lippincott, 1992, p. 221.)

cardiac and respiratory actions. Electrodes must be placed properly to obtain accurate readings of the cardiac and pulmonary systems. The skin is cleansed with alcohol to remove oil, dirt, lotions, and powder. Alarms are set to maximum and minimum settings above and below the child's resting rates. The electrode sites must be checked every 2 hours for skin redness or irritation and to determine that the electrodes are secure. The child's cardiac and respiratory status must be checked immediately when the alarm sounds.

Neurologic Assessment

Increased intracranial pressure often is caused by a head injury. It also may be caused by certain metabolic conditions, such as diabetes mellitus, or by drug ingestion, severe hemorrhage, dehydration, and seizures. To determine the level of the child's neurologic functioning, the nurse must perform a neurologic assessment. The most frequently used neurologic assessment tool is the Glasgow coma scale. The use of a standard scale for testing permits the comparison of results from one time to another and from one examiner to another. Neurologic assessment is performed every 1 or 2 hours to observe for significant changes (Figure 3-6).

Regulation of Body Temperature

Significant alterations in body temperature can have severe consequences for all children. "Normal" body temperature varies from 37°C (98.6°F) orally to 38°C (100.4°F) rectally. The body temperature generally is desired to be maintained below 38.3°C (101°F) orally or 38.9°C (102°F) rectally, although the health care facility or physician may set lower limits. Excess coverings should be removed from the child with fever to permit additional cooling through evaporation. Methods used to reduce the fever are the following:

- Giving a tepid sponge bath
- Maintaining hydration (encouraging fluids)
- Administering acetaminophen
- Using a hypothermia pad or blanket

Sponge baths and hypothermia treatments should not be maintained for longer than 20 to 30 minutes at one time, otherwise vasoconstriction occurs, resulting in further increases in the child's core temperature. Because many children have a fever but do not need hospitalization, the family caregivers need instructions on fever reduction (Box 3-2).

Tepid Sponge Bath

When a sponge bath is administered, only tepid water should be used. Ice or alcohol should never be added to the water. Extreme cooling may be a shock to the immature nervous system, and alcohol may be absorbed through

GLASGOW COMA SCALES			MODIFIED COMA SCALE FOR INFANTS		
ACTIVITY	BEST RESPONSE		ACTIVITY	BEST RESPONSE	
Eye Opening	Spontaneous	4	Eye Opening	Spontaneous	4
	To speech	3		To speech	3
	To pain	2		To pain	2
	None	1		None	1
Verbal	Oriented	5	Verbal	Coos, babbles	5
	Confused	4		Irritable	4
	Inappropriate words	3		Cries to pain	3
	Nonspecific sounds	2		Moans to pain	2
	None	1		None	1
Motor	Follows commands	6	Motor	Normal spontaneous movements	6
	Localizes pain	5		Withdraws to touch	5
	Withdraws to pain	4		Withdraws to pain	4
	Abnormal flexion	3		Abnormal flexion	3
	Extend	2		Abnormal extension	2
	None	1		None	1

PUPIL SIZE:

6mm   5mm   4mm   3mm   2mm   1mm

REACTION: **N**–normal, **S**–sluggish, **F**–fixed

DATE	TIME	PUPIL SIZE		PUPIL REACTION		EXTREMITY MOVEMENT/ RESPONSE				GLASGOW COMA SCALE			VITAL SIGNS		
		R	L	R	L	RA	LA	RL	LL	VERBAL RESP.	MOTOR RESP.	EYE OPENING	BP	PULSE	RESP.

GUIDE TO NEUROLOGIC EVALUATION

Pupils
Pupils should be examined in dim light
1. Compare each pupil with the size chart and record pupil size.
2. Use a bright flashlight to check the reaction of each pupil. Hold the flashlight to the outer aspect of the eye. While watching the pupil, turn the flashlight on and bring it directly over the pupil. Record the reaction. Repeat for the other eye. Report if either pupil is fixed or dilated.

Extremities
1. Observe the child for quality and strength of muscle tone in each upper extremity. Have child squeeze nurse's hand. Have child raise arms. Ask child to turn palms up, then palms down. Infant is observed for movement and position of arms when stroked or lightly pinched.
2. The child should be able to move each leg on command, and push against nurse's hands with each foot. Infant is observed for movement of legs and feet when stroked or lightly pinched.
3. Score the extremities using the motor scale appropriate for age (below).

Glasgow Coma Scale
Assess each response according to age

Eye opening
4 Opens eyes spontaneously when approached
3 Opens eyes to spoken or shouted speech
2 Opens eyes only to painful stimuli (nail bed pressure)
1 Does not open eyes in response to pain

Verbal
5 Oriented to time, place, person; infant responds by cooing and babbling, recognizes parent
4 Talks, not oriented to time, place, person; infant irritable, doesn't recognize parent
3 Words senseless, unintelligible; infant cries in response to pain
2 Responds with moaning and groaning, no intelligible words; infant moans to pain
1 No response

Motor
6 Responds to commands; infant smiles, responds
5 Tries to remove painful stimuli with hands; infant withdraws from touch
4 Attempts to withdraw from painful stimuli; infant withdraws from pain source
3 Flexes arms at elbows and wrists in response to pain (decorticate rigidity)
2 Extends arms at elbows in response to pain (cerebrate rigidity)
1 No motor response to pain

Check infant's fontanelle for bulging and record results

Figure 3-6. Neurologic flow sheet and neurologic evaluation guide. (Neurologic flow sheet courtesy of Lewistown Hospital, Lewistown, PA.)

Box 3-2

Home Care Guide for Fever Reduction

1. Temperature for sponging bath should begin with warm water and gradually be lowered to 37°C (98.6°F) so that child becomes used to the cool water.
2. Do not place child in a tub for bath if it may be difficult to hold child securely.
3. Sponge for no longer than 30 minutes.
4. If tub is used, gently dribble water over child's body.
5. If child is in bed, uncover only one body part at a time. Use long strokes, and place extra washcloths in armpits and groin.
6. Never use alcohol in sponge bath.
7. Never use ice in the water for sponging.
8. Stop if child begins to shiver. Shivering raises body temperature.
9. When finished, dry child by gently rubbing skin to increase circulation.
10. When done, do not overdress or heavily cover child. Diaper, light sheet, or light pajamas are sufficient.
11. Do not repeat unless temperature is elevated and skin is warm.
12. Encourage child to drink fluids.
13. Keep room environment cool.
14. Use acetaminophen or other antipyretic according to directions of physician.
15. Wait for 30 minutes to take temperature again.
16. Call physician at once if child's temperature is 40.6°C (105°F) or higher.
17. Call physician if child has history of febrile seizures.

the skin or the fumes can be inhaled, further complicating the child's problems. The child should not be permitted to shiver because the process of shivering raises the temperature. The temperature, pulse, and respiration measurements are taken at the beginning of the procedure. Extra washcloths are needed to place in the axilla and groin. Long, gentle strokes are used during the procedure, starting from the head and working down the body, exposing only one part of the body at a time. A tub bath may be given unless contraindicated by the child's condition. The sponge bath is continued for 20 to 30 minutes but should be stopped if the child begins to shiver. After the bath, the child is dried and can be dressed in light pajamas or covered lightly with a sheet. The temperature is taken 30 minutes after the bath is completed. If the temperature is not falling, the procedure may need to be

repeated. Documentation includes the time the procedure was started, the length of the bath, the initial temperature, the temperature taken 30 minutes after the procedure, and the child's reaction to the procedure.

Therapeutic Application of Cold

In addition to reducing body temperature, the local application of cold also may help prevent swelling, control hemorrhage, and provide an anesthetic effect. Intervals of approximately 20 minutes are recommended, both for dry cold (ice bag and commercial instant-cold preparation) and moist cold (compress, soak, and bath) treatments. Dry cold applications should be covered lightly to protect the child's skin from direct contact. Because cold decreases circulation, prolonged chilling may result in frostbite and gangrene. The child's skin must be inspected before and after the cold application to detect skin redness or irritation. Documentation includes the application, the beginning time, the length of time, and the condition of the skin before and after the application.

Detailed instructions for the therapeutic application of cold and heat may be obtained in the procedure manuals of individual hospitals and from manufacturers of commercial devices.

Therapeutic Application of Heat

The local application of heat increases circulation by vasodilation and promotes muscle relaxation, thereby relieving pain and congestion. It also speeds the formation and drainage of superficial abscesses.

Artificial heat should never be applied to the skin of a child without a physician's order. Tissue damage can occur, particularly in fair-skinned people or those who have suffered sensory loss or impaired circulation. These children should be closely monitored, and none should receive heat treatments longer than 30 minutes at a time, unless specifically ordered by the physician.

Moist heat produces faster results than does dry heat and is usually in the form of a warm compress or soak.

Dry heat may be applied by means of an electric heating pad, a K-pad (a unit that circulates warm water through plastic enclosed tubing), or a hot water bottle. Many children have been burned because of improper use of hot water bottles; therefore, these devices are not recommended. Electric heating pads and K-pads should be covered with a pillowcase, towel, or stockinette. As with the application of cold, documentation includes the application, the beginning time, the length of time, and the condition of the skin before and after the application.

Assisting with Diagnostic and Treatment Procedures

Many procedures in highly technologic health care facilities may be frightening and painful to children. The nurse can be an important source of comfort to children who must undergo these procedures, even though it is difficult to assist with or perform procedures that cause pain. The child who is old enough to understand the purpose of the procedure and the expected benefit must have the procedure explained and be encouraged to ask questions and given complete answers. Infants can be soothed and comforted only before and after the procedure.

The nurse caring for toddlers has a greater opportunity to explain procedures than when caring for infants, but at best the nurse will be only imperfectly understood. Even when toddlers grasp the words, they have little meaning. The reality is the pain that occurs.

Sometimes children's interest can be diverted so that they may forget their fear. They must be allowed to cry if necessary, and they should always be listened to and have their questions answered. It takes maturity and experience on the nurse's part to know exactly which questions are stalling techniques and which call for firmness and action. Children need someone to take charge in a kind, firm manner that tells them the decision is not in their hands. They are too young to take this responsibility for themselves.

Nurses have conflicting feelings about the merit of giving some reward after a treatment. Careful thought is necessary. Children given a lollipop or a small toy following an uncomfortable procedure tend to remember the experience as not totally bad. This has nothing to do with their behavior. It is not a reward for being brave or good or big; it is simply a part of the entire treatment. The unpleasant part is mitigated by the pleasant. An older person's reward is contemplating the improvement in health the procedure may provide, but the child does not have sufficient reasoning ability to understand future benefits.

Blood Tests

Blood tests are part of almost every hospitalization experience. Although the specimens usually are obtained by laboratory personnel or a physician, the nurse needs to be familiar with the general procedure in order to explain it to the child and may be asked to help restrain the child during the procedure. Blood specimens are obtained either by pricking the heel, the great toe, the earlobe, or the finger or by venipuncture. In infants, the jugular or scalp veins are most commonly used; at times, the femoral vein is used (Figure 3-7**A** and **B**). In older children, the veins in the arm are used.

Urine Tests

Equipment needed to obtain a urine specimen is assembled, including sterile water, soap or antiseptic solution, sterile cotton balls or gauze squares, urine collector, specimen container, and nonsterile gloves. The procedure is explained to the child who is old enough to comprehend. The infant or child is positioned so that the genitalia are exposed. The nurse washes his or her hands,

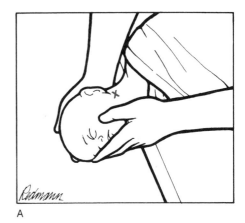

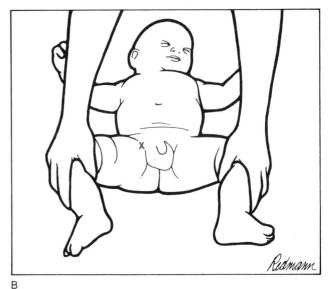

Figure 3-7. **A**, Position of infant for jugular venipuncture. **B**, Position of infant for femoral venipuncture.

puts on gloves, and cleanses the genitalia. On the male patient, the tip of the penis is wiped with a soapy cotton ball, followed by a rinse with a cotton ball saturated with sterile water. In the female patient, the labia major is cleansed front to back, using one cotton ball for each wipe. The labia minor are then exposed and cleansed in the same fashion. The area is rinsed with a cotton ball saturated with sterile water. The male or female genitalia are permitted to air-dry. The paper backing is removed from the urine collection container, and the adhesive surface is applied over the penis in the male and the vulva in the female. The child may be diapered. The nurse completes the procedure with careful handwashing. The specimen may be sent to the laboratory in the plastic collection container or in a specimen container preferred by the laboratory. Appropriate documentation includes the time of specimen collection, the amount and color of the urine, the test to be performed, and the condition of the perineal area. Occasionally, the child may need to be catheterized to obtain a specimen. An older child may be able to cooperate in the collection of a midstream specimen, if needed.

Stool Tests

Stool specimens are tested for various reasons, including the presence of occult blood, ova and parasites, bacteria, glucose, or excess fat. The nurse puts on gloves and collects these specimens from a diaper or bedpan using a tongue blade and places them in clean specimen containers. Stool specimens must not be contaminated with urine, and they must be labeled and delivered to the laboratory promptly. Documentation includes the time the specimen is collected; the color, the amount, the consistency, and the odor of the stool; the test to be performed; and the skin condition.

Cerebrospinal Fluid Tests

When analysis of cerebrospinal fluid is necessary, a lumbar puncture is performed. During this procedure, the nurse must restrain the child in position as shown in Figure 3-8 until the procedure is completed. The nurse holds the child's hands with the hand that has passed under the child's lower extremities and holds the child snugly against his or her chest. This position enlarges the intervertebral spaces for easier access with the aspiration needle. Children undergoing this procedure may be too young to understand the nurse's explanation. The nurse should tell the child, however, that it is important to hold still and the child will have help to do this. The lumbar puncture is performed with strict asepsis. A sterile dressing is applied when the procedure is complete. The child needs to remain quiet for 1 hour after the procedure. Vital signs, level of consciousness, and motor activity should be monitored frequently for the first several hours after the procedure.

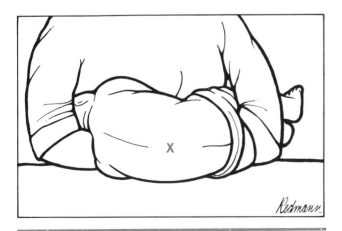

Figure 3-8. Position of infant for lumbar puncture.

Infection Control in the Pediatric Setting

Infection control is an important aspect of caring for children in the pediatric setting. The child who is ill may be especially vulnerable to **pathogenic** (disease-carrying) **microorganisms**. Isolation precautions must be taken to protect the children, families, and personnel. Microorganisms are spread by contact (direct, indirect, or droplet), vehicle (food, water, blood, or contaminated products), airborne (dust particles in the air), or vector (mosquitoes, vermin) means of transmission. Each type of microorganism is transmitted in a specific way; thus, isolation precautions are tailored to specifically prevent the spread of microorganisms of that type.

The following are seven categories of isolation that the Centers for Disease Control has identified and examples of reasons they must be implemented:

- Universal precautions—to protect health care workers and patients from spread of diseases such as hepatitis B virus, human immunodeficiency virus, and other blood-borne pathogens
- Strict isolation—congenital rubella, diphtheria, herpes zoster, and chicken pox (varicella)
- Respiratory isolation—measles, mumps, meningitis, and pertussis
- Enteric isolation—gastroenteritis, amebic dysentery, and enteroviral infections
- Drainage and secretion precautions—draining abscesses, cellulitis, skin infections, and impetigo
- Blood and body fluids—acquired immunodeficiency syndrome, syphilis, scabies, tuberculosis, and rat bite fever
- Respiratory syncytial virus (RSV) precautions—pneumonia caused by RSV or influenza virus, acute respiratory infections such as bronchiolitis, bronchitis, croup, and common colds.

Table 3-3 provides a summary of precautions used with each type of isolation (see Nursing Care Plan for the Child in Protective Isolation).

Handwashing is the cornerstone of all infection control. The nurse must wash his or her hands conscientiously between seeing each patient. Even when gloves are worn for a procedure, the nurse *must* wash hands between patients.

Medication Administration

Caring for children who are ill challenges every nurse to function at the highest level of professional competence. Giving medications is one of the most important nursing

Table 3-3. Summary of Infection Control Measures

Isolation Type	Private Room	Mask/Gown	Gloves	Dishes	Linen	Garbage	Comments
Strict	Yes—usually special ventilation required	Yes/Yes	Yes	Yes	Yes	Yes	Toys must be decontaminated before reuse.
Respiratory	Yes	Yes/No	No	No	No	Yes	No special consideration for toys.
Enteric	Patients with same organism may share a room	No/No*	Yes	Yes	Yes	Yes	Clean grossly contaminated toys with an antimicrobial agent.
Contact (wound and skin)	No	No/No*	Yes	Yes	Yes	Yes	Clean grossly contaminated toys with an antimicrobial agent.
Blood or body (universal)	Yes—if patient's hygiene is poor	No/No*	Yes	Yes	Yes	Yes	Clean grossly contaminated toys with an antimicrobial agent.
RSV	Yes—cohorting is suggested during outbreaks	Yes/No*	Yes	No	No	Yes	Toys must be decontaminated before reuse.
Protective	Yes	Yes (including shoe cover)	Yes	Yes	Yes	Yes	Games and toys must be decontaminated prior to being taken into the room.

* If soiling with secretions is likely, a gown is required.
RSV, respiratory synctial virus.
Adapted from Skale N. Manual of Pediatric Nursing Procedures. Philadelphia: JB Lippincott, 1992, p. 112.

responsibilities, calling for accuracy, precision, and considerable psychological skill. Basic to administering medications to a person of any age are the following five "rights" of medication administration:

- The right child—the identification bracelet must be checked *each* time a medication is given to confirm identification of the child.

- The right drug—check the drug label to confirm it is the correct drug; do not use a drug that is not clearly labeled; check the expiration date of the drug.

- The right dose—always double-check the dose when in doubt; question the order if it is not clear; have another qualified person double-check any time a divided dosage is to be given, or for insulin, digoxin, and other agents governed by policy of the facility; use drug references, or check with a physician or pharmacist for the appropriateness of the dose; orders must be questioned *before* the drug is given.

- The right route—give the drug only by the route indicated; question the order if it is unclear or confusing.

- The right time—administering a drug at the correct time helps maintain the desired blood level of the drug.

Administering medications to children, however, is much more complex than these guidelines indicate. Accurate administration of medications to children is especially critical because of the variable responses to drugs that children have as a result of immature body systems. The nurse must understand the factors that influence or alter how the child absorbs, metabolizes, and excretes the medication and any allergies that the child has. The nurse is responsible for the administration of medications and therefore is legally liable for errors of medication.

Nine rules to guide the nurse in administering medications are presented in Box 3-3. The nurse should evaluate each child from a developmental point of view to successfully administer medications. Understanding, planning, and implementing nursing care that considers the child's developmental level and coping mechanisms contribute to administering medications with minimal trauma to the child (Table 3-4).

Computing Dosages

Commercial unit-dose packaging often does not include dosages for children, so the nurse must calculate the correct dosage. The most reliable formula to calculate dosages is the **body surface area (BSA) method**. The **West nomogram** (a graph with several scales arranged so that when two values are known, the third can be plotted by drawing a line with a straightedge), commonly used to calculate BSA, may be found in most pediatric

Nursing Care Plan
for the Child in Protective Isolation

Nursing Diagnosis
Social isolation related to required isolation precautions

Goal: Promote social contact

Nursing Interventions	*Rationale*	*Evaluation*
Identify ways to help the child communicate with others through means other than physical contact (eg, telephone, letters, etc.)	The child needs to feel connected to family and friends.	The child interacts with nursing staff and maintains meaningful interaction with family and friends through the telephone or written contact.

Nursing Diagnosis
High risk for altered growth and development related to separation from significant others and inadequate sensory stimulation

Goal: Provide age-appropriate stimulation

Nursing Interventions	*Rationale*	*Evaluation*
Provide games, books, puzzles, and other activities appropriate for the child's age, developmental stage, and interests. Ask family members to bring in the child's favorite objects or games. Be sure to replace items on a routine basis before the child becomes bored with them.	Interesting activities can occupy the child for stretches of time but may contribute to the child's feelings of boredom if left around for too long.	Child engages in age-appropriate activities as illness and isolation precautions allow.
Consult the play therapist for ideas on special projects the child might do independently.	A hospital play therapist often has new and unusual ideas, resources, and materials for play that are age-appropriate and interesting.	
Encourage the child to get out of bed frequently, if physically able, and teach some age-appropriate exercises to maintain physical shape.	The child needs physical as well as cognitive and emotional stimulation in order to continue normal growth and development.	

Nursing Diagnosis
Diversional activity deficit related to monotony of confinement

Goal: Promote sensory stimulation

Nursing Interventions	*Rationale*	*Evaluation*
Spend some time each day to visit with the child, play a board game, or just talk.	Reassures the child that you value his or her company even though family and friends are not allowed to visit or can visit only on a limited basis.	Child engages in age-appropriate activities and conversation with caregivers.

(continued)

Nursing Care Plan
for the Child in Protective Isolation (Continued)

Nursing Interventions	Rationale	Evaluation
If the child has any special audiotapes, ask family members to bring these and a tape recorder to the hospital. In addition, family members might make tapes for the child or ask friends to make a tape filling the child in on activities going on at school or home. The child could respond with a tape of his or her own.	Keeps the child closer in touch with significant others and provides a fun activity that can last through the period of isolation.	
Make routine care procedures fun within the limits of child's developmental stage and energy level. Use this time to talk about things going on outside or activities the child enjoys when well.	Provides some diversion from the routine and gives the child something to look forward to.	

Nursing Diagnosis
Powerlessness related to required isolation precautions

Goal: Promote feeling of control

Nursing Interventions	Rationale	Evaluation
Include child in planning for daily routine, such as, when bath is scheduled or food choices and timing for meals.	Gives child some control over day's activities.	Child makes decisions within age constraints, concerning daily activities.
Plan some special activity with the child for each day, and keep your promise.	Gives the child something to look forward to and reinforces child's feeling of control.	

settings (Figure 3-9). The child's weight is marked on the right scale, and the height is marked on the left scale. A straightedge is used to draw a line between the two marks. The point at which it crosses the column labeled *SA* (surface area) is the BSA expressed in square meters (m^2). The average adult BSA is 1.7 m^2, thus the formula to calculate the appropriate dosage for a child is

$$\text{Estimated child's dose} = \frac{\text{Child's BSA } (m^2)}{1.7 \text{ (Adult BSA)}} \times \text{Adult dose}$$

For example, a child is 37 inches (95 cm) tall and weighs 34 lb (15.5 kg). The usual adult dose of the medication is 500 mg. Place and hold one end of a straightedge on the first column at 37 inches and move it so that it lines up with 34 lb in the far right column. On the column marked SA, the straightedge falls across 0.64 (m^2). You are ready to do the calculation

$$\frac{.64}{1.7} = 0.38$$

You now know that the child's BSA is 0.38 as great as the average adult. You are ready to calculate the child's dose by multiplying 0.38 times 500 mg

$$0.38 \times 500 = 190$$

The child's dose is 190 mg.

Calculating Fractional Dosage
It may be necessary to calculate a fractional dosage when full-strength drugs must be diluted to achieve the concentration ordered by the physician. The simplest way to determine the amount needed of a full-strength drug is to divide the desired strength (the dose ordered) by the strength of the drug on hand. The nurse then gives the

Box 3-3

Nine Rules in Medication Administration in Children

1. Never give a child a choice of whether or not to receive medicine. The medication is ordered and is necessary for recovery; therefore, there is no choice to be made.
2. Do give choices that allow the child some control over the situation, such as the kind of juice, the number of bandages, or the injection site.
3. Never lie. Do not tell a child that a shot will not hurt.
4. Keep explanations simple and brief. Use words that the child will comprehend.
5. Assure the child that it is all right to be afraid and that it is OK to cry.
6. Do not talk in front of the child as if the child were not there. Include the child in the conversation when talking to family caregivers.
7. Be positive in approaching the child. Be firm and assertive when explaining to the child what will happen.
8. Keep the time between explanation and execution to a minimum. The younger the child, the shorter the time should be.
   Keep the explanation simple.
   Preparations such as setting up injection, solutions, or instrument trays should be done out of the child's sight.
9. Obtain cooperation from family caregivers. They may be able to calm a frightened child, persuade the child to take the medication, and achieve cooperation for care.

From Skale N. Manual of Pediatric Nursing Procedures. Philadelphia: JB Lippincott, 1992.

required fraction of the standard amount. The formula is the following:

$$\frac{\text{Dose Desired}}{\text{Dose on Hand}} \times \frac{\text{Quantity}}{\text{(Diluent)}} = \frac{\text{Amount to}}{\text{be Given}}$$

For example, elixir of phenobarbital contains 20 mg of phenobarbital in each 5 mL of the elixir. If the order reads "elixir of phenobarbital 4 mg po (by mouth)," the desired dose (dose ordered) is 4 mg and the dose on hand is 20 mg/5 mL. The problem is set up as follows:

$$\frac{4 \text{ mg}}{20 \text{ mg}} \times 5 \qquad \frac{1}{5} \times 5 = 1$$

The correct dose is 1 mL.

Because this medication is in elixir form, it should be well diluted with water before giving it to a child, as discussed later.

After computing the dosage, the nurse should *always* have the computation checked by another staff person qualified to give medication, or someone in the department who is delegated for this purpose. Errors are easy to make and easy to overlook. A second person should do the computation separately, then both results should be compared.

Errors in Medications

Medication errors can occur because nurses are human and not perfect. To admit an error is often difficult, especially if there has been carelessness concerning the rules. A person may be strongly tempted to adopt a "wait and see" attitude, which is the gravest error of all. Nurses must accept responsibility for their own actions. Serious consequences for the child may be avoided if a mistake is disclosed promptly.

Oral Medication

Small babies are not too particular about the taste of food if they are hungry. Almost anything liquid may be sucked through a nipple, including liquid medicines, unless it is bitter. Medications that are available in syrup or fruit-flavored suspensions are easily administered this way. Another method of administering oral medications is to drop them slowly into the baby's mouth with a plastic medicine dropper or oral syringe (Figure 3-10).

Elixirs contain alcohol and are apt to cause choking unless they are diluted. Syrups and suspensions do not need dilution, but they are thick and may need dilution to ensure that the child gets the full dose. Always check with the pharmacist before diluting any medication.

When a child is old enough to swallow a pill, make sure that the pill is actually swallowed before you leave. Usually the child cooperates so well when asked to open his or her mouth that you are confronted with a mouth opened up so wide that tonsils can be inspected. This opening of the mouth also gives you the opportunity to look under the tongue. Chewable tablets work well for the preschool child.

It usually is best to give medicine in solution form to a small child. If you must use a tablet, dissolve it in water. Do not use orange juice for a solvent unless specifically ordered to do so—the child may always associate the taste of orange juice with the unpleasant medicine. If the medicine is bitter, honey or corn syrup may disguise the taste. The child may develop a dislike for corn syrup, but that is not as important as a lifelong dislike of orange juice.

There is little excuse for restraining a small child and forcing a medication down the child's throat. The child can always have the last word and bring it up again. The

Table 3-4. Developmental Considerations in Medication Administration

Age	Behaviors	Nursing Actions
Birth–3 months	Reaches randomly toward mouth and has a strong reflex to grasp objects	The infant's hands must be held to prevent spilling of medications.
	Poor head control	The infant's head must be supported while medications are being given.
	Tongue movement may force medication out of mouth	A syringe or dropper should be placed along the side of the mouth.
	Sucks as a reflex with stimulation	Use this natural sucking desire by placing oral medications into a nipple and administering in that manner.
	Stops sucking when full	Administer medications before feeding when infant is hungry. Be aware that some medications' absorption will be affected by food.
	Infant responds to tactile stimulations	The likelihood that the medication is taken will increase if the infant is held in a feeding position.
3–12 months	Begins to develop fine muscle control and advances from sitting to crawling	Medication must be kept out of reach to avoid accidental ingestion.
	Tongue may protrude when swallowing	Administer medication with a syringe.
	Responds to tactile stimuli	Physical comfort (holding) given after a medication will be helpful.
12–30 months	Advances from independent walking to running without falling	Allow the toddler to choose position for taking medication.
	Advances from messy self-feeding to proficient feeding with minimal spilling	Allow the toddler to take medicine from a cup or spoon.
	Has voluntary tongue control. Begins to drink from a cup	Disguise medication in a small amount of food to decrease incidence of spitting out medication.
	Develops second molars	Chewable tablets may be an alternative.
	Exhibits independence and self-assertiveness	Allow as much freedom as possible. Use games to gain confidence. Use a consistent firm approach. Give immediate praise for cooperation.
	Responds to sense of time and simple direction	Give directions to "Drink this now" and "Open your mouth."
	Responds to and participates in routines of daily living	Involve the family caregivers and include the toddler in medicine routines.
	Expresses feelings easily	Allow for expression through play.
30 mo–6 years	Knows full name	Ask the child his or her name before giving medicine.
	Is easily influenced by others when responding to new foods or tastes	Approach the child in a calm positive manner when giving medications.
	Has a good sense of time and a tolerance of frustration	Use correct immediate rewards for the young child and delayed gratification for the older child.
	Enjoys making decisions	Give choices when possible.
	Has many fantasies	Give simple explanations. Stress that the medication is not being given because the child is bad.
	Has fear of mutilation	
	Is more coordinated	Can hold cup and may be able to master pill-taking.
	Begins to lose teeth	Chewable tablets may be inappropriate because of loose teeth.
6–12 years	Strives for independence	Give acceptable choices. Respect the need for regression during hospitalization.
	Has concern for bodily mutilation	Give reassurance that medication given, especially injectables, will not cause harm. Reinforce that medications should only be taken only when given by nurse or family caregiver.
	Can tell time	Include the child in daily schedule of medication. Make the child a poster of medications and time due so he or she can be involved in care.
	Is concerned with body image and privacy	Provide private area for administration of medication, especially injections.
	Peer support and interaction are important	Allow child to share experiences with others.

(continued)

Table 3-4. Developmental Considerations in Medication Administration (*Continued*)

Age	Behaviors	Nursing Actions
12 + years	Strives for independence	Write a contract with the adolescent, spelling out expectations for self-medication.
	Is able to understand abstract theories	Explain why medications are given and how they work.
	Decisions are influenced by peers	Encourage teens to talk with their peers in a support group. Work with teens to plan medication schedule around their activities. Differentiate pill-taking from drug-taking.
	Questions authority figures	Be honest and provide medication information in writing.
	Is concerned with sex and sexuality	Explain relationship between illness, medications, and sexuality. For example, emphasize that "This medication will not react with your birth control pills."

From Skale N. Manual of Pediatric Nursing Procedures. Philadelphia: JB Lippincott, 1992, p. 118.

danger of aspiration is real. Of even greater importance are the antagonism and helplessness built up in the child by such a procedure. A child's sense of dignity needs to be respected as much as that of an adult's. Refer to Table 3-4 to review the developmental characteristics to be considered at each age.

Intramuscular Medication

Children have the same fear of needles as do adults. Students are reluctant to hurt the child and often cause the pain they are trying to prevent by inserting the needle slowly. A swift, sure thrust and insertion is nearly painless, but the nurse must stay calm and sure and be prepared for the child's squirming. It is best to plan to have a second nurse present to help hold the child if the child is younger than school age or if this is the first time the child has had an injection.

Injections should be given to a child in the treatment room rather than in bed or in the playroom. The bed and playroom should be "safe" places for the child. The nurse may have a ready Band-Aid to cover the injection site. This technique prevents young children from worrying that they might "leak out" of the hole, and the bandage serves as a badge of courage or bravery for the older child. Table 3-5 describes intramuscular injection sites, how to locate them, and the suggested needle size and amount of medication. Figures 3-11 through 3-14 illustrate each of these sites and how to locate them.

Other Routes of Medication Administration

The principles of administering medications by other routes are much the same as those for administering to adults, with a few variations. Eye, ear, and nose drops should be warmed to room temperature before being administered. The infant or young child may need to be restrained for safe administration. This restraint may be accomplished with a mummy restraint or the assistance of a second person. The nurse must realize that these are invasive procedures and that the young child may be resistant. Approaching the child with patience, explanations, and praise for cooperation aids in gaining the child's cooperation. Documentation must be completed after the administration of any medication.

Eye Drops or Ointment

The child is placed in a supine position. To instill the drops, the lower lid is pulled down to form a pocket, and the solution is dropped into the pocket. The eye is held shut briefly, if possible, to aid in distribution of the medication to the conjunctiva. Ointment is applied from the inner to the outer canthus, with care not to touch the eye with the tip of the dropper or tube.

Ear Drops

The infant or young child is placed in a side-lying position with the affected ear up. The infant's or toddler's pinna (the outer part of the ear) is pulled *down* and back to straighten the ear canal. The pinna of the child older than 3 years of age is pulled *up* and back, as with adults, to straighten the canal. After instillation of the drops, the area in front of the ear may be gently massaged. The child should be kept in a position with the affected ear up for 5 to 10 minutes. A cotton pledget may be loosely inserted into the ear to prevent leakage of medication, but care should be taken to avoid blockage of drainage from the ear.

Nose Drops

Before nose drops are instilled, the nostrils should be wiped free of mucus. For nose drop instillation, the infant may be held in the nurse's arms with the head tilted over the arm. The toddler's or older child's head may be placed over a pillow while the child is lying flat. The infant or child should maintain the position for at least 1 minute to ensure distribution of the medication.

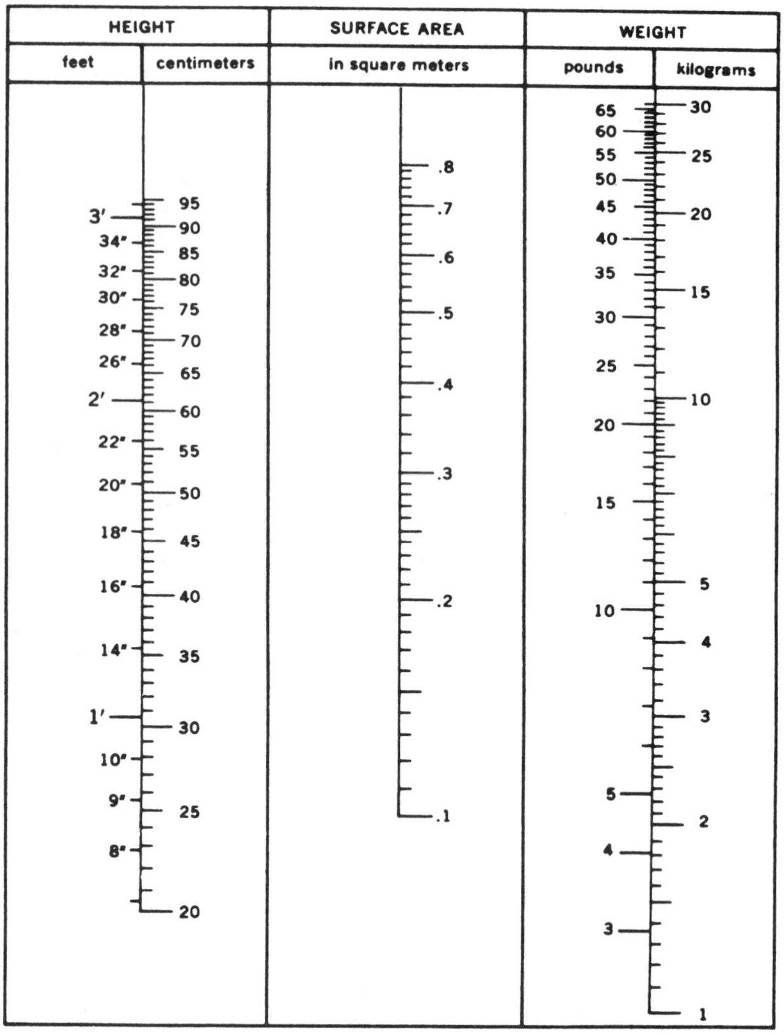

HEIGHT		SURFACE AREA	WEIGHT	
feet	centimeters	in square meters	pounds	kilograms

Figure 3-9. West nomogram for estimating surface area of infants and young children. To determine the body surface area, draw a straight line between the point representing the child's height on the left scale to the child's weight on the right scale. The point at which this line intersects the middle scale is the child's body surface area in square meters. (Courtesy of Abbott Laboratories, Chicago, IL.)

Rectal Medications

For the administration of rectal medications, the child is placed in a side-lying position, and the nurse must wear gloves or a finger cot. The suppository is lubricated and then inserted into the rectum, followed by a finger, up to the first knuckle joint. The little finger should be used for insertion in infants. After the insertion of the suppository, the buttocks must be held tightly together for 1 or 2 minutes until the child's urge to expel the suppository passes.

Intravenous Therapy

Fluids and medications are often administered intravenously to infants and children. Planning nursing care for the child receiving intravenous therapy requires knowledge of the physiology of fluids and electrolytes as well as the child's developmental level and an understanding of the emotional aspects of intravenous therapy for the pediatric patient. Intravenous therapy is commonly administered in the pediatric patient for the following reasons:

- To maintain fluid and electrolyte balance
- To administer antibiotic therapy
- To provide nutritional support
- To administer chemotherapy or anticancer drugs
- To administer pain medication

Candidates for intravenous therapy include children who have poor gastrointestinal absorption caused by diarrhea, vomiting, and dehydration; those who need a high serum concentration of a drug; those who have resistant infections that require intravenous medications; those with emergency problems; and those who need continuous pain relief.

Fundamentals of Fluid Balance

Maintenance of fluid balance in the body tissues is essential to health. Severe imbalance, when uncorrected, causes death, as exemplified in patients with serious dehydration resulting from severe diarrhea or vomiting or from the loss of fluids in extensive burns. The fundamental concepts of fluid and electrolyte balance in body tissue are reviewed briefly to help the student understand the importance of adequate fluid therapy for the sick child.

Water

A continuous supply of water is necessary for life. At birth, water accounts for approximately 77% of body weight. This proportion decreases to the adult level of approximately 60% between 1 and 2 years of age.

In health, the body's water requirement is met through the normal intake of fluids and foods. Intake is regulated by the person's thirst and hunger. Normal body losses of fluid occur through the lungs (breathing) and the skin (sweating) and in the urine and feces. In the normal state of health, intake and output amounts balance each other, and the body is said to be in a state of homeostasis.

Homeostasis, meaning a uniform state, signifies biologically the dynamic equilibrium of the healthy organism. This balance is achieved by appropriate shifts in fluid and electrolytes across the cellular membrane and by elimination of the end products of metabolism and excess electrolytes.

Body water, which contains electrolytes, is situated within the cells, in the spaces between the cells, and in the plasma and blood. **Imbalance** (the failure to maintain homeostasis) may be the result of some pathologic

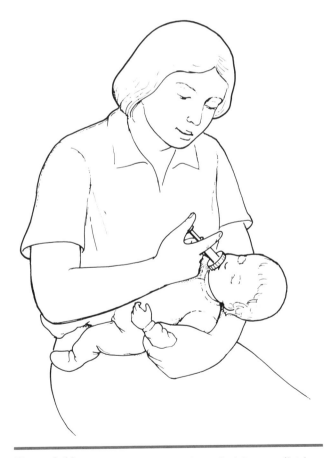

Figure 3-10. Common device used to administer pediatric oral medications.

process in the body. Some of the disorders associated with imbalance are pyloric stenosis, high fever, persistent or severe diarrhea and vomiting, and extensive burns. Retention of fluid may occur through impaired kidney action or altered metabolism.

Intracellular Fluid. **Intracellular fluid** is that fluid contained within the body cells. Nearly half the volume of body water in the infant is intracellular. Intracellular fluid accounts for about 40% of body weight in both infants and adults. Each cell must be supplied with oxygen and nutrients to keep the body in a healthy state. In addition, the body's water and salt levels must be kept constant within narrow parameters.

Cells are surrounded by a semipermeable membrane that retains protein and other large constituents within the cell. Water, certain salts and minerals, nutrients, and oxygen enter the cell through this membrane. Waste products and useful substances produced within the cell are excreted or secreted into the surrounding spaces.

Extracellular Fluid. **Extracellular fluid** is situated outside the cells. It may be **interstitial fluid** (situated within the spaces or gaps of body tissue) or **intravascular fluid** (situated within the blood vessels or blood plasma). **Blood plasma** contains protein within the walls of the blood vessels and water and mineral salts that flow freely from the vascular system into the surrounding tissues.

Interstitial fluid (also called intercellular or tissue fluid) has a composition similar to plasma except that it contains almost no protein. This reservoir of fluid outside the body cells decreases or increases easily in response to disease. An increase in interstitial fluid results in edema. Dehydration depletes this fluid before the intracellular and plasma supplies are affected.

In the infant, about 25% to 35% of body weight is due to interstitial fluid. In the adult, interstitial fluid accounts for only approximately 15% of body weight (Figure 3-15). Infants and children become dehydrated much more quickly than do adults. In part, this dehydration occurs because of a greater fluid exchange caused by the rapid metabolic activity associated with infants' growth and because of the relatively larger ratio of skin surface area to body fluid volume, which is two or three times that of adults.

Because of the factors just discussed, the infant who is taking in no fluid loses an amount of body fluid equal to the extracellular volume in about 5 days, or twice as rapidly as does the adult. The infant's relatively larger volume of extracellular fluid may be designed to partially compensate for this greater loss.

Electrolytes

Electrolytes are chemical compounds (minerals) that break down into **ions** when placed in water. An ion is an atom having a positive or a negative electrical charge.

Table 3-5. Intramuscular Injection Sites

Muscle Site	Needle Size	Maximum Amount	Procedure
Vastus lateralis (Figure 3-11**A** and **B**)	Infant: 25 gauge, ⅝ inch or 23 gauge, 1 inch Older: 22 gauge, 1–1½ inch	1 mL 2 mL	This main thigh muscle is used almost exclusively in infants for IM injections but is used frequently in children of all ages. Locate the trochanter (hip joint) and knee as landmarks. Select a site midway between these landmarks, using the lateral aspect. Inject at a 90-degree angle, or a 45-degree angle, directing the needle toward the knee
Ventrogluteal (Figure 3-12)	Assess child's muscle mass, and choose from those listed for the ventrogluteal, 22–25 gauge, ⅝–1 inch	Infant: ½–¾ mL Toddler: 1 mL School age and older: 1½–2 mL	With thumb facing the front of the child, place forefinger on the anterior superior iliac spine (see Figure 3-13), middle finger on the iliac crest with the palm centered over the greater trochanter. Inject at 90-degree angle below the iliac crest within the triangle defined. No important nerves are in this area
Gluteal (Figure 3-13**A**)	This site is not recommended in children who have not been walking for at least 1 yr, 20–25 gauge, ½–1½ inch	Not recommended for infant or toddler School age and older: 1½–2 mL	Because of the location of the sciatic nerve, this site is discouraged in younger children. Place child on abdomen, with toes pointing in (Figure 3-13**B**). This relaxes the gluteus. Locate the posterior superior iliac crest and the greater trochanter of the femur. Draw an imaginary line between the two. Give the injection above and to the outside of this line. The needle should be inserted at a 90-degree angle
Deltoid (Figure 3-14)	Not recommended for infants Older: 22–25 gauge, ½–1 inch	Small muscle limits amount to ½–1 mL	Expose entire arm. Locate the acromion process at the top of the arm. Give the injection in the densest part of the muscle, below the acromion process and above the armpit. Not recommended for repeated injections. Can be used for one-time immunizations. Angle needle slightly toward the shoulder

IM, intramuscular.

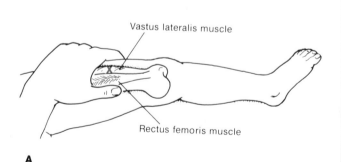

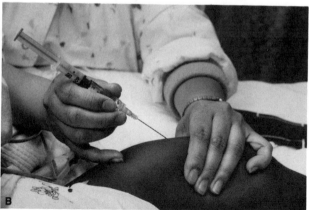

Figure 3-11. **A**, Vastus lateralis muscle. **B**, Intramuscular injection into the vastus lateralis—note the angle of the needle and syringe. (From Skale N. Manual of Pediatric Nursing Procedures. Philadelphia: JB Lippincott, 1992, p. 124.)

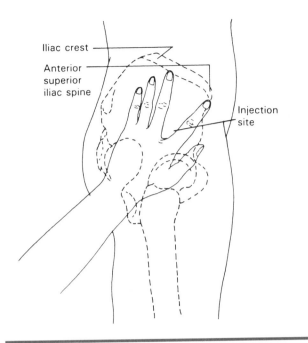

Figure 3-12. Locating the ventrogluteal intramuscular injection site. (From Skale N. Manual of Pediatric Nursing Procedures. Philadelphia: JB Lippincott, 1992, p. 124.)

Important electrolytes in body fluids are sodium (Na^+), potassium (K^+), magnesium (Mg^{2+}), calcium (Ca^{2+}), chloride (Cl^-), phosphate (PO_4^{3-}), and bicarbonate (HCO_3^-). Electrolytes have the important function of maintaining acid–base balance. Each water compartment of the body has its own normal electrolyte composition.

Acid–Base Balance

Acid–base balance is a state of equilibrium between the acidity and the alkalinity of body fluids. The acidity of a solution is determined by the concentration of hydrogen (H^+) ions. Acidity is expressed by the symbol pH. Neutral fluids have a pH of 7.0, acid fluids lower than 7.0, and alkaline fluids higher than 7.0. Normally, body fluids are slightly alkaline. Internal body fluids have a pH ranging from 7.35 to 7.45. Body excretions, however, are products of metabolism and become acid in character. The normal pH of urine, for example, is 5.5 to 6.5.

Defects in the acid–base balance result either in acidosis or alkalosis. **Acidosis** may occur in conditions such as diabetes, kidney failure, and diarrhea. Hypochloremic alkalosis may occur in pyloric stenosis because of the decrease in chloride concentration and increase in carbon dioxide.

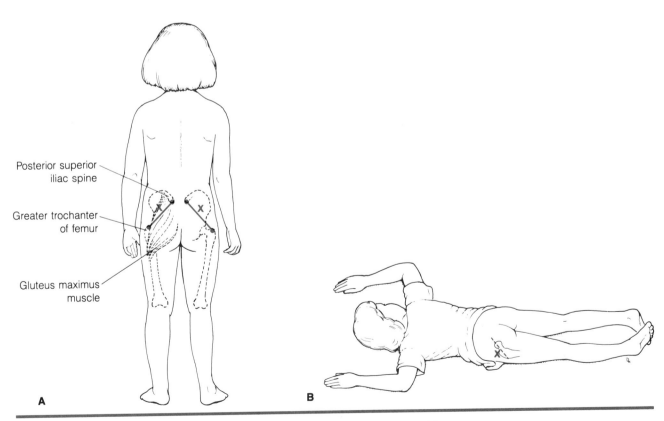

Figure 3-13. **A,** Locating the gluteus intramuscular injection site. **B,** Child in position for gluteus intramuscular injection. Site marked by X. (From Skale N. Manual of Pediatric Nursing Procedures. Philadelphia: JB Lippincott, 1992, p. 125.)

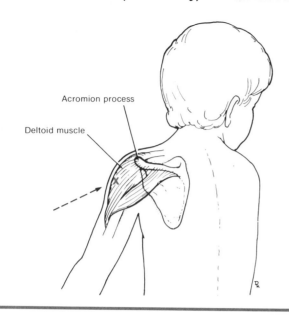

Figure 3-14. Location of deltoid intramuscular injection site. Site marked by X. (From Skale N. Manual of Pediatric Nursing Procedures. Philadelphia, JB Lippincott, 1992, p. 126.)

In normal health, the fluid and electrolyte balance is maintained through the intake of a well-balanced diet. The kidneys play an important part in regulating concentrations of electrolytes in the various fluid compartments. In illness, the balance may be disturbed because of excessive losses of certain electrolytes. Replacement of these minerals is necessary to restore health and maintain life. When the infant or child is able to take sufficient fluids orally, that is the preferred route, but often it is necessary to administer fluids intravenously.

Intravenous Fluid Administration

Intravenous fluids are administered to provide water, electrolytes, and nutrients that the child needs. **Total parenteral nutrition (TPN)**, chemotherapy, and blood products also are administered intravenously. TPN, often called **hyperalimentation**, is the administration of dextrose, lipids, amino acids, electrolytes, vitamins, minerals, and trace elements into the circulatory system to meet the nutritional needs of the child whose needs cannot be met through the gastrointestinal tract. These solutions often are given through a central venous line. Medications are not given by the central venous line but must be given through a peripheral site. A central venous line passes directly into the subclavian vein through the jugular vein or subclavian vein. The line is inserted by surgical technique. Caring for a child with a central venous line calls for skilled nursing care because of the danger of complications such as contamination, thrombosis, dislodgement of the catheter, and **extravasation** (fluid es-

capes into surrounding tissue). The infant or child must be closely monitored for hyperglycemia, dehydration, or **azotemia** (nitrogen-containing compounds in the blood). Peripheral vein hyperalimentation may be used on a short-term basis. Extra care must be taken to avoid infiltration because tissue sloughing may be severe.

For long-term administration of TPN, a venous access device such as a Hickman or Broviac catheter may be inserted into the jugular or subclavian vein in a surgical procedure under anesthesia. These catheters may exit through a tunnel in the subcutaneous tissue on the right chest. Children can be discharged from the hospital on TPN therapy after family caregivers have been instructed in the care of the device, thus reducing hospitalization time and expense.

Dressing changes are routinely performed on the external site of a central venous device. This is a sterile procedure, and the nurse must have adequate space to place the equipment and wear sterile gloves to use sterile forceps. All application is done in a circular motion working from the insertion site to the outer edge in a "clean-to-dirty" fashion. A commonly used procedure begins with cleaning the skin with acetone to clean the site, followed by tincture of iodine for antibacterial action, and finishing with alcohol to clean off the iodine to prevent skin irritation. Topical antimicrobial ointment (bacitracin) is applied to the insertion site, followed by two small gauze

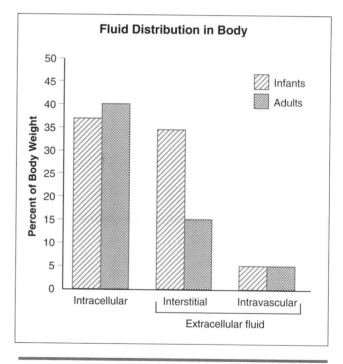

Figure 3-15. Graph indicating distribution of fluid in body compartments. Comparison between the infant and adult fluid distribution in body compartments shows that the adult total is about 60% of body weight, but the infant total is more than 70% of body weight.

sponges. The skin around these small sponges is sprayed with tincture of benzoin to toughen the skin. When the skin is dry, a large dressing is placed over the site and the edges are securely taped. Documentation includes the dressing change and skin condition, including redness, swelling, drainage, irritation, and any unusual reaction.

Intravenous Medication

Intravenous medications often are administered to pediatric patients. Some drugs must be administered intravenously to be effective, and in some patients the quick response gained from intravenous administration is important. Delivering medications by the intravenous route is actually less traumatic than administering multiple intramuscular injections. The nurse must be careful to double-check the medication label before hanging the intravenous fluid bottle to determine that the medication is correct for the correct patient, that it is being administered at the correct time, and that it is not outdated.

Intravenous Sites

Site selection in the pediatric patient varies with the age of the child. The best site in infants and toddlers is the scalp because there is an abundant supply of superficial veins. Other sites include the hand, the foot, and the antecubital fossa. When a scalp vein is used, the infant's hair is shaved over a small area. The family caregivers can be reassured that the infant's hair will grow back quickly. An inverted medicine cup, or paper cup with the bottom cut out, is often taped over the site to protect it. The needle is stabilized with U-shaped taping and a loop of the tubing is taped so that if the child pulls on the tubing, the loop will absorb the pull and the site will remain intact. The older infant's hands may need to be restrained. This restraint may be accomplished by pinning the shirt sleeves to the bed or diapers. If a site in the hand, foot, or arm is used, the limb should be stabilized on a board before the insertion is attempted. These latter sites restrict the child's movement much more than the scalp site, therefore they are less preferred (Figure 3-16). The use of a plastic cannula or winged small-vein needle has made surgical cutdowns much less frequently needed. In a surgical cutdown, a small incision is made, usually in the foot or the hand, providing access to a vein. The cutdown procedure is performed by a physician under sterile conditions.

Older children may be permitted some choice of site, if possible. The child should be involved in all aspects of the procedure within age-appropriate capabilities. The preschool child often is able to cooperate if given adequate explanation. Play therapy in preparation for intravenous therapy may be helpful. Honesty is essential with children of any age. The older school-age child and adolescent may have many questions that should be answered with explanations at their level of understanding.

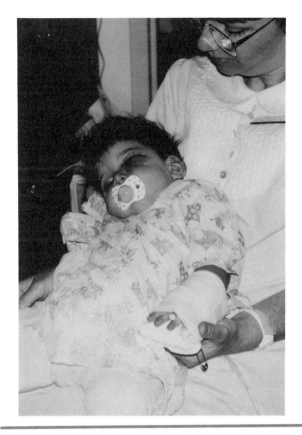

Figure 3-16. A peripheral site for intravenous infusion. A medicine cup protects the site, "wings" on the armboard are pinned to the bed. (Courtesy of Department of Medical Photography, Children's Hospital, Buffalo, NY.)

Family caregivers also need explanations and should be included in the preparation for the procedure. By their presence and reassurance, family caregivers may provide the emotional support the child needs and help the child maintain calm throughout the procedure.

In preparation for starting an intravenous line, the nurse must collect all the equipment that may be needed, including the intravenous tubing, any extension tubing that may be needed, the container of solution, the equipment to stabilize the site, a tourniquet, cleansing supplies such as povidone-iodine or alcohol swabs, sterile gauze, adhesive tape, cling roll gauze, an intravenous pole, an infusion pump or controller, and a plastic cannula or winged small-vein needle, usually between a 21-gauge and 25-gauge size (depending on the size of the child). The nurse who starts an intravenous infusion in the pediatric patient should be skilled in the procedure. The small veins of children are sometimes difficult to access and may easily be blown. Venipuncture is a procedure that requires practice and expertise. An unskilled nurse should not attempt to start an intravenous infusion in a child unless under direct supervision of a person who is skilled in pediatric intravenous administration. The staff nurse may serve as the child's advocate when the physician or intravenous nurse comes to start an infusion. The staff nurse who has cared for the child has the child's confidence and knows the child's preferences.

Infusion Control

There are numerous intravenous infusion pumps suitable for pediatric use. The rate of infusion for infants and children must be carefully monitored. The intravenous drip rate must be slow for the small child to avoid overloading the circulation and inducing cardiac failure. Various adapting devices are available that decrease the size of the drop to a "mini" or "micro" drop of 1/50 or 1/60 mL, thus delivering 50 to 60 minidrops or microdrops per milliliter rather than the 15 drops per milliliter of a regular set (Figure 3-17). Many intravenous sets also contain a control chamber (or burette) that contains 100 to 150 mL of fluid and is designed to deliver controlled volumes of fluid, avoiding the accidental entrance of too great a volume of fluid into the child's system. Regardless of the control systems and safeguards, the child and the intravenous infusion should be monitored as frequently as every hour. The intravenous site must be checked to see that it is intact and observed for redness, pain, **induration** (hardness), rate of flow, moisture at the site, and swelling. Documentation is done on an intravenous flow sheet on which is recorded the rate of flow, the amount in the bottle, the amount in the burette, the amount infused, and the condition of the site.

For the administration of an intravenous medication, a heparin lock may be used. This method allows the child more freedom and permits the child to be free of intravenous tubing between medication administrations. The veins on the back of the hand are often used for heparin lock insertion. Medication is administered through the lock, and when the administration is completed, the needle and tubing are removed and the heparin lock is flushed. A self-healing rubber stopper closes the heparin lock so that it does not leak between administrations. This method also may be used for a child who must have frequent blood samples drawn. The heparin lock is flushed every 4 to 8 hours with saline or heparin, according to the facility's procedure.

The Child Undergoing Surgery

Surgery frightens most adults, even though they understand why it is necessary and how it helps correct their health problem. Young children do not have this understanding and may become frightened of even a minor surgical procedure. Older children and adolescents are capable of understanding the need for surgery and what it will accomplish, if they are properly prepared.

Many hospitals have outpatient surgery facilities (surgicenters) that are used for minor procedures and permit the patient to return home the day of the operation. These facilities help reduce or eliminate the separation of parents and children, one of the most stressful factors in surgery for infants and young children. Whether hospitalized for less than 1 day or for several weeks, the child who has surgery needs sympathetic and thorough preoperative and postoperative care. When the child is too young to benefit from preoperative teaching, explanations should be directed to family caregivers to help relieve their anxiety and prepare them to participate in the child's care after surgery.

Preoperative Care

Specific physical and psychological preparation of the child and the family varies according to the type of surgery planned. General aspects of care include patient teaching, preparation of the skin, preparation of the gastrointestinal and urinary systems, and preoperative medication.

Patient Teaching

The child admitted for planned surgery probably has had some preadmission preparation by the physician and family caregivers. Many families, however, may have an

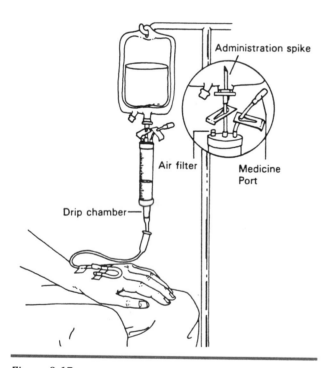

Figure 3-17. Secondary administration through a volume control set. (From Earnest V. Clinical Skills in Nursing Practice, 2d ed. Philadelphia, JB Lippincott, 1993.)

unclear understanding of the surgery and what it involves, or they may be too anxious to be helpful. The health professionals involved in the child's care must determine how much the child knows and is capable of learning, help correct any misunderstandings, and explain the preparation for surgery and what the surgery will "fix" as well as how the child will feel after surgery. This preparation must be based on the child's age, developmental level, previous experiences, and parental support. All explanations should be clear and honest, expressed in terms the child and the family caregivers can understand. Questions should be encouraged to be sure all information is understood correctly. If possible, preoperative teaching should be conducted in short sessions rather than trying to discuss everything at once.

Therapeutic play, discussed in Chapter 2, is useful in preparing the child for surgery. Identifying the area of the body to be operated on with drawings helps the child have a better understanding of what is going to happen (Figure 3-18).

Children need to be prepared for standard preoperative tests and procedures, such as radiographs and blood and urine tests. Nurses may explain the reason for withholding food and fluids before surgery so children do not feel that they are being neglected or punished when others receive meal trays.

Children sometimes interpret surgery as punishment and should be reassured that they did not cause the condition. They also fear mutilation or death and need to be able to explore those feelings, recognizing them as acceptable fears. Children deserve careful explanation that the physician is going to repair only the affected body part.

It is important to emphasize that the child will not feel anything during surgery because of the special sleep that anesthesia causes. Describing the postanesthesia care unit (PACU, or wake-up room) and any tubes, bandages, or appliances that will be in place after surgery lets the child know what to expect. If possible, the child should be able to see and handle the anesthesia mask (if this is the method to be used) and equipment that will be part of the postoperative experience.

Role playing, adjusted to the child's age and understanding, is helpful. This approach may include a trip on a stretcher, pretending to go to surgery. The nurse or play leader can pretend to be the patient, if the child makes such a request.

The older child or adolescent may have a greater interest in the surgery itself, what is wrong and why, how the repair is done, and the expected postoperative results. Models of a child's internal organs, or individual organs such as a heart, are useful for demonstration, or the patient may be involved in making the drawing.

A child needs to understand that several people will be involved in preoperative, surgical, and postoperative care. If possible, staff members from the anesthesia department and the operating room, recovery room, or the intensive care unit (ICU) areas should visit the child preoperatively. Explaining what the people will be wearing (caps, masks, and gloves), the equipment, and that

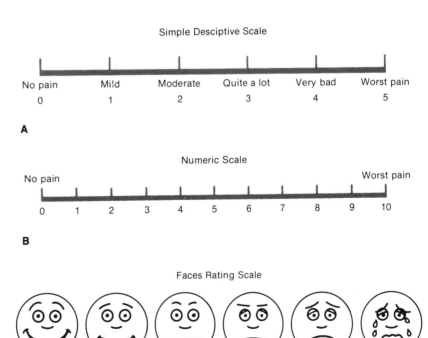

Figure 3-18. Pain scales: **A**, Simple descriptive scale; **B**, Numeric scale; **C**, Faces rating scale. (From Skale N. Manual of Pediatric Nursing Procedures. Philadelphia: JB Lippincott, 1992, p. 153.)

the lights will be bright helps make the operating room experience less frightening. A preoperative tour of the PACU or ICU is also helpful.

Most patients experience postoperative pain, and children should be prepared for this experience. They also need to know when they may expect to be allowed to have fluids and food after surgery.

Children should be taught to practice coughing and deep-breathing exercises. Deep-breathing practice may be done with games that encourage blowing. Teaching them to splint the operative site with a pillow helps reassure them that the sutures will not break and let the wound open.

Children should be told where their family will be during and after surgery, and every effort should be made to minimize separation. Family caregivers should be encouraged to be present when the child leaves for the operating room.

Skin Preparation

Depending on the type of surgery, skin preparation may include a tub bath or shower and certainly includes special cleaning and inspection of the operative site. If shaving is needed as part of the preparation, it usually is performed in the operating room. If fingers or toes are involved, the nails are carefully trimmed. The operative site may be painted with a special antiseptic solution as an extra precaution against infection, depending on the physician's orders and the procedures of individual hospitals.

Gastrointestinal and Urinary System Preparation

The surgeon may order a cleansing enema the night before surgery. This enema is an intrusive procedure and needs to be explained to the child before it is given. If old enough, the child should understand the reason for the enema.

Children usually receive nothing by mouth (NPO) 4 to 12 hours before surgery because food or fluids in the stomach may cause vomiting and aspiration, particularly during general anesthesia. The child should be told that food and drink are being withheld to prevent an upset stomach. The NPO period varies according to the age of the child; infants become dehydrated more rapidly than older children do and thus require a shorter NPO period before surgery. Loose teeth are also a potential hazard and should be counted and recorded according to hospital policy.

In some instances, urinary catheterization may be performed preoperatively, but usually it is done while the child is in the operating room. The catheter is often removed immediately after surgery but can be left in place for several hours or days. Children who are not catheterized before surgery should be encouraged to void before the administration of preoperative medication.

Preoperative Medication

Depending on the physician's order, preoperative medications usually are given in two stages: a sedative is administered about 1 1/2 to 2 hours before surgery, and an analgesic–atropine mixture may be administered immediately before the patient leaves for the operating room. When the sedative has been given, the lights should be dimmed, and noise should be minimized to help the child relax and rest. Family caregivers and the child should be aware that atropine can cause a blotchy rash and a flushed face.

Preoperative medication should be brought to the child's room when it is time for the administration. At that time, the child is told that it is time for medication and that another nurse has come along to help the child hold still. Medication should be administered carefully and quickly because delays only increase the child's anxiety.

If hospital regulations permit, family caregivers should accompany the child to the operating room and wait until the child is anesthetized. If this is not possible, the nurse who has been caring for the child can go along to the operating room and introduce the child to personnel there.

Postoperative Care

During the immediate postoperative period, the child is cared for in the PACU or the surgical ICU. Meanwhile, the room in the pediatric unit should be prepared with appropriate equipment for the child's return. Depending on the type of surgery performed, it may be necessary to have suctioning, resuscitation, or other equipment at the bedside.

When the child has been returned to the room, nursing care focuses on careful observation for any signs or symptoms of complications: shock, hemorrhage, or respiratory distress. Vital signs are monitored according to postoperative orders and recorded. The child is kept warm with blankets as needed. Dressings, intravenous apparatus, urinary catheters, and any other appliances are noted and observed. An intravenous flow sheet is begun that documents the type of fluid, the amount of fluid to be absorbed, the rate of flow, any additive medications, the site, and the appearance and condition of the site. The intravenous flow sheet may be separate or incorporated into a general flow sheet for the pediatric patient. The first voiding is an important milestone in the child's postoperative progress because it indicates the adequacy of blood flow, and should be noted, recorded, and reported. Any irritation or burning also should be noted, and the physician should be notified if **anuria** (absence of urine) persists longer than 6 hours.

Postoperative orders may provide for ice chips or clear liquids to prevent dehydration; these may be administered with a spoon or in a small medicine cup. Frequent repositioning is necessary to prevent skin breakdown, orthostatic pneumonia, and decreased circulation. Coughing, deep breathing, and position changes are performed at least every 2 hours.

Pain Management

Pain is a concern of postoperative patients in any age group. Most adult patients are able to verbally express the pain they feel and request relief. However, infants and young children are not able to adequately express themselves and need help to tell where or how great the pain is. Longstanding beliefs that children do not have the same amount of pain that adults have, or that they tolerate pain better than adults, have contributed to the undermedication of infants and children in pain. Recent research has shown that children do experience pain as keenly as adults.

The nurse must be alert to indications of pain, especially in young patients. Careful assessment is necessary, noting changes in behavior such as rigidity, thrashing, facial expressions, loud crying or screaming, flexion of knees (indicating abdominal pain), restlessness, and irritability. Physiologic changes, such as increased pulse rate and blood pressure, sweating palms, dilated pupils, flushed or moist skin, and loss of appetite, also may indicate pain. Some children may try to hide pain because they fear an injection or because they are afraid that admitting to pain will increase the time they have to stay in the hospital.

Various tools have been devised to help children express the amount of pain they feel. These tools include the faces scale, the numeric scale, descriptive scales, and the color scale. The first three scales are useful primarily with children 7 years of age and older (Figure 3-18). To use the color scale, the young child is given crayons ranging from yellow to red or black. Yellow represents no pain, and the darkest color (or red) represents the most pain. The child selects the color that represents the amount of pain felt.

Pain medication may be administered orally, by routine intramuscular or intravenous routes, or by **patient-controlled analgesia** (**PCA**). PCA is a programmed intravenous infusion of narcotic analgesia that the child may control within set limits (Figure 3-19**A** and **B**). A low-level dose of analgesia may be administered with the child having the capability of administering a bolus as needed. PCA may be used for children 7 years of age or older who have no cognitive impairment and meet a careful evaluation for its use. Intramuscular injections are avoided, if possible. Vital signs must be monitored, and the child's level of consciousness must be documented at least every 4 hours.

Comfort measures should be employed along with the administration of analgesics. The child is encouraged to become involved in activities that may provide distraction. The activities need to be appropriate to the child's age, level of development, and interests. No child should be allowed to suffer pain unnecessarily.

Surgical Dressings

Postoperative care includes close observation of any dressings for signs of drainage or hemorrhage and reinforcement or changing dressings as ordered by the physician. Wet dressings can increase the possibility of contamination; clean, dry dressings increase the child's comfort. If there is no physician's order to change the dressing, the nurse is expected to reinforce the moist original dressing by covering it with a dry dressing and taping the second dressing in place. If bloody drainage is present, the nurse should draw around the outline of the drainage with a marker and mark it with the time and date.

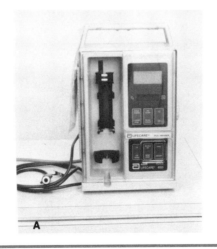
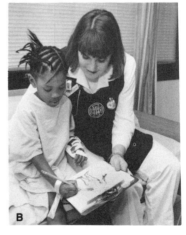

Figure 3-19. **A**, PCA pump. **B**, Distraction supplements pain control while child is using PCA. (From Skale N. Manual of Pediatric Nursing Procedures. Philadelphia, JB Lippincott, 1992, p. 153.)

In this way the amount of additional drainage can be assessed when the dressings are inspected later.

Supplies needed for changing dressing vary according to the wound site and the physician's orders, which specifies the sterile or antiseptic technique to be used. Detailed procedures for these techniques and the supplies to be used can be found in the procedure manuals of individual health care facilities.

As with all procedures, the nurse must explain to the child what will be done and why before beginning the dressing change. Some dressing changes may be painful; if so, the child should be told that it will hurt and should be praised for behavior that shows courage and cooperation.

Patient Teaching

Postoperative patient teaching is as necessary as teaching that helped prepare the patient. Some explanations and instructions given earlier need to be repeated during postoperative care because the patient's earlier anxiety may have prevented thorough understanding. Now that tubes, restraints, and dressings are part of the child's reality, they need to be discussed again: why they are important and how they affect the child's activities.

Family caregivers want to know how they can help care for the child and what limitations are placed on the child's activity. If caregivers know what to expect and how to aid in their child's recovery, they will be cooperative during the postoperative period.

As the child recuperates, the caregivers and child should be encouraged to share their feelings about the surgery, any changes in body image, and their expectations for recovery and rehabilitation.

When it is time for the sutures to be removed, the nurse should reassure the child that the opening has healed and the child's "insides will not fall out" when the sutures are removed. This idea is a common fear that children have.

Before the child is discharged from the hospital, teaching focuses on home care, use of any special equipment or appliances, medications, diet, restrictions on activities, and therapeutic exercise (Figure 3-20). The nursing process is used to assess the needs of the child and the family to plan appropriate postoperative care and teaching.

Gavage Feeding

Sometimes infants or children who have had surgery are too weak to tolerate adequate food and fluid by mouth and must receive nourishment by means of gavage feedings. **Gavage feedings** provide nourishment directly through a tube passed into the stomach. This procedure is particularly appropriate in infants. If gavage feedings are not well tolerated, the nurse should report it and await alternate orders from the physician.

Whether the tube is inserted nasally or orally, the measurement is the same: from the tip of the child's nose

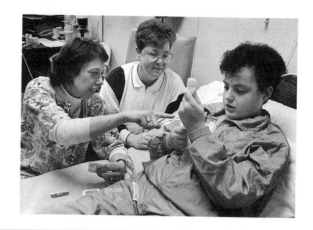

Figure 3-20. Incorporating the entire family into the teaching process increases learning effectiveness. (From Jackson DB, Saunders RB. Child Health Nursing. Philadelphia: JB Lippincott, 1993, p. 4. Photo courtesy of Kathy Sloane/ Courtesy of Children's Hospital, Oakland, CA.)

to the earlobe and down to the tip of the sternum (Figure 3-21). This length may be marked on the tube with tape or a marking pen. The end of the tube to be inserted should be lubricated with sterile water or water-soluble lubricating jelly, *never* an oily substance because of the danger of oil aspiration into the lungs.

To prepare the child for gavage feeding, elevate the head and place a rolled-up diaper behind the neck. Turn the head and align the body to the right.

After the tube is inserted, its position is verified by aspirating stomach contents or by inserting 1 to 5 mL of air (using a syringe with an adapter) and listening with a stethoscope. If the tube is properly placed, gurgling or

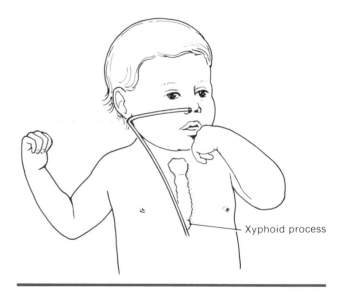

Xyphoid process

Figure 3-21. Measurement of tubing for nasogastric tube insertion. (From Skale N. Manual of Pediatric Nursing Procedures. Philadelphia: JB Lippincott, 1992, p. 407.)

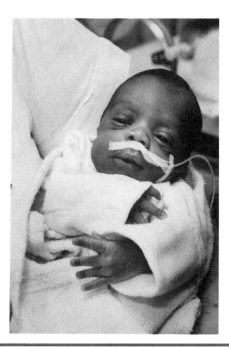

Figure 3-22. Nasogastric tube taped to infant's cheek. (From Skale N. Manual of Pediatric Nursing Procedures. Philadelphia: JB Lippincott, 1992, p. 409.)

growling sounds are heard as air enters the stomach. If stomach contents are aspirated, these should be measured and replaced, and in a very small infant, subtracted from the amount ordered for that particular feeding.

The nurse may hold the tube in place if it is going to be removed immediately after the feeding. If the tube is left in position for further use, it should be secured with tape (Figure 3-22). The correct position must be verified before each feeding.

The feeding syringe is inserted into the tube, and its plunger is pushed gently to start the flow of formula, which has been warmed to room temperature. The plunger is then removed, and the feeding is allowed to flow by gravity only. The entire feeding should take 15 to 20 minutes, after which the infant will need to be burped and to be positioned on the right side for at least 1 hour to prevent regurgitation and aspiration.

The type and amount of contents aspirated by the nurse, the amount of formula fed, the infant's tolerance for the procedure, and the positioning of the infant after completion should be recorded on the chart. The feeding tube and any leftover formula should be discarded at the completion of the procedure.

Gastrostomy Feeding

Children who must receive tube feedings over a long period may have a **gastrostomy tube** surgically inserted through the abdominal wall into the stomach. This procedure is performed under general anesthesia. It also is used in children who have obstructions or surgical re-

pairs in the mouth, pharynx, esophagus, or cardiac sphincter of the stomach or who are respirator-dependent.

The surgeon inserts a catheter (plain, Foley, or mushroom [Pezzer] catheter with the tip removed) that is left unclamped and connected to gravity drainage for 24 hours. Meticulous care of the wound site is necessary to prevent infection and irritation. Until the area has healed, it must be covered with a sterile dressing. Ointment, Stomadhesive, or other skin preparations may be ordered for application to the site. The child may need to be restrained to prevent pulling on the catheter that may cause leakage of caustic gastric juices.

Procedures for positioning and feeding the child with a gastrostomy tube are similar to those for gavage feedings. The residual stomach contents are aspirated, measured, and replaced at the beginning of the procedure. The child's head and shoulders are elevated during the feeding. After each feeding, the child is placed on the right side or in Fowler's position.

When regular oral feedings are resumed, the tube is surgically removed, and the opening usually closes spontaneously.

For long-term gastrostomy feedings, a gastrostomy button may be inserted. Among the advantages of buttons are that they are more desirable cosmetically, simple to care for, and cause less skin irritation.

Summary

Whether a child is 6 months, 6 years, or 16 years old, illness and hospitalization make a significant impact on growth and development. Even with the most attractive, best-equipped surroundings and the most competent medical and surgical treatment, the child's recovery and rehabilitation require effective, well-planned nursing care. Each nurse who gives competent, comforting care helps make hospitalization a positive growth experience for the child.

Administering medications to children is challenging. An attitude of friendly persuasion may be the most useful plan. Children should know that the nurse is in charge but not be overwhelmed by oppressive authority. Accuracy in administration and dosage calculations is essential. Drugs that are administered intravenously require careful observation and conscientious nursing care.

Superb skills and technologic advances help surgeons achieve almost miraculous results in treating children's health problems. To the child facing surgery, however, and often to family caregivers, the operating room is an overwhelming place filled with masked faces, sharp instruments, and countless, nameless terrors. Teaching children and family caregivers what to expect and explaining what is going to happen before, during, and after procedures help reduce the fears and anxieties and make the child part of the team working toward restoration of optimum health. Teaching is part of all nursing care, and at no time is it more important than for the child who must have surgery. Even the most remarkable surgical treatment is incomplete without nurses who offer skilled physical care and sensitive attention to the emotional needs of the child and his or her family.

Review Questions

1. Tell step-by-step how you would take vital signs on a young infant. Explain the order in which you would do them and why.
2. When counting respirations of an infant or young child, what besides rate must you observe?
3. Chastity is a 3-year-old girl with a fever of 104.4°F (40.2°C). You must give her a sponge bath. Describe exactly what you would do. Include all explanations to the child.
4. What effects may result from the local application of cold?
5. Jason is a 5-year-old boy who dashed into the street and was hit by the side of a passing car. He has been admitted with possible head injuries. What is one of your primary concerns? What nursing care will he need? Describe this care.
6. Catlin weighs 28.5 lb (13 kg) and measures 35.5 inches (90 cm). Find her BSA using the West nomogram. Calculate the dose of a medication for her if the adult dosage is 750 mg.
7. The physician ordered elixir of phenobarbital 15 mg every 12 hours for seizure activity. If the available supply was labeled 20 mg/mL, how many milliliters would you give?
8. How would you approach each of the following children when giving oral medications? intramuscular medications?
   a. 6-month-old Kristi
   b. 18-month-old Jared
   c. 3-year-old Sarah
   d. 4½-year-old Miguel
   e. 8-year-old Nicole
   f. 16-year-old Jon
9. Name each of the intramuscular injection sites. Show how to locate the sites, and name the landmarks used.
10. Why does an infant become seriously dehydrated much faster than an adult?
11. Why is the scalp vein commonly used as an intravenous site in infants?
12. Hong is a 4½-year-old child scheduled for a tonsillectomy and adenoidectomy. You have the opportunity to prepare him for surgery before and after admission. Detail the appropriate preparation.
13. You are observing 2-year-old Kent postoperatively after abdominal surgery. What signs would you look for to indicate he is having pain?
14. When preparing to give 6-month-old Kristi a tube feeding, what should you do first after setting up the equipment? How would you do this?
15. How would you position Kristi after the tube feeding? Why?

Bibliography

Baird SC, White NE, Basinger M. Can you rely on tympanic thermometers? RN 55(8):48–51, 1992.

Barnes LP. Don't forget to play. MCN 17(4):183, 1992.

Bender LH, Weaver K, Edwards K. Postoperative patient-controlled analgesia in children. Pediatr Nurs 16(6):549–554, 1990.

Broome ME. Preparation of children for painful procedures. Pediatr Nurs 16(6):537–541, 1990.

Broome ME, Slack JF. Influences on nurses' management of pain in children. MCN 15(3):158–166, 1990.

Carabott JA, Javaheri Z, Keilty K, et al. Oral fluid intake in children following tonsillectomy and adenoidectomy. Pediatr Nurs 18(2):124–127, 1992.

Castiglia PT, Harbin RE. Child Health Care: Process and Practice. Philadelphia: JB Lippincott, 1992.

Danek GD, Noris EM. Pediatric IV catheters: Efficacy of saline flush. Pediatr Nurs 18(2):111–113, 1992.

Elander G, Lindberg T, Quarnstrom B. Pain relief in infants after major surgery. J Pediatr Surg 26(2):128–131, 1991.

Ellett M, Beckstrand J, Wech J, et al. Predicting the distance for gavage tube placement in children. Pediatr Nurs 18(2):119–121, 1992.

Favaloro R, Touzel B. A comparison of adolescents' and nurses' postoperative pain ratings and perceptions. Pediatr Nurs 16(4):414–416, 1990.

Gildea JH. When fever becomes an enemy. Pediatr Nurs 18(2):165–167, 1992.

Gureno MA, Reisinger CL. Patient-controlled analgesia for the young pediatric patient. Pediatr Nurs 17(3):251–254, 1991.

Manssoon ME, Fredrikson B, Rosberg B. Comparison of preparation and narcotic-sedative premedication in children undergoing surgery. Pediatr Nurs 18(4):337–342, 1992.

Neal J, Slayton D. Neonatal and pediatric PEG tubes. MCN 17(4):184–191, 1992.

Pillitteri A. Maternal and Child Health Nursing. Philadelphia: JB Lippincott, 1992.

Skale N. Manual of Pediatric Nursing Procedures. Philadelphia: JB Lippincott, 1992.

Stevens B. Development and testing of a pediatric pain management sheet. Pediatr Nurs 16(6):543–548, 1990.

Whaley LF, Wong DL. Nursing Care of Infants and Children, 4th ed. St. Louis: Mosby-Year Book, 1991.

A Child Is Born

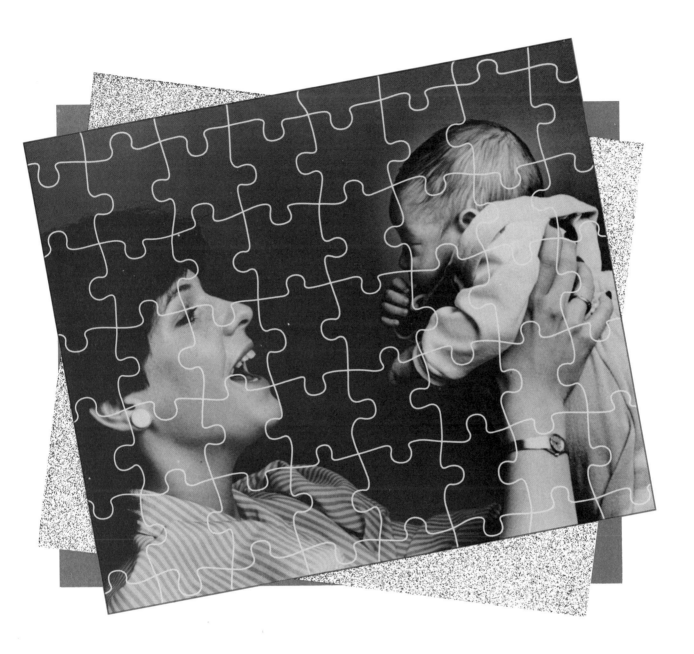

Unit II

The Prenatal Period

Chapter 4

Student Objectives

Upon completion of this chapter, the student will be able to:

1. Define the vocabulary terms listed in the key terms section.
2. Identify the three stages of prenatal development that occur during the first 8 weeks following conception.
3. State three bits of information that can be obtained from an amniocentesis.
4. State how many pairs of chromosomes there are in each human cell.
5. List the kind of information that a karyotype can provide.
6. Describe how the sex of the child is determined at the time of conception.
7. Draw a diagram illustrating the inheritance of an autosomal recessive inheritance in which both parents are carriers of the disease. Explain the pattern.
8. List three primary goals of genetic counseling.
9. Identify the factors that may create problems for the pregnant teenager.
10. State the primary dietary goal for the pregnant woman.
11. List three maternal habits that may be harmful to the fetus.
12. Describe the danger that rubella presents for the unborn fetus, and discuss preventive procedures.
13. Name three types of childbirth preparation.

Marks MG: BROADRIBB'S INTRODUCTORY PEDIATRIC NURSING, 4th ed. © 1994 J.B. Lippincott Company.

amniocentesis

amniotic sac

autosomal dominant trait

autosomal recessive trait

autosome

centromere

chromosome

conception

differentiation

dominant gene

elderly primigravida

embryo

fertilization

fetus

genes

genetic code

genetic counseling

genotype

gestation

growth

heterozygous

homozygous

karyotype

mutation

organogenesis

placenta

recessive gene

sex chromosome

teratogen

trimester

umbilical cord

viability

zygote

*F*rom the moment of conception until full maturity, human life proceeds in an orderly pattern of growth and development. This pattern and the person that results from it are shaped by various factors that precede and follow conception. Genetic influences help determine a child's physical and intellectual characteristics, as do environmental influences. Once conception has occurred, a child's genetic heritage does not change. The environment can be altered, however, with either positive or negative effects on the child and the family. Fortunately, a great deal of knowledge is now available to prospective parents to help them provide a favorable environment in which their child may grow and develop.

Prenatal Growth and Development

Conception occurs when a sperm cell reaches and penetrates an ovum. This process is also called **fertilization**, and it produces a fertilized ovum, or **zygote**. During the first 10 days to 2 weeks of life, the zygote becomes implanted in the lining of the uterus. Once implanted, the growing organism is referred to as an **embryo**. After it acquires a human likeness, usually about the eighth week of life, it is termed a **fetus**.

At no other time in a person's life is growth more rapid than during the intrauterine period. The microscopic zygote increases in size more than 200 billion times during the 9 months before birth. Two distinct but related processes take place during the transformation of zygote to infant: growth and differentiation. **Growth** is the result of cell division and is marked by an increase in size and weight. **Differentiation** changes the dividing cells, creating specialized tissues necessary to form an organized, coordinated person.

Gestation

Gestation is the period between conception and birth. The normal time required for a child to grow from a single cell to a newborn infant is 9 calendar months, or 10 lunar months (Figure 4-1). A baby born before the sixth month is considered at risk and may not survive, even with the special life-support systems available in modern intensive care nurseries. The age of **viability** is the earliest gestational age at which a fetus can survive outside the uterine environment. Deviation in the gestational age of newborn babies is normal, but the closer the infant comes to the full 9 months' gestation, the greater the chances are for a healthy neonatal period.

Trimesters

Gestation is divided into **trimesters** (periods of 3 months). **Organogenesis**, the process by which cells differentiate into major organ systems, commences shortly after conception and is almost completed by the end of the eighth week. Even the 4-week-old embryo shows evidence of beginning organs and organ systems (Figure 4-2). After the eighth week of life, the major changes are the growth and development of organs and organ systems. The first

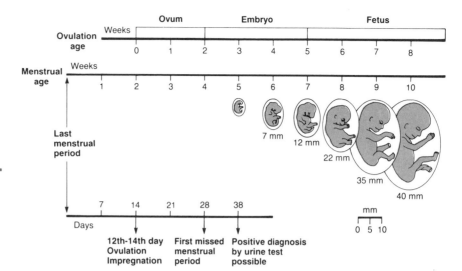

Figure 4-1. Growth of the ovum, embryo, and fetus during the early weeks of pregnancy. (From Martin LL, Reeder SR. Essentials of Maternity Nursing, 16th ed. Philadelphia: JB Lippincott, 1991, p. 54.)

trimester is the time when the fetus is most vulnerable to any hazard in the intrauterine environment.

The second trimester is a period of continuing growth and development. All reflexes are present by the end of the fourth month, except for functional respiration and vocal response. All nerve cells are present by the fifth month, although not functionally mature.

If circumstances cause premature birth during the third trimester, the child has developed sufficiently to survive, assuming that constant, expert care is provided. During this last trimester, the fetus stores iron for postnatal use and develops subcutaneous fat, which enables it to begin independent life. Figure 4-3 summarizes the month-by-month growth and development of the fetus.

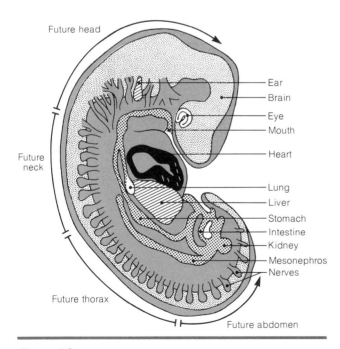

Figure 4-2. Four-week-old embryo.

Intrauterine Development

The child develops within the protection of a fluid environment surrounded by the **amniotic sac**. This strong translucent membrane is large and elastic enough to permit the fetus to move about and turn at will during most of its intrauterine life. The amniotic sac usually contains about 1000 mL of amniotic fluid, which is a clear, neutral to slightly alkaline (pH 7.0 to 7.25) liquid. This fluid protects the fetus from direct impact on the mother's abdomen, separates the fetus from the membranes, aids symmetric growth and development, helps maintain a constant body temperature by preventing heat loss, provides oral fluid for the fetus, and acts as an excretion collection system.

Ultrasound examination is a noninvasive procedure that is commonly performed during pregnancy. Through the use of high-frequency sound waves directed toward the mother's uterus, a visual image is formed on a monitor. Intrauterine pregnancy can be verified. The fetus' breathing, cardiac action, and movement may be seen. Fetal measurements may be made, multiple fetuses identified, excessive or inadequate amounts of amniotic fluid noted, and early identification of problems such as polycystic kidneys, limb abnormalities, hydrocephalus intestinal obstructions, and myelomeningocele is possible.

Analysis of amniotic fluid through **amniocentesis** reveals much about the fetus, including sex, state of fetal health, and fetal maturity. A sample of amniotic fluid is withdrawn for early diagnosis of possible disorders, such as chromosomal abnormalities, blood disorders, and respiratory problems. Performed under local anesthesia, the procedure is done by inserting a needle through the abdominal and uterine walls into the amniotic sac and withdrawing a small amount of fluid (10 to 20 mL) through a syringe. Although amniocentesis carries a slight risk to the mother and fetus, it is a recommended procedure when the mother is older than 35 years of age or when there is a known risk to the fetus of inheriting a serious

Fetal Development

1st Lunar Month

The fetus is 0.75 cm to 1 cm in length.

Trophoblasts embed in decidua.

Chorionic villi form.

Foundations for nervous system, genitourinary system, skin, bones, and lungs are formed.

Buds of arms and legs begin to form.

Rudiments of eyes, ears, and nose appear.

4 weeks

2nd Lunar Month

The fetus is 2.5 cm in length and weighs 4 g.

Fetus is markedly bent.

Head is disproportionately large, owing to brain development.

Sex differentiation begins.

Centers of bone begin to ossify.

8 weeks

3rd Lunar Month

The fetus is 7 cm to 9 cm in length and weighs 28 g.

Fingers and toes are distinct.

Placenta is complete

Fetal circulation is complete.

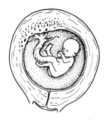

3 months

4th Lunar Month

The fetus is 10 cm to 17 cm in length and weighs 55 g to 120 g.

Sex is differentiated.

Rudimentary kidneys secrete urine.

Heartbeat is present.

Nasal septum and palate close.

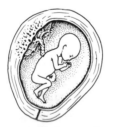

4 months

5th Lunar Month

The fetus is 25 cm in length and weighs 223 g.

Lanugo covers entire body.

Fetal movements are felt by mother.

Heart sounds are perceptible by auscultation.

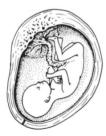

5 months

6th Lunar Month

The fetus is 28 cm to 36 cm in length and weighs 680 g.

Skin appears wrinkled.

Vernix caseosa appears.

Eyebrows and fingernails develop.

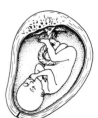

6 months

7th Lunar Month

The fetus is 35 cm to 38 cm in length and weighs 1200 g.

Skin is red.

Pupillary membrane disappears from eyes.

The fetus has an excellent chance of survival.

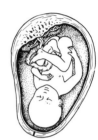

7 months

8th Lunar Month

The fetus is 38 cm to 43 cm in length and weighs 2.7 kg.

Fetus is viable.

Eyelids open.

Fingerprints are set.

Vigorous fetal movement occurs.

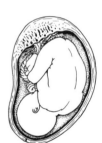

8 months

9th Lunar Month

The fetus is 42 cm to 49 cm in length and weighs 1900 g to 2700 g.

Face and body have a loose wrinkled appearance because of subcutaneous fat deposit.

Lanugo disappears

Amniotic fluid decreases.

9 months

10th Lunar Month

The fetus is 48 cm to 52 cm in length and weighs 3000 g.

Skin is smooth.

Eyes are uniformly slate colored.

Bones of skull are ossified and nearly together at sutures.

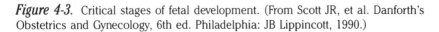

Figure 4-3. Critical stages of fetal development. (From Scott JR, et al. Danforth's Obstetrics and Gynecology, 6th ed. Philadelphia: JB Lippincott, 1990.)

genetic defect. Later in pregnancy, this test also may be used to determine fetal lung and kidney maturity before early cesarean delivery or induction of labor.

During intrauterine development, the **placenta**, or what will be the afterbirth, links the fetus to the mother. This organ performs four functions for the developing fetus: respiration, nutrition, excretion, and protection. The placenta is a reddish, disk-shaped organ, connected to the fetus by the **umbilical cord** (Figure 4-4). Blood from the placenta brings food, oxygen, hormones, and protective antibodies to the fetus by way of the umbilical vein. The umbilical arteries carry deoxygenated fetal blood and waste products back to the placenta. The placenta normally emerges soon after delivery of the baby, hence the term afterbirth.

Many drugs, viruses, and infections cross the placental barrier from the mother to the fetus. These hazards to the developing fetus are discussed in the section on environmental influences.

Genetic Influences

The science of genetics studies the ways in which normal and abnormal traits are transmitted from one generation to the next. The basic principles of genetics were discovered in 1865 by an Austrian monk named Gregor Mendel through his experimentation with common garden peas. Only in the 20th century have Mendel's principles been rediscovered and employed in science and medicine.

Before Mendel's time it was believed that the characteristics of parents were blended in their children. Mendel's experiments proved that this blending does not occur but rather that the parent's individual characteristics could reappear unchanged in later generations.

All living organisms are composed of living cells that contain all the material necessary for the maintenance and propagation of the particular species. Each cell contains a number of small bodies called **chromosomes**. Chromosomes are threadlike structures that occur in pairs; each pair is attached at the center by a **centromere**. Threaded along these chromosomes are **genes**, the units that carry genetic instructions from one generation to another. Like chromosomes, genes also occur in pairs. The instructions they carry are called the **genetic code**, the blueprint for the development of the individual organism. Each person's unique set of genes is called his or her **genotype**.

Each human cell contains 46 chromosomes, consisting of 23 essentially identical or homologous pairs. One member of each pair is contributed by the father, and one by the mother, to the single cell formed by the union of sperm and egg at conception, which determines the sex and inherited traits of the new organism.

Twenty-two of these pairs are alike in the male and the female and are called **autosomes**. The remaining pair is a pair of **sex chromosomes**, which differ in the male and the female. When the form or number of autosomes is altered, birth defects or abnormalities result.

Karyotypes

Modern technology has made it possible to photograph the nuclei of human cells and enlarge them to show the chromosomes. The chromosomes are cut from the photographs, matched in pairs, and grouped. The resulting picture is a **karyotype** and is used to locate chromosomal malformations and translocations (the change in position of a segment of chromosome to another location on the chromosome or to another chromosome). Karyotypes of normal chromosomes are properly paired (Figure 4-5). In some abnormal conditions, translocations occur. In other conditions, such as in trisomy 21 (Down syndrome), three chromosomes occur in the 21 or 22

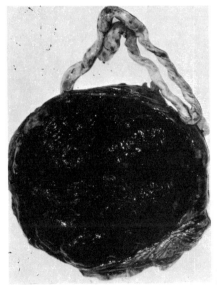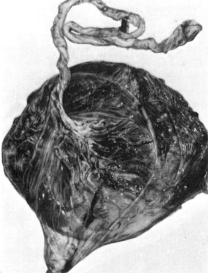

Figure 4-4. **Left,** The maternal surface of the placenta is rough and irregular. **Right,** The fetal surface is smooth and shiny. (From Bethea DC. Introductory Maternity Nursing, 5th ed. Philadelphia: JB Lippincott, 1989.)

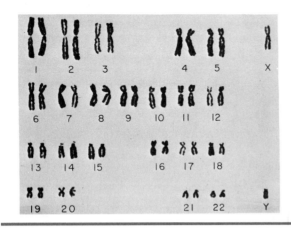

Figure 4-5. Arrangement of normal chromosomes into a standard karyotype. (Courtesy of Dr. Kurt Hirschhorn.)

position (Figure 4-6), producing a total of 47 chromosomes instead of the normal 46.

Determination of Sex

All egg cells from the female carry a pair of female chromosomes called the X chromosomes. Sperm cells, however, carry one X (female) and one Y (male) chromosome. It appears to be a matter of chance whether or not the egg, which always has an X chromosome, is fertilized by a sperm carrying an X chromosome or by one carrying a Y chromosome. In the former instance, the offspring is a girl. The Y chromosome is dominant over the X, so that if the Y enters into the union, the result is always a male child. Thus, it is the father's sex cell that determines the child's sex (Figure 4-7).

Cells reproduce by division; each parent cell produces two daughter cells, each of which in turn produces two new cells. In this manner, the single cell produced by the union of the sperm and the ovum eventually multiplies to produce an infant.

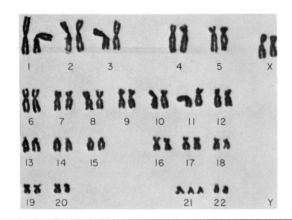

Figure 4-6. Karyotype showing trisomy 21. Note three chromosomes in the 21 position. (Courtesy of Dr. Kurt Hirschhorn.)

Determination of Inherited Traits

The ultramicroscopic bodies called genes carry genetic instruction from one generation to another with mathematic regularity. Any gene can be altered, however, by mutation or chromosomal rearrangement. **Mutation** in a gene means that a fundamental change has taken place in its structure, resulting in the transmission of a trait different from that normally carried by the particular gene. Much remains to be learned about the causes of mutations, most of which result in undesirable traits.

When any two members of a pair of genes carry the same genetic instructions, the person carrying these genes is said to be **homozygous** for that particular trait. When each member of a pair of genes carries different instructions, the person is **heterozygous** for the trait. One member of a heterozygous pair of genes is the dominant gene. Thus, a trait or condition appearing in a heterozygous person is called an **autosomal dominant trait**. A **dominant gene** may be defined as one that is expressed in only one of a chromosome pair. Huntington's disease, neurofibromatosis, and osteogenesis imperfecta are examples of dominantly inherited diseases.

A gene carrying different information for the same trait that is not expressed (eg, blue eyes versus brown eyes) is called a **recessive gene**. A recessive gene is detectable only when present on both chromosomes. Inheritance patterns for **autosomal recessive traits** are shown in Figure 4-8. However, if both parents express the recessive trait, all their children will have the same trait or condition because each parent must have two genes for the trait, and the children cannot possibly escape inheriting two also. Some examples of recessively inherited diseases are thalassemia and cystic fibrosis.

Genetic Counseling

Knowledge about genetics and the causes of specific birth defects continues to increase rapidly. One of the benefits of this increased knowledge is **genetic counseling**. Couples who are concerned about transmitting a specific disease to their children may consult a genetic counselor for screening and counseling. The counselor, a geneticist, studies the family history of both partners and may perform tissue analysis to determine chromosome patterns. This counseling is particularly important to people who may think they are carriers of hereditary disorders such as Tay-Sachs disease and sickle cell anemia. It is also helpful to people whose family history includes one or more members who are mentally retarded.

Genetic counseling has four primary goals: (1) to identify malformations and diseases that can be transmitted genetically and determine the probability of their recurrence; (2) to help couples make informed choices about future reproduction; (3) to identify potential problems for the fetus or neonate and to ensure early diagnosis and management; and (4) to ultimately reduce the number of children born with hereditary disorders. Health profes-

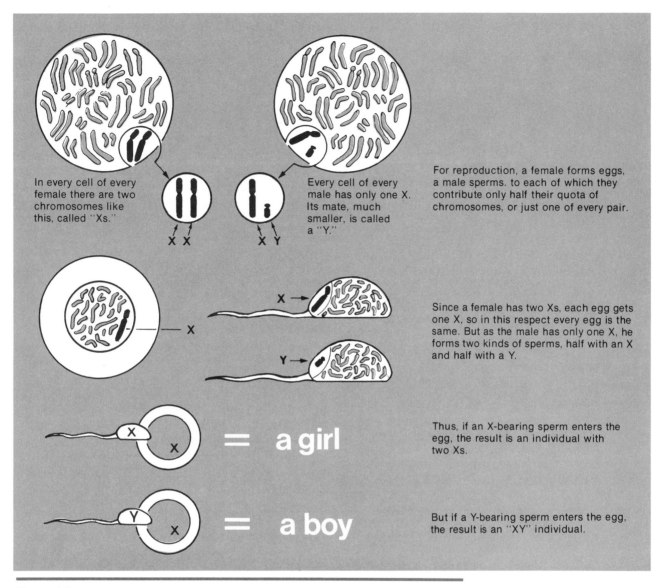

In every cell of every female there are two chromosomes like this, called "Xs."

Every cell of every male has only one X. Its mate, much smaller, is called a "Y."

X X   X Y

For reproduction, a female forms eggs, a male sperms. to each of which they contribute only half their quota of chromosomes, or just one of every pair.

X

X →

Y →

Since a female has two Xs, each egg gets one X, so in this respect every egg is the same. But as the male has only one X, he forms two kinds of sperms, half with an X and half with a Y.

X   X   = a girl

Thus, if an X-bearing sperm enters the egg, the result is an individual with two Xs.

Y   X   = a boy

But if a Y-bearing sperm enters the egg, the result is an "XY" individual.

Figure 4-7. Sex is determined at the time sperm and ovum unite. (From Scheinfeld A. Your Hereditary and Environment. Philadelphia: JB Lippincott, 1965.)

sionals can provide only information and support; the final decision concerning whether or not to have a child remains with one or both members of the couple.

Environmental Influences

Although it is recognized that the genetic material furnishes the building blocks for a new person, the old controversy concerning the importance of heredity versus environment (nature versus nurture) has lost its significance, at least in relation to intrauterine life. Current knowledge indicates that hereditary and environment influence and modify each other.

Because the mother's body is the environment for the developing fetus, nothing is more important to the successful outcome of a pregnancy than the mother's health,

both physical and emotional. Although it is no longer believed that a mother who attends art exhibitions will have a child who appreciates art, it is known that some of her reactions influence the child. Emotions such as fear and anxiety cause epinephrine to be released into the blood stream, which passes through the placenta to the fetus, triggering a physical reaction similar to that of the mother's. There is growing evidence that extreme, prolonged stress in the mother may interfere with the supply of blood to the fetus, which may have an effect on the unborn child or lead to preterm labor.

Maternal Age

Statistics indicate that the most favorable time for a woman to bear children is between the ages of 20 and 34 years. Mothers younger than age 20 experience difficulties, such

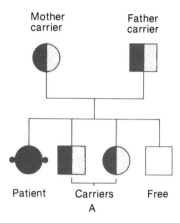

A

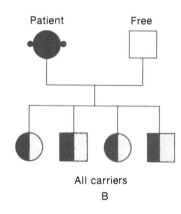

B

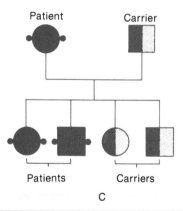

C

Figure 4-8. Autosomal recessive pattern inheritance. **A,** Both parents carriers—ratio of one patient, two carriers, one free from disease. **B,** One patient—one parent free from disease, all children carriers—no clinical disease. **C,** One parent carrier, one parent has disease—ratio of two children with disease, two carriers.

as excessive weight gain, toxemia, and prolonged labor, more often than do older mothers. Teenage pregnancies produce infants of low birth weight, increasing the risk of neonatal morbidity and mortality. In addition to the physical problems encountered by teenage mothers, emotional and financial complications often occur. A young adolescent still has growing and maturing of her own to do. Issues of independence versus dependency of an unborn child or infant may result in resentment. This resentment may be reflected in neglect of her own health and, later, in neglect or abuse of the infant. Very young couples often are limited in their earning capacity, and the additional expense of a baby places additional burdens on an already strained financial situation.

The unmarried teenage mother presents special problems. She often has no one to support her emotionally or financially or anyone with whom to share the wondrous changes that are happening within her body. She may deny the need or find it difficult to obtain the prenatal care and advice necessary for a normal birth and healthy development of the infant. Should she decide to give up her baby for adoption, she needs counseling and guidance to rebuild her changed life. It is important that nurses who care for these young women do so in a supportive, nonjudgmental manner so as not to contribute to their guilt and emotional insecurity.

An increasing number of women are delaying their childbearing to the later part of their reproductive years. It was once thought that women who became mothers after 35 years of age would be subject to a host of pregnancy complications. But with early prenatal care, the **elderly primigravida** is not likely to experience more complications than her younger counterpart, aside from a slightly greater chance of hypertension, varicosities, and hemorrhoids. However, older women do have a greater likelihood of bearing children with Down syndrome or other congenital anomalies. For instance, the incidence of Down syndrome is five times as great for mothers older than 35 years of age as for those aged 30, but currently only 20% of infants with Down syndrome are born to mothers older than 35, possibly because of early prenatal diagnoses and intervention.

Maternal Nutrition

The unborn child has a comfortable nutritional arrangement with the mother. In general, a prospective mother who follows a sensible diet and augments it correctly to fit the needs of the child provides adequately for both herself and her child. The primary goal should be optimum growth and development of the fetus. A weight gain of 25 to 35 lb currently is considered desirable. During the first part of pregnancy, about 2300 cal/day is required by pregnant women between 23 and 50 years of age. The pregnant girl younger than 15 years of age should have an intake of 2700 cal/day to fulfill both her own and her baby's growth needs. The pregnant woman's caloric intake should include nutritious foods, selected from the basic food groups, and ample liquids, including 6 to 8 glasses of water each day.

Maternal dietary allowances of protein, iron, vitamins A, B, C, and D, and calcium need to be increased during pregnancy. The infant needs to receive sufficient iron to build up an iron store for the first few months after

Table 4-1. Quantities of Food Necessary During Pregnancy

Food Group	Nonpregnant Woman	Pregnant Woman
Meat	2 servings of meat, fowl, or fish daily; 3 eggs per week	4 servings of meat, fowl, or fish daily; 3 eggs per week
Vegetables		
Dark green or deep yellow	1 serving (at least 3 times per week)	2 servings daily
Other vegetables	1 serving or more daily	1 serving or more daily
Fruits		
Citrus, melon, tomato, strawberries	1 serving daily	1 serving or more daily
Other fruits	1 serving daily	1 serving or more daily
Breads and Cereals	4 or more servings daily	4 servings daily
Dairy		
Milk	2 8-oz glasses daily	4 8-oz glasses daily
Additional fluid	Ad lib	At least 2 glasses daily

From Pillitteri A. Maternal and Child Health. Philadelphia: JB Lippincott, 1992, p. 283.

birth. The pregnant adolescent needs careful guidance because she may be accustomed to eating a lot of non-nutritious "fast foods." She needs sound nutritional teaching and guidance to provide her baby with adequate nourishment (Table 4-1).

Maternal Infections

A mother's infections represent distinct hazards for the unborn child. One example is that of maternal rubella (German measles). Although a mild disease in adults, rubella produces a high percentage of congenital malformations in the fetus when the mother is infected during the first trimester. Congenital cataracts, deafness, mental retardation, and congenital heart disease are abnormalities resulting most often from this virus.

A live-virus rubella vaccine is used to vaccinate young children, which has markedly reduced the incidence of rubella in pregnant women and thus the number of newborns affected by the virus. In addition, newly pregnant mothers are tested for rubella titer during their early prenatal examinations, and those who are not adequately protected are given the rubella vaccine after delivery to protect subsequent pregnancies. The vaccine must not be administered to a pregnant woman, therefore caution must be used when giving the vaccine to adolescent girls and women of childbearing age to determine that they are not pregnant.

Another virus encountered with increasing frequency is herpes simplex virus, hominus type 2. A primary first-episode infection during the first trimester may result in serious congenital anomalies; a recurrence during pregnancy is not as harmful, but if vaginal lesions are present at the time of delivery, a cesarean delivery is necessary to prevent the newborn from a possibly fatal direct exposure to the virus. In addition, babies born to mothers with untreated syphilis may be born with congenital syphilis.

Of increasing concern is the human immunodeficiency virus (HIV), which may be transmitted to the unborn children of infected mothers. HIV-positive infants usually have no major symptoms when born but develop symptoms of acquired immunodeficiency syndrome (AIDS) within the first 24 months of life. At the present time, there is no cure for AIDS, and these children ultimately die from complications of the disease.

Teratogens

As mentioned earlier, the placenta makes possible the transfer of food and oxygen from the mother to the developing child, but the placenta is not selective in the materials transferred. Therefore, many illicit, prescribed, or over-the-counter drugs taken by the mother also reach the fetus and can produce birth defects. Drugs taken by the pregnant woman that are known to disrupt prenatal growth processes are called **teratogens** (from the Latin *terato*, meaning monster, and *genesis*, meaning birth). The effect of a teratogen depends on when it enters the fetal system and in what stages of differentiation the various organs and organ systems are at that time. Generally, the fetus is most vulnerable to teratogens during the first trimester.

Alcohol. During recent years, alcohol consumption has increased among the population in the United States, particularly among those younger than 25 years of age. Use of alcohol has been shown to interfere with pregnancy, causing permanent damage to the fetus. No safe amount of alcohol consumption has been determined because the degree of toxicity is controlled by the ability of the mother's liver to detoxify the alcohol. Ingestion of alcohol during pregnancy may retard fetal growth and produce fetal alcohol syndrome. This syndrome is characterized by a flat facial profile, short eye slits, a smaller brain with mental retardation, poor coordination, and irritability as infants and hyperactivity as children.

Every woman of childbearing age needs to understand the potential damage that her use of alcohol and other drugs may inflict on her unborn child because the most serious damage can occur during the first 4 weeks of life before pregnancy is suspected.

Smoking. A recent Surgeon General's report on smoking and health estimates that one in four pregnant women smokes cigarettes throughout her pregnancy. Smoking during pregnancy has been proved to retard the growth of the fetus, reduce birth weights by an average of 200 g, and double the chance of the baby being low birth weight. The rate of fetal and infant death is 25% to 50% higher among women who smoke during pregnancy than among those who do not. Women who stop smoking cigarettes in the first 3 or 4 months of pregnancy and abstain for the rest of their pregnancy give birth to babies of normal weight, as do women who stop smoking before they become pregnant. Reduction of the amount of smoking, however, has been shown to provide little benefit, if any. Only stopping completely can reverse the risks.[1]

Many organizations provide educational materials that point out the hazards of smoking during pregnancy and help people to quit. Among these groups are the National Foundation of the March of Dimes and the American Lung Association.

Prescription and Over-the-Counter Medications. Studies have shown that certain medications taken by the mother during the first 12 weeks of pregnancy may produce structural changes in the embryo. The thalidomide tragedy of the 1960s focused international attention on this problem. This drug, a sedative and tranquilizer, had been used widely in Germany and other parts of Europe for only a few years when its teratogenic effects became apparent. In Germany alone, more than 4000 children were born with severe malformations of the extremities (phocomelia or amyelia) as well as abnormalities of the face, heart, and viscera.

Bendectin, a drug prescribed in the 1970s and early 1980s for pregnant women who experienced "morning sickness," was also thought to have teratogenic effects and as a result was taken off the market.

Some hormones also may cause fetal abnormalities. Because they are often administered as drugs, in addition to being present in both mother and fetus, the increased supply may cause a harmful imbalance or interaction with other drugs. Diethylstilbestrol is a drug that was given in large doses to many pregnant women from the 1940s through the 1960s to prevent abortion. When the offspring of these women reached young adulthood, the girls experienced increased risk for vaginal cancer and the men experienced infertility caused by sperm changes.

Pharmaceutical companies are required to conduct research on drugs before their approval by the Food and Drug Administration for general use. Drugs are classified by the degree of teratogenic risk; however, new information sometimes reveals that a drug formerly thought safe may have effects not known earlier. The best advice for any pregnant woman is to ask her physician's advice before taking *any* medication, even those she has been accustomed to taking, including aspirin. Caution is the best policy when medications are involved.

Cocaine and Other Illicit Drugs. Cocaine is the number one illicit drug in the United States. With the advent of crack, an inexpensive form of cocaine, drug use has increased among all socioeconomic groups. The resulting increase in infants affected adversely has reached 11%, or 375,000, each year nationwide.[2] This drug use results in many new challenges in the care of infants.

The effects of cocaine on the circulatory system of the mother cause constriction of the uterine blood vessels, thus creating complications, such as first-trimester abortions, premature deliveries, premature placental separation, intrauterine growth retardation (IUGR), and numerous congenital abnormalities.

Other illicit drugs that affect the fetus include heroin, phencyclidine piperidine (PCP), and narcotics, such as meperidine (Demerol). Most of these cause IUGR, passive addiction, and possible neurologic impairment. Although methadone is a prescribed drug (used for treatment of heroin addiction), it also falls into this group of drugs because it is a synthetic drug with many of the same properties as heroin and morphine and affects the fetus adversely.

Radiation. Since the atomic bombs fell on Hiroshima and Nagasaki, Japan, evidence has clearly shown that radiation causes genetic mutation and birth defects. Irradiation of the abdomen of a pregnant woman may arrest embryonic development and cause malformations. Natural background radiation, occupational exposure, and diagnostic or therapeutic procedures are a few sources of irradiation. Because the most sensitive period of organogenesis begins within a week or two after conception, radiographic examination of the abdomen of any woman of childbearing age should be done only during the first 2 weeks after a regular menstrual period.

Mechanical Factors. Moving freely within the fluid of the amniotic sac, the fetus is protected from physical trauma. During the latter part of pregnancy, however, the fetus may be large enough to crowd the uterine cavity, which may result in certain positional abnormalities such as metatarsus varus (clubfoot), torticollis, and dislocation of the hip.

Occasionally, bands of amniotic tissue can constrict fetal limbs and inhibit growth. If the production of amniotic fluid decreases as intrauterine space becomes more limited, malformations of the jaw, asymmetry of the head, and compression marks on the body may result. Although the fetus is safeguarded within the uterus, its protection is not perfect. If the mother suffers severe abdominal trauma, spontaneous abortion, or premature delivery, a disabling injury to the child may result.

Education for Parenthood

Parenthood is probably one of the most difficult tasks anyone can assume because its difficulties are more complex than ever before. Despite our "affluent" society, the United States still has a high infant mortality rate, a large number of mentally retarded infants and children, a continuing breakdown in family structure, many culturally deprived families, increasing neglect or abuse of children, and an increasing number of illegitimate pregnancies. Education for parenthood thus becomes a primary need.

Much of the education for parenthood focuses on prenatal care of the mother and on the mechanics of the birth process. These topics are and should be paramount concerns because they are the foundation from which the child grows. Complete education for parenthood must be an ongoing venture, helping parents cope with children at all stages of development. Nurses are providing more of that education as they assume an increasingly important role in the care of children and families. .

Prenatal Care

As stated earlier, proper prenatal care is the best method to protect the health of the mother and her infant. Ideally, prenatal visits to the physician, nurse midwife, or clinic should begin soon after the woman's last menstrual period. For a normal pregnancy, these visits should be monthly until the 32nd week, every 2 weeks until the 36th week, and weekly thereafter until delivery. Visits may be more frequent in a high-risk pregnancy.

The health care provider in prenatal care has the following goals: to ensure that the pregnancy is proceeding normally, to answer questions and concerns of patient and family, and to teach parenting skills. Continuing care permits diagnosis of any maternal health problems that existed before the pregnancy or that develop during gestation and monitoring of the growth and health of the fetus.

Prenatal Clinics

Those in greatest need of prenatal care and other preparation for parenthood often have the least awareness about the need for or the availability of such services. National attention has been directed toward the importance of locating and assisting women in the high-risk pregnancy group. These are women in particular need of prenatal care because of socioeconomic factors, poor health, history of previous difficulties in childbirth, and lack of knowledge of prenatal development.

Particular attention has been focused on providing adequate prenatal clinics. A prenatal clinic is inadequate if it cannot serve the population for which it is intended. An adequate prenatal clinic should be located in the area where it is needed. The amount of money and time involved in reaching a clinic that is far away discourages early and regular attendance.

A clinic is inadequate if it is too small or deficient in personnel. Women are not encouraged to attend if they have to wait hours for attention that is often routine, impersonal, and inadequate.

Successful clinics need adequately trained personnel representing the various disciplines involved in healthy childbearing. Competent obstetricians and registered nurses are necessary. Nutritionists, social workers, and family counselors should be readily available for consultation. An atmosphere of caring, interest, and support is essential for a successful clinic.

Prepared Childbirth

Pregnancy affects more than the prospective mother; it touches the lives of the father-to-be, other children in the family, grandparents, and other relatives. Although it is often a time of joyous anticipation, pregnancy holds potential problems for everyone involved. "Pregnancy is more than simply a biologic event; it is a time of crisis for those involved, a time when identities are changing and new roles are being explored."[3] Each person reacts in a unique way, based on his or her needs and interpretations of the event.

Preparation for childbirth includes consideration of total family involvement, particularly the "pregnant" father. He should be included in as much of the prenatal activity as possible, especially classes concerning prenatal care and hygiene, fetal development, and the mechanics of birth. These classes are offered by many hospitals and other groups in most communities.

Classes also have been developed specifically for pregnant teenagers, including the birth father whenever possible. Sibling and grandparent classes also are offered by many hospitals. The emphasis of a family-centered experience is the primary concern of most childbirth educators.

Natural Childbirth

Never has more knowledge about pregnancy, labor, and birth been available to prospective parents. Many couples have taken advantage of this information and have come to regard pregnancy and birth as natural rather than pathologic processes. These couples often choose "natural" childbirth, that is, birth unassisted by maternal anesthesia because they are aware that no drug can be considered completely safe for the unborn baby. They attend classes that emphasize the Lamaze or other prepared childbirth methods, including pain control through proper breathing (Figure 4-9). Fathers or other support people learn how to coach the mothers during labor and how to support more effectively the emotional and physical needs of the mother throughout the pregnancy. These classes offer couples the opportunity to share experiences, emotions, and concerns with each other as well as with the instructor. Two of the principal organizations fostering these kinds of prenatal education programs are the International Childbirth Education Association and the American Society for Psychoprophylaxis in Obstetrics.

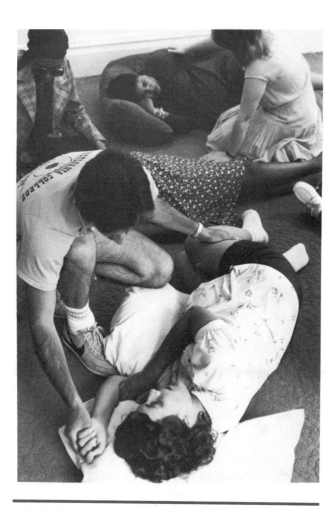

Figure 4-9. Couples practicing various methods of pushing, muscle relaxation, and breathing in preparation for labor. (From May KA, Mahlmeister MR. Comprehensive Maternity Nursing, 2nd ed. Philadelphia: JB Lippincott, 1990, p. 557. Courtesy of John B. Franklin Maternity Hospital, formerly Booth Maternity Center, Philadelphia)

Cesarean Birth

Not all women have the option of natural childbirth or even a vaginal delivery in the traditional delivery room. Certain maternal problems, such as a contracted pelvis, a weak or defective uterine scar, preeclampsia, eclampsia, placental disorders, difficult labor, cephalopelvic disproportion, pelvic tumors, gonorrhea, and herpes type 2 infections, necessitate cesarean delivery (delivery of the infant through a uterine incision). Some of these problems may be apparent early in the pregnancy, and the couple is therefore aware that cesarean delivery is a certainty. This couple has as great a need for educational preparation for their particular birth experience as does the couple planning natural childbirth. Classes for these parents are being offered by most hospitals and often are taught by women who have experienced cesarean delivery.

When cesarean delivery is performed as an emergency procedure owing to fetal or maternal distress, there is little time to psychologically prepare the couple. However, most childbirth preparation classes cover this possibility. In some hospitals, the father may not be permitted in the operating room to witness the birth unless he has attended cesarean birth preparation classes. This policy may lead to feelings of inadequacy and disappointment for the mother and feelings of exclusion for the father. This couple needs postdelivery counseling and reassurance to be sure that they understand and accept the reason for the cesarean delivery.

Summary

Life from conception to birth is a remarkable process. The sex and genetic makeup of the baby-to-be are established at conception. From zygote to embryo to fetus to newborn, the infant is shaped by the interaction of genetic and environmental influences. A healthy infant begins with healthy parents. During the 9 months of gestation, many environmental factors interplay to determine the final outcome. A knowledgeable mother who conscientiously cares for herself during pregnancy increases the probability of producing a healthy newborn. Nurses can play a vital role in helping to educate the mother-to-be. Parenthood is a great responsibility for which couples should begin preparing by attending childbirth classes. Couples may desire to gain control over their birth experience, and health care personnel should listen to their requests. By trying to understand these needs, the nurse can help the couple have an enriching birthing experience.

Review Questions

1. Laurie is the 15-year-old daughter of your cousin. Laurie has just confided to you that she thinks she is

pregnant. What advice would you want to give her first? Why?

2. Laurie's pregnancy has been confirmed. Her knowledge of anatomy and physiology is weak. Starting with conception, what would you teach her about the growth and development of her fetus?

3. Laurie says she hopes the baby is a boy. What response would you give her to help her understand the sex determination of the fetus?

4. What would you want to tell Laurie concerning the impact her age has on the pregnancy?

5. What health teaching would you want to give Laurie concerning nutrition? drugs? smoking?

6. What types of prenatal classes are available in your local hospital? in your community?

7. What recommendation would you make to Laurie concerning prenatal classes?

8. Your 38-year-old neighbor is thinking about having a baby. What can you tell her about the hazards of pregnancy in the woman older than 35 years of age?

References

1. Educator update: It still pays to quit smoking now. Childbirth Instructor 1:6, 1991.
2. Jacques JT, Snyder N. Newborn victims of addiction. RN 4:47, 1991.
3. Colman AD, Colman LL. Pregnancy: The Psychological Experience. New York: Herder and Herder, 1971.

Bibliography

Bobak IM, Jensen MD, Zalar MK. Maternity and Gynecologic Care, 4th ed. St. Louis: CV Mosby, 1989.

Eschleman MM. Introductory Nutrition and Diet Therapy, 2nd ed. Philadelphia: JB Lippincott, 1991.

Martin LL, Reeder SJ. Essentials of Maternity Nursing. Philadelphia: JB Lippincott, 1991.

Pillitteri A. Maternal and Child Health Nursing. Philadelphia: JB Lippincott, 1992.

Schuster C, Ashburn S. The Process of Human Development, 3rd ed. Philadelphia: JB Lippincott, 1992.

Whaley L, Wong D. Nursing Care of Infants and Children, 4th ed. St. Louis: Mosby-Year Book, 1991.

The Normal Newborn

Chapter 5

Student Objectives

Upon completion of this chapter, the student will be able to:

1. Describe how a newborn is assessed at birth for a patent airway.
2. Discuss the circulatory changes that take place at birth.
3. Describe molding of the head, and explain why it occurs.
4. Explain the Apgar scoring system.
5. Identify the reason for eye care at birth, and name three effective medications.
6. Describe the common means of identification of the neonate in the delivery room.
7. List three reasons why the newborn regulates body heat poorly.
8. List four mechanisms of heat loss in the newborn, and give an example of each.
9. State the average weight and length of a newborn.
10. List three advantages and three disadvantages of circumcision.
11. Describe the general appearance of the newborn's a) Head; b) Skin; c) Genitalia.
12. Describe six normal neonatal reflexes.
13. Explain physiologic jaundice (icterus neonatorum).
14. State seven advantages of breastfeeding.
15. Explain the need for vitamin K in the newborn.
16. List two metabolic conditions for which newborns are screened in most states.
17. List four purposes of the newborn bath.

Marks MG: BROADRIBB'S INTRODUCTORY PEDIATRIC
NURSING, 4th ed. © 1994 J.B. Lippincott Company.

Key Terms

acrocyanosis

areola

babinski reflex

bonding

caput succedaneum

cavernous hemangioma

cephalhematoma

circumcision

colostrum

conduction

convection

cradle cap

ductus arteriosus

ductus venosus

en face position

erythema toxicum

evaporation

fontanelle

foramen ovale

forceps marks

gag reflex

lanugo

meconium

milia

mongolian spots

moro reflex

mother–baby nursing

mutual gazing

neonate

palmar grasp reflex

petechiae

phimosis

physiologic jaundice

pseudomenses

pseudostrabimus

radiation

regurgitation

rooting reflex

smegma

startle reflex

step reflex

sucking reflex

suture

tonic neck reflex

vascular nevus

vernix caseosa

*B*irth is hard work for the mother and the baby; therefore, calling it labor is accurate. As the uterus prepares for birth, the infant is slowly squeezed against the bony areas of the mother's pelvis and movement is restricted. Uterine contractions propel the infant down, into, and around through the birth canal with the head serving as a dilator.

The head pushes repeatedly against the mother's perineum before finally emerging.

After 9 months in the warm, dark security of the uterus, the newborn suddenly enters a strange, bright, cooler world. Is it any wonder that a cry is forthcoming? The cry fulfills a biologic need: by the drawing of air into the lungs with the first breath, the breathing process is initiated, which is one big step for the infant toward maintaining life.

Although totally helpless in comparison with other baby mammals, the human infant is physically equipped to survive outside the uterus—to regulate temperature, eat, sleep, and respond to certain stimuli—provided that someone else is ready to meet all the infant's needs.

The newborn is also ready to develop social relationships, usually beginning with the parents. Research has shown that the first hour after birth is critically important to future family relationships. Hospitals and birthing centers have responded to this knowledge and to parents' requests by providing settings in which the father may be fully involved with the birthing experience.

Transition Period

The transition period from intrauterine life to extrauterine existence is a period of instability. During the first 24 hours of life, the infant is highly vulnerable and needs intensive observation because this is the time when many of the physiologic adjustments required for extrauterine life are completed (Table 5-1).

Respiration Begins

Secretions of mucus and amniotic fluid fill the nose and mouth of the newborn. As soon as the head is delivered, the secretions should be suctioned gently with a bulb syringe, first from the mouth and then from the nose (Figure 5-1). After delivery is completed, the **neonate** (the term used to describe a newborn in the first 28 days of life) should be held for a few seconds with the head lower than the body to facilitate drainage.

Failure to breathe within 1 minute after birth is an indication that some method of resuscitation is needed. Complications during labor often may be used as an

Table 5-1. Comparison of Physiologic Changes Between Fetal and Neonatal Life

Area of Change	Fetal Period	Neonatal Period
Environmental	Warm, stable, watery, fluid absorber of shock. Stable temperature, twilight lighting. Minimal sensory stimulations	Bright, noisy, dry atmosphere; temperature changes, much sensory stimulation
Circulatory	Ductus venosus—arterialized blood from umbilical vein goes to inferior vena cava	Ductus venosus becomes occluded and is known as the *ligamentum venosum*. Anatomic closure completed at end of 2 months
	Ductus arteriosus—blood from right ventricle bypasses lung into descending aorta	Ductus arteriosus becomes occluded, is known as *ligamentum arteriosum*. Functional closure within 3–4 days; anatomic closure completed by 3 weeks
	Foramen ovale—permits major portion of oxygenated blood entering the heart to go directly from the right atrium to the left atrium, left ventricle, and out the ascending aorta	Foramen ovale closes, but closure is reversible for several days. Pulmonary circulation increases and more blood is returned from the lung to the left atrium
Umbilical blood supply	Oxygenated blood travels to fetus by way of the umbilical vein—returns to placenta via the umbilical arteries	Placenta circulation ceases when cord is tied. Umbilical vein becomes obliterated
Blood composition	High numbers of red blood cells and high hemoglobin level necessary to provide adequate oxygenation in utero	Decrease in red blood cells and hemoglobin levels during first day of life
Respiratory	Respiratory movements begin during 4th month of fetal life. Amniotic fluid moves in and out of lungs as result of these movements. Lungs are collapsed, oxygenation via placental circulation	Lungs start to expand at first breath, full expansion takes several days. Placental oxygenation ceases with severance of umbilical cord
Neurologic	Fetus responds to stimulation as a whole. Neurologic activity seen at about 8 weeks' gestation; isolated muscular reactions seen in response to stimulation. By 9 weeks, swimming motions and some spontaneous movements are present. By 13–14 weeks, movement may be perceptible to mother	Infant responds to stimulation by certain discrete reflexes, such as rooting, plantar, and moro reflexes

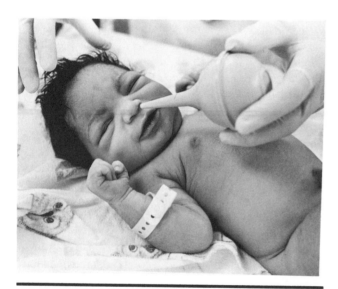

Figure 5-1. A bulb syringe is used to suction mucus from the newborn's nose and mouth. (From May KA, Mahlmeister LR. Comprehensive Maternity Nursing, 2nd ed. Philadelphia: JB Lippincott, 1993, p. 971. Photo: Kathy Sloane)

indicator of possible respiratory problems at birth. Signs of respiratory distress include delayed respiration or irregular, gasping breath, sternal retractions, and cyanosis. Fetal distress; meconium-stained amniotic fluid; maternal medical complications, such as diabetes, hypertension, and cesarean birth; prematurity; and postmaturity all contribute to the potential for respiratory complications.

In the event of airway obstruction after secretions are cleared from the nose and mouth, gentle stimulation, such as rubbing the infant's back, may be helpful. If further measures are required, suctioning may be necessary.

When respirations are delayed or depressed, the use of an Ambu bag may be helpful (Figure 5-2). Measures used for the relief of serious respiratory problems are intubation, oxygen, and mouth-to-mouth resuscitation. These measures require the serious attention of the physician, the anesthesiologist, and the obstetric team. Infants manifesting severe distress are transferred to the neonatal intensive care unit (NICU).

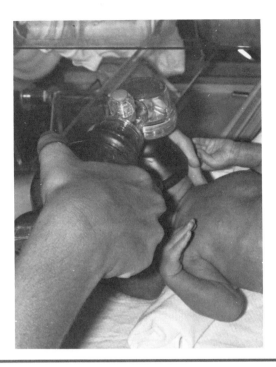

Figure 5-2. Use of Ambu-bag portable resuscitator may be necessary when respirations are delayed or depressed. (From Oehler JM. Family-Centered Neonatal Nursing Care. Philadelphia: JB Lippincott, 1981.)

Circulation Changes

During fetal life, the lungs are inactive, requiring only a small amount of blood to nourish their tissues. Blood is circulated through the umbilical arteries to the placenta, where waste products and carbon dioxide are exchanged for nutrients. The blood then is returned to the fetus through the umbilical vein.

At birth, the umbilical cord is cut and the infant establishes an independent system. Certain fetal circulatory bypasses, such as the ductus arteriosus, the foramen ovale, and the ductus venosus, are no longer necessary after birth. They close and atrophy gradually through the first weeks of life (Figure 5-3).

The **foramen ovale** (an opening between the right and left atria) closes with the first breath, but the closure is reversible for the first few days of life, with fusion of tissue taking 6 to 8 weeks. The **ductus arteriosus** (the prenatal blood vessel between the pulmonary artery and the aorta) closes functionally within 3 or 4 days, but the **ductus venosus** (the prenatal blood vessel between the umbilical vein and the inferior vena cava) does not achieve complete closure until the end of the second month of life.

The cord stump is examined immediately after being cut to determine the presence of one vein and two arteries. If only one artery is present, the newborn needs to be further examined for congenital defects of the internal organs.

Care in the Delivery Room

The first few minutes of life are a critical period in which the immediate needs of establishing and maintaining an open airway and keeping the newborn warm take priority. The newborn's condition is assessed by means of Apgar scoring at 1 and 5 minutes of life. Identification of the newborn and eye care also are completed within these first hours of birth.

Apgar Score

Within 1 minute after birth, and again at 5 minutes, the general condition of all infants should be assessed according to the Apgar scoring method introduced by the physician Virginia Apgar in 1958 (Table 5-2). The infant is given a score of 0, 1, or 2 for each of five specific signs: heart rate, respiratory rate, muscle tone, reflex irritability, and color. A score of 10 indicates that the infant is in the best possible condition. A score of 7 to 10 is considered good and usually requires no special treatment. A score of 4 to 6 indicates a moderately depressed neonate who needs close observation. A score lower than 4 indicates the need for immediate attention and treatment as well as careful and continuous observation in the NICU.

This score is documented in the infant's chart for immediate availability as a reliable index of the condition at birth and as an important guide for subsequent care.

Cord Care

The umbilical cord is clamped shortly after birth. The cord is clamped with two clamps, then it is cut between the two clamps. Some physicians and nurse midwives encourage the father to perform this cutting in order to involve the father in the birth process and to enhance the symbolism of freeing the newborn from the uterus and accepting responsibility for the infant's care. The end attached to the infant is clamped with a cord clamp or tied; the maternal clamp is then released. The cord appears to contain no nerve endings; neither the mother nor the infant show any discomfort when it is cut. The stump is left without a dressing and should be inspected daily. The cord stump may be treated with an antiseptic agent, which also may encourage drying of the stump. The cord stump is usually dry enough in 24 hours that the clamp may be removed. The cord stump is inspected daily, and alcohol is applied several times daily until the stump falls off.

Eye Care

Prophylactic eye treatment against gonococcal ophthalmia neonatorum is mandatory in the United States. Because gonorrhea in a woman may be asymptomatic, this disease was once a frequent cause of neonatal blindness,

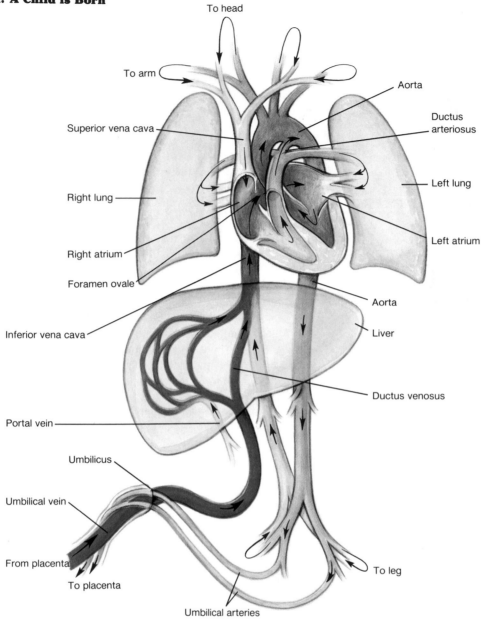

Figure 5-3. Fetal circulation. (From Pillitteri A. Maternal and Child Health Nursing. Philadelphia: JB Lippincott, 1992.)

infecting the infant during passage through the birth canal of the infected mother.

The drugs approved for instillation into the eyes of the neonate are 1% silver nitrate solution, erythromycin 0.5% ophthalmic ointment in single-use tubes, or tetracycline 1% ointment. Erythromycin is believed to be more effective against *Chlamydia* infections, therefore many hospitals have switched to using it. Another advantage of the ointment is that it does not cause the chemical conjunctivitis that is common with silver nitrate solution. However, silver nitrate is a more economical method of treatment.

Because of the sensitive parent–infant attachment, or **bonding**, period during the early hours after birth, some authorities recommend waiting 1 hour before instilling eye medication. Some state health codes, however, require instillation "immediately" after birth. Additional studies are needed to provide more conclusive evidence on the need for immediate treatment versus the value of uninterrupted bonding during the first hour of life.

Before the eyedrops are instilled, the infant's eyelids should be cleansed with sterile cotton moistened in sterile water. A separate pledget should be used for each eye, sponging from the nose outward until all blood or mucus is removed.

Next, the infant's eyes should be opened, one at a

Table 5-2. Apgar Scoring Chart

Sign	0	1	2	1 min	5 min
Heart rate (beats/min)	Absent	<100	>100	—	—
Respiratory rate (breaths/min)	Absent	Slow, irregular	Good, crying	—	—
Muscle tone	Limp	Some flexion of extremities	Active motion	—	—
Reflex irritability					
Response to catheter in nostril	No response	Grimace	Cough or sneeze	—	—
or					
Slap to sole of foot	No response	Grimace	Cry and withdrawal of foot	—	—
Color	Blue, pale	Body pink, extremities blue	Completely pink	—	—

Developed by Dr. Virginia Apgar.

time, using gentle pressure on the upper and lower lids. One or two drops of solution or 1/4-inch ointment should be dropped into each eye onto the conjunctival sac, never onto the cornea. If silver nitrate is used, the eyelids are held open for 30 to 60 seconds to allow the solution to flow from the inner to the outer aspect of the eye.

Formerly, the practice was to flush the eyes with sterile water or sterile saline solution following the instillation of silver nitrate. This practice has been discontinued in many hospitals because studies showed that the rinse did not reduce conjunctival irritation and may have diluted the effectiveness of the prophylactic eyedrops. Parents should be warned that eye irritation may occur in the next 24 hours, with swelling and drainage, if silver nitrate is used.

Identification

Before the infant is transferred from the delivery room or the birthing room, identification bracelets with identical numbers are placed on the mother's wrist and the baby's wrist and ankle. In some hospitals, handprints or footprints are also taken and become part of the infant's chart, sometimes with the addition of the mother's right index fingerprint.

Prevention of Heat Loss

From a stable intrauterine temperature of 37°C (98.6°F), the wet neonate emerges into a world almost 30°F cooler. With an immature temperature-regulating system, a proportionately large body surface area relative to weight, a larger surface area for size than an adult's, and just a thin layer of subcutaneous fat, the neonate is subject to heat loss at birth. Unable to regulate body temperature by shivering, the neonate exposed to cool air kicks and cries, thereby increasing the metabolic rate and oxygen consumption, which may lead to metabolic acidosis. Conversely, in an overheated environment, the newborn has

difficulty dispersing heat and may suffer from hyperthermia.

Newborns may lose heat through four processes: evaporation, radiation, conduction, and convection. **Evaporation** is heat loss through conversion of a liquid to a vapor. To prevent the rapid loss of heat from evaporation of the amniotic fluid, it is imperative that the infant be dried rapidly and gently with a warm towel and placed into a warm environment. In settings where skin-to-skin contact between the infant and the mother is encouraged, an overhead radiant warmer may be used to reduce heat loss. Some hospitals and birthing rooms use stockinette caps on neonates because so much heat is lost through the neonate's wet head. If the infant is not placed skin-to-skin with the mother, a soft, warm blanket is used to wrap the newborn, who is either given to the mother to hold or placed in a warm crib or infant warmer.

Heat loss through **radiation** is the transfer of body heat to cooler solid objects that are not in direct contact with the infant. The temperature of the surrounding air has no effect on heat loss through radiation; therefore, the infant should not be examined until he or she is moved as far as possible from the walls of the delivery room, which tend to be colder than the air.

Conduction heat loss occurs when the neonate's skin is in direct contact with a cooler solid object. To avoid this, the infant should be placed on a padded surface and should be insulated with clothes and blankets.

Convection heat loss is similar to conduction but is increased by moving air currents. Transporting the infant in a crib with solid sides reduces convection heat loss.

Observation and Documentation

During this critical transitional period, close observation of the infant is essential. In addition to the Apgar score, the nurse records the exact time of birth, the skin condition, the quality of the infant's cry, the presence of any congenital anomalies or evidence of birth injuries, and the type of forceps (if any) used to extract the infant. Weight and length of the infant are noted before transfer from the delivery room or immediately on admission to the nursery. The first urination and defecation must be noted and recorded; usually this happens after transfer to the nursery or the mother's room. Failure to urinate during the first 24 hours or to defecate during the first 36 hours may indicate a serious problem.

Physiologic Characteristics of the Newborn

Approximately 95% of newborn infants born at term weigh between 2.5 to 4.6 kg (5½ to 10 lb) and measure 45 to 55 cm (18 to 23 inches) in length. Normal head circumference measures about 33 to 35 cm (12 to 14 inches). Crown-to-rump measurements average 31 to 35 cm and are about equal to the head circumference.

Head and Skull

The six bones of the newborn's skull are not united but can mold and overlap to permit the large head to pass through the birth canal. These bones are divided by narrow bands of connective tissue called **sutures**. At the juncture of these bones are small spaces called **fontanelles**. At birth, the two palpable fontanelles, or soft spots, are the anterior fontanelle at the juncture of the frontal and parietal bones and the posterior fontanelle at the juncture of the parietal and occipital bones (Figure 5-4).

During delivery, the head had molded along the suture lines and may appear to be asymmetric or elongated (Figure 5-5). Usually, normal shape is assumed after a few days. The sections of the bony skull calcify and join during the first months of life. The posterior (triangle-shaped) fontanelle closes in about 1½ to 3 months of

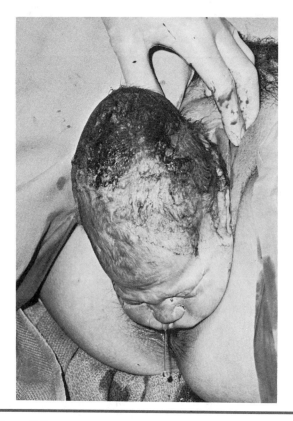

Figure 5-5. The head of this newborn is elongated owing to the pressure applied by forceps.

life; the anterior fontanelle (diamond-shaped) closes between 12 and 18 months.

The brain is covered with a tough membrane, making it difficult to injure the child's head through the fontanelles by ordinary handling. Mothers need to be reassured that the baby's scalp may be washed with soap and water (*not* baby oil) over these areas without harm, and ordinary cleansing may be helpful to prevent cradle cap (seborrheic dermatitis). **Cradle cap** is an accumulation

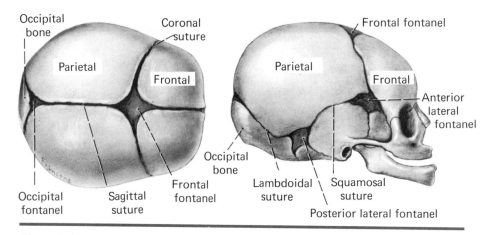

Figure 5-4. Infant skull showing fontanelles and cranial sutures.

of oil, serum, and dirt that often forms on an infant's scalp.

Chest

The chest of the newborn has a smaller circumference than the head. The breasts of both male and female newborns may be engorged as a result of maternal estrogens in the bloodstream, and a pale, milky fluid called witches' milk may be secreted. This condition disappears within 4 to 6 weeks. Meanwhile, the breasts should be handled gently and not manipulated in any way.

Bony Structure

The arms and legs of the newborn are short in comparison with the trunk. Prenatal development proceeds in a cephalocaudal (head-to-toe) progression and in a proximal (nearest to center) to distal (remote) sequence (Figure 5-6). This process means that the head and trunk are well developed, but the distal areas (arms, hands, legs, and feet) develop later. Development always proceeds from the general to the specific, the gross muscle control coming before fine muscle control.

Body Temperature

At delivery, the infant's body temperature is generally the same as the mother's but drops rapidly after entering the cooler environment. As mentioned earlier, a warm, stable

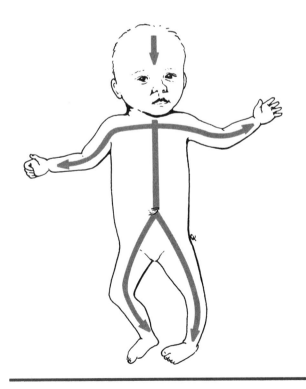

Figure 5-6. **Arrows** indicate the cephalocaudal and proximodistal progress of infant development.

environment is necessary until the neonate has adjusted to independent living. In the delivery room, the infant is usually wrapped in a warm blanket or placed in a heated crib. Body temperature varies after birth according to the environment, with a range of 36.4° to 37°C (97.5° to 98.6°F), owing to the immature nervous system. It usually stabilizes in a few days. Normal newborn axillary temperature, after stabilization, varies between 36° and 37.2°C (96.8° and 99°F).

The newborn's temperature may be taken by rectum, axilla, or tympanic membrane. In most newborn nurseries, the first temperature is taken rectally to determine the patency of the anal opening. There may be a shallow opening in the anus, however, with the rectum ending in a blind pouch. In this instance, the ability to insert a thermometer into the rectum does not signify a patent rectum. When a temperature is measured rectally, care must be taken to insert the thermometer only just beyond the bulb of the thermometer. Axillary and tympanic temperatures are obtained following the procedure outlined in Chapter 3.

Respiratory System

The first and most important task of the neonate is the oxygenation of the red blood cells, which occurs with the first cry. Although respiratory movements appear in fetal life, there is no *functional* respiration before birth. Breathing in the healthy newborn is quiet and shallow, but variations in rate and rhythm are normal. In normal infants, the rate may vary from 20 to 100 breaths per minute, according to whether the infant is sleeping or awake, crying, lying passively, or vigorously moving the arms and legs. Because the rate fluctuates rapidly, the respirations should be counted for 1 full minute. The overall rate for the period of 1 minute is usually 30 to 50 breaths per minute. Persistent rates higher than 60 or less than 30 breaths per minute should be called to the physician's attention because they may indicate cardiac or pulmonary difficulty. Sternal retractions are considered abnormal and also should be reported.

The newborn infant's breathing is diaphragmatic–abdominal, therefore respirations may be counted most easily by watching the rise and fall of the abdomen rather than the chest. Parents should be informed of this characteristic to prevent any alarm about what may seem to them to be abnormal breathing.

Circulatory System

The changes that occur in the circulatory system at birth are primarily due to oxygenating the blood through the pulmonary system and to discarding the placenta, umbilical vein, and arteries. Shortly after birth, the blood flows through the infant's circulatory system in the same manner as that of an adult. **Acrocyanosis** (cyanosis of the hands and feet) is common and occurs because of the immature peripheral circulatory system. When the infant cries, however, the skin color becomes rosy red.

At birth, the infant's heart rate may reach 180 beats per minute, then decrease to 100 to 120 beats per minute. Usually by the second day of life, the pulse varies between 90 and 160 beats per minute, depending on whether the infant is asleep or awake and active. Blood pressure is difficult to measure in the newborn unless it is taken with specialized equipment using ultrasonography, such as a Doppler and an oscillometer. An initial blood pressure measurement should be taken, however, to provide a baseline and serve to alert the staff to any cardiac problems.

Gastrointestinal Tract

The gastrointestinal tract is functional at birth, and meconium usually is passed within 8 to 24 hours. **Meconium** is a sticky, greenish black substance composed of bile, mucus, cellular waste, intestinal secretions, fat, hair, and other materials swallowed during fetal life, together with amniotic fluid. The time of the first stool should be noted and recorded to confirm anal patency. If no stool is passed during the first 24 hours after birth, the physician should be notified because some obstruction may exist in the intestinal tract.

The neonate is able to digest the fat, protein, and carbohydrates in breast milk or in a modified formula. **Regurgitation**, spitting up of small quantities of milk, occurs rather easily in the young infant and is different from vomiting. It may be caused by an air bubble in the infant's stomach, too rapid nursing, or overfeeding.

Vomiting is differentiated from regurgitation in that there is an expulsion of an appreciable amount of fluid. Although this also may result from rapid feeding or inadequate burping, frequent or persistent vomiting may signal an abnormal condition and should be reported to the physician.

The neonate hiccups easily; this is most likely caused by feeding too rapidly. However, hiccupping does occur in fetal life. Burping the infant to bring up swallowed air or nursing for another minute usually controls the hiccups. In any instance, they eventually stop without treatment.

Genitourinary Tract

The kidneys secrete urine before birth, and some urine collects in the bladder after birth. A record of the first urination is important to confirm adequate kidney function and the absence of severe constrictions somewhere in the urinary system.

The male testes are usually descended into the scrotum at birth, but occasionally one or both are in the process of descending or remain in the abdomen. These testes usually descend spontaneously during the first year of life.

The prepuce of the penis in the male newborn child is normally tight. **Phimosis**, or adherence of the foreskin to the glans penis, is normal in early infancy. Forceful retraction should not be attempted. The foreskin usually becomes retractable by 3 years of age. If minor irritations develop, cleansing with soap and water is all that is needed. One danger of forceful retraction of the foreskin during early infancy is that the elastic fibers at the tip of the foreskin may tear and bleed. The result will be that the foreskin heals by scarring, perhaps making circumcision necessary later.

In 1975, the American Academy of Pediatrics opposed the routine **circumcision** of the newborn, stating that there is no sound medical reason for the procedure and that good personal hygiene is adequate without surgical risk. The Academy changed its position in 1989, stating that circumcision for the newborn has potential medical advantages and benefits as well as disadvantages and risks. Parents should be thoroughly informed by the physician about both the risks and benefits of the procedure (Table 5-3). Circumcision of the newborn male is performed frequently for religious reasons, most notably by those of Jewish faith. Circumcision does prevent the ac-

Table 5-3. Advantages and Disadvantages of Neonatal Circumcision

Advantages	*Disadvantages*

Prevention of
    Penile cancer
    Inflammation of glans and prepuce
    Complications of later circumcision
	Complications of
	    Hemorrhage
	    Infection
	    Dehiscence

Possible decrease of
    Urinary tract infections in males
    Sexually transmitted disease
	Meatitis from loss of protective foreskin
	Adhesions
	Concealed penis
	Urethral fistula

Preserves male body image
    To be same as circumcised father
        or peers when older
	Meatal stenosis
	
	Pain at time of procedure

cumulation of the secretions collectively called **smegma**. If the foreskin of the newborn male is so tight that it obstructs the urinary system, circumcision is performed at once.

In the female neonate, the labia are prominent owing to the effect of the mother's estrogens during intrauterine life. The infant may have a slight red-tinged vaginal discharge called **pseudomenses**, which results from a decline in the hormonal level compared with the higher concentration in the maternal hormone environment. Unless the mother understands why this happens, she may become alarmed. She should be told that although it does not appear in all newborn female infants, it is a natural manifestation resulting from hormonal transfer and it will disappear in a few days. It should be particularly emphasized that this discharge is not due to any trauma or infection.

Nervous System: Reflexes

The neonate exhibits a number of normal reflexes triggered by an immature nervous system. Research findings indicate that infants follow their reflexes for the first 3 months of life. For example, all newborns smile, even if they are blind, and all infants tightly grasp objects placed in their palms. Most of the reflexes disappear during the first year of life. Infants should be tested for the most common ones because their absence may indicate a disturbance in the nervous system.

The **rooting reflex**, present at birth, is seen when the cheek is stroked and the infant responds by turning the head toward the side that was stroked. Thus, when the mother or the nurse places a hand on the infant's cheek to turn the head toward the breast, the infant turns instead toward the person's hand.

The **sucking reflex** is so well developed at birth that personnel in the delivery room are often startled by the loud sucking noises coming from the newborn's crib.

Present at birth, the **gag reflex** continues throughout life. Any stimulation of the posterior pharynx by food, suction, or passage of a tube causes gagging.

Pressure on the palms of the hands or soles of the feet near the base of the digits causes flexion of hands and toes. The **palmar grasp reflex** is so strong in a healthy infant that the infant can be lifted off the examining table (Figure 5-7). The palmar grasp reflex diminishes after 3 months; the plantar grasp reflex persists until 9 to 12 months of age.

When the lateral plantar surface is stroked, the toes flare open. Called the **Babinski** (or plantar) **reflex**, this reaction usually disappears by the end of the first year. Until 6 weeks of age, most normal infants, when held in an upright position, make stepping movements (Figure 5-8). This movement is called the **step**, or dance, **reflex**.

Any sudden jarring or abrupt change in equilibrium

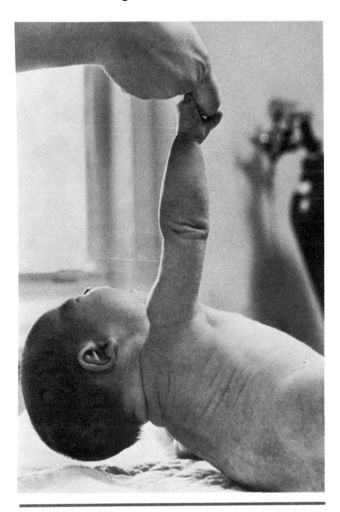

Figure 5-7. Grasp reflex present in all normal newborns is sufficiently strong to lift them from the examining table. (Courtesy of Mead Johnson Laboratories, Evansville, IN.)

elicits the **Moro reflex** in the normal newborn. It consists primarily of abduction and extension of the arms. All digits extend except the index finger and the thumb, which are flexed to form a C-shape (Figure 5-9). If the response is not immediate, bilateral, and symmetric, possible injury to the brachial plexus, the humerus, or the clavicle may be present. Persistence of this reflex after 6 months of age may indicate brain damage.

Similar to the Moro reflex, the **startle reflex** follows any loud noise and consists of abduction of the arms and flexion of the elbows. Unlike in the Moro reflex, the hands remain clenched. Absence of this reflex may indicate hearing impairment.

Not always apparent during the first weeks of life, the **tonic neck reflex**, also called the **fencing reflex**, may be observed when the infant lies on the back, with the head turned to one side, the arm and leg on the same side extended, and the opposite arm flexed as if in a fencing position (Figure 5-10). Usually, this reflex disappears between 3 and 4 months of age.

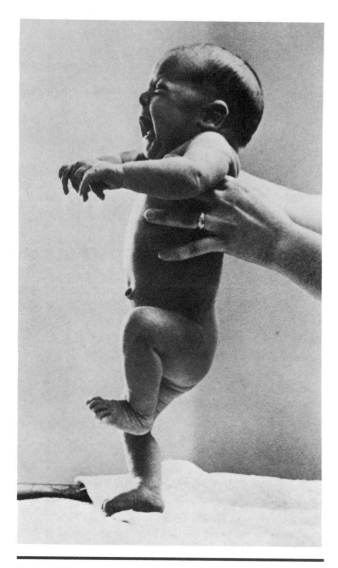

Figure 5-8. Step, or dance, reflex simulates walking when infant is held so that the sole of the foot touches examining table. (Courtesy of Mead Johnson Laboratories, Evansville, IN.)

Special Senses

Sight

Research has shown that the unborn baby is able to distinguish light from dark and at birth can see. The rod cells in the retina of the eyes, which are responsible for light perception, are functional at birth; but the retina, the newborn's special organ of visual perception, is not fully developed until about 16 weeks of age. The neonate's head turns toward a light, and the neonate blinks and closes his or her eyes at a bright light. The infant follows a bright moving object momentarily, but fixation of coordination comes much later. The nerves and muscles that control focusing and coordination are not completely developed until the sixth month, accounting for the cross-eyed look called **pseudostrabismus** that babies sporadically show. Parents have no cause for alarm if their infant's eyes are not coordinated in their movements occasionally, but if lack of focusing remains at 4 months, the baby's pediatrician should be alerted.

Most dark-skinned infants have brown eyes at birth, whereas most light-skinned newborn's eyes are slate gray or dark blue. Tears are produced constantly at birth but are completely disposed of through the nasolacrimal duct until about 2 or 3 months of age, when tear production increases.

Newborns have approximately 20/500 vision as compared with a normal-seeing adult's vision of 20/20. This means that most distant objects appear very fuzzy. Close vision is much better, and the infant can see most of the features of a human face clearly at a distance of 7 to 15 inches (17.78 to 38.10 cm). This is one reason why the **en face position** (the caregiver and the infant establish eye contact in the same vertical plane) is so important to parent–infant attachment during the period immediately after birth.

Hearing

A newborn stops crying momentarily at the sound of a soothing voice and is startled and cries at a loud noise. Immediately after birth, the infant can distinguish the mother's voice from that of a male physician. The sense of hearing certainly contributes to the infant's emotional reactions to fear and to comforting. It is not known exactly how early the infant hears soft voices and other faint sounds, but infants 2 or 3 days old stop crying momentarily when talked to soothingly.

Smell

The sense of smell is not highly developed at birth, but research has shown that the newborn infant does turn toward the mother's breast because of the smell of breast milk. Neonates can differentiate the smell of their mothers' breast milk from that of other females. Strong smells also bring about reaction, and a newborn turns away from smells such as vinegar and alcohol.

Taste

Because much of taste depends on the sense of smell, it is likely that the infant's sense of taste is not highly developed at birth. Some studies have shown, however, that breathing, sucking, and swallowing patterns are different when infants are fed formula than when they are fed breast milk. In addition, neonates have produced the expected reaction of distaste for sour or bitter solutions and pleasure at a sweet solution. They definitely prefer glucose and water more than unflavored (sterile) water.

Touch

Sensitivity to touch is present from birth, particularly in the lips and tongue. The sense of pain is also present at birth; but, like adults, infants vary in their sensitivity to pain. Newborns react to painful pinpricks. Sensitivity

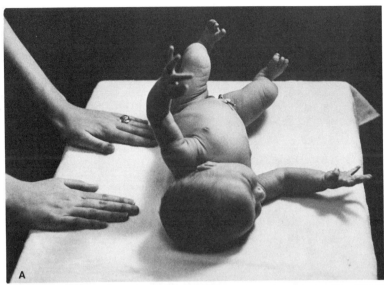

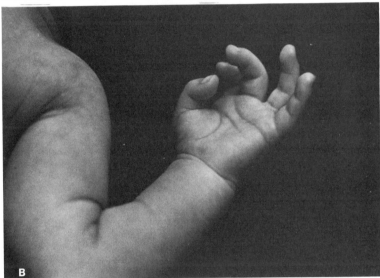

Figure 5-9. Moro reflex is elicited by sudden jarring or change in equilibrium. **A,** Arms abduct at the shoulder and extend at the elbow. **B,** All digits extend except the index finger and the thumb, which curve into a C-shape. (Courtesy of Mead Johnson Laboratories, Evansville, IN.)

appears to increase during the first few days of life as part of individual development. The infant cries lustily when suffering gastrointestinal discomfort.

Skin

Normal Appearance

Sluggish peripheral circulation and vasomotor instability are manifested in the deep red color the infant acquires when crying as well as in the pale hands and feet of many newborns. The skin is usually red to dark pink in white newborns. African American newborns have reddish brown skin, and Hispanic infants have an olive or yellowish tint to the skin. The skin should feel elastic when picked up between the examiner's fingers.

Fine, downy hair, called **lanugo**, covers the skin of the fetus. It is usually not present in a full-term infant but may be seen on an infant born prematurely.

A greasy, cheeselike substance called **vernix caseosa** protects the skin during fetal life. Vernix caseosa is an oil and water mixture containing cells flaked from the skin and fatty substances secreted by the sebaceous glands. At birth, vernix may cover the skin or remain only in the folds of the skin. In most hospitals, not all of the vernix is removed with the first bath, but it is left on as a protective agent. It eventually is absorbed or rubs off.

Skin Blemishes

A variety of temporary skin blemishes may be found on newborns. One of the most common of these is a **vascular nevus**, known as a "strawberry mark." A **nevus** is defined as a circumscribed new growth of the skin of congenital origin; it may be either vascular or nonvascular. The strawberry mark is a slightly raised, bright-red collection of blood vessels that does not blanch completely on pressure. It may be present at birth or may

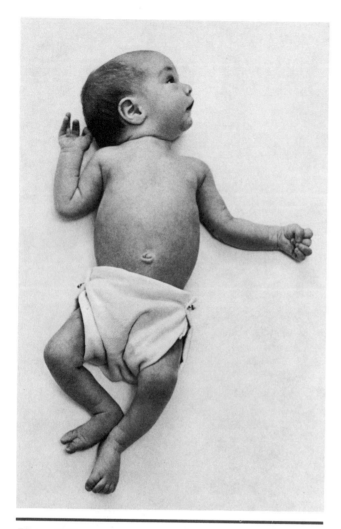

Figure 5-10. Tonic neck reflex is present when the infant lies on his or her back with the head turned to one side, with the arm and leg on the same side extended and the arm on the opposite side flexed. (Courtesy of Mead Johnson Laboratories, Evansville, IN.)

appear during the first 6 months of life. This blemish may enlarge during the first 6 months of life, but eventually when it ceases to grow, fibrosis replaces the capillaries and the lesion shrinks. Treatment is not usually indicated because most of these marks regress and disappear by 10 years of age. If the lesion is so large as to cause emotional trauma in the child, the physician may suggest removal of the blemish.

Erythema toxicum (fine rash of the newborn) may appear over the trunk, back, abdomen, and buttocks. It appears in about 24 hours and disappears in several days. It is not infectious and does not need treatment.

Vascular nevi sometimes are present in **cavernous hemangiomas**, subcutaneous collections of blood vessels with bluish, overlying skin. Although these lesions are benign tumors, they may become so large and extensive as to interfere with the functions of the body part on

which they appear. Small hemangiomas called "stork bites" often are seen on the eyelids or back of the neck. They disappear within 6 to 12 months without treatment.

In infants of African, Mediterranean, Native American, or Asian descent, **mongolian spots** (areas of bluish black pigmentation) resembling bruises may be seen most often over the sacral or gluteal region. They usually fade within a year or two.

Milia are pearly white cysts appearing on the faces of about 40% of newborn infants. They are usually retention cysts of sebaceous glands or hair follicles and disappear in a few weeks without treatment.

Petechiae are small, bluish purple spots caused by tiny broken capillaries. These spots may be seen on the face as a result of the excess pressure on the head when the delivery has been rapid or difficult. They disappear in a day or so.

Forceps marks may be noticeable on the infant's face if the delivery was assisted with the use of forceps. These marks ordinarily disappear in a day or two. After a difficult delivery, bruises and edema may be present on the head or scalp, or if a breech delivery, on the buttocks and the genitalia. Although these gradually clear up without treatment, such bruises may be distressing to the parents, who may not understand the relative insignificance of these marks. The nurse may carefully and simply explain that they are minor bruises and will fade quickly. Occasionally, the infant's head is misshapen by its passage through the birth canal. The mother is naturally distressed and needs to know that this is temporary, owing to the ability of the head to accommodate to the narrow passage. The head acquires a normal rounded shape in a few days.

Caput succedaneum is an edematous swelling of the soft tissues of the scalp caused by prolonged pressure of the occiput against the cervix during labor and delivery. The edema disappears in a few days.

Cephalhematoma is a collection of blood between the periosteum and the skull (Figure 5-11). The swelling of the overlying scalp usually is not visible until several hours after birth. This swelling also may frighten the mother, who may think some injury has occurred. The edema of caput succedaneum may spread across the scalp, but the swelling of cephalhematoma is contained within the suture lines because it is contained by the periosteum and cannot cross suture lines. Most cephalhematomas are reabsorbed within 2 weeks to 3 months, depending on their size. Because the only serious complication may be the introduction of infection, aspiration, incision, or any other treatment is contraindicated.

Physiologic jaundice (icterus neonatorum) occurs in a large number of newborn infants, has no medical significance, and is believed to be the result of the breakdown of fetal red blood cells. It must, however, be carefully observed and reported in an effort to distinguish it from a serious jaundice condition. A simple heel stick

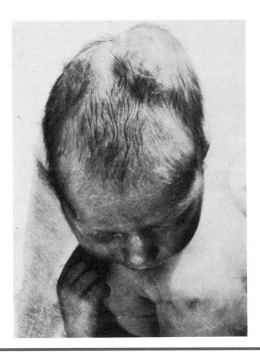

Figure 5-11. Cephalhematoma of left parietal hemisphere.

may be done by the nursing staff to perform a micro-bilirubin examination in the nursery. This study may confirm or disprove that the newborn's bilirubin level is elevated. Physiologic jaundice, with yellowing of the skin, does not appear until after the second day of life, which may be after the newborn goes home with the family. *Family caregivers should be advised to report to the physician any jaundice appearing during the first 3 days.*

Newborn-Parent Behavior

Newborn Activity

The healthy newborn, if placed face down, lifts or turns his or her head to one side to clear the airway. The infant exercises in uncoordinated, random movements, involving the entire body in the activity. The muscles are taut, and it is difficult to manually extend the extremities. The infant momentarily ceases activity at the sound of a nearby voice.

The newborn may sneeze to clear the nasal passages, yawn, hiccup, stretch, blink, and cough. The fetus learned to suck and swallow in intrauterine life.

The infant's only way of expressing tension from hunger, cold, pain, or other discomfort is by crying. Prompt comforting and attention to the infant's needs usually will restore composure and alleviate the discomfort. It is often with these first moments of comforting and soothing that the parent-child attachment process begins.

Mother-Infant Interaction

Even though infant and mother have been physically inseparable for 9 months, their emotional togetherness and the beginning of mutual love and attachment start after delivery, ideally in the first few hours. Many babies are alert for a short time after delivery, offering a good opportunity for sensory contact with the mother.

Pioneering research by Klaus and Kennell indicates that early attachment activities have a significant effect on the long-term parent-child relationship.[1] This conclusion does not mean that early attachment guarantees a satisfactory lifetime relationship or that lack of opportunity for early attachment threatens seriously the family's chances for a strong relationship. It simply indicates that the family relationship is given the best possible start if the mother, the father, and the infant may be together during this early sensitive period in their new life as a family.

Touch is a highly significant part of the attachment process. Many hospitals and birthing rooms offer the opportunity for skin-to-skin contact between the mother and the infant (and sometimes the father and the infant). Shortly after delivery, the nude infant may be placed on the mother's abdomen and chest and held to the mother's breast if the mother plans to breastfeed (Figure 5-12). Touching provides warmth, comfort, and a sense of security, all vital needs of the vulnerable newborn.

Studies have shown that the mother is likely to follow a predictable pattern of touching her new baby, first using only the fingertips to touch the extremities, then gradually moving her fingers over the infant's entire body, and finally using her entire hand to massage the trunk of the body. Next, she tries to reposition herself and the baby in

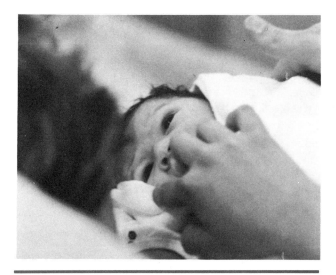

Figure 5-12. Touch is important in the attachment process. (Photo: BABES, Inc.) (From May MA, Mahlmeister LR. Comprehensive Maternity Nursing. Philadelphia: JB Lippincott, 1990, p. 974.)

the en face position. This is also referred to as **mutual gazing**.

The attachment process is affected by many factors, among them the mother's physical and emotional condition after labor, the infant's condition and behavior, the comparison of the real infant with the "fantasy" infant that the mother has imagined since she became aware of her pregnancy. The mother who had a difficult labor or heavy sedation may not be alert enough to participate effectively. If the infant has a problem that requires immediate transfer to the special care nursery or NICU, there will be no time for early attachment.

Every woman during her pregnancy imagines what her baby will look like, how he or she will act, what the child will eventually accomplish, and how she and others in the family will be affected by this new person. This imaginary baby is likely different from the real infant she meets soon after delivery.

At first sight, the infant seldom presents the chubby, well-formed baby pictured by the world in general. The head is large in proportion to the body and may be misshapen by the process of being born. Blood and vernix still cling to body, and the neonate probably is crying. Is this the baby the mother has dreamed about and planned for? The newborn may appear completely self-centered, displeased over this abrupt introduction to the world. Such a first impression may summon feelings of guilt in the mother that she does not feel the expected gush of love and tenderness. If the baby is quiet and passive and she had imagined an awake, alert, active child, she may be disappointed, giving less attention and stimulation than she would to an infant who more closely resembles the imagined child. It is important that both parents understand that each infant is unique, with individual characteristics and developmental potential. Studies have shown that pointing out to parents their child's unique characteristics may help develop a more positive attitude, reduce feeding and sleeping problems, and bring about greater activity and alertness in the infant. One widely used guide for assessing neonatal activity is the Brazelton Neonatal Behavioral Assessment Scale (Figure 5-13). Special training is necessary to use the test. The Brazelton criteria also helps the parents to "tune in" to their baby and learn more about this budding personality and the how their responses affect their adjustment to each other.

Father–Infant Interaction

Fathers who are involved during the pregnancy, delivery, and postpartum period develop an attachment as strong as the mother's attachment.[2]

The father's attachment behavior is similar to that of the mother: touching; holding the infant in the en face position; observing the beauty of the child, particularly any features that resemble the father; and expressing feelings of elation and satisfaction (Figure 5-14). Many

---

BRAZELTON SCALE CRITERIA

1. Response decrement to light
2. Response decrement to rattle
3. Response decrement to bell
4. Response decrement to pinprick
5. Orientation response—inanimate visual
6. Orientation response—inanimate auditory
7. Orientation—animate visual
8. Orientation—animate auditory
9. Orientation—animate-visual and auditory
10. Alertness
11. General tonus
12. Motor maturity
13. Pull-to-sit
14. Cuddliness
15. Defensive movements
16. Consolability with intervention
17. Peak of excitement
18. Rapidity of buildup
19. Irritability (to aversive stimuli: uncover, undress, pull-to-sit, prone, pinprick, TNR, Moro, defensive reaction)
20. Activity
21. Tremulousness
22. Amount of startle during exam
23. Lability of skin color
24. Lability of states
25. Self-quieting activity
26. Hand to mouth facility
27. Smiles

Figure 5-13. Brazelton Neonatal Behavioral Assessment Scale. (From Clinics in Developmental Medicine 50, England, Spastics International Publications, 1974.)

fathers indicate that they want to share the responsibility of raising the baby.

Some cultures dictate that men not show emotion; thus, some fathers may need encouragement to express their feelings about their infant. Nurses should reinforce any positive attachment behavior displayed by either parent and should show, whenever necessary, the soothing effect of cuddling, stroking, rocking, and talking to the baby.

Care in the Hospital Nursery or the Mother's Room

After a careful assessment of the newborn has been made and the family has had time together, the infant is transferred either to the newborn nursery or to the mother's room. Many maternity units have a receiving or recovery nursery in which the infant is cared for and carefully watched for the first hours of life. Other units may set

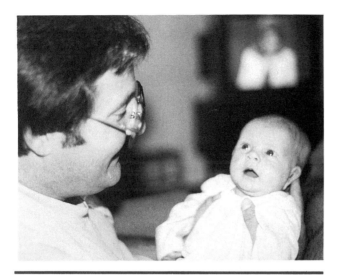

Figure 5-14. Attachment: father and newborn communicating. (From Castiglia PT, Harbin RE. Child Health Care: Process and Practice. Philadelphia: JB Lippincott, 1992, p. 185.)

aside a portion of the general newborn nursery as a receiving area.

Prematurely born infants are transferred to a premature unit or a NICU. In the NICU, infants with serious congenital anomalies or birth defects also receive special care. Infants of diabetic mothers may be placed in the specialized unit because they need to be carefully observed, even though they are generally large for gestational age. Often, newborns with serious problems who are born in smaller hospitals or birthing centers may need to be transferred to a tertiary hospital where they can receive intensive specialized care.

Every maternity unit must have a means available to segregate infants who have been exposed to any sort of infection before, during, or after birth. Infants born outside the hospital or infants born to mothers whose membranes were ruptured longer than 24 hours are kept in segregation to protect the other newborns in the nursery.

Mother–Baby Nursing

One of the options that many hospitals offer their mothers is **mother–baby nursing**. In mother–baby nursing, postpartum and nursery nurses are cross-educated, so that one nurse takes care of both the mother and the infant. After the infant's condition has stabilized, the infant's bassinet is kept beside the mother, who participates in caring for her newborn while being carefully guided and taught by their nurse. Some hospitals have individual labor-delivery-recovery-postpartum (LDRP) suites into which the mother is initially admitted. Labor and delivery take place in this suite, and the mother and infant stay here for the entire hospitalization. Nurses who staff these units are completely cross-educated; that is, they are educated and skilled in providing nursing care through-

out labor, delivery, recovery, and postpartum periods, including care of the newborn. The LDRP suite approach and mother–baby nursing offer many of the following advantages that were found desirable with rooming in:

1. It provides maximum opportunity for maternal–infant interaction while the mother and the newborn are still in the care of maternity personnel.
2. It fosters infant feeding on a permissive (demand) schedule.
3. It offers a fine opportunity to teach the mother, father, or other support persons about infant care and gives supervised experience in caring for the infant.
4. It provides an opportunity for sibling and grandparent visiting in privacy.
5. It reduces the incidence of cross-infection.

Admission to the Nursery

On admission, the infant's identification is verified, the Apgar score is reported, the cord stump is inspected, and the delivery room record is reviewed. The infant is placed on his or her side in a bassinet or isolette to facilitate mucus drainage from the nose and the mouth. In many hospitals, vitamin K is administered at this time to prevent hemorrhage and promote clotting, if it has not been administered in the delivery room. The neonate usually is unable to produce adequate vitamin K because the intestine of the newborn is sterile and the flora needed to help produce vitamin K in the body are not available. Vitamin K is administered intramuscularly in the vastus lateralis. By the second week of life, after the infant has ingested food and normal flora is produced, the infant manufactures sufficient vitamin K.

Until the newborn is given his or her first bath, the nurse must wear gloves for protection from blood and body fluids during any contact with the neonate. The infant's temperature is taken, the vital signs are assessed, and then the infant is allowed to rest. Bathing, weighing, and dressing may be postponed until the infant's condition and temperature are stabilized. However, close observations are made, and vital signs are assessed at 15- to 30-minute intervals (Figure 5-15). The nursery temperature should be approximately 24°C (75°F), and the humidity should be lower than 50%. The neonate is bundled to maintain body heat and, if necessary, additional external heat may be used in the form of heat lamps or warmers. When stable, the infant may be weighed, sponge bathed, and dressed.

Routine Nursing Care

Newborns are highly susceptible to infection. Newborns, removed from the protection of the uterus, have not developed any defenses against disease; therefore, particular

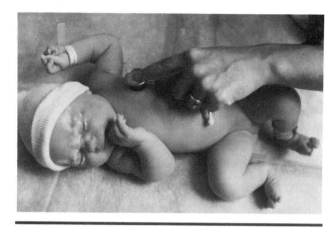

Figure 5-15. Heart sound, rate, and rhythm are evaluated periodically after admission to the nursery. (From May KA, Mahlmeister LR, Comprehensive Maternity Nursing, 2nd ed. Philadelphia: JB Lippincott, 1990.)

attention to hygiene is essential when the infant is handled. Except for weighing, all care, including bathing, examinations, and taking temperatures, is given inside the bassinet. The nursery scale should be covered with a disposable liner or paper towel that is discarded after each infant is weighed. The scale is sprayed or wiped with a germicidal, fungicidal solution and freshly covered before the next infant is put on the scale.

Handwashing

Undoubtedly, the most important of all precautions is that of handwashing before handling any infant. This principle applies to all nurses, physicians, laboratory personnel, parents, or anyone handling a newborn.

Before entering the nursery, remove any wristwatches, rings, and bracelets. After entering the handwashing area, clean under the fingernails with an orangewood stick. Wash the hands with disposable sponge brushes under running water, using an antiseptic preparation. Wash between the fingers, the palms, the backs of the hands, and the wrists and arms up to the elbows with a circular motions for 3 minutes. Rinse and dry with a paper towel. Turn the faucet off with a paper towel. Between handling babies, wash thoroughly for 30 seconds. In most obstetric units, attendants must wear scrub gowns or suits.

Anyone suffering from any respiratory condition, intestinal upset, skin rash or cuts, elevated temperature, or any sign of illness should not enter the nursery or participate in the care of the infants.

Mothers should be taught to use a thorough handwashing technique after toileting and before handling her baby. Fathers, siblings, grandparents, or other visitors who are in the room when the baby is in the mother's room should put on long-sleeved gowns over their clothing. An area where these persons may wash, with appropriate brushes, antiseptic solution, and paper towels as well as clean gowns, should be available in the room. Directions for handwashing and putting on gowns should be displayed prominently in a clearly visible place.

Bathing

Daily sponge baths are given using warm water and, if needed, a bland soap. As with all infants, cleansing proceeds from the head downward. If the scalp needs cleansing, it should be washed with water and soap and then rinsed with a washcloth, taking care not to get water in the infant's eyes.

A mild soap may be used in cleansing the infant. Some nurseries prefer to use "dry" skin care, in which only the head, face, and body folds are cleansed with cotton balls moistened with sterile water, leaving the remainder of the skin untouched unless it is very dirty. The diaper area is cleansed after each bowel movement. In some nurseries, complete sponge baths are given every other day instead of daily.

An antiseptic is applied to the stump of the cord each day. Inspection of the stump for infection should be performed daily while the infant is undressed. The stump may be painted with an antiseptic or cleansed several times a day with 70% alcohol to prevent infection and promote drying. The stump is exposed to the air to allow it to dry. The diaper should be turned down and the shirt turned up so that the cord is not closely covered.

If the infant has been circumcised, the penis should be checked for bleeding. Sterile gauze with sterile petroleum jelly may be applied to the area. The mother may be taught to apply Vaseline or other recommended ointment to the surgical site with each diaper change for about 2 weeks until healing is complete. Retraction of the foreskin in the uncircumcised infant should not be attempted because phimosis is normal in the newborn.

Temperature

The infant is weighed once daily in most nurseries, although some physicians prefer that it be done every other day. At this time, the infant's temperature is taken by the axillary method (Figure 5-16). The thermometer is placed in the center of the armpit, taking care to have skin on skin, with no clothing in the way. The arm and the thermometer should be held securely in place while the temperature is being taken. Electronic tympanic thermometers have been used recently with success. Usually, only the initial temperature is taken rectally because of the danger of irritation to or puncturing of the rectal mucosa.

Phenylketonuria Testing

Laboratory screening for phenylketonuria (PKU) is mandatory in most states for all newborn infants. A simple procedure is used in which the heel is pricked and three drops of blood are placed on filter paper, which is all that is necessary.

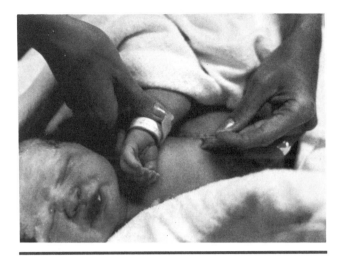

Figure 5-16. Taking axillary temperature in the newborn. (From May MA, Mahlmeister LR. Comprehensive Maternity Nursing. Philadelphia: JB Lippincott, 1990, p. 934.)

PKU testing is essential to prevent the mental retardation that may occur owing to a congenital lack of an enzyme necessary for the metabolism of phenylalanine, an essential amino acid. Once detected, this disorder may be completely corrected by dietary regulation. See Chapter 7 for further discussion.

Newborn Feeding

Feeding time is an occasion that provides stimulation and builds confidence. The infant makes eye-to-eye contact with the mother and touches her, while the mother looks, touches, explores, and talks to the infant. The infant learns to trust through repeated touch, fondling, and warm physical comfort. The infant's response to her comforting care gives the mother a sense of satisfaction and confidence. Eventually, when the infant learns that signals of need are answered promptly, the infant is able to wait after crying for the response. The infant should not be made to wait too long because the newly developed sense of trust is fragile if it is not reinforced soon.

At one time, mothers were told, "Put the baby on a feeding schedule and never deviate from it. When the baby cries, check to see if there is anything disturbing him or her; then put him or her down and let him or her cry." Unfortunately, the infant did not know about being trained to conform to a schedule. The baby knew only that hunger demanded satisfaction. The infant's discomfort and sense of aloneness needed comfort and reassurance. Routine did nothing to satisfy needs, but it did potentially shake the infant's trust and belief that the world was a safe and caring place. Attitudes have changed, and infants are now fed primarily on a demand schedule. While in the hospital, the formula-fed newborns are basically fed on a

4-hour schedule, but this may be adjusted by the mother when the infant is taken home. Both breast-fed and formula-fed infants have a need to suck. Sometimes this need is not satisfied by feeding. Pacifiers may be given to the infant to help satisfy this need. This decision depends on the attitudes of the parents, but often the use of pacifiers is considered more desirable than having the infant sucking his or her fingers or thumb. Families should be alerted to the danger in the use of makeshift pacifiers. Pacifiers constructed from nipples and plastic collars from infant formula bottles are dangerous. Deaths of infants have occurred from the aspiration of such nipples. Only commercial pacifiers should be used.

The nurse should inform the mother that a weight loss of 5% to 10% in the infant normally occurs during the first few days of life. This loss is to be expected and should be regained within about 2 weeks.

Breastfeeding

Breastfeeding is the ideal form of infant nutrition. Whether to breastfeed or formula feed, however, is the decision of the mother or the couple, unless there is a valid reason against either method. Many mothers will have already decided during pregnancy, often consulting with her mate, family, or other persons with whom she can review the advantages and possible disadvantages of breastfeeding (Table 5-4).

When breastfeeding is chosen, the infant is usually put to the breast shortly after birth in the delivery or birthing room. The infant's sucking promotes early secretion of milk, is a source of security and comfort to the infant and a satisfaction to the mother, and is a stimulant of uterine contractions. During this time, the infant is often placed skin-to-skin with the mother, enhancing the bonding process.

Nursing on demand seems to work best for most infants. The mother should be instructed to expect to nurse every 2 to 3 hours for the first few days. The nursing should be limited to 5 minutes on each breast. The time may be increased gradually until the infant nurses 10 to 15 minutes on the first breast (to empty it) and as the infant desires on the second.

The mother must wash her hands before each feeding. If this is the mother's first child, she will need help and support when she first attempts to nurse her infant. At first it is usually easier for the mother to nurse while lying flat with a pillow under her head and cradling the infant's head. The nurse may instruct the mother to turn to one side, place her nipple between her index and third finger, and bring it toward the infant's mouth. As she brushes her nipple near the newborn's lips, the baby will actively seek it (Figure 5-17).

A considerable portion of the **areola** (the darkened area around the nipple) should be drawn into the infant's mouth because this stimulates the mammary glands and

Table 5-4. Advantages and Disadvantages of Breastfeeding

Advantages	*Disadvantages*
1. Nutritionally best for baby	1. Mother may be sensitive to nursing when others are around
2. Provides protection against allergies	2. Neonatal jaundice may occur from inadequate fluid intake
3. Provides antibodies against illness	3. Mother needs to watch what medications she takes
4. Helps to develop a special bond between mother and infant	4. Mother needs to be careful about diet, limiting caffeine intake and other foods that may upset the infant
5. Promotes **involution of uterus** (return of uterus to its prepregnant state)	5. Mother cannot take oral contraceptive
6. Easily digested	6. Mother's nipples may become sore and cracked
7. Convenient, always ready, inexpensive, sterile	7. Breastfeeding makes demands on mother's time
8. Correct temperature	
9. Provides times for mother to rest while nursing	
10. Mother gains a sense of accomplishment and satisfaction	
11. Obesity is infrequent in breast-fed children	

helps prevent sore nipples. If the mother's breasts are large and soft, the infant's nose may be obstructed by pressing against the breast while trying to nurse. The mother may be shown how to press her breast away from the infant's nose with her finger so that breathing is comfortable (Figure 5-18). The mother may find that she prefers sitting in bed with a pillow support for her arm or in a chair with arms at a comfortable level (many hospitals provide comfortable rocking chairs for this purpose). The infant is held in a position lying entirely on the side facing the mother, with the mother's nipple directly in front of the infant's mouth.

Nearly all mothers experience some discomfort when the infant is first put to the breast. The nurse may reassure the mother that this discomfort is normal and does not last. For the first 2 or 3 days, the mother's breasts secrete **colostrum**, a yellowish, watery fluid, which has a higher protein, vitamin A, and mineral content, and a lower fat and carbohydrate content than breast milk. It also contains antibodies that may play a part in the immune mechanism of the newborn child. Its laxative effect helps promote evacuation of meconium from the infant's bowel.

Until lactation begins, both breasts should be used at each feeding to stimulate secretion of milk. Later, when the breasts are full, one breast is generally sufficient at a feeding. A reminder of which breast to use each time may be needed, such as a safety pin on the brassiere strap of the side to be used next. It is important that a breast be emptied at one feeding to stimulate refilling. Many physicians do not want the infants to have any supplemental

feedings during this initial period, so that the infant will be hungry and nurse vigorously to stimulate the production of the mother's milk.

Whether the infant is breast or formula fed, some air is swallowed during nursing, and the infant needs burping to help expel the swallowed air. After feeding, the infant may be held up on mother's shoulder, sat upright on her lap with the head supported, or laid face down across the mother's lap while she gently rubs the infant's back in any of these positions. Some infants who nurse eagerly may need more than one burping during a feeding.

The mother who wishes to have support for breastfeeding after leaving the hospital may appreciate a referral to the LaLeche League, if she has not already had contact with them. The LaLeche League is a national organization dedicated to helping breastfeeding mothers have a successful experience. Most hospitals have names of local members who are happy to consult with new mothers.

Formula Feeding

If the mother does not breastfeed her infant, for whatever reason, she still may provide all the necessary nutrients through a formula. She also may furnish the same comfort and security as she holds the infant (Figure 5-19). The mother should be warned of the problems created by "propping" the bottle. This practice deprives the infant of the comfort and security of being held and may cause aspiration if the infant is left unattended. Infants who

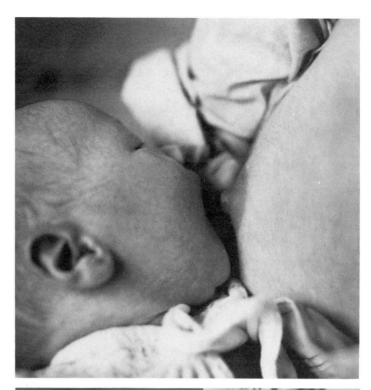

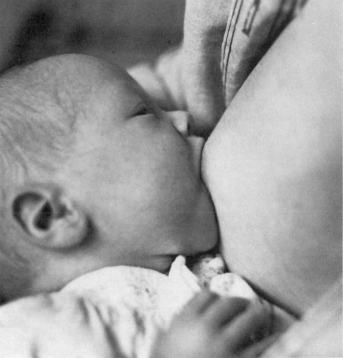

Figure 5-17. When offered a nipple, the newborn responds immediately and vigorously owing to the rooting and sucking reflexes. (Photo by Imaginique Productions; Waechter EH, Blake FG. Nursing Care of Children, 9th ed. Philadelphia: JB Lippincott, 1976.)

nurse from propped bottles become more prone to develop middle ear infections as a result of formula pooling in the infant's mouth and pharynx and thereby providing a medium for bacterial growth.

Formula may be purchased already prepared in individual bottles, but this can be quite expensive. More economical formulas are prepared from dry powder or cans of formula that may be mixed with water. Water to be

used to mix the formula should be boiled. The person preparing the formula must wash his or her hands before starting the preparation. All equipment to be used must be washed and rinsed thoroughly. Disposable bottles are available but add to the cost of infant feeding. The best plan is to prepare one bottle at a time and use it immediately. Formula may be given to the infant at room temperature but may be warmed, if desired. Bottles should

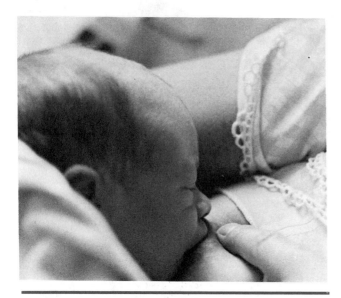

Figure 5-18. The mother presses her breast away from the infant's nose to enable more comfortable breathing while feeding. (Photo by Marcia Lieberman.) (From Waechter EH, Blake FG. Nursing Care of Children, 9th ed. Philadelphia: JB Lippincott, 1976.)

never be warmed in a microwave oven because of the danger of burns from bottles that may explode or from formula that is too hot. Formula remaining in the bottle should not be saved from one feeding to the next because of the risk of bacterial growth. Open cans of formula may be covered and refrigerated until the next feeding.

The bottle-fed infant should be burped after every ½ to 1 oz they consume. The newborn takes approximately 2 oz at each feeding. After the feeding, the infant should be positioned on the right side to minimize regurgitation and allow air that was swallowed to rise above the level of fluid and escape. The feeding should take about 15 to 20 minutes. If the bottle is tilted so that formula fills the nipple, the amount of air swallowed is reduced. The new mother should be encouraged to find a comfortable position with arm support when preparing to feed the infant. Her comfort transfers to the infant and makes the feeding time more pleasant for both of them. The father or other support person should be encouraged to help with feeding. They need the same support and instructions that the mother requires.

Teaching the New Parent

Nurses have a major responsibility for patient teaching, so it is of the utmost importance that they are well-informed. Most new parents are eager to learn all they can about their new roles. Many realize suddenly that they have taken on a tremendous task: that of raising a healthy, well-adjusted child. Although many may have attended paren-

tal classes, the situation has changed from a theoretical study to serious business.

Some mothers and fathers who have older children feel comfortable in their ability to care for a new infant. Others may want a review to update on infant care. Some parents have definite ideas about how they want to care for their infants, so nurses should be objective in the way they present information. Information and instruction should be made available to all the infant's prospective caretakers, if possible.

The most effective teaching often occurs on an individual basis when the nurse and the mother and father or support person are together with the infant. In addition to determining how much the parent already knows, the nurse needs to know what anxieties the family has and perhaps any misunderstandings and misinformation that need to be corrected. Mother–baby nursing is ideal for this, offering both parents (or mother and support person) a chance to care for the infant under the guidance of the nurse.

Short stays have created additional problems in finding time to teach infant care. Audiovisual materials, such as slide-tape programs and videocassettes, are being used in many hospitals. Often the videocassette programs are set up on an in-hospital television channel or on separate patient teaching carts (equipped with a videocassette recorder and monitor) that the patient may view in her own room with other members of her support system. Care must be taken to follow up these programs with an opportunity to encourage questions to clarify any misunderstandings. The nurse must be familiar with these materials so that questions can be handled effectively. In

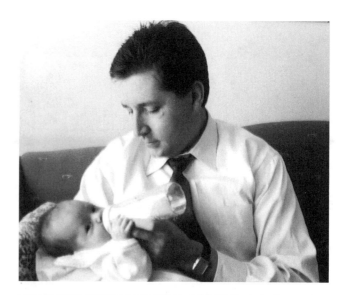

Figure 5-19. Formula-fed babies need the warmth and closeness of the mother or other caregiver. (From Jackson DB, Saunders RB. Child Health Nursing. Philadelphia: JB Lippincott, 1993, p. 228.)

addition, the mother and support person (particularly with a first baby) need to observe a newborn bath and bathe the infant under the supervision and guidance of the nurse, if at all possible, within the time constraints of short hospitalizations. Written materials are also widely used. The nurse must be particularly careful in assuming that all patients are able to read and understand these materials. Reading abilities and language differences of a family may create difficulties about which the nurse must be sensitive so that the infant care information is made clear to all (see the Parent Teaching displays on Skin Rashes—Points to Cover; Infections—Points to Cover; Stools—Points to Cover; Newborn Bath; and Sponge Bath).

Family Adjustment

The family is reshaped each time an infant is born because every member of that family is affected by the presence of this new person. By the same token, the family shapes the child. Those who are parents for the first time probably have the greatest anxieties because they have totally new roles to learn. Early research on parent–infant attachment studied the "mothering" aspect of the relationship; more recent studies of neonatal behavior indicate that the infant has a definite role in the attachment process. Fathers also have been the subject of increasing research, all of which has aided the understanding of how relationships are formed, the factors that help or hinder the process, and how to avoid potential problems. However, although early contact has been carefully studied, no definite conclusions have been reached, and parents and families should not be made to feel that all is lost if early bonding does not take place for one reason or another.

The Parent's Adjustment

Regardless of how much preparation the mother has had for her new role, it is still a totally new experience. She is prepared to love her child, but the fact remains that she has a new child who needs total care 24 hours a day. It looms as a terrific responsibility.

She perhaps has expected that a surge of motherly love instinctively will enable her to love and care for her baby without any doubt or trouble. This does not happen on the first day, or even after a week, but it does develop over time. If she has had a previous child, she may find that this child does not "measure up" in the same way that the previous child did. This reaction may contribute to feelings of guilt and self-doubt. When she feels inadequate, exhausted, and discouraged—as many people do when confronted with a new and seemingly overwhelming responsibility—she is likely to feel resentment, followed by feelings of guilt over actually resenting the new baby. Although she loves the baby, no one has prepared her for the normal resentment that the respon-

Parent Teaching

Skin Rashes—Points to Cover

1. The infant may break out with heat rash when dressed too warmly. Dress infant with only light covering or diapers only.

2. Disposable diapers may cause some infants to develop a rash from the plastic in them. Observe infant for rash if using disposable diapers. Switching brands may sometimes help, but if the rash persists, cloth diapers may be necessary.

3. Cloth diapers may also cause a rash. Keep the infant as dry as possible. If cloth diapers are used, care must be taken to close the safety pins when removed and to insert them into the diaper with points outward.

4. Good laundry practices are important.
   a. Wash baby's clothing separate from the rest of your laundry. Use a mild soap, rinse well, twice if possible.
   b. Avoid use of softeners or strong detergents on baby's clothes.
   c. White vinegar ($2/3$ cup) may be added to the final wash rinse as a fabric softener. It softens the clothes without leaving an odor.

5. If the infant develops a diaper rash, keep dry and expose to air, if possible. Urine irritates diaper rash. A soothing ointment (such as A&D or lanolin) may be used to protect the skin. If the rash persists, notify the physician, who may order a special ointment.

6. Dry skin may be soothed with an soothing ointment. This may be bought over-the-counter in stores.

sibility of total care for a helpless, demanding infant often brings.

Rather than trying to deny her resentment and what she considers as unworthy feelings, the mother needs help to admit them and, furthermore, to understand that resentment is a normal reaction. She needs to understand that as she grows into her task and as she and her child begin to adjust to each other, resentment and feelings of inadequacy will fade away. Those who can learn to admit that they are normal women with a right to normal emotions have come a long way toward reaching equilibrium.

Another way to help is to find some way in which the mother may be relieved of some of the burden until her strength rises to the occasion. The father or other support person may be helpful by giving her some relief from care responsibilities each day and encouraging the mother to rest or get out of the house for a short period. If there are older children, she needs to have some time to spend with

Parent Teaching

Infections—Points to Cover

1. One way infants get infectious diseases is through handling by other people. Be careful who handles the baby. No one with any type of infection should visit. Avoid taking the baby into crowded places for the first month or so. Newborns have low resistance to disease.

2. If you think your infant is getting sick, note symptoms. Take the temperature and call the baby's physician.

3. Check with the baby's physician before giving any medications to be certain of the type and amount of medicine to use.

4. Handwashing carried out by anyone who is going to handle the infant is one of the most important ways to avoid infections.

5. Anything that is going into the infant's mouth should be washed before being given to the child.

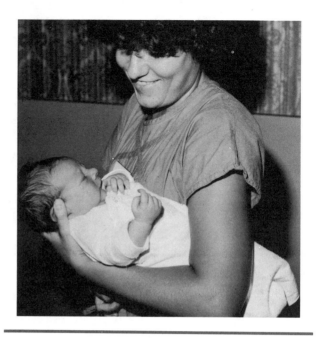

Figure 5-20. The football hold is only one correct method of holding the newborn. (From Martin L, Reeder SJ. Maternity Nursing, 17th ed. Philadelphia: JB Lippincott, 1991.)

them, perhaps while the newborn is sleeping, but she still needs time completely for herself.

Even a father who loves his new baby very much may feel left out and neglected when the mother and the baby come home and all her time and attention seem to be devoted to the baby. He may resent the fact that she seems

Parent Teaching

Stools—Points to Cover

1. Breastfed infants—average 2–4 stools a day, with a range of 1 to 7 for the first few months. Occasionally, an infant may have one movement every few days and still be comfortable and normal. After breastfeeding is established, the stool will be yellow to golden with a consistency of liquid paste and an odor described as that of sour milk.

2. Bottle-fed infants—average 1–4 stools per day. An infant may have more or less and still be normal. The color of the stool may range from pale yellow to light brown, and the consistency may be firmer and more solid than breast-fed stools.

3. When solid food is added, stools tend to become darker, firmer, and stronger in odor.

4. Constipation is rare. Consistency, not frequency, is the sign of constipation. If the stool is hard or dry and difficult for the infant to pass, constipation is present. Notify the physician for treatment.

exhausted, unless he understands just how much effort it takes to care for a helpless infant. This is especially true of the first-time father. Like the mother, he needs to be encouraged to admit his feelings because they are normal reactions to the situation. He also needs to be encouraged to give the mother a break or to help arrange for someone to come in to give her a break. If they can find a family member or other person who will relieve them for short periods regularly, they should plan to take advantage of this and do something together, even if it is only to take a walk. These little "breathers" can do much to "refresh the spirit."

The Infant's Adjustment

Each infant uniquely affects and reacts to the family environment. The infant's primary developmental task, according to Erikson, is to develop a sense of trust. After 9 months of security, the infant has been thrust into a world in which needs must be made known, with no assurance that they will be met. At birth, the infant embarked in a strange country where the language, customs, and rules are unknown. Now another move (to home) occurs, and the difference is noticeable. The infant is sensitive to attitudes that alter the touch or the tone of voice of the caretakers. Likewise, the caretakers are affected by the infant's reactions and characteristics. The infant needs reassurance that this is a friendly world. Throughout the process, the nurse must be aware of the variety of life situations into which the infant is born and must adjust teaching and nursing care appropriately.

Parent Teaching

Newborn Bath

Purposes of the Bath Procedure

1. The bath removes waste products from the infant's skin and removes odors.
2. This is a time when the bathgiver has the opportunity to inspect the infant's body carefully and note any changes such as rashes, discolorations, and abnormal movements of the extremities.
3. The infant has the opportunity to kick and exercise.
4. This is a time to be alone with the infant and become acquainted. It is also a time for the baby to begin to feel more secure. Talking, cooing, cuddling, and stroking are an important part of the bath procedure. The more the bathgiver can relax and enjoy the infant, the happier the time will be for both of them.

Some Topics Most Often Covered in a Bath Demonstration

1. *Picking up and holding a young baby*. Slide an arm under the baby up toward the head; with hand under head, lift the infant up. One comfortable method of holding a baby is the *football hold*, in which the infant's head rests in the palm of the holder's hand, and the body lies along the inside of the holder's arm, with the infant resting on the holder's hip (Figure 5-20).
2. *Types of baths appropriate for the young baby*. Until the cord stump falls off and the navel is healed, the baby should have sponge baths only because the cord stump should be kept as dry as possible. Many parents like to give their baby a daily bath, but it is not really necessary. Every other day is adequate. On the nonbathing day, wipe off the baby's face with water and a clean cloth, and cleanse the diaper area at each change.
3. *Use of baby powders and lotions*. Generally, use of baby powders and lotions is discouraged, because they can irritate the infant's skin. They should be used only after consultation with the infant's physician.
4. *Temperature taking*. During the bath the nurse can demonstrate how to take the infant's temperature and how to read the thermometer. The mother should practice reading the thermometer. The nurse should make clear that the infant's temperature needs to be taken only when the infant is ill in order to be able to report it to the physician. When the temperature is to be taken rectally, lubricate the bulb end of the rectal thermometer. With the infant in a dorsal recumbent position, grasp the ankles in one hand and raise the legs toward the head with knees bent outward. This will expose the rectum so that the end of the thermometer can slip in easily. The thermometer should not be inserted more than 2 cm (0.8 inch). Continue to hold the infant's legs and the thermometer for about 3 minutes if a mercury thermometer is used. Normal rectal temperature for a neonate is 37° to 37.8°C (98.6° to 100°F).
5. *Use of bulb syringe*. Some hospitals provide bulb syringes for each newborn for use in clearing the nares and mouth of excess mucus. This is a good time to teach the use of the bulb syringe.
6. *Cord care and circumcision care in circumcised males*. These topics are appropriate to discuss even if the circumcision care has already been covered. New families can be quite anxious about taking care of these two "wounds" as they heal.
7. *Cradle cap*. After the infant's face is washed, the scalp should be washed. The nurse can point out the "soft spot" and reassure that it is not easily injured. The importance of regular shampooing to prevent cradle cap should be stressed. The hair can be combed at the end of the bath.
8. *Positioning of infant*. This is a good time to explain the importance of positioning the infant on either side or on the back but not on the abdomen. This is recommended until the infant is older than 6 months of age as a measure to prevent sudden infant death syndrome.
9. *Good hygiene measures*. Anyone who is going to handle the infant should wash their hands and arms well before touching the baby. Anyone with any type of infection should be discouraged from visiting.

Parent Teaching

Sponge Bath

Assemble the necessary articles on the bathing table. Any sturdy table covered with a clean cloth can be used. Articles needed are the following:

Basin of warm water, warm to the elbow, 37.8° to 40.6°C (100° to 105°F). It is preferable that the basin be used for this purpose only.

Cake of mild, unscented soap to be used only if needed.

Soft washcloth; towel for drying baby; large soft towel or cotton blanket on table on which to lay baby.

Alcohol—70% (rubbing)

Cotton balls

Comb and/or brush

Ointment such as A&D for dry skin

Clean clothes for baby

Procedure

Have everything ready before picking up the baby. *Never* leave the baby on the table unattended: small infants can easily roll off the table; keep one hand on the infant at all times. Place the baby on the blanket or towel and wash the face with clear water. If eyes have been draining, sponge them with a clean piece of cotton, wiping from the inner canthus outward and using clean cotton for each eye. Wash the outer folds of the ears and behind them, but do not poke in the infant's ear because serious harm can be done.

Remember, "Nothing smaller than your elbow in the ear."

If the infant has a nasal discharge, wash the edge of his or her nostrils with cotton but do not poke in his or her nose. To dislodge dried mucus that is just inside the nostril, cleanse with a small piece of cotton dipped in water. This will usually make the infant sneeze and dislodge any mucus lodged further up in the nose.

Pick up the baby and hold like a football. Wet the head, lather well with soap and rinse well and dry. Combing the hair gently with a fine-tooth comb helps to loosen and rid the scalp of debris that could cause cradle cap if not removed. *Do not* use shampoo until the infant is 1 month old.

Undress the baby. Cleanse the diaper area with clean wet cloth if the diaper is soiled. Always clean from front to back to avoid contamination of the urinary system with fecal material. Wash hands before continuing the bath. (It is a good idea to have another small basin of water handy for handwashing.)

Wash the baby's arms, trunk, and legs. Lather the baby's body with soap, getting into skin folds, such as in the neck and underarms. Rinse soap from the skin and dry thoroughly, making certain to dry well in the skin folds and in the groin.

Wash the genital area, getting into the creases. Gently cleanse around the labia of girls, but do not try to retract the foreskin in an uncircumcised boy unless under the specific direction from the pediatrician. Circumcision care should be performed on circumcised boys.

Dry the infant, then turn him or her on his or her abdomen and wash the back of the neck, the trunk, and lastly the buttocks, cleansing around the rectum.

Wet a cotton ball with alcohol, and wipe the cord stump and the skin immediately around it. This should be done until the cord falls off. The cord may take 3–4 weeks to dry and fall off. If a few drops of blood appear when the cord falls off, simply wipe the area with alcohol. There should not be any drainage the next day.

Remove the wet towel on which the baby had been lying, and dress the baby.

Dress the infant according to the season. Fold the undershirt up and the diaper down so that the cord is exposed to the air to promote drying.

The Sibling's Adjustment

Sibling attachment and adjustment are as important as those of other family members. Increased knowledge about sibling rivalry and the detrimental effects of separation anxiety make including the other children in the events surrounding the birth of a new family member important. Much controversy surrounds the practice of including siblings in witnessing the actual birth. However, much more liberal practices have been evolving that include sibling visitation after the birth. Many hospitals provide prenatal sibling classes in which the prenatal instructor talks about feelings of new babies, how they look, how they behave, how to handle them, the amount of care they take, and feelings of rivalry. The classes often include a tour of the obstetric department to see where their mother will be. Studies indicate that newborns who have direct contact with their siblings have no higher incidence of infection than do those who have contact only with adults. Maternity units do need to monitor the siblings to prevent those with possible infections from visiting.

Anderberg says that after the birth of a baby, siblings are more concerned about reunion with their mothers than acquaintance with the newborn.[3] However, after reassurances from the mother, the child accepts the new infant. Children who had established prenatal relationships with the fetus demonstrate a higher frequency of attachment behavior with the newborn than do those siblings who have not established such a relationship.

Summary

The neonate is an intriguing, exciting being entering a world in which the care of the newborn has changed dramatically in recent years. Although helpless and vulnerable, this infant is complex and capable of responding to and eliciting responses from caregivers. The trauma of birth and abrupt changes in environment make the first day of life a time of stabilization for the neonate, demanding careful observation for any possible complications. All of the newborn's systems are immature, but they begin the process of maturing immediately after birth, some systems more slowly than others. The new family has much to learn, and the nurse has a great responsibility to assist in that process. The changes in obstetric care with shortened stays has made the learning process one that is intense, but it should be thorough. Family-centered care has created a positive atmosphere in which the infant's family is assisted in learning about, caring for, appreciating, and enjoying their infant. The family will find that adjustments must be made in their lives as the infant and the family learn to live in contentment with each other.

Review Questions

1. Draw a simple sketch of a newborn's circulatory system, indicating the changes that occur at birth or within the first weeks of life.
2. The parent of a dark-skinned infant questions you about a large area on the infant's right buttock that appears to be a bruise. What response will you give to this parent to provide reassurance?
3. What is the single most important method of infection control in the newborn nursery?
4. Ms. Smith needs guidance with breastfeeding. Describe in detail what you will tell her.
5. Tonya, a young mother, indicates that she is worried that she might hurt her baby's soft spot. What will you say to her?
6. Jack, the father of a newborn, raises questions about the rash that he notices on his new daughter's abdomen. What can you say to reassure him?
7. You walk by Mary Greene's room and notice that her baby is crying loudly while Mary apparently is watching a television soap opera. What would you do and say?
8. If a Greene family member asks about the "funny shape" of the baby's obviously molded head, what will you tell him or her?
9. What teaching will you give to the Greenes concerning the prevention of cradle cap?
10. What will you tell Mary about positioning her baby after feeding?
11. You are teaching Rosa about caring for her baby. The baby has caput succedaneum. What will you tell her about it?
12. You hear Mr. Quiroga, a first-time father, complain that his wife holds the baby all the time and barely lets him touch the baby. How might you approach this couple to help solve this problem? What could you say to them that would help this father engage in bonding with his baby?

References

1. Klaus MH, Kennell JH. Parent–Infant Bonding, 2nd ed. St Louis: CV Mosby, 1982.
2. Schuster CS, Ashburn SS. The Process of Human Development: A Holistic Life-Span Approach, 3rd ed. Philadelphia: JB Lippincott, 1992.
3. Anderberg GJ. Initial acquaintance and attachment behavior of siblings with the newborn. J Obstet Gynecol Neonatal Nurs 17:49–54, 1988.

Bibliography

Castiglia PT, Harbin RE. Child Health Care: Process and Practice. Philadelphia: JB Lippincott, 1992.

DiFlorio I. Mothers' comprehension of terminology associated with the care of a newborn baby. Pediatr Nurs 17(2):193–196, 1991.

Edgehouse L, Radzuminski SG. A device for supplementing breastfeeding. MCN 15(1):34–35, 1990.

Evans CJ. Description of a home follow-up program for child-bearing families. J Obstet Gynecol Neonatal Nurs 20(2):113–118, 1991.

Greenspan S, Greenspan N. First Feelings. New York: Viking Press, 1986.

Hill PD. The enigma of insufficient milk supply. MCN 16(6): 313–315, 1991.

Klaus MH, Klaus PH. The Amazing Newborn. Reading, MA: Addison-Wesley, 1985.

Pillitteri A. Maternal and Child Health Nursing. Philadelphia: JB Lippincott, 1992.

Schuster CS, Ashburn SS. The Process of Human Development, 3rd ed. Philadelphia: JB Lippincott, 1992.

Shrago L, Bocar D. The infant's contribution to breastfeeding. J Obstet Gynecol Neonatal Nurs 19(3):209–220, 1990.

Spadt SK, Martin KR, Thomas AM. Experiential classes for siblings-to-be. MCN 15(3):184–186, 1990.

Whaley LF, Wong DL. Nursing Care of Infants and Children, 4th ed. St Louis: Mosby-Year Book, 1991.

The High-Risk Newborn

Student Objectives

Upon completion of this chapter the student will be able to:

1. State four possible causes of prematurity.
2. Differentiate between prematurity and small for gestational age.
3. Identify the characteristics of the preterm infant.
4. List eight systems and the symptoms that are most likely to cause problems in the preterm infant.
5. Discuss hydration and feeding of the preterm infant.
6. Describe phototherapy.
7. Discuss the emotional aspects that confront the parents of a preterm infant.
8. Describe common symptoms of necrotizing enterocolitis.
9. Describe the postterm infant.
10. List six possible problems of an infant born to a diabetic mother.
11. Describe what happens to red blood cells in hemolytic disease of an infant.
12. State which mothers are at risk for having an infant with erythroblastosis fetalis.
13. Explain how erythroblastosis fetalis may be prevented.
14. List the criteria for giving RhoGAM.
15. State the signs and symptoms of sepsis neonatorum.
16. State two problems that occur that place the postterm infant in danger.
17. State why newborns of HIV-positive mothers test positive for HIV antibodies.
18. Describe precautions the nurse must use when caring for the newborn of an HIV-positive mother.
19. List the handicaps to which an infant born to an alcoholic mother are prone.
20. Describe the symptoms of addiction in the newborn.
21. List three drugs used to treat the newborn affected by addiction.

Marks MG: BROADRIBB'S INTRODUCTORY PEDIATRIC NURSING, 4th ed. © 1994 J.B. Lippincott Company.

Key Terms

amniocentesis

antigen

antigen–antibody response

apnea

erythroblastosis fetalis

fiberoptic blanket

hemolysis

hyaline membrane disease

hydrops fetalis

hyperbilirubinemia

hyperthermia

kernicterus

lecithin

necrotizing enterocolitis

phototherapy

postterm (postmature) infant

preterm (premature) infant

priapism

pulse oximeter

respiratory distress syndrome (RDS)

retinopathy of prematurity (ROP)

retrolental fibroplasia (RLF)

RhoGAM

small for gestational age (SGA)

surfactant

swaddling

term infant

thermoregulation

tissue perfusion

A high-risk neonate is defined as any neonate who is in danger of serious illness or death as a result of prenatal, perinatal, or neonatal conditions, regardless of birth weight or gestational age. Only technologically advanced expert care by skilled health professionals and a controlled environment can offer them hope of realizing a normal life potential. A number of factors may place a fetus at risk (Box 6-1).

The largest number of high-risk newborns are small infants. About two thirds of these are preterm or premature; the rest are term infants of low birth weight, or **small for gestational age (SGA)**. Classifications of newborns are shown in Box 6-2. These tiny beings and their parents

often have multiple problems to deal with before they can be together as a family.

Immediate physical survival of the infant is not the only factor to be considered. Research indicates that nearly 40% of infants hospitalized for a long time at birth are later victims of neglect or abuse; several reasons are suggested for this tragic statistic. The small infant, preterm or SGA, appears unlike the "fantasy baby" of their dreams, and parents may feel guilty about this. The need for the high-risk newborn to be in the neonatal intensive care unit (NICU) means that the early bonding is interrupted, and the infant has little chance to be held, cuddled, and comforted, even though emotional needs of the high-risk newborn are probably more acute than those of a normal term infant. Unmet emotional needs may make the infant irritable, unstable, and easily stressed, which is an added source of great tension for the infant's family. To try to alleviate some of these problems, visits by family members are encouraged. The family often is encouraged to bring in clothing for the infant to wear to help the family feel that the infant is an individual and to encourage parent–infant attachment. Pictures of the infant's family members may be taped to the infant's unit, and small visual toys may be placed near the infant. Health professionals who are aware of the potential problems may contribute much to the prevention of child abuse.

Box 6-1

Factors that Place a Fetus at Risk

Age of mother <17 or >35 years

Unmarried mother

Prenatal care—none or late

Poor maternal nutrition

Maternal illness—diabetes, hypertension, cardiac disease

Genetic abnormalities

Multiple births

Maternal history of complications of pregnancy—placental abnormalities, premature rupture of membranes, long period of infertility

Maternal addiction

Box 6-2

Terms Used to Describe
Newborns According to Size

SGA—small for gestational age, newborns in the lowest 10th percentile of weight for gestational age

AGA—appropriate for gestational age, newborns between the 10th and 90th percentile of weight for gestational age

LGA—large for gestational age, newborns in the top 10th percentile of weight for gestational age

IUGR—intrauterine growth retardation, used to describe fetus who is small for gestational age

LBW—low birth weight, newborn weighing less than 2500 g but more than 1500 g, regardless of reason

VLBW—very low birth weight, newborn whose birthweight was less than 1500 g, regardless of gestational age

Preterm (premature)—any infant born before the end of the 37th week of gestation, regardless of cause

Postterm (postmature)—any infant born after the end of the 42nd week of gestation

NICU nurses are highly skilled in the use of complicated mechanical equipment and are especially sensitive to even the most subtle change in the infant. These specially educated nurses are also sensitive to the emotional needs of both the infant and the family. In addition, they serve as teachers to the family in the care of the infant after discharge or as support for the family in the event of the death of the infant.

The Preterm Infant

At one time, prematurity was defined only on the basis of birth weight: any live infant weighing 2500 g (5 lb, 8 oz) or less at birth. Time proved this definition inadequate because some infants born at full term weigh less than 2500 g and others weigh more than that even though delivered prematurely.

The American Academy of Pediatrics has adopted the use of the term **preterm (premature) infant** to mean any infant of less than 37 weeks' gestation. A **term infant** is one born between the beginning of the 38th week and the end of the 42nd week of gestation, regardless of birth weight, and a **postterm (postmature) infant** is one born after completion of the 42nd week of gestation, regardless of birth weight. The Dubowitz scoring system was devised as an assessment tool based on external and neurologic development. Variations of the system are currently in use in many hospitals (Figure 6-1). The newborn

is evaluated by the criteria on the chart, and the gestational age of the infant is calculated from the score. This assessment usually is performed within the first 24 hours of life and at least by the time the newborn is 42 hours old.

The preterm infant's untimely departure from the uterus may mean that various organs and systems are not sufficiently mature to adjust to extrauterine life. Small community hospitals are often not equipped to care adequately for the preterm infant. When premature delivery is expected, the mother often is taken to a facility with a NICU before delivery, if possible. However, unexpected problems arise, and transportation of a newborn may be necessary. Teams of specially trained personnel may come from the NICU to transport the neonate by ambulance, van, or helicopter. The newborn is transported in a unit that is self-contained, providing for warmth and oxygen and operating on auxiliary (battery) power. Intravenous fluids, monitors, and other emergency equipment also may be used during the transport of the newborn.

Characteristics of the Preterm Infant

Compared with the term infant, the preterm infant is tiny, scrawny, and red (Figure 6-2). The extremities are thin, with little muscle or subcutaneous fat. Head and abdomen are disproportionately large, and the skin is thin, relatively translucent, and usually wrinkled. Veins of the abdomen and scalp are more visible. Lanugo is plentiful over the extremities, back, and shoulders. The ears have soft, minimal cartilage and thus are extremely pliable. The soft bones of the skull have a tendency to flatten on the sides, and the ribs yield with each labored breath. Testes are undescended in the male; the labia and clitoris are prominent in the female. The soles of the feet and the palms of the hands have few creases. Many of the typical newborn reflexes are weak or absent (Figure 6-3).

Problems of the Preterm Infant

The preterm infant's physiologic immaturity causes many difficulties (Box 6-3), the most critical of which is respiratory. Typically, respirations are shallow, rapid, and irregular, with periods of **apnea** (temporary interruption of the breathing impulse). Respirations may become so labored that the chest wall, and perhaps even the sternum, is retracted.

Pediatrician and nursery staff should be alerted to an impending birth of a preterm infant so that equipment for resuscitation and emergency care is ready. If the birth occurs in a facility without a NICU, plans should be made to transport the newborn immediately after birth.

Respiratory Distress Syndrome
Respiratory distress syndrome (RDS), also known as **hyaline membrane disease**, occurs in about 50,000 of the 250,000 premature infants born in the United States each year. It occurs because the lungs are too immature to

ESTIMATION OF GESTATIONAL AGE BY MATURITY RATING
Side 1

Symbols: X - 1st Exam   O - 2nd Exam

NEUROMUSCULAR MATURITY

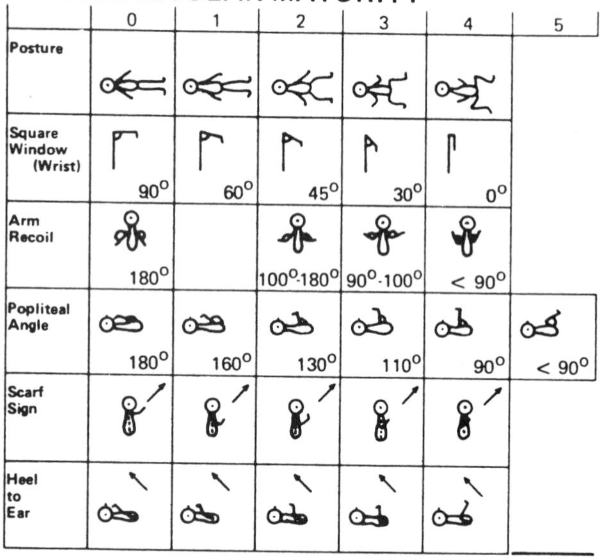

	0	1	2	3	4	5
Posture						
Square Window (Wrist)	90°	60°	45°	30°	0°	
Arm Recoil	180°		100°-180°	90°-100°	< 90°	
Popliteal Angle	180°	160°	130°	110°	90°	< 90°
Scarf Sign						
Heel to Ear						

Gestation by Dates _____ wks

Birth Date _____ Hour _____ am / pm

APGAR _____ 1 min _____ 5 min

MATURITY RATING

Score	Wks
5	26
10	28
15	30
20	32
25	34
30	36
35	38
40	40
45	42
50	44

PHYSICAL MATURITY

	0	1	2	3	4	5
SKIN	gelatinous red, transparent	smooth pink, visible veins	superficial peeling &/or rash, few veins	cracking pale area, rare veins	parchment, deep cracking, no vessels	leathery, cracked, wrinkled
LANUGO	none	abundant	thinning	bald areas	mostly bald	
PLANTAR CREASES	no crease	faint red marks	anterior transverse crease only	creases ant. 2/3	creases cover entire sole	
BREAST	barely percept.	flat areola, no bud	stippled areola, 1–2 mm bud	raised areola, 3–4 mm bud	full areola, 5–10 mm bud	
EAR	pinna flat, stays folded	sl. curved pinna, soft with slow recoil	well-curv. pinna, soft but ready recoil	formed & firm with instant recoil	thick cartilage, ear stiff	
GENITALS Male	scrotum empty, no rugae		testes descending, few rugae	testes down, good rugae	testes pendulous, deep rugae	
GENITALS Female	prominent clitoris & labia minora		majora & minora equally prominent	majora large, minora small	clitoris & minora completely covered	

SCORING SECTION

	1st Exam=X	2nd Exam=O
Estimating Gest Age by Maturity Rating	_____Weeks	_____Weeks
Time of Exam	Date _____ am / Hour _____pm	Date _____ am / Hour _____pm
Age at Exam	_____ Hours	_____ Hours
Signature of Examiner	M.D.	M.D.

Figure 6-1. Estimation of gestational age by maturity rating. (Scoring system: Ballard JL, Kazmaierk K, Driver M. A simplified assessment of gestational age. Pediatr Res, 11:374, 1977. Figures adapted from Sweet AY. Classification of the low-birth-weight infant. In Kalus MH, Fanaroff AA, et al. eds: Care of the High-Risk Infant. Philadelphia: WB Saunders, 1977.)

function properly. Normally, the lungs remain partially expanded after each breath, owing to a substance called **surfactant**, a biochemical compound that reduces surface tension inside the air sacs. The premature infant's lungs are deficient in surfactant and thus collapse after each breath, greatly reducing the infant's vital supply of oxygen. This damages the lung cells, and these damaged cells combine with other substances present in the lungs to form a fibrous substance called hyaline membrane. This membrane lines the alveoli and blocks gas exchange in the alveoli.

Surfactant replacement therapy with surfactant made

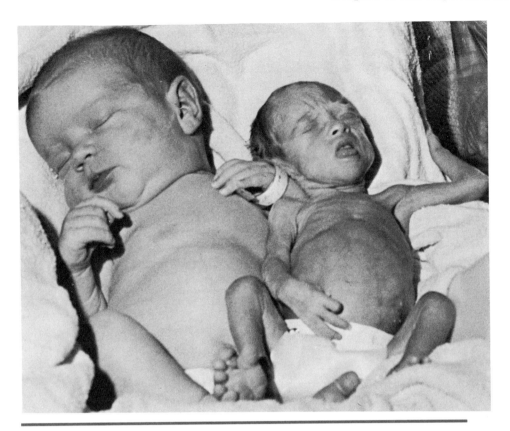

Figure 6-2. The difference between full-term and premature infants is striking. The premature infant has a relatively large head and loose skin. Sometimes loops of intestine are visible through the thin abdominal wall.

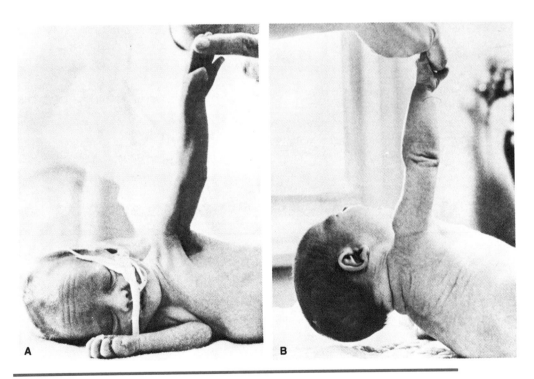

Figure 6-3. The grasp reflex present in the premature newborn (**A**) is much weaker than that noted in the full-term infant. (**B**) (Courtesy of Mead Johnson Laboratories, Evansville, IN.)

Box 6-3

Systems and Situations that are Most Likely to Cause Problems in the Premature Infant

The premature infant has altered physiology due to immature and often poorly developed systems. The severity of any problem that occurs depends on the gestational age of the infant.

Respiratory System

Alveoli begin to form at 26–28 weeks' gestation; therefore, lungs are poorly developed.

Respiratory muscles are poorly developed.

Chest wall lacks stability.

Production of surfactant is reduced.

There is reduced compliance and low functional residual capacity of the lung.

Breathing may be labored and irregular with periods of apnea and cyanosis.

Infant is prone to atelectasis.

Gag and cough reflexes are poor; thus, aspiration may be a problem.

Digestive System

The stomach is small, and vomiting is likely to occur because of poor muscle tone at the cardiac sphincter. It is difficult to provide caloric requirement in the early days.

Tolerance is decreased related to decreased enzymes.

Lacks bile salts that aid digestion of fats and absorption of vitamin D and other fat-soluble vitamins.

Limited ability to convert glucose to glycogen and break down glycogen to glucose.

Limited and immature ability to release insulin in response to glucose.

Lacks coordinated sucking-swallowing reflex before 32–34 weeks' gestational age; immature esophageal motility.

Poor Thermal Stability

Has little subcutaneous fat; thus, there is no heat storage or insulation; poor glycogen and lipid stores.

Limited ability to shiver; has poor vasomotor control of blood flow to skin capillaries.

There is relatively large surface area in comparison to body weight.

Sweat glands are decreased; infant cannot perspire before 32 weeks' gestational age.

Has reduced muscle and fat deposits that restrict metabolic rate and heat production.

    Brown fat is deposited after 28 weeks' gestation in adipose tissue around axillae, kidneys, scapula, neck, and adrenal glands.

Usually is less active.

Posture flaccid—increasing surface area exposed.

Renal Function

Sodium excretion is probably increased, which may lead to hyponatremia; there is difficulty in excreting potassium.

Ability to concentrate urine decreases; thus, when vomiting or diarrhea occurs, dehydration is likely to follow. Decreased ability to conserve or excrete fluid.

Ability to acidify urine decreases.

Glomerular tubular imbalance accounts for sugar, protein, amino acids, and sodium present in urine.

Nervous System

Response to stimulation is slow.

Suck, swallow, and gag reflexes are poor; therefore, feeding and possible aspiration are problems.

Cough reflex is weak or absent.

Centers that control respirations, temperature, and other vital functions are poorly developed.

Infection

Actively formed antibodies are lacking at birth (active immunity).

No immunoglobulin M is present at birth.

Limited chemotaxis (reaction of cell to chemical stimuli).

Decreased opsonization (preparation of cells for phagocytosis).

Limited phagocytosis (digestion of bacteria by cells).

Hypofunctioning adrenal gland contributes to a decreased antiinflammatory response.

Liver Function

Does not have adequate ability to handle and conjugate bilirubin.

Does not store or release glucose well; thus, there is a tendency toward hypoglycemia.

There is a steady decrease in hemoglobin after birth and in the production of blood; therefore, anemia may occur.

Does not make or store vitamin K; thus, infant is susceptible to hemorrhagic disease.

(continued)

Box 6-3 (Continued)

Systems and Situations that are Most Likely to Cause Problems in the Premature Infant

Eyes

Oxygen may cause retinal arteries to constrict, resulting in anoxic damage.

The retinae detach from the surface of posterior chambers, and a fibrous mass forms, resulting in an inability to receive visual stimulation. This is *retrolental fibroplasia* (RLF).

The exact amount and level of oxygen needed to produce RLF is unknown. An infant weighing less than 1000 g is at high risk for RLF. It is also related to conditions such as sepsis, transfusions, chronic disease, and hypoxia.

Skin

Sensitive because of permeability and collagen instability.

Decreased cohesion between epidermis and dermis.

Decreased thickness of stratus corneum (outer layer of epidermis).

Delayed skin pH recovery to acidity following washing with alkaline-based soaps, creams, and emollients.

Increased risk of toxicity from topical application and percutaneous absorption of drugs and substances.

Adapted from Suddarth D. Lippincott Manual of Nursing Practice, 6th ed. Philadelphia: JB Lippincott, 1991.

synthetically, obtained from animal sources, or extracted from human amniotic fluid has proved successful in the treatment of RDS. Surfactant is administered as an inhalant through a catheter inserted into an endotracheal tube, immediately at or soon after birth. The therapy may be used as preventive treatment ("rescue") to avoid the development of RDS in the infant at risk. Infants with RDS usually receive additional oxygen through continuous positive airway pressure (CPAP), using intubation or a plastic hood. This helps the lungs to remain partially expanded until they begin producing surfactant, usually within the first 5 days of life.

If premature delivery is expected, an attempt may be made to prevent RDS. Through amniocentesis, the amount of **lecithin**, the major component of surfactant, may be measured to determine lung maturity. If insufficient lecithin is present 24 to 48 hours before delivery, the mother may be given a glucocorticosteroid drug (Betamethasone) that crosses the placenta and causes the infant's lungs to produce surfactant. The infant begins to produce surfactant about 72 hours after birth, therefore the critical time comes within these first several days. Those infants who survive the first 4 days have a much improved chance of recovery unless other problems are overwhelming.

Heat Loss

Cold stress is a greater threat to the preterm newborn than it is to the term infant. The preterm infant cannot shiver and has no integration of reflex control of peripheral blood vessels. Cold stress may result in hypoxia, metabolic acidosis, and hypoglycemia. Therefore, to prevent heat loss and to control other aspects of the premature infant's environment, an isolette or radiant warmer is used (Figure 6-4). The isolette has a clear Plexiglas top

that allows a full view of the infant from all aspects. The isolette maintains ideal temperature, humidity, and oxygen concentrations and isolates the infant from infection. Portholes at the side afford access to the infant with minimal temperature and oxygen loss. The temperature of the isolette or the radiant warmer is controlled by a heat-sensing probe attached to the infant's skin. If oxygen is administered through an oxygen hood, it must be warmed and moisturized before it is administered.

Other Problems

The preterm infant desperately needs nourishment but has a digestive system that may be unprepared to receive and digest food. The stomach is small, with a capacity that may be less than 1 to 2 oz. The sphincters at either end of the stomach are immature, causing regurgitation or vomiting if feedings distend the stomach. The immature liver is unable to manage all the bilirubin produced by **hemolysis** (destruction of red blood cells with the release of hemoglobin), making the infant prone to jaundice and high blood bilirubin levels, or **hyperbilirubinemia**, that may result in brain damage.

The preterm infant does not receive enough antibodies from the mother and cannot produce them. This characteristic makes the infant particularly vulnerable to infection.

Muscle weakness in the premature infant contributes to nutritional and respiratory problems and to a posture distinct from that of the term infant (Figure 6-5). The infant may not be able to change positions and is prone to fatigue and exhaustion, even from eating and breathing. Skilled, gentle, intensive care is needed for the infant to survive and develop.

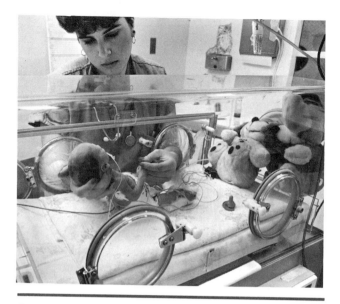

Figure 6-4. Isolette infant incubator. (From Reeder SJ, Martin LL, Koniak D. Maternity Nursing: Family, Newborn, and Women's Health Care, 17th ed. Philadelphia: JB Lippincott, 1992.)

Nursing Process in the Care of the Preterm Infant

The physical condition of a preterm infant demands the skilled assessment and planning of nursing care, emphasizing maintenance of adequate oxygenation, continuous electronic cardiac and respiratory monitoring, frequent manual monitoring of vital signs, **thermoregulation** (regulation of the infant's temperature), infection control, hydration, and provision of adequate nutrition, sensory stimulation for the infant, and emotional support for the parents.

ASSESSMENT

The initial assessment focuses on the status of the respiratory, circulatory, and neurologic systems to determine the immediate needs of the infant.

NURSING DIAGNOSIS

Based on the initial assessment, some of the nursing diagnoses that may be included are the following:

- Ineffective breathing patterns related to an immature respiratory system
- Ineffective thermoregulation related to immaturity and transition to extrauterine life
- High risk for infection related to an immature immune system and environmental factors
- High risk for altered nutrition, less than body requirements related to an inability to suck adequately because of weakness
- High risk for impaired skin integrity related to urinary

excretion of bilirubin and exposure to phototherapy light

- Activity intolerance related to poor oxygenation and weakness
- High risk for parental anxiety related to an unpredictable prognosis
- High risk for altered parenting related to separation from the infant and difficulty accepting an impaired infant
- Altered family process related to the effect of prolonged hospitalization on the family
- Parental grieving related to the infant's serious condition or death (discussed in a later section)

PLANNING AND IMPLEMENTATION

The premature infant is cared for by highly skilled nurses in a NICU. Nursing goals are formulated and implemented to address each of the nursing diagnoses indentified for the individual infant.

Improving Respiratory Function. Not all preterm infants need extra oxygen but many do. Isolettes are made with oxygen inlets and humidifiers for raising the oxygen concentration in the incubator from 20% to 21% (room air) to a higher percentage. Also, clear plastic hoods placed over the infant's head supply humidified oxygen at the concentration desired. Oxygen saturation of the blood may be monitored by pulse oximetry, or the oxygen and carbon dioxide levels may be measured by transcutaneous monitoring. Both of these methods aid in establishing the desirable oxygen concentration in the infant.

High blood concentrations of oxygen are associated with a disease of the blood vessels of the eye, **retinopathy of prematurity (ROP)**. ROP begins with vasoconstriction of the eye vessels. In later stages, there is an increase of capillaries that, for some infants, results in scarring, causing retinal detachment. This final stage is called **retrolental fibroplasia (RLF)**. Although associated with high oxygen levels (higher than 40% is considered dangerous), the exact reason for the mechanism is not known. Usually, the younger the preterm, the higher the probability of ROP. Recent information indicates that ROP is a complex disease of prematurity that has many causes and is therefore difficult to prevent. Observations should be made of the pulse and respiratory rates, retractions, skin color, muscle tone, alertness, and activity. In the absence of lung pathologic changes, it is safer to keep the oxygen concentration lower than 40%, unless hypoxia is documented. For the infant's protection, incubators are constructed so that it is difficult to get concentrations higher than 40% without special maneuvers.

Observation of the preterm infant's respirations is obviously of utmost importance (Figure 6-6). Measuring the rate of respiration and identifying retractions are essential to determining proper oxygen concentrations. One of the most hazardous characteristics of the preterm in-

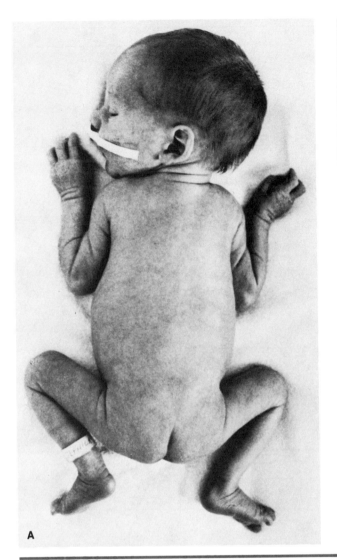 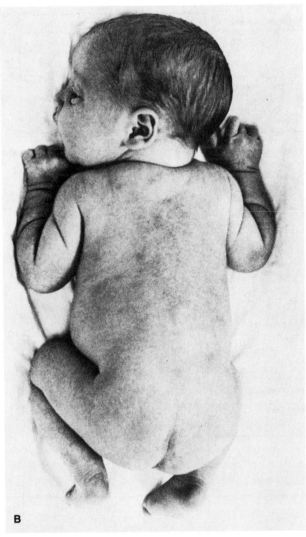

Figure 6-5. It is easy to distinguish the premature newborn from the term infant when both are in the prone position. **A**, The premature infant lies with pelvis flat and legs spread in a froglike position. **B**, Term infant lies with limbs flexed, pelvis raised, and knees drawn up under abdomen. (Courtesy of Mead Johnson Laboratories, Evansville, IN.)

fant is the tendency to stop breathing periodically (apnea). The hypoxia caused by this apnea and general respiratory difficulty may cause mental retardation or other neurologic problems.

Electronic apnea alarms are used routinely. Electrodes are placed across the infant's chest with leads to the apnea monitor outside the isolette, providing a continuous reading of the respiratory rate. Visual and audio alarms may be set to alert the nurse when the rate goes too high or too low or if the infant waits too long to take a breath.

It is a nursing responsibility to place, check, and replace the leads from the infant. The electrodes should be removed and relocated slightly at least daily to protect the infant's sensitive skin from being damaged by the electrode paste and adhesive. The skin should be cleansed

carefully between applications of the electrodes. Many false alarms are the result of leads coming loose. Some of these alarms may be prevented by using a small amount of electrode paste and being careful to keep the paste inside the circle of adhesive on the electrode.

Respiratory assistance may be used to handle apnea. Usually, a gentle stimulation, such as wiggling a foot, is enough to remind the infant to breathe. However, there are times when respirations need to be assisted by a bag and mask. Every nursery nurse should know how to "bag" an infant. The principles of this form of assisted respirations are similar to those of mouth-to-mouth artificial respirations. The neck must be slightly extended to open the airway. The mask covers the infant's mouth and nose. A tight seal between the mask and the infant's face must be maintained. The small bag, filled with oxygen or air, is

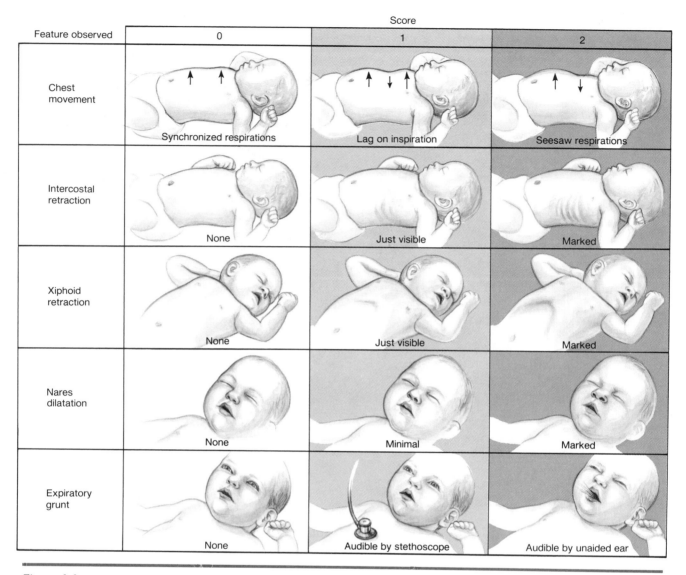

Feature observed	Score		
	0	1	2
Chest movement	Synchronized respirations	Lag on inspiration	Seesaw respirations
Intercostal retraction	None	Just visible	Marked
Xiphoid retraction	None	Just visible	Marked
Nares dilatation	None	Minimal	Marked
Expiratory grunt	None	Audible by stethoscope	Audible by unaided ear

Figure 6-6. Grading of neonatal respiratory distress based on Silverman-Anderson index. (From Pillitteri A. Maternal and Child Health Nursing. Philadelphia: JB Lippincott, 1992, p. 664.)

squeezed quickly. The quantity of air needed is relatively small, and the pressure is gentle.

Maintaining Body Temperature. The high-risk infant must be monitored closely and continuously. Monitors that record temperature, pulse, respirations, and blood pressure, transcutaneous oxygen and carbon dioxide monitors, and **pulse oximeters** (measure oxygen saturation) are all part of the equipment routinely used in the high-risk nursery, but close observation by the nurse who is regularly assigned to the same infant is still an essential part of the infant's care. The nurse observes the monitoring and life support equipment, making sure that it is functioning properly, and systematically assesses the infant. Assessment and other procedures should be timed so that the infant is disturbed as little as possible to conserve his or her energy.

Most isolettes are equipped with a control system for temperature regulation. A temperature-sensitive electrode is attached to the infant's abdomen and connected to the isolette thermostat. The unit may then be set to turn the heater on and off according to the infant's skin temperature. Open units with overhead radiant warmers provide maximum access to the infant when use of sophisticated equipment or frequent manipulation for treatment and assessment is necessary. The temperature remains more constant than in the closed unit, which is constantly having the door or portholes opened and the atmosphere breached. Care must be taken not to overheat the infant, a condition called **hyperthermia**, because this causes consumption of oxygen and calories and may jeopardize the infant. Clothing, a head covering (such as a stockinette cap), and blankets should be used when the infant is removed from the warm environment of the isolette or radiant warmer to be held for feeding or cuddling. It is still standard practice to take and record axillary temperatures when the infant is being monitored by either of these methods.

Although monitoring equipment provides a continual reading of the heart rate, apical pulses are taken periodically, listening to the heart through the chest using a stethoscope for 1 full minute not to miss an irregularity in rhythm. Observations should include rate, rhythm, and strength. The pulse rate is normally rapid (120 to 140 beats per minute) and unstable. Premature infants are subject to dangerous periods of bradycardia (as low as 60 to 80 beats per minute) and tachycardia (as high as 160 to 200 beats per minute). The nurse's observations of the pulse rate, rhythm, and strength are essential to understanding how the infant is tolerating treatments, activity, feedings, and the temperature and oxygen concentration of the isolette.

Preventing Infection. Infection control in the care of the high-risk newborn is an urgent concern. The preterm infant does not have the ability to resist bacterial invasions; the caretakers of the infant must provide an atmosphere that protects from such attacks. The primary means of preventing infection is handwashing. All persons who come in contact with the newborn must practice good handwashing immediately before touching the infant and when moving from one infant to another. Studies show that handwashing is the most important aspect of infection control.

Other points of "good housekeeping" that are important include regular cleaning or changing of humidifying water, intravenous tubings, suction equipment, respiratory equipment, and monitoring equipment. The high-risk nursery is a separate area from the normal newborn nursery and usually is staffed by its own personnel. This separation helps eliminate sources of infection. Personnel in this area usually wear scrub suits or gowns. Personnel from other departments (radiology, respiratory therapy, or laboratory) put a cover gown over their uniforms while working with the high-risk infant.

Maintaining Adequate Nutrition. When born, a preterm infant may be too weak to suck or not yet have adequate sucking and swallowing reflexes. For several hours or even 1 day the preterm infant may be able to manage without fluids, but soon intravenous fluids will be necessary. In many instances, an intravenous "life line" is established immediately after delivery. Fluids are infused through a catheter passed into the umbilical vein in the stub of the umbilical cord if it is still fresh. Intravenous fluids may be given through other veins, particularly the peripheral veins of the hands or feet. Extremely small amounts of fluid are needed, perhaps as little as 5 to 10 mL/h or even less. They may be measured accurately and administered at a steady rate by using an infusion pump. Accurate and complete records of intravenous fluids are kept, and careful, frequent observations for infiltration or overhydration are essential. All urinary output is measured and recorded by weighing the diapers before and after they are used. The normal range of urine volume is between 35 and 40 mL/kg per 24 hours during the first few days, increasing to between 50 and 100 mL. The nurse also should observe and record the number of urinations, the color of the urine, and edema. Edema changes the loose, wrinkled skin to tight, shiny skin.

At first, some preterm infants receive all their fluid, electrolyte, vitamin and caloric needs by intravenous routes. Others are able to start with a nipple and bottle (Figure 6-7). Premature infants are likely to have problems with aspiration because the gag reflex does not develop until about the 32nd to 34th week of gestation. Many infants need gavage feedings. The frequency and quantity of the gavage feedings are determined for each infant. Usually, feedings are given every 2 hours. Care should be taken not to extend the feeding time too long because this may tire the infant. A feeding should be completed in less than 30 minutes, or the next feeding should be given by gavage to allow the infant to rest. If the stomach is not being emptied by the next feeding, more time needs to be allowed between feedings or smaller feedings need to be given. Usually, the quantity given is just as much as the infant can tolerate and is increased milliliter by milliliter as quickly as tolerated. Starting an infant on 5 to 10 mL per feeding is not unusual. Special premature infant nursers are used that are calibrated in 1-mL markings. The feeding is not too large if the infant's stomach is not so distended that it causes respiratory difficulty, vomiting, or regurgitation and if there is not much formula left in the stomach by the next feeding.

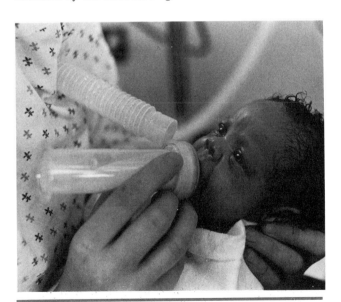

Figure 6-7. This preterm infant with chronic lung disease still requires a small amount of supplementary oxygen but is able to be out of the isolette for short periods to be held for feedings. (Photo by Marcia Lieberman.) (From Waechter EH, Blake FG. Nursing Care of Children, 9th ed. Philadelphia: JB Lippincott, 1976.)

The breast milk of mothers of preterm infants is thought to be higher in protein, sodium and chloride, and immunoglobulin A. Mothers may be encouraged to pump their breast milk and freeze it to use for bottle or gavage feedings until the infant is strong enough to breast feed. The use of her own milk to nourish her newborn is a tremendous boost to the emotional satisfaction of the mother.

The most common premature infant formula has 13 cal/oz (often called half-strength formula). A formula with 20 cal/oz (the usual strength for newborns) also may be used. If the formula is too rich (too high in carbohydrates and fats), the infant may experience vomiting and diarrhea. If the infant does not gain weight after an initial postnatal weight loss, the calories may not be enough. Breast milk for the preterm infant is a preferred source of nutrition.

When an infant who is being gavage fed begins to suck vigorously on fingers, hands, pacifier, or gavage tubing, along with demonstrating evidence of a gag reflex, nipple feeding should be tried. The infant who can take the same quantity of formula by nipple that was tolerated by gavage without becoming too tired is ready. Some infants need alternating gavage and nipple feedings to see them through the transition period. The nipple for a preterm infant is of softer rubber than the regular nipple. It is also smaller but no shorter than the regular nipple.

Preterm infants need to be burped often during and after feedings. Sometimes simply changing the infant's position is enough assistance. At other times it may help to rub or pat the infant's back gently. At all times during feedings, caution must be used to prevent aspiration. The infant should be held for the feeding with oxygen supply available as needed. After a feeding, the best position is probably on the infant's left side with the head of the mattress slightly elevated.

There are other methods by which preterm infants may be fed if neither gavage or nipple feeding is tolerated and if intravenous fluids are inadequate. Some babies do better if fed with a rubber-tipped medicine dropper. For other babies, it is necessary to provide gastrostomy feedings. Nonnutritive sucking opportunities, such as a pacifier, should be given to the infant who is not receiving nipple feedings.

The infant should be weighed daily at the same time each day. These daily weights give an indication of the infant's overall health and indicate whether or not enough calories are being consumed. The physicians and parents probably will want to know the infant's current weight each day. Weighing the infant on the same scales in the same clothing at the same time helps ensure accurate, comparable data.

Caring for the Infant Undergoing Phototherapy. Jaundice is a common occurrence in prematurity. The bilirubin level may be measured noninvasively with transcutaneous bilirubinometry or by a heel stick, results of which may be interpreted by the nursery nurse with specialized equipment. Babies with elevated bilirubin levels are exposed to specially designed fluorescent lights to prevent bilirubin levels from reaching the danger point of 20 mg/dL, beyond which **kernicterus** (severe brain damage from excessive bilirubin levels) is a threat. The criteria for treatment with **phototherapy** varies with the infant's size and age. The lights are placed above and outside the isolette. The infant is nude, and the eyes are shielded from the ultraviolet light (Figure 6-8). The eye patches may promote infection if they are not clean and changed frequently, or they may cause eye damage if they are not applied so that they stay in place. Nurses should be aware that the light may cause the infant to have skin rashes; "sunburn" or tanning; loose, greenish stools; hyperthermia; increased metabolic rate; increased evaporative loss of water; and **priapism**, a perpetual abnormal erection of the penis. Infants undergoing phototherapy treatment need as much as 25% more fluids to prevent dehydration. The serum bilirubin level is monitored routinely when the infant is receiving phototherapy. A **fiberoptic blanket** (a specialized pad with plastic fibers that are illuminating, covered with a disposable protective cover) is available that, when wrapped about the infant, disperses therapeutic light to the infant. These blankets may help make home phototherapy more common, thus cutting hospitalization costs for the infant with hyperbilirubinemia and reducing the separation time for the infant and family.

Promoting Energy Conservation and Sensory Stimulation. The preterm newborn uses the most energy to breathe and pump blood. The nurse should plan the infant's day to avoid exhaustion from constant handling and moving about. The infant's energy may be con-

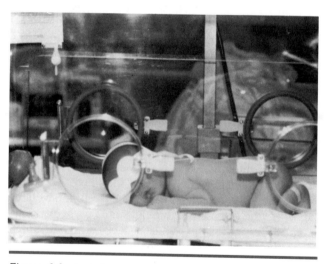

Figure 6-8. An infant's eyes are shielded from the ultraviolet light when receiving phototherapy. (From May KA, Mahlmeister LR. Comprehensive Maternity Nursing: Nursing Process and The Childbearing Family, 2nd ed. Philadelphia: JB Lippincott, 1990.)

served by eliminating regular bathing but giving only "face and fanny" care as needed. Preterm infants usually are dressed in only a diaper, if anything. This practice conserves energy, provides more freedom of movement, and allows a better opportunity to observe the infant. However, it should not mislead the nurse into ignoring or avoiding the infant or discouraging contact essential to establishing a normal relationship.

Older preterm infants have a special need for sensory stimulation. Mobiles hung over the isolette and toys placed in or on the infant unit may provide visual stimulation. A radio with the volume turned low, a music box, or a wind-up toy in the isolette may provide auditory stimulation. An excellent form of auditory stimulation comes from the voices of the infant's family, physician, and nurses talking and singing. Being bathed, held, cuddled, and fondled provides needed tactile stimulation. Contact is essential to the infant and the family. Some NICUs have a program of "foster grandparents" who regularly visit long-term NICU infants and provide them with sensory stimulation—cuddling, loving, crooning, and talking. These programs have proven beneficial to both the infants and the volunteer grandparents.

The nurse must position the preterm infant carefully and change the position periodically. The infant may be positioned from side to side. If the infant is placed on his or her back, special care must be taken to see that aspiration of vomitus does not occur. Preterm infants have a knack of wriggling into corners and cracks from which they cannot extract themselves, therefore close observation is necessary.

Reducing Parental Anxiety. The birth of a preterm infant creates a crisis for the family caregivers. Their long-awaited baby is whisked away from them, sometimes to a distant neonatal center, and hooked up to a maze of machines. Parents feel anxiety, guilt, fear, depression, and perhaps anger. They cannot share the early sensitive attachment period. Establishing touch and eye contact ordinarily achieved in 10 minutes with a normal-term infant may take weeks. Parents often leave the hospital empty-handed, without the perfect, healthy infant of their dreams. How can they learn to know and love the strange, scrawny creature who now lives in that plastic box? These feelings are normal, but studies have shown that if these feelings are not expressed and resolved, they can damage the long-term relationship of parents and child, even resulting in child neglect or abuse.

The mother's condition also must be considered. If the infant was delivered by cesarean birth, or if the labor was difficult or prolonged, she may feel abandoned or too weak to become involved with the baby.

Nurses who work with high-risk infants can do much to help families cope with the crisis of prematurity and early separation. To help ease some of the apprehensions of the family caregivers, transport teams prepare the infant for transportation, then take the infant in the transport incubator into the mother's room so that they may see (and touch, if possible) the infant before the child is whisked away. Instant photos also are taken by nursery staff in many instances, so that the family has some concrete reminder of the infant until they can visit in person. Explaining what is happening to their infant in the NICU and reporting periodically on the infant's condition (through phone contact if the NICU is not in the same hospital) reassures the family that their child is receiving excellent care and that they are being kept informed. Listening to the family and encouraging them to express their feelings may help them support one another. As soon as possible, the family should see, touch, and help care for their infant (Figure 6-9). Most NICUs do not restrict visiting hours for parents or support persons, and they encourage families to visit their infants often, whenever it is convenient for the family. Many hospitals offer 24-hour phone privileges to families so that they are never out of touch with their infant's caregivers.

Before the mother is discharged from the hospital, plans are made for both parents or other support persons to visit the infant and to participate in the care. They need to feel that the infant belongs to them, not to the hospital. To help foster this feeling and strengthen the attachment, nurses work closely with families to help them progress toward successful parenthood (Figure 6-10). Siblings should be included in the visits to see the infant. The monitors, warmers, ventilators, and other equipment may be frightening to siblings and family caregivers. Nurses must make the infant's family feel welcome and comfortable when they visit. A primary nurse assigned to care for the infant gives the family a constant person to contact, increasing their feelings of confidence in the care the infant is receiving.

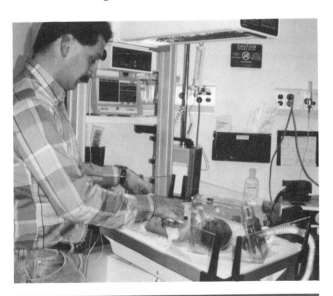

Figure 6-9. Parents should be encouraged to visit and participate in the care of their high-risk newborn as soon and as often as possible.

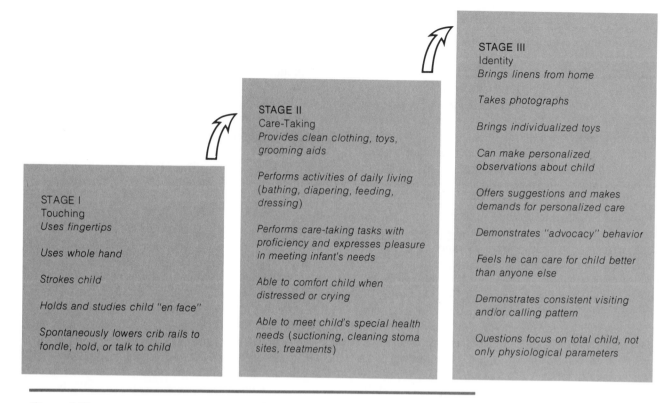

STAGE I
Touching
Uses fingertips

Uses whole hand

Strokes child

Holds and studies child "en face"

Spontaneously lowers crib rails to fondle, hold, or talk to child

STAGE II
Care-Taking
Provides clean clothing, toys, grooming aids

Performs activities of daily living (bathing, diapering, feeding, dressing)

Performs care-taking tasks with proficiency and expresses pleasure in meeting infant's needs

Able to comfort child when distressed or crying

Able to meet child's special health needs (suctioning, cleaning stoma sites, treatments)

STAGE III
Identity
Brings linens from home

Takes photographs

Brings individualized toys

Can make personalized observations about child

Offers suggestions and makes demands for personalized care

Demonstrates "advocacy" behavior

Feels he can care for child better than anyone else

Demonstrates consistent visiting and/or calling pattern

Questions focus on total child, not only physiological parameters

Figure 6-10. Stage's of parenting behaviors observed in parents of high-risk infants. (Adapted from the work of Rubin R, Schaeffer Jay S, Schraeder B. *In* Schraeder BD. Attachment and parenting despite lengthy intensive care. Am J Matern Child Nurs 5:37–41, 1980.)

Support groups of families who have experienced the crisis that a preterm infant causes are of great value to new families of high-risk infants. Members of these groups visit new high-risk families in the hospital and at home. These groups are successful in helping high-risk parents deal with their feelings and solve the problems that may arise when their infant is ready to come home or if the infant dies.

As the time for discharge of the infant comes closer, the family of the infant is understandably apprehensive. The NICU nurses must teach the mother and her support persons those skills they need to care for the infant. This knowledge gives them confidence that they are capable of taking care of the infant. Some hospitals allow persons to stay overnight before the infant's discharge so that they can participate in round-the-clock care. The knowledge that they can telephone their physician and nurse at any time after discharge to have questions answered is reassuring.

Before discharge, most preterm infants will have successfully made the transition from isolette to open crib, thriving without artificial support systems. In addition to the feeding, bathing, and general care of the infant, many families of premature infants need to learn infant cardiopulmonary resuscitation and the use of an apnea monitor before the infant is discharged from the hospital. High-risk infants are being sent home in some instances with oxygen, gastrostomy feeding tubes, and many other kinds of sophisticated equipment. This approach helps place the infant in the home much earlier, but it requires intensive training and support of the family members who need to care for the infant. After the baby goes home, a nurse, usually a community health nurse, visits the family to check on the health of mother and the baby. The nurse provides additional support and teaching about the infant's care, if necessary, and answers any questions or concerns the family might have.

EVALUATION

The evaluation of the preterm infant is an ongoing process that demands continual adjustment and readjustment of the nursing diagnoses, planning, and implementation. Goals for the nursing diagnoses include:

- Respiratory rate remains less than 60 breaths per minute; no grunting or retractions noted; breath sounds clear; no episodes of apnea

- Infant's temperature is maintained at greater than 36.5°C (97.7°F)

- No signs of infection as evidenced by vital signs within normal limits; breath sounds clear

- Infant gains weight daily; skin turgor improves
- Infant's skin is free of redness, rashes, and irritation; eyes are protected from damage as a result of photo-therapy
- Infant's energy is conserved as evidenced by long periods of rest for the infant; sensory stimulation needs are met
- Family caregivers express feelings and anxieties concerning the infant's condition
- Family caregivers visit and establish relationship with the infant; hold and help care for the infant
- Family caregivers demonstrate knowledge of care infant needs
- Family contacts a support group for high-risk infants

Other High-Risk Conditions

The Infant of a Diabetic Mother

The severity of the mother's diabetes has a direct relationship to the risk factor for the infant. The diabetic woman who is able to closely control her blood glucose level before conception and throughout pregnancy, particularly the early months, will be able to avoid having an infant with congenital anomalies commonly associated with diabetes.

Infants of mothers with poorly controlled diabetes have a distinctive appearance (Figure 6-11). They are large for gestational age, plump and full-faced, and coated with vernix caseosa. Both the placenta and the umbilical cord are oversized. Infants of mothers with poorly controlled, long-term, or severe diabetes actually may suffer from intrauterine growth retardation.

Infants of diabetic mothers often are at risk for hypoglycemia in the first few hours after birth. In the uterus, the high blood glucose levels of the mother increase the blood glucose level of the fetus before birth and cause the fetal pancreas to secrete increased amounts of insulin. This process leads to the increased intrauterine growth of the fetus. After birth, however, the high levels of glucose are suddenly cut off, and the pancreas of the infant cannot readjust quickly enough, thus hypoglycemia (or hyperinsulinism) occurs. This may jeopardize the infant's life if not detected quickly and treated with oral or intravenous glucose to raise the level of the infant's blood glucose. Hypoglycemia, if left untreated, may cause severe, irreversible damage to the central nervous system. The usual range of blood glucose levels for newborns is 45 to 90 mg/dL. If the newborn's blood glucose level is 25 mg/dL or lower, the infant is treated with intravenous fluids, early feedings, and intravenous or oral glucose. The newborn's blood glucose level is checked by heel stick on a frequent schedule for the first 24 hours of life.

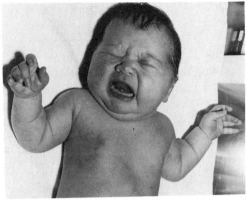
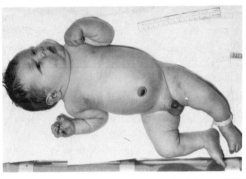

Figure 6-11. Infant of diabetic mother. (From Avery GB. Neonatology, 2nd ed. Philadelphia, JB Lippincott, 1981.)

These infants are subject to many other hazards, including congenital anomalies, hypocalcemia, hyperbilirubinemia, and hyaline membrane disease. Infants of diabetic mothers require especially careful observation.

The Infant with Hemolytic Disease of the Newborn

Hemolytic disease of the newborn is another name for **erythroblastosis fetalis**, a condition in which the infant's red blood cells are broken down (hemolyzed) and destroyed, producing severe anemia and hyperbilirubinemia. This rapid destruction of red blood cells may produce heart failure, brain damage, and death.

Before the mid-1960s, hemolytic disease was largely the result of Rh incompatibility between the blood of the mother and the blood of the fetus. The introduction of Rho immune globulin, or **RhoGAM**, in the mid-1960s has markedly reduced the incidence of this disorder. Hemolytic disease occurring today is principally the result of ABO incompatibility and is generally much less severe than the Rh-induced disorder.

Rh Incompatibility

The Rh factor is a protein substance that is called an **antigen** and is found on the surface of red blood cells. It is called Rh because it was first identified in the blood of rhesus monkeys. Those persons who possess the factor are referred to as Rh positive (D), and those lacking it as Rh negative (d). The blood type of a person is inherited, following the same hereditary rules regarding dominant and recessive traits. Rh positive is dominant. If both members of a couple are Rh negative, there will be no hemolytic disorder with their children. However, if the mother is Rh negative, the father is Rh positive, and the child inherits Rh positive blood, the disorder may occur.

If the father is homozygous positive, then both of his genes carry the D (dominant) trait, but if he is heterozygous positive, one of the genes is a D and the other a d. Thus, if the father is heterozygous positive and the mother Rh negative, there is a 50% probability of their having a baby who is Rh negative (without hemolytic disease). Because of the mechanism by which the mother is sensitized to the Rh factor, there is little chance of the first baby being affected.

Pathophysiology. The mechanism is based on the principles of the **antigen–antibody response**. Although fetal and maternal circulations are completely separated, a break in the placental barrier may allow some of the fetal red blood cells to escape into the maternal circulation. The break often occurs at the time the placenta separates during delivery, or it may take place after an abortion. The Rh-positive fetal cells entering the maternal circulation act as a "mini transfusion," causing the mother to form protective antibodies. It may take some time, however, for the antibodies to form, thus the first baby is rarely affected.

With the next pregnancy, if any of the baby's red blood cells enter the maternal circulation, antibodies form rapidly. Consequently, the maternal antibodies enter the fetal circulation and begin to hemolyze the baby's red blood cells (Figure 6-12).

The rapid destruction of red blood cells causes excretion of bilirubin into the amniotic fluid. The body of the fetus makes a valiant attempt to replace the red blood cells being destroyed by sending out large amounts of immature red blood cells called erythroblasts into the blood stream. For this reason, the disease is called **erythroblastosis fetalis**. As the process of rapid destruction of the red blood cells continues, anemia develops. If the anemia is severe enough, heart failure and death of the fetus in utero may result.

Treatment. All expectant mothers should have their blood tested for blood group and Rh type at the initial prenatal visit. If the woman is found to be Rh negative, she should then be followed closely throughout her pregnancy.* At periodic intervals, she should have blood titers performed as a screening method to detect the presence of anti-

---

* The father's blood also should be typed, and if he is Rh positive, a genotype may be done to determine if he is homozygous or heterozygous.

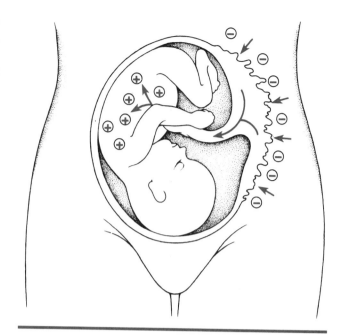

Figure 6-12. In Rh incompatibility, antibodies from the mother enter the child and begin destroying its blood cells.

bodies. This allows the attending physician to evaluate the health of the fetus and plan for the infant's delivery and care.

When titers show the presence of antibodies, the physician then tries to determine how much the fetus is affected. Because there is no direct way to sample the fetus' blood to find out the degree of anemia, indirect means must be used. Diagnosis may be made through the use of **amniocentesis**. By inserting a needle into the amniotic sac, 10 to 15 mL of amniotic fluid is removed. The fluid is sent to the laboratory for spectrophotometric analysis, which shows the amount of bile pigments (bilirubin) in the amniotic fluid. Thus, it can be determined if the fetus is mildly, moderately, or severely affected.

If analysis of the amniotic fluid shows that the fetus is severely affected, the obstetrician will either perform an intrauterine transfusion of Rh-negative blood or, if the fetus is beyond 32 weeks' gestation, induce labor or perform cesarean delivery. After delivery, the baby is turned over to a pediatrician, who will arrange for exchange transfusions.

Prevention. The dramatic reduction in the incidence of erythroblastosis fetalis is due largely to the introduction of RhoGAM. It is effective only in mothers who do not have Rh antibodies, and it must be injected into the mother within 72 hours after delivery of an Rh-positive infant or after abortion of an Rh-positive fetus. Most obstetricians also give the mother an injection of RhoGAM in the 28th week of pregnancy to prevent any sensitization occurring during the pregnancy. RhoGAM essentially neutralizes any Rh-positive cells that may have escaped into the mother's system, preventing isoimmunization. As mentioned earlier, RhoGAM also must be given to the Rh-negative mother after an abortion. It is *never* given to an infant or to a father.

The use of RhoGAM on all patients who are candidates for it offers the hope of eliminating hemolytic disease caused by Rh incompatibility. The criteria for giving RhoGAM are that

- The mother must be Rh negative.
- The mother must not be sensitized by an earlier pregnancy.
- The infant must be Rh positive.
- The direct Coombs' test, a test for antibodies performed on cord blood at delivery, is weakly reactive or negative.

Erythroblastosis Fetalis

Infants with known incompatibility to the mother's blood are examined carefully at birth for pallor, edema, jaundice, and an enlarged spleen and liver. In the instance of inadequate or absence of prenatal care, a severely affected infant may be stillborn or have **hydrops fetalis**, with extensive edema, marked anemia and jaundice, and enlargement of the liver and spleen. These babies are in critical condition and need exchange transfusions at the earliest possible moment.

The severely affected infants who are not treated are at risk of severe brain damage or kernicterus from excess bilirubin levels. Death occurs in about 75% of infants with kernicterus; those who survive may be mentally retarded or develop spastic paralysis or nerve deafness. Exchange transfusions are given at once to those infants who have signs of neurologic damage when first seen, although there is no proof that the damage is reversible. Fortunately, current ability to detect and treat hemolytic disease has reduced the number of infants who become permanently damaged to just a few.

A severely affected newborn usually is transfused without waiting for laboratory confirmation. All other suspected infants have a sample of cord blood sent to the laboratory for a Coombs' test for the presence of damaging antibodies, Rh and ABO typing, hemoglobin and red blood cell levels, and measurement of plasma bilirubin. A positive direct Coombs' test indicates the presence of antibodies on the surface of the infant's red blood cells. A negative direct Coombs' test indicates that there are no antibodies on the infant's red blood cells.

Treatment. A positive Coombs' test indicates presence of the disease but not the degree of severity. If bilirubin and hemoglobin levels are within normal limits, the infant is watched carefully; frequent laboratory blood tests are performed. A nurse may perform a microbilirubin screening doing a heel stick and using specialized equipment in the nursery. Phototherapy also may be ordered (see ear-

lier section). Exchange transfusions are performed at the discretion of the physician. The infant is cared for in a NICU.

Any infant admitted to the newborn nursery should be examined for jaundice during the first 36 hours or more. The nurse must keep in mind that early development of jaundice (within the first 24 to 48 hours) is a probable indication of hemolytic disease.

Infants whose bilirubin has been restored to normal levels may be discharged to routine home care like any well newborn. The nurse should be sensitive to the parents' feelings of guilt and anxiety. They may feel that they caused the condition and need to ventilate their feelings. They never must be made to feel that they are responsible for the condition.

ABO Incompatibility

The major blood groups are A, B, AB, and O, and each has antigens that may be incompatible with those of another group. The most common incompatibility in the newborn occurs between an infant with type O blood and a mother with type A or B. Although the reactions are usually less severe than in Rh incompatibility, the clinical manifestations are similar, including jaundice and enlarged liver and spleen, but usually without severe anemia. Treatment is also similar; however, no preventive measures exist.

The Infant with Neonatal Sepsis

Newborns are at increased risk for infections because their immune systems are immature and they are not able to localize infections. High-risk infants are even more susceptible than normal newborns. A primary responsibility of the nursing staff is to prevent infection in these high-risk infants. Infections may be acquired prenatally from the mother (through the placenta), during the intrapartum period (during labor and delivery) from maternal vaginal infection or inhalation of contaminated amniotic fluid, and after birth from cross contamination with other infants, health care personnel, or contaminated equipment. The newborn often does not have any specific signs of illness. A variety of signs such as cyanosis, pallor, thermal instability (difficulty keeping temperature within normal range), convulsions, lethargy, apnea, jaundice, or just "not looking right" may be the clue that alerts the nurse to possible problems. Treatment consists of intensive antibiotic therapy, intravenous fluids, respiratory therapy, and other supportive measures.

The Infant with Necrotizing Enterocolitis

Necrotizing enterocolitis (NEC), an acute inflammatory disease of the intestine, occurs most often in small preterm infants, but it may occur in full-term neonates. The cause is not clearly defined. Precipitating factors are hypoxia causing poor **tissue perfusion** (filling with blood) to the bowel, bacterial invasion of the bowel, and feedings of formula that provide material on which bacterial enzymes can work.

Clinical manifestations are distention of the abdomen, return of more than 2 mL of undigested formula when the gastric contents are aspirated before a feeding, and occult blood in the stool. NEC usually occurs within the first 10 days of life. Diagnosis is confirmed by abdominal radiographs of the abdomen.

Treatment begins with the discontinuation of oral feedings, nasogastric suction, and intravenous fluids and antibiotics. There is danger of rupture of a necrotic area causing peritonitis. A temporary colostomy may be needed to relieve the obstruction, and surgical removal of the necrotic bowel may be necessary.

The infant suffering from NEC is gravely ill and must be cared for in a NICU.

The Postterm Infant

When pregnancy lasts longer than 42 weeks, the infant is considered to be postterm, or postmature, regardless of birth weight. Approximately 12% of all infants are postterm, and the causes of delayed birth are not known. Some have an appearance similar to term infants, but others look like infants 1 to 3 weeks old. Little lanugo or vernix remains, scalp hair is abundant, and fingernails are long. The skin is dry, cracked, wrinkled, peeling, and whiter than that of the normal newborn. The infants have little subcutaneous fat, and they appear long and thin.

These infants are threatened by failing placental function and are at risk for intrauterine hypoxia during labor and delivery. It is customary, therefore, for the physician or nurse midwife to induce labor or perform a cesarean delivery when the baby is markedly overdue. Many physicians believe that pregnancy should be terminated by the end of 42 weeks.

Often, the postterm infant has expelled meconium in utero. At birth, the meconium may be aspirated into the lungs, obstructing the respiratory passages and irritating the lungs, which may lead to pneumonia. Whenever meconium-stained amniotic fluid is detected in any delivery, oral and nasopharyngeal suctioning often is performed as soon as the head is born. After delivery, gastric lavage also may be performed to remove any meconium swallowed and to prevent aspiration of vomitus.

The Infant of a Human Immunodeficiency Virus–Positive Mother

The newborn of a human immunodeficiency virus (HIV)–positive mother may not show any signs of infection at birth and appears much the same as any other newborn. HIV may be transmitted to the fetus across the placenta, from the mother's body fluids during birth, or through breast milk. If the mother is known to be positive for HIV, she should not breastfeed her newborn. The infant's test results are positive for HIV antibodies for as long as 15 months because they have passively acquired antibodies from the mother. Only 20% to 40% of infants born to known HIV-infected mothers are infected themselves.[1] Signs of HIV infection usually are not seen in infants younger than 4 to 6 months of age, and by 1 year of age, about half of those who are infected are symptomatic. By 2 years of age, most HIV-infected infants become symptomatic. Prognosis is poor for infants who have symptoms before 1 year of age and those who develop *Pneumocystis carinii* pneumonia. Bacterial infections, such as pneumonia, meningitis, and bacteremia, are common in infected newborns. These infants also commonly have thrush, mouth sores, and severe diaper rash. Gloves must be worn by personnel when they are performing the first bath on every newborn. Gloves also must be worn by the nurse when performing any procedure in which the nurse could be exposed to blood or body fluids that may contain blood (see Chapter 17 for further discussion of HIV-infected children).

The Infant of an Addicted Mother

As mentioned in Chapter 4, alcohol is one of the many teratogenic substances that crosses the placenta to the infant. No amount of alcohol is believed to be safe, and women who plan to become pregnant are advised to stop drinking at least 3 months before they plan to become pregnant. Fetal alcohol syndrome (FAS) is often apparent in infants of mothers with chronic alcoholism and sometimes in those whose mothers who are low to moderate consumers of alcohol. The ability of the mother's liver to detoxify the alcohol is apparently of greater importance than the actual amount consumed. FAS is characterized by low birth weight, smaller height and head circumference, short palpebral fissures (eyelid folds), reduced ocular growth, and a flattened nasal bridge. These infants are prone to respiratory difficulties, hypoglycemia, hypocalcemia, and hyperbilirubinemia. Their growth continues to be slow and their mental development retarded, despite expert care and nutrition.

Infants of mothers addicted to cocaine, heroin, methadone, or other narcotics are born addicted, and many of those infants suffer withdrawal symptoms during the early neonatal period. These symptoms include tremors, restlessness, hyperactivity, disorganized reflexes, increased muscle tone, sneezing, tachypnea, and a shrill cry. Ineffective sucking and swallowing reflexes create feeding problems, and regurgitation and vomiting occur often after feeding. Typical treatment is the administration of chlorpromazine, diazepam, paregoric, or phenobarbital intramuscularly, orally, or both. Many of these babies respond favorably to movement and close body contact with their caregivers; therefore, some nurseries place the infants in special carriers that hold them close to the nurse's chest while moving about the nursery. **Swaddling** (wrapping securely in a small blanket) the infant with arms across the chest also is recommended as a method of quieting the agitated infant.

Unfortunately, identifying the pregnant woman who abuses alcohol or drugs may be difficult. Many of these women do not have prenatal care or have only periodic care. They may not keep appointments because of apathy or simply because they are not awake during the day but rather stay awake at night. As a result, many of these infants have suffered prenatal insults that result in intrauterine growth retardation, congenital abnormalities, and premature birth. (For further discussion of the problems of drug abuse, see Chapters 17 and 18).

The Death of a Fetus or Newborn

When a child dies, either before birth or in the first weeks after birth, parents are faced with the crisis of mourning someone they never had a chance to know. They had expected a joyous event; they experienced a devastating loss. Nurses who work with these families need to understand the grieving process and their own feelings about death to help parents cope with this crisis.

Mothers sometimes are aware that the fetus is dead long before any signs of labor appear, yet many mothers deny that something could be wrong until they are informed by their physicians. Parents, particularly the mothers of a stillborn infant or one who dies immediately after birth, may need to see and touch the infant to accept the reality of the infant's death. This is an issue that should be decided by each parent *individually*, after discussing it with the nurse, physician, social worker, or pastoral counselor. Before seeing the infant, parents need to be prepared for the infant's appearance—the temperature, color, size, and any deformities or bruises. The mother must be able to mourn this baby as a real person, without such well-meaning comments such as "You can have another baby," comments that deny this baby as an individual.

Many maternity units have set procedures in which photos are taken of the infant. Parents are given the opportunity to hold their infant in a private manner. Memory books with footprints, bracelets, locks of hair, and photos are given to the parents. If the parents do not want these mementos at the time of delivery, they are kept for a period (sometimes for 5 years) and are available for the parents whenever they choose. Parents are encouraged to name the child to add to the reality of the life. Both parents need to feel that the nurse has the time and interest to listen and that it is important for them to express their feelings. Attempts to cheer them up do not aid the grieving process but strike a note of insincerity and

insensitivity. Nurses need to know that it is all right for them to grieve with the parents, to touch or hold them, and to cry with them.

The crisis of stillbirth or neonatal death is another instance when parent support groups may be effective. No one is able to better understand the feelings and problems of this tragic situation than parents who have lived through it and managed to rebuild their lives. They are proof that life can go on, even though it seems impossible at the time of crisis. Compassionate Friends and SHARE are two support groups with chapters throughout the United States and Canada. Most maternity units have information about and may make referrals to support groups that are locally active. In addition, parents who have previously experienced such a loss sometimes volunteer to contact these families to provide personal support. These people often provide the maternity nurses with their phone number so that they may be contacted when their support is desired.

The mother whose infant dies often questions, "Why me?" "What did I do wrong?" "It's not fair." The family may be upset and confused. Nurses often have difficulty facing their own feelings about the death of a newborn. One of the most important aspects of caring for the parent whose newborn has died is to provide the parent with the opportunity to talk about the death. Friends and other relatives may try to talk about everything else to distract the parents, but often their need to talk is great. The nurse may say, "Do you want to talk about your baby?" The nurse must be careful to use active listening techniques and avoid pat reassurances. It does hurt; it is devastating; it is overwhelming. The parents need to be allowed to express these feelings in a nonjudgmental atmosphere, and the nurse can encourage this outpouring.

Summary

The high-risk infant starts extrauterine life with many problems, regardless of the cause for the high-risk classification. Breathing, feeding, and regulating temperature are difficult, if not impossible, for the infant without skilled medical and nursing intervention. A number of factors may have contributed to the infant's compromised condition, including prematurity, substance abuse or addiction, postmaturity, maternal conditions such as diabetes or HIV infection, and neonatal sepsis. The infant may need to be transported to a distant facility with a specialized NICU. The separation of the infant and the family and the concern for the infant's condition cause added stress for the family. In addition to the urgent need for skilled physical care, the infant has emotional needs that must be responded to with sensitivity. The infant's family also must be counseled and supported to deal with this crisis. If the infant survives, the family may need long-term support and assistance in caring for the infant after discharge. In the event of the infant's death, the family needs care, understanding, guidance, and support in mourning their loss.

Review Questions

1. Describe the appearance of the preterm (premature) infant.
2. What is missing in the lungs of the newborn who has RDS? What treatment is helpful in RDS?
3. What specific treatment may be used to try to prevent RDS? Explain the theory behind this treatment.
4. Why is cold stress dangerous for the high-risk newborn?
5. What is the most essential practice for infection control in the care of the high-risk infant?
6. What are some indications that the gavage-fed infant is ready to start nipple feeding?
7. Mike sees his baby daughter under the phototherapy lights for the first time. He is very upset and demands to know why her eyes are covered. What explanation will you give him about the treatment and about the eye covering?
8. How does the nurse conserve the energy of the premature infant?
9. In which ways can the nurse help the parents of a preterm infant?
10. Your friend Kati, a diabetic, tells you that she has decided that she is ready to start a family and is planning to get pregnant. What advice will you give her that will help ensure a healthy baby?
11. Describe the neonate whose mother has diabetes mellitus.
12. Sue is Rh negative and pregnant with her first baby. The father of her baby is Rh positive. She asks you why she needs to have RhoGAM. How will you explain to her how RhoGAM works?
13. Teenager Carla admits to drinking at parties. She is pregnant now. What can you tell her that will help her understand the impact of drinking on her unborn child?
14. What are the characteristics of fetal alcohol syndrome?
15. What are the symptoms of narcotic withdrawal in the neonate?
16. How can the nurse help the parents after delivery of a stillborn or when an infant dies soon after birth?
17. Inquire at the facility in which you have your clinical experience in maternity care to determine the procedure used when a neonatal death takes place.

Reference

1. Lambert J. Maternal issues regarding HIV infection. Pediatr Ann 19(7):468, 1991.

Bibliography

Bell J, Esterling LS. What Will I Tell The Children? Child Life Department. Omaha: University of Nebraska Medical Center, and Meyer Children's Rehabilitation Institute, 1986.

Bradford LS. Pediatric Aids in Nurse Review, Vol 3. Springhouse, PA: Springhouse Corporation, 1989.

Carlson GE. Retinopathy of prematurity: Nursing interventions. Pediatr Nurs 17(4):348–351, 1991.

Carpenito LJ. Handbook of Nursing Diagnosis, 4th ed. Philadelphia: JB Lippincott, 1991.

Castiglia PT, Harbin RE. Child Health Care: Process and Practice. Philadelphia: JB Lippincott, 1992.

Chasnoff IJ. Cocaine and pregnancy. Childbirth Educator 4: 37–42, 1987.

Gennaro S, Zukowsky K, Brooten D, et al. Concerns of mothers of low–birth weight infants. Pediatr Nurs 16(5):459–462, 1990.

Green A. Intravenous immunoglobulin for neonates. MCN 16(4): 208–211, 1991.

Heery K. Getting high-risk infants out of the hospital. RN 54(6): 58, 1991.

Hill AS, Cochran CK, Dickerson C. Nursing care of the infant with erythroblastosis fetalis. J Pediatr Nurs 4(6):395–402, 1989.

Jacques JT, Snyder N. Newborn victims of addiction. RN 54(4): 47–52, 1991.

Kelley SJ, Walsh JH, Thompson K. Birth outcomes, health problems, and neglect with prenatal exposure to cocaine. Pediatr Nurs 17(2): 130–135, 1991.

Ladden M. The impact of preterm birth on the family and society. I. Psychological sequelae of preterm birth. Pediatr Nurs 16(5): 515–518, 1990a.

Ladden M. The impact of preterm birth on the family and society. II. Transition to home. Pediatr Nurs 16(6):620, 1990b.

Long CA. Cryotherapy: A new treatment for retinopathy of prematurity. Pediatr Nurs 15(3):269–272, 1989.

Nolan ED. Infants at risk: A time for action. Pediatr Nurs 17(2): 175–178, 1991.

Pillitteri A. Maternal and Child Health Nursing. Philadelphia: JB Lippincott, 1992.

Read-Sisti D. A dream dies. MCN 15(4):258, 1990.

Ross T, Dickason EJ. Vertical transmission of HIV and HBV. MCN 17(4):193–195, 1992.

Schraeder BD, Heverly MA, Rappaport J. The value of early home assessment in identifying risk in children who were very low birth weight. Pediatr Nurs 16(3):268–273, 1990.

Small M, Engler AJ, Rushton CH. Saying goodbye in the intensive care unit: Helping caregivers grieve. Pediatr Nurs 17(1):103–105, 1991.

Whaley LF, Wong DL. Nursing Care of Infants and Children, 4th ed. St. Louis: Mosby-Year Book, 1991.

Wheeler SR, Limbo RK. Blue print for a perinatal bereavement support group. Pediatr Nurs 16(4):341, 1990.

The Newborn with Special Needs

Chapter 7

Student Objectives

Upon completion of this chapter, the student will be able to:

1. Differentiate between cleft lip and cleft palate.
2. Identify the early signs that indicate the presence of an esophageal fistula.
3. Name the greatest preoperative danger for infants with tracheoesophageal atresia.
4. List and describe the five types of hernias that infants have.
5. Differentiate the three types of spina bifida that may occur.
6. Name the type of spina bifida that is most difficult to treat, and state why it is.
7. Describe the two types of hydrocephalus that may occur.
8. State the most obvious symptoms of hydrocephalus.
9. Describe two types of shunting performed for hydrocephalus.
10. State the signs and symptoms of congestive heart failure in the child with congenital heart disease.
11. List five common types of congenital heart defects, and trace the blood flow of each defect, indicating if blood is oxygen poor or oxygen rich.
12. State the two most common skeletal deformities in the newborn.
13. Discuss the importance of early treatment for clubfoot.
14. List three signs and symptoms of congenital dislocation of the hip.
15. Describe the treatment for congenital dislocation of the hip.
16. Describe congenital rubella, and discuss its prevention.
17. State the cause of gonorrheal ophthalmia neonatorum.
18. State the effect of herpes simplex virus on the newborn.
19. Identify the test to detect phenylketonuria in the newborn.
20. Describe the treatment for phenylketonuria.
21. Name the tests performed on newborns to detect congenital hypothyroidism.
22. State the one serious outcome that is common to untreated conditions of phenylketonuria, congenital hypothyroidism, and galactosemia.

Marks MG: BROADRIBB'S INTRODUCTORY PEDIATRIC NURSING, 4th ed. © 1994 J.B. Lippincott Company.

Key Terms

atresia	overriding aorta
bilateral	phenylketonuria
chordee	pulmonary stenosis
congenital hip dysplasia	right ventricular hypertrophy
congestive heart failure	spina bifida
cyanotic heart disease	supernumerary
ductus arteriosus	talipes equinovarus
ductus venosus	unilateral
foramen ovale	ventricular septal defect
galactosemia	ventriculoatrial shunting
hernia	ventriculoperitoneal shunting
hypothermia	
imperforate anus	
interstitial keratitis	

*L*ike other high-risk infants, the birth of an infant with a congenital defect or birth injury represents a crisis for parents and caregivers. Depending on the defect, immediate or early surgery may be necessary. Early, continuous skilled observation and highly skilled nursing care are required. Rehabilitation of the infant and education of the family caregivers in the care of the infant are essential. The emotional needs of the infant and the family must be integrated into the plans for nursing care. Many of these infants will have a brighter future as a result of increased diagnostic and medical knowledge and advances in surgical techniques.

Family caregivers experience a grief response whether the infant's defect is a result of injury at birth or of abnormal intrauterine development. They mourn the loss of the perfect child of their dreams, question why it happened, and possibly wonder how they will show the infant to family and friends without shame or embarrassment.

This grief may interfere with the process of parent–infant attachment. Parents need to understand that their response is normal and that they are entitled to honest answers to their questions about the infant's condition. Other children in the family should be informed gently but honestly about the infant and should be allowed to visit the infant accompanied by adult family members. Care must be taken to devote sufficient time and attention to the older siblings to avoid jealousy toward the infant.

Congenital Anomalies

Congenital anomalies may be caused by genetic or environmental factors. These anomalies include facial deformities, such as cleft lip and palate, and defects of the gastrointestinal, central nervous, cardiovascular, skeletal, and genitourinary systems. Defects such as the facial deformities and severe neural tube defects are apparent at birth, but others may be discovered only after a complete physical examination. Congenital anomalies account for a large percentage of the health problems seen in infants and children.

Facial Deformities

The birth of an infant with a facial deformity may change the atmosphere of the delivery from one of joyous anticipation to one of awkward tension. The most common facial malformations, cleft lip and cleft palate, occur either alone or in combination. Cleft lip occurs in about 1 in 1000 live births and is more frequent in males. Cleft palate occurs in 1 in 25,000, more frequently in females. Its cause is not entirely clear; it appears to be genetically influenced but does occur in isolated instances with no genetic history.

Cleft Lip and Palate

Parents and family are naturally eager to see and hold their newborn infant and must be prepared for the shock of seeing the disfigurement of a cleft lip. Their emotional reaction to such an obvious malformation is usually much greater than to a "hidden" defect such as congenital heart disease. They need encouragement and support as well as considerable instruction about the feeding and care of this infant. The child born with a cleft palate (but with an intact lip) does not have the external disfigurement that may be so distressing to the new parent, but the problems are more serious. Although a cleft lip and a cleft palate often appear together, either defect may appear alone. In embryonic development, the palate closes at a later time than does the lip, and the failure to close occurs for different reasons.

The cleft lip and palate defects result from failure of the maxillary and premaxillary processes to fuse during the fifth to eighth week of intrauterine life. The cleft may be a simple notch in the vermilion line, or it may extend up into the floor of the nose (Figure 7-1). It may be either **unilateral** (one side of the lip) or **bilateral** (both sides). Cleft palate occurs with a cleft lip about 50% of the time, most often with bilateral cleft lip. Cleft palate, which develops sometime between the 7th and 12th weeks of gestation, often is accompanied by nasal deformity and dental disorders such as deformed, missing, or **supernumerary** (excessive in number) teeth.

When the embryo is about 8 weeks old, there is still no roof to the mouth: the tissues that are to become the palate are two shelves running from the front to the back of the mouth and projecting vertically downward on either side of the tongue. The shelves move from a vertical position to a horizontal position, their free edges meeting and fusing in midline. Later, bone forms within this tissue to form the hard palate.

Normally, the palate is intact by the 10th week of fetal life. Exactly what happens to prevent this closure is not known with certainty. It occurs more frequently in near relatives of people with the defect than in the general population, and there appears to be some evidence that environmental and hereditary factors may each play a part in this defect.

Clinical Manifestations and Diagnosis. The physical appearance of the infant sufficiently confirms the diagnosis of cleft lip. Diagnosis of cleft palate is made at birth with the close inspection of the newborn's palate. To be certain that a cleft palate is not missed, the examiner must insert a gloved finger into the newborn's mouth to feel the palate to determine that it is intact. If a cleft is found, consultation is set up with a clinic specializing in cleft palate repair.

Treatment. Surgery, usually performed by a plastic surgeon, is a major part of the treatment of a child with a cleft lip, palate, or both. Total care involves many other specialists, including pediatricians, nurses, orthodontists, prosthodontists, otolaryngologists, speech therapists, and occasionally, psychiatrists. Long-term, intensive, multidisciplinary care is needed for infants with major defects.

Plastic surgeons' opinions differ as to the best time for repair of the cleft lip. Some surgeons are in favor of early repair, before the infant is discharged from the hospital, believing that they can alleviate some of the family's feelings of rejection of the infant; other surgeons prefer to wait until the infant is 1 or 2 months old, weighs about 10 lb, and is increasing steadily in weight. Infants who are not born in large medical centers with specialists on the staff are discharged from the birth hospital and referred to a center or physician specializing in cleft lip and palate repair.

If early surgery is contemplated, the infant should be healthy and of average or above average weight. The infant also must be observed constantly because a newborn has greater difficulty dealing with excess mucus than does an older infant. These infants must be cared for by competent plastic surgeons and experienced nurses.

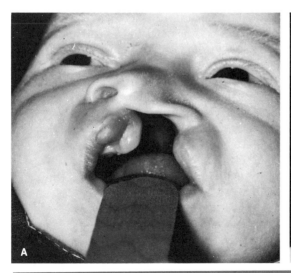 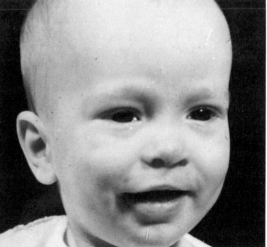

Figure 7-1. **A**, A 2-week-old infant with unilateral cleft lip. **B**, Same child at age 14 months, showing surgical repair. (From Pillitteri A. An introduction to clinical embryology. Chicago: Year Book, 1974.)

The goal in repairing the cleft palate is to give the child a union of the cleft parts that would allow intelligible and pleasant speech and to avoid injury to the maxillary growth. The timing of cleft palate repair is individualized, according to the size, placement, and degree of deformity. The surgery may need to be done in stages over several years to achieve the best results. The optimal time for surgery to repair the cleft palate is considered to be between the ages of 6 months and 5 years. Because the child is not able to make certain sounds when starting to talk, undesirable speech habits are formed that are difficult to correct. If surgery must be delayed beyond the third year, a dental speech appliance may help the child develop intelligible speech.

Nursing Process for the Infant with Cleft Lip and Palate

ASSESSMENT

One of the primary concerns in the nursing care of the infant with a cleft lip, with or without a cleft palate, is the emotional care of the infant's family. Assessment of the infant must include exploration of the family's acceptance of the infant. The nurse must practice active listening with reflective responses, accept the family's emotional responses, and demonstrate complete acceptance of the infant.

The family caregivers who return to the hospital with the young infant for the beginning repair of a cleft palate already have been faced with the challenges of feeding their infant. The nurse should conduct a thorough interview with the caregivers, including the methods they found to be most effective in feeding their infant.

Physical assessment of the infant includes temperature, apical pulse, and respirations. The nurse must listen to breath sounds to detect any pulmonary congestion. Skin turgor and color are evaluated, noting any deviations from the normal state. Neurologic assessment, alertness, and responsiveness also are noted. An assessment and description of the cleft are documented.

NURSING DIAGNOSES

Formulation of nursing diagnoses depends partly on the timing of the initial cleft lip surgery. If the infant is to be discharged from the hospital before surgery, the nursing diagnoses are directed to the emotional care of the family and the feeding and nutrition of the infant. If the newborn is to have lip repair surgery before discharge, nursing diagnoses also include the preoperative aspects. The nursing diagnosis is based in part on the operative plans.

Nursing diagnoses for the newborn infant may include the following:

- High risk for inadequate nutrition: less than body requirements related to inability to suck secondary to cleft lip

- High risk for inadequate bonding related to visible physical defect
- Anxiety of family caregivers related to lack of knowledge about surgery

Before admission for either cleft lip or palate repair, the infant should be gradually accustomed to elbow restraints. Some preoperative and postoperative nursing diagnoses applicable to the infant admitted for surgical repair may include the following:

- High risk for aspiration related to a reduced level of consciousness postoperatively
- Ineffective breathing pattern related to anatomic changes
- High risk for fluid volume deficit related to NPO status postoperatively
- Altered nutrition: less than body requirements related to difficulty in feeding postoperatively
- High risk of injury to the operative site related to infant's desire to suck thumb or fingers and anatomic changes
- High risk for altered oral mucous membranes related to surgical incision
- High risk for infection related to postoperative period
- Pain related to surgical procedure
- High risk for altered growth and development related to hospitalizations and surgery
- Anxiety related to physical restraints
- Family caregivers' health-seeking behaviors related to long-term aspects of cleft palate

PLANNING AND IMPLEMENTATION: PREOPERATIVE CARE

Planning and implementation must be modified to adapt to the surgical plans. If the infant is to be discharged from the birth hospital to have surgery a month or two later, the nurse may focus on preparing the family to care for the infant at home and help the family cope with their emotions. The major nursing goals include teaching the family adequate methods of feeding the infant, reducing the parental guilt and anxiety regarding the infant's physical defect, and preparing for the future repair of the cleft lip and cleft palate.

Assuring Adequate Nutrition. The nutritional condition of the infant is important to the planning of surgery because the infant must be in good condition before surgery can be scheduled. Feeding the infant with a cleft lip before repair is a challenge. The procedure may be time consuming and tedious. The infant's ability to suck is inadequate, making feeding difficult. Breastfeeding may be successful because the breast tissue may mold to close the gap. If the infant is unable to breastfeed, the mother's breast milk may be expressed and used instead of formula until after the surgical repair is healed. Use of various nipples may be tried to find the method that works best for the individual infant. A soft nipple with a crosscut made to promote easy flow of milk or formula may work well. Lamb's nipples (extra-long nipples) have been used with success, as well as specialized cleft palate nipples that are molded to fit into the open palate area to close the gap. Perhaps one of the simplest and most effective methods is the use of an eye dropper or an asepto syringe with a short piece of rubber tubing on the tip (Breck feeder). The dropper or syringe, when carefully used, drips formula into the infant's mouth at a rate slow enough to allow the infant to swallow. As the infant learns to eat, much coughing, sputtering, and choking may occur. The nurse or family caregiver feeding the infant must be alert for signs of aspiration.

Whatever feeding method is used, the experience may be frustrating for both the feeder and the infant. Family caregivers who will be involved in caring for the infant after discharge should have an opportunity to practice the feeding techniques under the supervision of the nurse. During the teaching process, the caregivers need ample opportunity to ask questions and be reassured that they are able to adequately care for the infant (see Parent Teaching Tips for Cleft Palate).

Promoting Family Coping. The family of the infant must be encouraged to verbalize their feelings regarding the defect and their disappointment. The nurse must convey to the family that their feelings are acceptable and normal. While caring for the infant, the nurse must demonstrate behavior that clearly displays acceptance of the infant. The nurse has a responsibility to serve as a model for the family caregivers' attitudes toward the child.

Reducing Family Anxiety. Family caregivers should be given information about cleft repairs. Pamphlets are available that present photographs of before-and-after corrections that will answer some of their questions. They should be encouraged to ask questions and be reassured that any question is valid. The families of infants with cleft palates (with or without cleft lips) will have had a lot of information provided to them before the infant is actually admitted for repair, but all families need additional support throughout such a procedure. The usual routine of preoperative, intraoperative, and postoperative care is explained. Written information is helpful, but the nurse must be certain that the parents understand the information. Simple things, such as showing them where they may wait while their baby is in surgery, how long the surgery should last, the postanesthesia care unit (PACU) procedure, and where the surgeon will expect to find them to report on the surgery are important (see Nursing Care Plan for the Infant with Cleft Lip/Palate).

PLANNING AND IMPLEMENTATION: POSTOPERATIVE CARE

Major nursing goals for the postoperative care of the infant who is hospitalized for surgical repair of cleft lip or palate include preventing aspiration, easing respiratory effort,

Parent Teaching
Cleft Lip/Cleft Palate

1. Sucking is important to speech development.
2. Holding the baby upright while feeding helps avoid choking.
3. Burp the baby frequently, because a lot of air is swallowed during feeding.
4. Don't tire the baby. Limit feeding times to 20 to 30 minutes maximum. If necessary, feed the baby more often.
5. Feed strained foods from the side of the spoon in small amounts, slowly.
6. Don't be alarmed if food seeps through cleft and out nose.
7. Have baby's ears checked any time he or she has a cold or upper respiratory infection.
8. Talk normally to baby (no "baby" talk). Talk a lot, repeat baby's babbling and cooing. This helps in speech development.
9. Try to understand early talking without trying to correct baby.
10. Good mouth care is a must.
11. Early dental care is essential to observe teething and prevent caries.

preventing injury to the surgical site, preventing infection, relieving pain, and increasing the family caregivers' knowledge about the long-term care of the child.

Preventing Aspiration. After a cleft lip repair, the infant may be positioned on his or her side to facilitate drainage of mucus and secretions. In the case of a cleft palate repair, the infant may be positioned on his or her side or abdomen postoperatively to aid in the drainage of mucus and secretions. The infant must be closely watched in the immediate postoperative period. Nothing should be put into the infant's mouth to clear mucus because of the danger of damage to the surgical site, particularly in the case of a palate repair.

Improving Respiratory Function. Immediately after a palate repair, the infant needs to change from a mouth-breathing pattern to nasal breathing. This change may frustrate the infant, but if positioned to ease breathing and given encouragement, the infant should be able to adjust quickly.

Monitoring Fluid Volume. In the immediate postoperative period, the infant needs to have parenteral fluids. All the precautions, including placement, discoloration of the site, swelling, and flow rate, should be checked every 2 hours. Documentation of intake and output levels and use of restraints are necessary. Paren-

Nursing Diagnosis

High risk for altered nutrition: less than body requirements related to inability to suck effectively secondary to cleft lip

Goal: *Maintain adequate food and fluid intake*

Nursing Interventions	Rationale	Evaluation
Try a variety of feeding methods to find the one that works best for this infant.	The cleft lip anomaly varies from infant to infant, and there is no one technique that works best for all; it is essential, however, to find the appropriate feeding method so that the infant does not become malnourished.	Infant ingests at least 50 cal/lb in 24 hours and loses no more than 10% of birth weight.

Nursing Diagnosis

High risk for altered parenting related to visible physical defect

Goal: *Encourage Parent–Infant Bonding*

Nursing Interventions	Rationale	Evaluation
Encourage caregivers to verbalize their feelings regarding their child's defect and convey to them that these feelings are acceptable.	Caregivers need the opportunity to express their disappointment to each other before facing family and friends outside the hospital; recognizing that such feelings are normal will help them to begin to deal with their emotions in a healthy way and begin the bonding process.	Caregivers talk about child's defect with each other and ask questions regarding their child's care.
Encourage caregivers to interact with infant through feeding and holding and simple care measures.	The more caregivers interact with their infant, the more they will grow accustomed to the defect, which will allow them to get to know their child's other characteristics.	Caregivers look at infant's face while feeding and begin to talk about their child's personality or other physical traits.

Nursing Diagnosis

Anxiety of parents related to lack of knowledge about surgery

Goal: *Reduce parental anxiety*

Nursing Interventions	Rationale	Evaluation
Provide caregivers with written and oral information about cleft repair.	Explaining the procedure in person allows the caregivers to ask questions and express concerns; later, when they've had time to digest some of the information, they can consult the written material for specifics—and go back to the nurse with more questions, if necessary. Also by explaining things in person, the nurse is able to determine whether the information has actually been understood.	Family caregivers ask questions about the surgery and postoperative care procedures. Caregivers state correctly what they expect from the procedure in terms of timing and surgical results.

teral fluids are continued until the infant is able to take oral fluids without nausea.

Maintaining Adequate Nutrition. As soon as the infant is no longer nauseated (vomiting must be avoided if possible), the surgeon usually permits clear liquids.

If the infant does not have a cleft lip, or if the lip has had an early repair, sucking may be learned more easily even though the suction generated is not as good as in the infant with an intact palate. A large nipple, with holes that allow the milk to drip freely, makes sucking easier for this baby. Sucking is an important activity for the development of speech muscles, therefore it should be encouraged. If the cleft is unilateral, the nipple should be aimed at the nonaffected side.

In the case of an infant who has had a palate repair, no nipples, spoons, or straws are permitted, just a drinking glass or cup. A favorite cup from home may be reassuring to the infant. Clear liquids such as flavored gelatin water, apple juice, and synthetic fruit-flavored drinks are offered. No red juices should be given because they may conceal bleeding. Usually, infants do not like broth. The diet is increased to full liquid, and the infant usually is discharged on a soft diet. Foods such as cooked infant cereals, ice cream, and flavored gelatin are often favorites with infants when they are allowed them. The surgeon determines the progression of the diet. Nothing hard or sharp should be placed in the infant's mouth.

Preventing Postoperative Injury. Continuous, skilled observation is essential. Swollen mouth tissues cause an excessive secretion of mucus that is poorly handled by a small infant. For the first few postoperative hours, the infant must *never* be left alone because aspiration of mucus occurs quickly and easily. Because it is necessary to keep anything from the infant's mouth, elbow restraints are necessary because that "beloved thumb" (or finger) is included in the things that may not go in the mouth. The thumb, although comforting, may quickly undo the repair or cause scarring along the suture line, which is not desirable. On this occasion, the infant's ultimate happiness and well-being must take precedence over immediate satisfaction. Therefore, elbow restraints must be properly applied and checked frequently (see Figure 2-9 in Chapter 2). Made with canvas and tongue blades, these restraints are tied firmly around the arm and pinned to the infant's shirt or gown to prevent them from sliding down below the elbow. The infant's arms can move freely but cannot bend at the elbows to reach the face. The restraints must be applied snugly but not allowed to hinder circulation. The older infant may need to be placed in a jacket restraint. Every effort must be made to prevent the infant with a lip repair from crying to prevent excessive tension on the suture line.

Restraints must be removed at least every 4 hours but should be removed only one at a time, and the released arm must be controlled so that the thumb or fingers do not "pop" into the mouth. The infant needs to be comforted, and additional means of comforting should be explored.

Talking to the infant continuously while caring for him or her and playing "Peek-a-Boo" and other baby games that divert ("Patty Cake" does not work well with elbow restraints) may be helpful. The skin should be inspected and massaged, lotion applied, and range of motion exercises performed. Restraints are replaced when they become soiled.

Promoting Healing. Gentle mouth care with tepid water or clear liquid may be recommended to follow the infant feeding. This care helps clean the suture area of any food or liquids to promote a cleaner incision for optimum healing.

CARE OF LIP SUTURE LINE. The lip suture line is left uncovered after surgery and must be kept meticulously clean and dry to prevent infection with subsequent scarring. A wire bow called a Logan bar or a butterfly closure is applied across the upper lip and attached to the cheeks with adhesive tape to prevent tension on the sutures caused by crying or other facial movement (Figure 7-2). The sutures are carefully cleaned after feeding and as often as necessary to prevent collection of dried formula or serum. Frequent cleaning is essential as long as the sutures are in place. The sutures are cleaned gently with sterile cotton swabs and saline or the solution of the surgeon's choice. An ointment such as bacitracin also may be ordered to be applied. Care of the suture line is of utmost importance because it has a direct effect on the cosmetic appearance of the repair. The family needs to be taught how to care for the suture line because the infant most likely will be discharged before the sutures are removed.

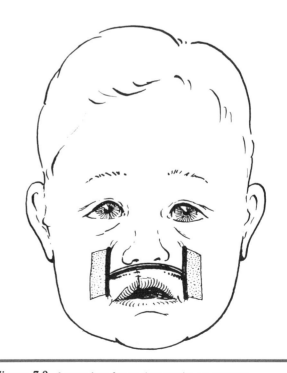

Figure 7-2. Logan bar for easing strain on sutures.

The sutures are removed 7 to 10 days after surgery. The infant probably will be allowed to suck on a soft nipple at this time. Following effective surgery and skilled, careful nursing care, the appearance of the baby's face should be greatly improved. The scar fades in time. Family caregivers need to know that the baby is probably going to need a slight adjustment of the vermilion line in later childhood, but they can expect a repair that is barely noticeable, if at all (Figure 7-3).

Preventing Infection. Aseptic technique is important throughout the care of the infant undergoing lip or palate repair. Good handwashing practices are essential, and the family caregivers should be instructed on the necessity for restriction of visiting by anyone with an upper respiratory infection. The caregivers of this infant must guard against any possible exposure to such a person. Observe for signs of otitis media that may occur from drainage into the eustachian tube.

Relieving Pain. The infant should be observed for signs of pain or discomfort from the surgery. Analgesics should be ordered for the infant and administered as needed. In addition to the desire to provide comfort for the infant, avoidance of crying is important because of the danger of disruption to the suture line.

Promoting Sensory Stimulation. The infant needs to have stimulating, safe toys in the crib. The nurse and family caregivers must use every opportunity to provide sensory stimulation. Talking to the infant, cuddling and holding him or her, and responding to the cries are all important interventions. Freedom from restraints within the limitations of safety must be provided. One caregiver should be assigned to provide stability and consistency of care. Family caregivers and health care personnel must encourage the older child to use speech and help enhance the child's self-esteem.

Providing Comfort Measures. The baby suffers emotional frustration because of the restraints, therefore satisfaction must be provided in other ways. Rocking, cuddling, and other soothing techniques are an important part of the nursing care. Family and other primary caregivers are the best people to supply this loving care.

Providing Family Teaching. Cleft lip and cleft palate centers provide teams of specialists who can give the services that the children and their families need through infancy, preschool, and school years. The caregivers should have information that explains the services of the pediatrician, plastic surgeon, orthodontist, speech therapist, nutritionist, and public health nurse. These professionals give explanations and counseling concerning the child's diet, speech training, immunizations, and general health. Family caregivers need to be encouraged to ask these people any questions they may have. The nurse must be alert to any evidence in conversation that the caregivers need additional information and arrange appropriate meetings.

Dental care for the child's deciduous teeth is of more than usual importance. The incidence of dental caries is high in children with a cleft palate, but the preservation of the deciduous teeth is important for the best results in speech as well as appearance.

EVALUATION

Outcome criteria for the preoperative infant include the following:

- The infant shows appropriate weight gain.
- The family demonstrates acceptance of the infant.
- The family asks appropriate questions about surgery and discusses their concerns.
- The family caregivers' level of anxiety is decreased, as evidenced by their cooperation with and confidence in the staff.

Outcome criteria for the postoperative infant include the following:

- No episodes of aspiration occur.
- The infant readjusts his or her breathing pattern with minimal frustration.
- Signs of adequate hydration are evident. There is no evidence of parenteral fluid infiltration.
- The infant retains and tolerates oral nutrition without nausea or vomiting; no red juices are given.

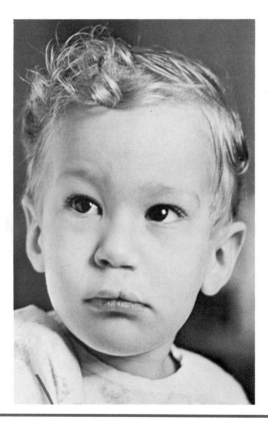

Figure 7-3. This child may need a revision of the vermilion line.

- The surgical site is not injured.
- The suture site is cleaned after each feeding.
- The infant remains infection free.
- The infant shows no signs of discomfort.
- The infant engages in age- and development-appropriate activities within the limits of restraints.
- The infant is content most of the time and responds appropriately to the caregiver and parents. The infant puts nothing into his or her mouth.
- The family caregivers' questions are answered promptly. The caregivers demonstrate an understanding of the infant's long-term treatment when responding to queries by the staff.

Digestive Tract Defects

Most digestive tract anomalies are apparent at birth or shortly thereafter. The anomalies are often the result of embryonic growth that was interrupted at a crucial stage. Many of these anomalies interfere with the normal nutrition and digestion that are essential to the normal growth and development of the infant. Many anomalies require immediate surgical intervention.

Esophageal Atresia

Atresia is the absence of a normal body opening or the abnormal closure of a body passage. **Esophageal atresia**, with or without fistula into the trachea, is a serious congenital anomaly and is among the most common anomalies causing respiratory distress. This condition occurs in about 1 in 2500 live births.

Although there are several types of esophageal atresia, more than 90% of them consist of the upper, or proximal, end of the esophagus ending in a blind pouch, with the lower, or distal, segment from the stomach connected to the trachea by a fistulous tract (Figure 7-4).

Clinical Manifestations and Diagnosis. Any mucus or fluid that an infant swallows goes into the blind pouch of the esophagus. This pouch soon fills and overflows, usually resulting in aspiration into the trachea. Few other conditions depend so greatly on careful nursing observation for early diagnosis and, therefore, improved chances of survival. The infant with this disorder has frothing and excessive drooling and periods of respiratory distress with choking and cyanosis. Many newborns have difficulty with mucus, but the nurse should be alert to the possibility of an anomaly and report such difficulties immediately. No feeding should be given until the infant has been examined.

If early signs are overlooked and feeding is attempted, the infant chokes, coughs, and regurgitates as the food enters the blind pouch. The newborn becomes deeply cyanotic and appears to be in severe respiratory distress. During this process, some of the formula may be aspirated, resulting in pneumonitis and making necessary surgery an increased hazard to the child. In a sense, this infant's life may depend on the careful observations of the nurse. If a fistula of the distal portion of the esophagus into the trachea exists, the infant is in danger of gastric contents refluxing into the lungs, causing a chemical pneumonitis.

Treatment. Surgical intervention is necessary to correct the defect. Timing of the surgery depends on the preference of the surgeon, the anomaly, and the condition of the infant. Aspiration of mucus must be prevented, and a continuous, gentle suction may be used. The infant needs intravenous fluids to maintain optimum hydration. The first stage of surgery may involve a gastrostomy and a method of draining the proximal esophageal pouch. A chest tube is inserted to drain chest fluids. An end-to-end anastomosis is sometimes possible. If the repair is complex, surgery may need to be done in stages.

Often these defects occur in premature infants; thus, additional factors may complicate the surgical repair and prognosis (Figure 7-5). If there are no other major problems, the long-term outcome should be good. Regular follow-up is necessary to observe for and dilate esophageal strictures that may be caused by scar tissue.

Imperforate Anus

In an infant with imperforate anus, the rectal pouch ends blindly at a distance above the anus, and there is no anal orifice. There may be a fistula between the rectum and the vagina in females or between the rectum and the urinary tract in males.

Early in intrauterine life, the membrane between the rectum and the anus should be absorbed, and a clear passage from the rectum to the anus should exist. If the membrane remains, blocking the union between the rectum and the anus, an **imperforate anus** results.

Diagnosis. In some newborn infants, only a dimple indicates the site of the anus (Figure 7-6**A**). When the initial rectal temperature is attempted, it is apparent that there is no anal opening. However, there may be a shallow opening in the anus, with the rectum ending in a blind pouch some distance higher (Figure 7-6**B**). For this reason, it is imperative to understand that the ability to pass a rectal thermometer into the rectum is not a reliable indication of a normal rectoanal canal.

More reliable presumptive evidence is obtained by watching carefully for the first meconium stool. If the infant does not pass a stool within the first 24 hours, the physician should be notified. Abdominal distention also occurs. Definitive diagnosis is made by radiographic studies.

Surgical Treatment. If the rectal pouch is separated from the anus by only a thin membrane, the surgeon may repair the defect from below. When a high defect is present, abdominoperineal resection is indicated. In these in-

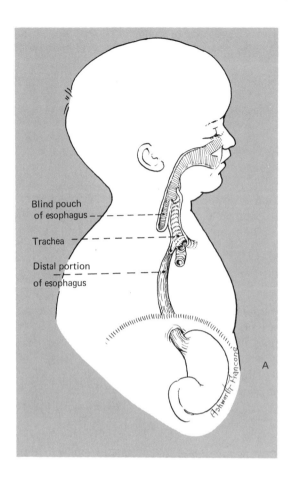

Blind pouch
of esophagus

Trachea

Distal portion
of esophagus

A

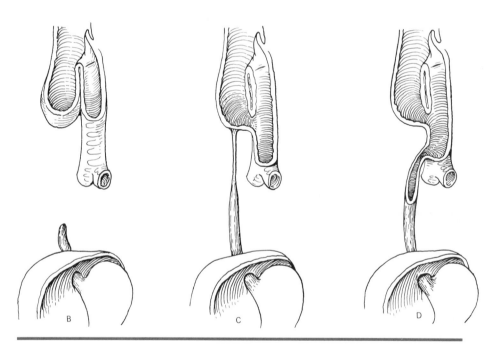

B   C   D

Figure 7-4. **A**, The most common form of esophageal atresia. **B**, Both segments of the esophagus are blind pouches. **C**, Esophagus is continuous but with narrowed segment. **D**, Upper segment of esophagus opens into trachea.

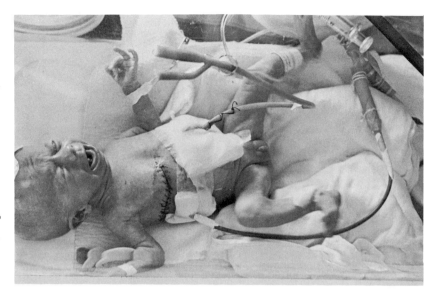

Figure 7-5. Repair of tracheal esophageal atresia and fistula showing chest incision and drainage tube. Gastrostomy tube is also in place.

fants, a colostomy is performed, and extensive abdominoperineal resection is delayed until the age of 3 to 5 months or later.

Home Care. When the infant goes home with a colostomy, the family will need to learn how to give colostomy care. The caregivers should be taught to keep the area around the colostomy clean with soap and water and to diaper the baby in the usual way. A protective ointment is useful for protection of the skin around the colostomy.

Hernias
A **hernia** is the abnormal protrusion of a part of an organ through a weak spot or other abnormal opening in a body wall. Complications occur depending on the amount of circulatory impairment involved and how much the herni-

ated organ impairs the functioning of another organ. Most hernias can be repaired surgically.

Diaphragmatic Hernia. In a congenital hernia of the diaphragm, some of the abdominal organs are displaced into the left chest through an opening in the diaphragm. The heart is pushed toward the right, and the left lung is compressed. Rapid, labored respirations and cyanosis are present on the first day of life, and breathing becomes increasingly difficult.

Surgery is essential and may be performed as an emergency procedure. During surgery, the abdominal viscera are withdrawn from the chest, and the diaphragmatic defect is closed.

This defect may be minimal and easily repaired or so extensive that pulmonary tissue has failed to develop

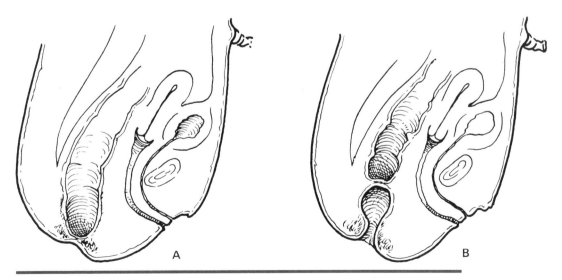

Figure 7-6. Imperforate anus (anal atresia). **A**, Membrane between anus and rectum. **B**, Rectum ending in a blind pouch at a distance above the perineum.

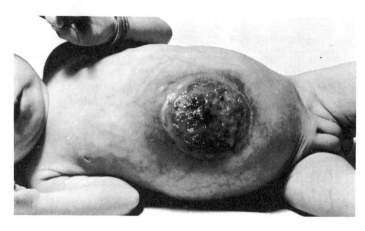

Figure 7-7. Omphalocele. (From Waechter EH, Blake FG. Nursing Care of Children, 9th ed. Philadelphia: JB Lippincott, 1976.)

normally. The outcome of surgical repair depends on the degree of pulmonary development, and prognosis in severe cases is guarded.

Hiatal Hernia. More common in adults than in newborns, hiatal hernia is caused when the cardiac portion of the stomach slides through the normal esophageal hiatus into the area above the diaphragm. This action causes reflux of gastric contents into the esophagus and subsequent regurgitation. If upright posture and modified feeding techniques do not successfully correct the problem, surgery is necessary to repair the defect.

Omphalocele. Omphalocele is a relatively rare congenital anomaly. Some of the abdominal contents protrude through into the root of the umbilical cord and form a sac lying on the abdomen (Figure 7-7). This sac may be small, with only a loop of bowel, or large and contain much of the intestine and the liver. The sac is covered with peritoneal membrane instead of skin. These defects may be detected during prenatal ultrasonography, so that prompt repair may be anticipated. At birth, the defect should be covered immediately with gauze moistened in sterile saline, which then may be covered with plastic wrap to prevent heat loss. Surgical replacement of the organs into the abdomen may be difficult with a large omphalocele because there may not be enough space in the abdominal cavity. Other congenital defects are present in many instances.

With large omphaloceles, surgery may be postponed and the surgeon will suture skin over the defect, creating a large hernia. The abdomen may enlarge enough as the child grows older so that replacement may be done.

Umbilical Hernia. Normally, the ring that encircled the fetal end of the umbilical cord closes gradually and spontaneously after birth. When this closure is incomplete, portions of omentum and intestine protrude through the opening. More common in preterm and African-American infants, umbilical hernia is largely a cosmetic problem, which is upsetting to parents but is associated with little or no morbidity (Figure 7-8). In rare instances, the bowel may strangulate in the sac, requiring immediate surgery. Almost all of these hernias close spontaneously by the

age of 3 years. Those hernias that do not should be surgically corrected before the child enters school.

Inguinal Hernia. More common in males, inguinal hernias occur when the small sac of peritoneum surrounding the testes fails to close off after the testes descend from the abdominal sac into the scrotum. This failure allows the intestine to slip into the inguinal canal, with resultant swelling. If the intestine becomes trapped (incarcerated) and the circulation to the trapped intestine is impaired

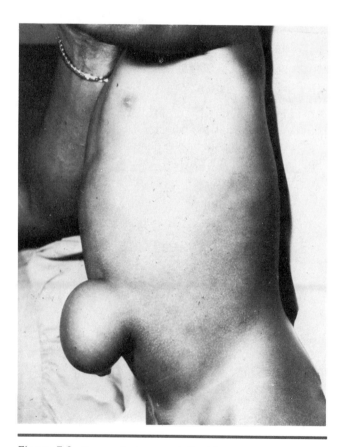

Figure 7-8. Unusually large umbilical hernia in infant. (Courtesy of Dr. Mark Ravitch.) (From Waechter EH, Blake FG. Nursing Care of Children, 9th ed. Philadelphia: JB Lippincott, 1976.)

(strangulated), surgery is necessary to prevent intestinal obstruction and gangrene of the bowel. As a preventive measure, inguinal hernias normally are repaired as soon as they are diagnosed.

Central Nervous System Defects

Central nervous system defects include disorders caused by an imbalance of cerebrospinal fluid, as in hydrocephalus and a range of disorders, often referred to as neural tube defects, resulting from malformations of the neural tube during embryonic development. These defects vary from the mild to severely disabling.

Spina Bifida

Caused by a defect in the neural arch, generally in the lumbosacral region, **spina bifida** is a failure of the posterior laminate of the vertebrae to close, leaving an opening through which the spinal meninges and spinal cord may protrude (Figure 7-9).

Clinical Manifestations. The occurrence of a bony defect without soft-tissue involvement is called spina bifida occulta. In most instances, it is asymptomatic and presents no problems. A dimple in the skin or a tuft of hair over the site may cause one to suspect its presence, or it may be entirely overlooked. When a portion of the spinal meninges protrudes through the bony defect and forms a cystic sac, the condition is termed spina bifida with meningocele. No nerve roots are involved; therefore, no paralysis or sensory loss below the lesion appears. The sac may, however, rupture or perforate, thus introducing infection into the spinal fluid and causing meningitis. For this reason, as well as for cosmetic purposes, surgical removal of the sac, with closure of the skin, is indicated.

Spina bifida with myelomeningocele signifies a pro-

trusion of the spinal cord and the meninges, with nerve roots embedded in the wall of the cyst (Figure 7-10). The effects of this defect vary in severity from sensory loss or partial paralysis below the lesion to complete flaccid paralysis of all muscles below the lesion. Complete paralysis involves the lower trunk and legs as well as bowel and bladder sphincters. It is not always possible, however, to make a clear-cut differentiation in diagnosis between a meningocele and a myelomeningocele on the basis of symptoms alone.

The condition myelomeningocele also may be termed meningomyelocele. The associated spina bifida is always implied but not necessarily named. Spina bifida cystica is the term used to designate either of these protrusions.

Diagnosis. Elevated maternal alphafetoprotein (AFP) levels followed up by ultrasonographic examination of the fetus may show an incomplete neural tube. An elevated AFP level in the maternal serum or amniotic fluid indicates the probability of central nervous system abnormalities. Further examination may confirm this and allow the pregnant woman the opportunity to terminate the pregnancy because the best time to perform these tests is between 13 to 15 weeks' gestation when peak levels are reached. AFP is currently performed by most obstetricians.

Diagnosis of the newborn with spina bifida is made from clinical observation and examination. Further evaluation of the extent of the defect may include magnetic resonance imaging (MRI), ultrasonography, computed tomography (CT) scanning, and myelograms. The newborn needs to be examined carefully for other associated defects, particularly hydrocephalus, genitourinary defects, and orthopedic anomalies.

Treatment. Many specialists are involved in the treatment of the infant, especially in the case of myelomeningocele.

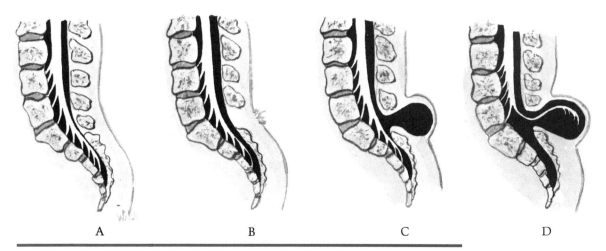

A B C D

Figure 7-9. Degrees of spinal cord anomalies. **A**, The normal spinal closure. **B**, Occulta defect. **C**, Meningocele defect. **D**, Myelomeningocele defect to clearly show the spinal cord involvement. (From Pillitteri A. Maternal Child Health Nursing. Philadelphia: JB Lippincott, 1992, p. 1169.)

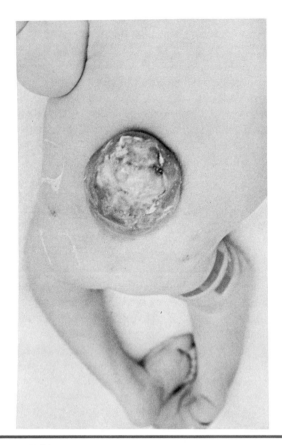

Figure 7-10. A myelomeningocele showing an additional defect of clubfeet.

These specialists may include neurologists, neurosurgeons, orthopedic specialists, pediatricians, urologists, and physical therapists. After a thorough evaluation of the infant is completed, a plan of surgical repair and treatment is developed. Highly skilled nursing care is necessary in all aspects of the infant's care. The child requires years of ongoing follow-up and therapy. Surgery is required to close the open defect but may not be performed immediately, depending on the decision of the surgeon. Waiting several days does not seem to cause additional problems, and this period gives the family an opportunity to adjust to the initial shock and become involved in the decision making.[1]

Nursing Process for the Infant with Myelomeningocele

ASSESSMENT

A routine newborn assessment is conducted with emphasis placed on the evaluation of the neurologic impairment of the infant. Observation of movement of the lower extremities, response to stimulus to the lower extremities, careful measurement of the head circumference, and examination of the fontanelles must be included. The

assessment must be thoroughly documented. When the infant is handled, great care must be taken to prevent any injury to the sac.

The family of this infant needs support and understanding throughout the initial care of the infant as well as for the many years of care during the child's life. The family's knowledge and understanding of the defect must be assessed, as well as their attitude concerning the birth of an infant with such serious problems.

NURSING DIAGNOSES

The nursing diagnoses suggested in this section are those that are appropriate for the newborn infant, but the nurse must be aware that this child will be hospitalized periodically throughout the child's lifetime, and suitable diagnoses will vary and need to be made at each admission after careful assessment. Possible nursing diagnoses are the following:

- High risk for infection related to vulnerability of the myelomeningocele sac
- High risk for impaired skin integrity related to exposure to urine and feces
- Impaired physical mobility related to lower limb impairments
- Family grieving related to the loss of the anticipated perfect newborn
- Family anxiety related to the complexities of caring for the infant with serious neurologic and musculoskeletal defects

PLANNING AND IMPLEMENTATION

The nursing goals for the care of the infant with myelomeningocele include prevention of infection and trauma, reduction of the family's anxiety, and support and education for the family about the condition.

Preventing Infection. The infant's vital signs, neurologic signs, and behavior should be monitored frequently to observe for any deviations from normal that may indicate an infection. Prophylactic antibiotics may be ordered. Routine aseptic technique must be carried out with conscientious handwashing, gloving, and gowning as appropriate. Until surgery is performed, the sac must be covered with a sterile dressing moistened in a warm sterile solution (often sterile saline). This dressing must be changed every 2 hours and must not be allowed to dry to avoid damage to the covering of the sac. The dressings may be covered with a plastic protective covering. The infant needs to be maintained in a prone position, so that no pressure is placed on the sac. After surgery, this positioning needs to continue until the surgical site is well healed. Diapering is not advisable with a low defect, but the sac must be protected from contamination with fecal material. This contamination may be prevented by placement of a protective barrier between the anus and the sac.

If the anal sphincter muscles are involved, the infant may have continual loose stools, adding to the challenge of keeping the sac infection free.

Promoting Skin Integrity. The nursing interventions that are discussed in the previous section on infection also are necessary to promote skin integrity around the area of the defect as well as the diaper area of the infant. As mentioned earlier, there may be continual leakage of stool as well as urine. This leakage causes skin irritation and breakdown if the infant is not kept clean and the diaper area is not free of stool and urine. Scrupulous perineal care must be carried out.

Improving Physical Mobility. Infants with spina bifida frequently have talipes equinovarus (clubfoot) and congenital hip dysplasia (dislocation of the hips), both of which are discussed later in this chapter. If there is loss of motion in the lower limbs owing to the defect, range of motion exercises should be conducted to prevent contractures. The infant should be positioned so that the hips are abducted and the feet are in a neutral position. The knees and other bony prominences should be massaged regularly with lotion, padded, and protected from irritation. When the infant is handled, care must be taken to prevent pressure on the sac.

Promoting Family Coping. The family of an infant with such a major anomaly is in a state of shock on first learning of the problems. The nurse needs to be especially sensitive to their needs and emotions. The family should be encouraged to express their emotions as openly as possible. The nurse must recognize that some families are able to express their emotions much more freely than others and adjust responses to the family with this in mind. The family may need privacy for a period to mourn together over their loss. The nurse must not avoid the family, however, because this only exaggerates their feelings of loss and depression. If possible, the family members are encouraged to cuddle or touch the infant with proper precautions for the safety of the defect. With permission of the physician, the infant may be held chest to chest to provide closer contact.

Providing Family Teaching. The family needs to be given factual information about the defect and encouraged to discuss their concerns and ask questions. Information about the infant's present state, the proposed surgery, and follow-up care need to be provided. The nurse must remember that anxiety may block the understanding and processing of knowledge, therefore repetition of information is required. Information should be reduced into small segments to facilitate comprehension. After surgery, the family needs to be prepared to care for the infant at home. The family may be taught to hold the infant's head, neck, and chest slightly raised in one hand during feeding. They also may be taught that stroking the infant's cheek helps stimulate sucking. Teaching the family how to care for the infant, allowing them to participate in the care, and guiding them in performing return demonstrations are all methods to use.

For long-term care and support, the family may be referred to the Spina Bifida Association. Materials concerning spina bifida should be made available to them. These children need long-term care involving many aspects of medical and surgical care as well as education and vocational training. Although children with spina bifida have many long-term problems, their intelligence is not affected. Many of these children grow into productive young adults who may live independently (Figure 7-11).

EVALUATION

- There are no signs of infection as evidenced by vital signs and neurologic signs within normal limits; there is an absence of signs of irritability or lethargy.

- The infant's skin remains clean and dry with no areas of reddening or other signs of irritation; bony prominences are protected from irritation.

- The lower limbs show no evidence of contractures.

- The family verbalizes anxieties and needs; holds, cuddles, and soothes infant as appropriate.

- The family demonstrates competence in performing care for the infant, verbalizes an understanding of the

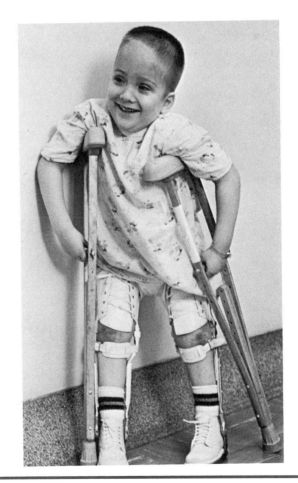

Figure 7-11. Learning to use new braces, this boy underwent successful surgery for repair of a myelomeningocele during infancy.

signs and symptoms that should be reported, and has referral information to helping agencies.

Hydrocephalus

Hydrocephalus is a condition characterized by an excess of cerebrospinal fluid within the ventricular and subarachnoid spaces of the cranial cavity. Normally, there is a delicate balance between the rate of formation and the absorption of cerebrospinal fluid. The entire volume is absorbed and replaced every 12 to 24 hours. In hydrocephalus, this balance is disturbed.

Cerebrospinal fluid is formed by the choroid plexus, mainly in the lateral ventricles. It is absorbed into the venous system through the arachnoid villi. Cerebrospinal fluid circulates within the ventricles and the subarachnoid space. It is a colorless fluid, consisting of water with traces of protein, glucose, and lymphocytes.

The noncommunicating type of congenital hydrocephalus occurs when there is an obstruction in the free circulation of cerebrospinal fluid. This blockage causes increased pressure on the brain or spinal cord. The site of obstruction may be at the foramen of Monro, the aqueduct of Sylvius, the foramen of Lushka, or the foramen of Magendie (Figure 7-12).

In the communicating type of hydrocephalus, there is no obstruction of the free flow of cerebrospinal fluid between the ventricles and the spinal theca. The condition is caused by defective absorption of the cerebrospinal fluid, thus causing pressure on the brain or spinal cord to increase. Congenital hydrocephalus is most often the obstructive or noncommunicating type.

Hydrocephalus may be recognized at birth, or it may not be evident until after a few weeks or months of life. The condition may not be congenital but may instead occur during later infancy or during childhood as the result of a neoplasm, a head injury, or an infection such as meningitis.

When hydrocephalus occurs early in life before the skull sutures close, the soft, pliable bones separate to allow head expansion. This condition is manifested by a rapid growth in head circumference. The fact that the soft bones are capable of yielding to pressure in this manner may partially explain why many of these infants fail to show the usual symptoms of brain pressure and may exhibit little or no damage in mental function until later in life. Other infants show severe brain damage, often occurring before birth.

Clinical Manifestations. An excessively large head at birth is suggestive of hydrocephalus. Rapid head growth with widening cranial sutures is also strongly suggestive of the malady. A rapidly enlarging head may be the first manifestation of this condition. An apparently large head in itself is not necessarily significant. Normally, every infant's head is measured at birth, and the rate of growth is checked at subsequent examinations. Any infant's head that appears to be abnormally large at birth or appears to be enlarging should be measured frequently.

As the head enlarges, the suture lines separate, and the spaces may be felt through the scalp. The anterior fontanelle becomes tense and bulging, the skull enlarges in all diameters, and the scalp becomes shiny and its veins dilate. If pressure continues to increase without intervention, the eyes appear to be pushed downward slightly, with the sclera visible above the iris, giving the so-called "setting sun" sign (Figure 7-13).

If the condition progresses without adequate drainage of excessive fluid, the head becomes increasingly heavy, the neck muscles fail to develop sufficiently, and the infant has difficulty raising or turning his or her head. Unless hydrocephalus is arrested, the infant becomes

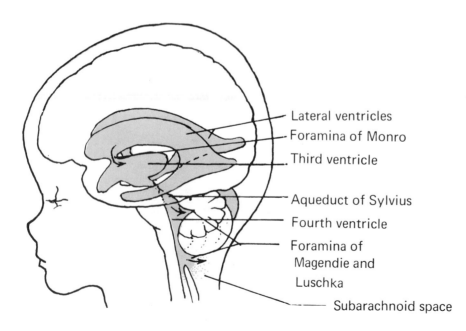

Lateral ventricles
Foramina of Monro
Third ventricle

Aqueduct of Sylvius
Fourth ventricle
Foramina of Magendie and Luschka
Subarachnoid space

Figure 7-12. Ventricles of the brain and channels for the normal flow of cerebrospinal fluid. (Courtesy of Dr. AJ Raimondi; Raffensberger J, Primrose R (eds). Pediatric Surgery for Nurses. Boston: Little, Brown, 1968.)

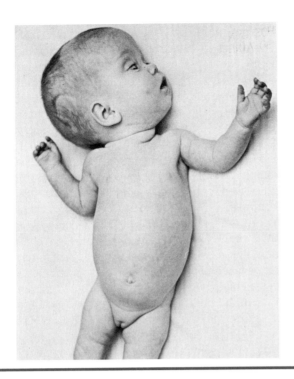

Figure 7-13. A child with hydrocephalus. Note the pull on the eyes giving the "setting sun" appearance. Note also the site of incision for a shunt.

increasingly helpless, and symptoms of increased intracranial pressure (ICP) develop. These symptoms may include irritability, restlessness, personality change, high-pitched cry, ataxia, projectile vomiting, failure to thrive, seizures, severe headache, changes in level of consciousness, and papilledema.

Diagnosis. Clinical manifestations, particularly excessive increase in the circumference of the head, are indications of hydrocephalus. Positive diagnosis is made with CT scan and MRI. Echoencephalography and ventriculograms also may be performed for further definition of the condition.

Treatment. Surgical intervention is the only effective means of relieving brain pressure and preventing further damage to the brain tissue. If minimal brain damage has occurred, the child may be able to function within a normal mental range. Motor function is usually retarded. In some instances, surgical intervention may remove the cause of the obstruction, such as a neoplasm, a cyst, or a hematoma, but for most children the procedure that must be done is placement of a shunting device that bypasses the point of obstruction, draining the excess cerebrospinal fluid into a body cavity. This procedure arrests excessive head growth and prevents further brain damage.

Shunting Procedures. All shunt procedures use a silicone rubber catheter that is radiopaque so that its position may be checked by radiographic examination. The silicone

rubber catheter reduces the problem of tissue reaction. A valve, or regulator, is an essential part of each catheter that prevents excess build-up of fluid or too rapid decompression of the ventricle. The most commonly used procedure, particularly for infants and small children is **ventriculoperitoneal shunting**, in which the cerebrospinal fluid is drained from a lateral ventricle in the brain, running subcutaneously, and emptying into the peritoneal cavity. This procedure allows the insertion of some excess tubing to accommodate growth. As the child grows, the catheter needs to be revised and lengthened (Figure 7-14).

Ventriculoatrial shunting drains cerebrospinal fluid into the right atrium of the heart. This procedure is not one that may be used in children with pathologic changes in the heart. The cerebrospinal fluid that is drained from the ventricle is absorbed into the blood stream.

Other pathways of drainage have been used with varying amounts of success. All types of shunts may have problems with kinking, blocking, moving, or shifting of tubing. The danger of infection in the tubing pathway is a constant concern. Children with shunts must be constantly observed for signs of malfunction or infection.

The long-term outcome for a child with hydrocephalus depends on a number of factors. Untreated, the outcome is very poor, often leading to death. With shunting, the

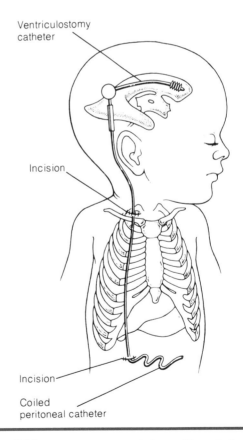

Ventriculostomy
catheter

Incision

Incision

Coiled
peritoneal catheter

Figure 7-14. Ventriculoperitoneal shunt. (From Jackson PL. Ventriculo-peritoneal shunts. Am J Nurs 80:1104, 1980.)

outcome depends on the initial cause of the increased fluid, the treatment of the cause, the brain damage sustained before shunting, complications with the shunting system, and continued long-term follow-up. It is possible for some of these children to lead relatively normal lives with follow-up and revisions as they grow.

Nursing Process for the Postoperative Infant with Hydrocephalus

ASSESSMENT

Complete assessment of vital and neurologic signs is necessary preoperatively and postoperatively. Measurement of the infant's head is essential. If the infant's fontanelles are not closed, they should be carefully observed for any signs of bulging. All signs of ICP should be observed for, reported, and documented. If this is a child who has returned for revision of an existing shunt, a complete history should be obtained preoperatively from the family so that a baseline of the child's behavior is available.

The family of the infant needs to be assessed for the level of knowledge individual members have about the condition. For the family of the newborn or young infant, the diagnosis most likely will come as an emotional shock. The nurse needs to conduct the assessment with sensitivity and understanding.

NURSING DIAGNOSES

Development of the nursing diagnoses varies with the results of the assessment, the age of the child, and whether this is the first placement of a shunt or a revision. Possible nursing diagnoses may include the following:

- High risk for injury related to increased intracranial pressure
- High risk for impaired skin integrity related to pressure from physical immobility
- High risk for infection related to the presence of a shunt
- High risk for altered growth and development related to impaired ability to achieve developmental tasks
- Family anxiety related to fear of surgical outcome
- High risk for altered health maintenance related to the family's insufficient knowledge about the child's condition and home care

PLANNING AND IMPLEMENTATION

The nursing goals for the postoperative care of the infant with shunt placement for hydrocephalus are directed at preventing complications, providing loving, supportive care to the infant, providing support for the family, and increasing the family's knowledge about the condition.

Preventing Injury. The nurse must regularly (every 2 to 4 hours) assess the level of consciousness, check the pupils for equality and reaction, assess the neurologic signs, and observe for a shrill cry, lethargy, or irritability. The occipitofrontal circumference must be measured and recorded daily. The nurse must carry out appropriate procedures to care for the shunt as directed. To prevent a rapid decrease in ICP, the infant must be kept flat. The infant must be observed for signs of seizure, and seizure precautions are initiated. Suction and oxygen equipment should be kept convenient at the bedside.

Promoting Skin Integrity. Following a shunting procedure, the infant's head is kept turned away from the operative site until the physician indicates that changing position is permitted. If the infant's head is enlarged, care should be taken to prevent pressure sores on the side on which the child rests. Care should be taken to support the head when the child is moved or picked up. Egg crate pads, lamb's wool, or a special mattress may be used, if necessary, to prevent pressure breakdown of the scalp. Reposition the infant at least every 2 hours as permitted. Immediately postoperatively, the dressings over the shunt site should be inspected frequently, then every 4 hours.

Preventing Infection. Infection is the primary threat that may complicate the postsurgical condition of the infant. Close observation for signs of infection is essential. Temperature elevation; redness, heat, or swelling along the surgical site; and signs of lethargy all may be indications of infection and must be monitored and reported promptly. Wound care should be meticulously performed as ordered. Antibiotics are administered as prescribed.

Providing Comfort Measures. Every infant has the need and the right to be picked up and held, cuddled, and comforted. An uncomfortable or painful experience increases the need for emotional support. An infant perceives such support principally through physical contact made in a soothing, loving manner.

The infant needs social interaction, to be talked to, played with, and given the opportunity for activity. Toys appropriate for the infant's physical and mental capacity must be provided. If the child has difficulty moving about the crib, toys must be within reach and vision, such as a cradle gym tied close enough for the infant to maneuver its parts.

Unless the infant's nervous system is so impaired that all activity increases irritability, the infant needs stimulation as much as any child does. If repositioning from side to side means turning the infant away from the sight of activity, the crib may be turned around so that vision is not obstructed.

An infant who is given the contact and support that all infants require develops a pleasing personality because of being nourished by emotional stimulation. The nurse's time for physical care is also a time for social interaction. Talking, laughing, and playing with the infant are all important aspects of the infant's care. Contacts should be frequent and should not be limited only to those times when physical care is being performed.

Reducing Family Anxiety. The family needs the condition and the anatomy of the surgical procedure explained in terms they can understand. The overall prognosis for the child needs to be discussed. The family must be encouraged to express their anxieties and questions. Accurate, nontechnical answers are extremely helpful. The family should be given information about support groups such as the National Hydrocephalus Foundation and encouraged to make contact with the group.

Providing Family Teaching. Care of the shunt must be demonstrated to the family, and members should perform a return demonstration. The family needs a list of those signs and symptoms that should be reported. The nurse should review these lists and make sure that the family understands them. Appropriate growth and developmental expectations for the child should be discussed, stressing realistic goals.

EVALUATION

- No signs of ICP are evidenced.
- The skin shows no evidence of pressure sores.
- There are no signs of infection, the vital signs are stable, and no redness or swelling is evidenced.
- The infant responds appropriately to growth and development tasks.
- The family expresses its fears and interacts appropriately with the infant.
- The family participates in the care of the infant and demonstrates an understanding of the equipment and signs and symptoms to report.

Cardiovascular System Defects

Cardiovascular system defects range from mild to severe. They may be detected immediately at birth or may not be detected for several months. Severe defects are among the leading causes of death in the first year of life.

Congenital Heart Disease

When a newborn infant is suspected of having a heart abnormality, the family is understandably upset. The heart is *the* vital organ; one can live without a number of other organs and appendages, but life itself depends on the heart. The family will have many questions, some of which may be answered by the nurse and others that must be answered by the physician. Many answers will not be available until after various evaluation procedures have been conducted.

Technologic advances have progressed rapidly in this field, making earlier detection and successful repair much more likely than was possible in the past. However,

heart defects are the leading cause of death from congenital anomalies in the first year of life.

A brief discussion of the development and function of the embryonic heart is useful to understanding the malformations that occur.

Pathophysiology. The heart begins beating early in the third to eighth week of intrauterine life. When first formed, the heart is a simple tube receiving blood from the placenta and pumping it out into its developing body. During this period, it rapidly develops into the normal, but complex, four-chambered heart.

Adjustments in circulation must be made at birth. During fetal life, the lungs are inactive, requiring only a small amount of blood to nourish their tissues. Blood is circulated through the umbilical arteries to the placenta, where waste products and carbon dioxide are exchanged for oxygen and nutrients. The blood is then returned to the fetus through the umbilical vein.

At birth, the umbilical cord is cut, and the infant's own independent system is established. Certain circulatory bypasses, such as the **ductus arteriosus**, the **foramen ovale**, and the **ductus venosus**, are no longer necessary. They close and atrophy during the first several weeks after birth. In addition, the pressure in the heart, which has been higher on the right side during fetal life, now changes so that the left side of the heart has the higher pressure (Figure 7-15; see also Figure 5-3 in Chapter 5).

During this period of complex development, any error in formation may cause serious circulatory difficulty. The incidence of cardiovascular malformations is about 8 in 1000 live births.

Etiology. Rubella in the expectant mother during the first trimester is a common cause of cardiac malformation. Maternal alcoholism, maternal irradiation, ingestion of certain drugs during pregnancy, maternal diabetes, and advanced maternal age (older than 40 years) also are known to increase the incidence. Maternal malnutrition and heredity are also contributing factors. Recent studies have shown that the offspring of mothers who had congenital heart anomalies have a much higher risk factor. If one child in the family has a congenital heart abnormality, later siblings have a very high risk factor for such a defect.

The newborn with a severe abnormality, such as a transposition of the great vessels, is cyanotic from birth, requiring oxygen and special treatment. A less seriously affected child, whose heart is able to compensate to some degree for the impaired circulation, may not have symptoms severe enough to call attention to the difficulty until he or she is a few months older and more active. Others may live a fairly normal life and not be aware of any heart trouble until a murmur or an enlarged heart is discovered on physical examination in later childhood. Some abnormalities are slight and allow the person to

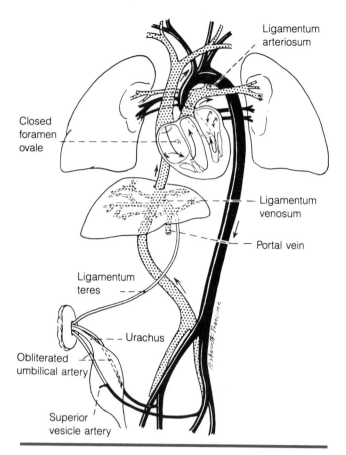

Closed foramen ovale

Ligamentum arteriosum

Ligamentum venosum

Portal vein

Ligamentum teres

Urachus

Obliterated umbilical artery

Superior vesicle artery

Figure 7-15. Normal blood circulation. **Arrows** show the direction of blood flow.

lead a normal life without correction. Others cause little apparent difficulty but need correction to improve the chance for a longer life and for optimum health. Some severe anomalies are incompatible with life for more than a short time, and others may be helped but not cured by surgery.

Clinical Manifestations. A cardiac murmur discovered early in life necessitates frequent physical examinations. This murmur may be a functional, "innocent" murmur that may disappear as the child grows older, or it may be the chief manifestation of an abnormal heart or an abnormal circulatory system. The most frequent parental complaint is that of feeding difficulties. Infants with cardiac anomalies severe enough to cause circulatory difficulties have a history of being poor eaters, tiring easily from the effort to suck, and fail to grow or thrive normally.

Manifestations of **congestive heart failure** (CHF) may appear the first year of life in infants with conditions such as large ventricular septal defects, coarctation of the aorta, and other defects that place an increased workload on the ventricles. One indication of CHF in infancy is easy fatigability, manifested by feeding problems. The infant tires, breathes hard, and refuses a bottle after 1 or 2 oz but soon becomes hungry again. Lying flat causes stress, and

the infant appears to be more comfortable if held upright over an adult's shoulder.

Other signs are failure to gain weight; a pale, mottled, or cyanotic color; a hoarse or weak cry; and tachycardia. Rapid respiration (with an expiratory grunt), flaring of the nares, and the use of accessory respiratory muscles with retractions at the diaphragmatic and suprasternal levels are other clinical manifestations of CHF. Edema is a factor, and the heart generally shows enlargement. Anoxic attacks (fainting spells) are common.

Diagnosis. The clinical symptoms of CHF are the primary basis for diagnosis. Chest radiographs that reveal an enlarged heart and electrocardiography indicate ventricular hypertrophy.

Treatment. Treatment of CHF includes digitalization to improve the contractility of the heart, angiotensin-converting enzyme (ACE) inhibitors to reduce the afterload on the heart, diuretics to reduce any edema, administration of oxygen, and the use of small doses of morphine for relaxation, if necessary. The infant should be placed in a position with the head elevated. Energy requirements should be kept to a minimum, easing the workload of the heart. Small, frequent feedings improve nutrition with minimal energy output.

Advances in medical technology are making possible the repair of the hearts in infants younger than 1 day old and other very young children. Miniaturization of instruments, earlier diagnosis through the use of improved diagnostic techniques, pediatric intensive care facilities staffed with highly skilled nurse specialists, and more sophisticated monitoring techniques all have contributed to these advances.

Most physicians now think it is important to operate as early as possible to repair defective hearts. Inadequate circulation may prevent adequate growth and development and cause permanent, irreparable physical, mental, and emotional damage. If the child is diagnosed early, before CHF failure occurs, correction may take place and CHF is avoided if effective repair is possible.

Care at Home Before Surgery. A child with congenital heart disease may show easy fatigability and retarded growth. If the child has a cyanotic type of heart disease with clubbing of the fingers or toes, periods of cyanosis and reduced exercise tolerance are evident. This young child may assume a squatting position, which reduces the return flow to the heart, thus temporarily reducing the workload of the heart.

Such a child should be allowed to lead as normal a life as possible. Families are naturally apprehensive and find it difficult not to overprotect the child. They often increase the child's anxiety and cause fear in the child about participating in normal activities. Children are rather sensible about finding their own limitations and usually limit their activities to their capacity if they are not made unduly apprehensive.

Some families are able to adjust well and provide guidance and security for their sick child. Others may become confused and frightened and show hostility, disinterest, or neglect, needing guidance and counseling. The nurse has a great responsibility to support the family. The primary goal of the nurse is reduction of the anxiety of child and family. This goal may be accomplished through open communication and ongoing contact.

Routine visits to a clinic or to a physician's office become a way of life, and the child may come to feel "different" from other people. Physicians and nurses have a responsibility both to the parents and the child to give clear explanations of the defect, using readily understandable terms and illustrating their explanations with appropriate diagrams, pictures, or models. A child who has knowledge of what is happening can accept much and continue with the business of living.

Cardiac Catheterization. Cardiac catheterization may be performed before heart surgery for more accurate information about the child's condition. The child or infant is sedated or anesthetized for this process, during which a radiopaque tube is inserted through a vein into the right atrium of the heart. In the infant or young child, the femoral vein often is used. Close observation of the child after the procedure is essential. The site used should be carefully monitored, and the extremity should be checked for pulses, edema, skin temperature and color, and any other signs of poor circulation or infection.

Preoperative Preparation. When a child enters the hospital for cardiac surgery, it is seldom a first admission. Generally, it has been preceded by cardiac catheterization or perhaps by other hospitalizations. Admission may be scheduled to precede surgery by a few days to allow time for adequate preparation. However, with the current stress on health care cost containment, many preoperative procedures are done on an outpatient status. Preoperative teaching should be intensive for the family and the child as appropriate to the age level. They should understand that blood may be obtained for typing and crossmatching and for other determinations as ordered. Additional roentgenograms may be made.

The apparatus to be used after surgery should be described with drawings and pictures. If possible, the parents and their child should be taken to a cardiac recovery room and should be shown chest tubes and an oxygen tent, meet the nursing personnel, and see the general appearance of the unit. Good judgment about the timing and the extent of such preparation is important because nothing is gained by arousing additional anxiety with premature or excessively graphic descriptions. A young child may become familiar with the surgical dress worn by personnel and with the oxygen tent and perhaps listen to the heart beat. The child should be taught how to

cough and should practice coughing. The child should understand that coughing is important after surgery and must be done regularly, even though it may hurt.

Cardiac Surgery. Open heart surgery, using the heart–lung machine, has made extensive heart correction possible for many children who, not long ago, would have otherwise spent a limited lifetime as disabled. Machines suitable for use with infants and small children are now available. In addition, complete heart transplants may be performed when no other treatment is possible.

Hypothermia—reducing the body temperature to 20° to 26°C (68° to 78.8°F)—is a useful technique that helps make early surgery possible. By gradually lowering the infant's or child's body temperature, physicians increase the time that the circulation may be stopped without causing brain damage. The temperature of the patient's blood is reduced by the use of cooling agents in the heart–lung machine. This maneuver provides a dry, bloodless, motionless field for the surgeon.

Postoperative Care. At the end of surgery, the child is taken to the pediatric intensive care unit to be skillfully nursed by specially trained personnel for as long as necessary. Children who have had closed chest surgery need the same careful nursing as those who have had open heart surgery.

By the time the child returns to the regular pediatric unit, chest drainage tubes usually have been removed and the child has started taking oral fluids and is ready to sit up in bed or in a chair. The child probably feels weak and helpless after such an experience and needs encouragement and reassurance. With recovery, however, a child is usually ready for activity. Improving health provides the incentive. Family caregivers usually need to reorient themselves and to accept their child's new status—an attitude that is not easy to acquire after what seemed like a long period of anxious watching.

The surgeon and the surgical staff evaluate the results of the surgery and make any necessary recommendations regarding the resumption of the child's activities. Plans should be made for follow-up and supervision as well as counseling and guidance.

Common Types of Congenital Heart Defects

Traditionally, congenital heart defects have been described as cyanotic or acyanotic conditions. **Cyanotic heart disease** implies an oxygen saturation of the peripheral arterial blood of 85% or less. This condition occurs when a heart defect allows any appreciable amount of oxygen-poor blood in the right side of the heart to mix with the oxygenated blood in the left side of the heart. Defects that permit right-to-left shunting may occur at the atrial, ventricular, or aortic level.

Many defects occur in combination, giving rise to complex situations. Many of the complex defects, and most of the rare, isolated defects may never be seen by

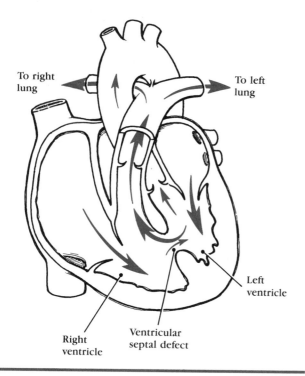

Figure 7-16. A ventricular septal defect is an abnormal opening between the right and left ventricle. Ventricular septal defects vary in size and may occur in the membranous or muscular portion of the ventricular septum. Owing to higher pressure in the left ventricle, a shunting of blood from the left to the right ventricle occurs during systole. If pulmonary vascular resistance produces pulmonary hypertension, the shunt of blood is then reversed from the right to the left ventricle, with cyanosis resulting. (From Bullock B. Pathophysiology: Adaptation and Alterations in Function, 3rd ed. Philadelphia: JB Lippincott, 1992, p. 525.)

most nurses. The conditions discussed here are common enough that the pediatric nurse needs to be familiar with their diagnosis and treatment.

Ventricular Septal Defect. This is the most common intracardiac defect. It consists of an abnormal opening in the septum between the two ventricles, allowing blood to pass directly from the left to the right ventricle. There is no leakage of unoxygenated blood into the left ventricle and thus no cyanosis (Figure 7-16).

Small, isolated defects are usually without symptoms and often are discovered during a routine physical examination. A characteristic loud, harsh murmur, associated with a systolic thrill, occasionally is heard on examination. There may be a history of frequent respiratory infections during infancy, but growth and development is not affected. The child leads a normal life.

Corrective surgery may be postponed until the age of 18 months to 2 years, when the surgical risk is less than that for infants. However, surgical techniques have improved to the degree that the repair may be made in the first year of life with high rates of success. The child is

observed closely and may be placed on prophylactic antibiotics to prevent frequent respiratory infections. If pulmonary involvement becomes a problem, the repair is done without further delay.

Atrial Septal Defects. In general, left-to-right shunting occurs in all true atrial septal defects. A patent foramen ovale, which is situated in the atrial septum, however, is present in a large number of healthy people and normally causes no problems. This is because the valve of the foramen ovale is anatomically structured to withstand left chamber pressure and makes the patent foramen ovale functionally closed (Figure 7-17).

True atrial septal defects are common heart anomalies and may occur as isolated defects or in combination with other heart anomalies.

Atrial septal defects are amenable to surgery, with a low surgical mortality risk. Since the advent of the heart-lung bypass machine, this repair may be performed in a dry field, replacing the older "blind" technique. The opening is either sutured or is closed with a nylon patch.

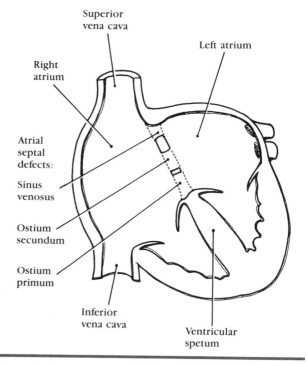

Figure 7-17. An atrial septal defect is an abnormal opening between the right and left atria. Basically, three types of abnormalities result from incorrect development of the atrial septum. An incompetent foramen ovale is the most common defect. The high ostium secundum defect results from abnormal development of the septum secundum. Improper development of the septum primum produces a basal opening known as an ostium primum defect, frequently involving the atrioventricular valves. In general, left to right shunting of blood occurs in all atrial septal defects. (From Bullock B. Pathophysiology: Adaptation and Alterations in Function, 3rd ed. Philadelphia: JB Lippincott, 1992, p. 525.)

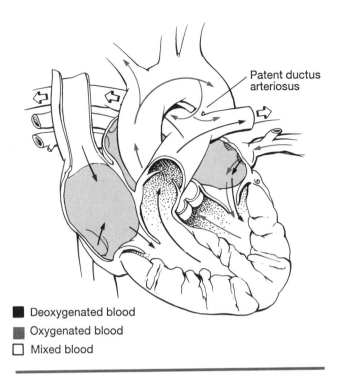

Patent ductus
arteriosus

■ Deoxygenated blood
▨ Oxygenated blood
☐ Mixed blood

Figure 7-18. The patent ductus arteriosus is a vascular connection that, during fetal life, short-circuits the pulmonary vascular bed and directs blood from the pulmonary artery to the aorta. Functional closure of the ductus normally occurs soon after birth. If the ductus remains patent after birth, the direction of blood flow in the ductus is reversed by the higher pressure in the aorta. (From Castiglia PT, Harbin RE. Child Health Care: Process and Practice. Philadelphia: JB Lippincott, 1992, p. 586.)

Patent Ductus Arteriosus. The ductus arteriosus is a vascular channel between the left main pulmonary artery and the descending aorta. In fetal life, this allows blood to bypass the nonfunctioning lungs and go directly into the systemic circuit. After birth, the duct normally closes, eventually becoming obliterated and forming the ligamentum arteriosum. If the ductus arteriosus remains patent, however, blood continues to be shunted from the aorta into the pulmonary artery. This situation overfloods the lungs and overloads the left heart chambers (Figure 7-18).

Normally, the ductus arteriosus is nonpatent after the first or second week of life and should be obliterated by the fourth month. Why it fails to close is not known. Patent ductus arteriosus is common in infants who exhibit the rubella syndrome, but most of the infants with this anomaly have no history of exposure to rubella during fetal life.

Symptoms of patent ductus arteriosus are often absent during childhood. Growth and development may be retarded in some children, with an easy fatigability and dyspnea on exertion. The diagnosis may be based on a characteristic, machinery-like murmur over the pulmonary area, a wide pulse pressure, and a bounding pulse.

Cardiac catheterization is diagnostic but is not required in the presence of classic clinical features.

Surgery is indicated in all diagnosed cases, even if they are asymptomatic. Some persons may live a normal life span without correction, but the risks involved far outweigh the surgical ones. Indomethacin (Indocin), a prostaglandin inhibitor, may be administered to premature infants with respiratory distress syndrome to promote closure of the ductus arteriosus with some success. If this fails to close the ductus, surgery is performed.

Surgical correction consists of closure of the defect by ligation or by division of the ductus. Division is the method of choice if the child's condition permits because the ductus occasionally reopens after ligation. The optimal age for surgery is before the age of 2 years, with earlier surgery for severely affected infants. Prognosis is excellent after a successful repair.

Coarctation of the Aorta. This is a congenital cardiovascular anomaly consisting of a constriction or narrowing of the aortic arch or of the descending aorta, usually adjacent to the ligamentum arteriosum (Figure 7-19).

Most children with this condition are asymptomatic until later childhood or young adulthood. A few infants have severe symptoms in their first year of life, showing dyspnea, tachycardia, and cyanosis, all signs of developing CHF.

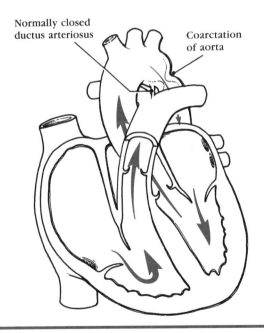

Normally closed
ductus arteriosus

Coarctation
of aorta

Figure 7-19. Coarctation of the aorta is characterized by a narrowed aortic lumen. It exists as a preductal or postductal obstruction, depending on the position of the obstruction in relation to the ductus arteriosus. Coarctations exist with great variation in anatomic features. The lesion produces an obstruction to the flow of blood through the aorta, causing an increased left ventricular pressure and work load. (From Bullock B. Pathophysiology: Adaptation and Alterations in Function, 3rd ed. Philadelphia: JB Lippincott, 1992, p. 526.)

In older children, the condition is easily diagnosed based on hypertension present in the upper extremities and hypotension in the lower extremities. The radial pulse is readily palpable, but the femoral pulses are weak or even impalpable. Blood pressure is normal or elevated in the arms and is low or undetectable in the legs. A high-pitched systolic murmur is usually present, heard over the base of the heart and over the interscapular area of the back. The diagnosis may be confirmed by aortography.

Obstruction to blood flow caused by the constricted portion of the aorta does not cause early difficulty in an average child because the blood bypasses the obstruction by way of collateral circulation. The bypass is chiefly from the branches of the subclavian and carotid arteries, which arise from the arch of the aorta. Eventually, the enlarged collateral arteries erode the rib margins, and the rib notching may be visualized by radiographic examination.

The uncorrected coarctation may cause hypertension and cardiac failure later in life. The optimal age for elective surgery is before the age of 2 years. Early surgery may be necessary for a gravely ill infant who may present with severe CHF. In early infancy, the mortality rate depends on the presence of other congenital heart problems.

Surgery consists of resection of the coarcted area with an end-to-end anastomosis of the proximal and distal ends of the aorta. Occasionally, a long defect may necessitate an end-to-end graft, using tubes of Dacron or similar material. Prognosis is excellent for the restoration of normal function after surgery.

Tetralogy of Fallot. This is a fairly common congenital heart defect, involving 50% to 70% of all cyanotic congenital heart diseases. It consists of a grouping of heart defects, the term "tetralogy" denoting four abnormal conditions. These are (1) **pulmonary stenosis**, (2) **ventricular septal defect**, (3) **overriding aorta**, and (4) **right ventricular hypertrophy**.

The pulmonary stenosis is usually of the infundibular type, in which there is a narrowing of the upper portion of the right ventricle; however, it may include stenosis of the valve cusps. Pulmonary stenosis results, in turn, in right ventricular hypertrophy.

The aorta appears to straddle the ventricular septum, overriding the ventricular septal defect. This defect allows a shunt of unsaturated blood from the right ventricle into the aorta or into the left ventricle (Figure 7-20).

The child with tetralogy of Fallot may be precyanotic in early infancy, with the cyanotic phase starting at from 4 to 6 months. Some severely affected infants, however, may show cyanosis earlier. As long as the ductus arteriosus remains open, enough blood apparently passes through the lungs to prevent cyanosis.

The infant presents with feeding difficulties and poor weight gain resulting in retarded growth and development. Dyspnea and easy fatigability become evident. Ex-

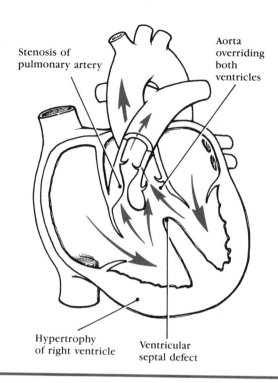

Figure 7-20. Tetralogy of Fallot is characterized by the combination of four defects: (1) pulmonary stenosis, (2) ventricular septal defect, (3) overriding aorta, and (4) hypertrophy of the right ventricle. It is the most common defect causing cyanosis in patients surviving beyond 2 years of age. The severity of symptoms depends on the degree of pulmonary stenosis, the size of the ventricular septal defect, and the degree to which the aorta overrides the septal defect. (From Bullock B. Pathophysiology: Adaptation and Alterations in Function, 3rd ed. Philadelphia: JB Lippincott, 1992, p. 525.)

ercise tolerance depends in part on the severity of the disease, some children becoming fatigued after little exertion. In the past on experiencing fatigue, breathlessness, and increased cyanosis, the child has been described as assuming a squatting posture for relief. Squatting apparently increased the systemic oxygen saturation. However, squatting rarely is seen because these infants' defects usually are repaired by the time they are 2 years old.

Attacks of paroxysmal dyspnea are common during infancy and early childhood. An anoxic spell is heralded by sudden restlessness, gasping respiration, and increased cyanosis, leading into a loss of consciousness and possibly convulsions. These attacks, called "tet spells," last from a few minutes to several hours and appear to be unpredictable, although stress does seem to trigger some episodes.

The history and clinical manifestations are usually sufficient to make a diagnosis. However, cardiac catheterization, electrocardiography, chest radiography, and laboratory tests to determine polycythemia and arterial oxygen saturation may be performed for further definition.

The preferred repair of these defects is total surgical correction. This procedure may be carried out only in a dry field, necessitating the use of a cardiopulmonary bypass machine. The heart is opened, and extensive resection is done. The septal defect is closed by use of a patch, and the valvular stenosis and infundibular chamber are resected.

Successful total correction apparently transforms a grossly abnormal heart into a functionally normal one. Most of these children are left without a pulmonary valve, however.

In those infants who are not able to withstand the total surgical correction until they are older, the Blalock-Taussig procedure is performed. This procedure is an end-to-end anastomosis of a vessel arising from the aorta, usually the subclavian artery, to the corresponding right or left pulmonary artery. The shunts are used with less frequency than previously because total surgical repair is meeting with much greater success and lower mortality rates.

Nursing Process for the Infant with Congestive Heart Failure

ASSESSMENT

The interview of the parent of an infant with CHF must include the gathering of information about the present illness and any previous episodes that the infant may have had. Questions should be asked about the problems the infant may have during feeding, episodes of rapid or difficult respirations, episodes of "turning blue," difficulty with lying flat, and how the infant has been gaining weight. Care must be taken to avoid causing any feelings of guilt in the caregiver.

The physical assessment of the infant includes a complete assessment of vital signs. Care should be taken to note the quality and rhythm of the apical pulse. Assessment of respirations is important and includes any use of accessory muscles, retractions, breath sounds, rate, and type of cry. Examination of the skin and extremities should include assessment of color, skin temperature, and evidence of edema. The nurse should closely observe the infant for signs of easy fatigability or an increase in symptoms on exertion.

NURSING DIAGNOSES

Some infants are so acutely ill on admission that they are admitted immediately to the pediatric intensive care unit, if one is available. The nursing diagnoses depend on the severity of the symptoms that determine the priority of care. Some diagnoses that may be useful include the following:

- Inadequate cardiac output related to structural defects of the heart

- Ineffective breathing pattern related to pulmonary congestion and anxiety
- Activity intolerance related to insufficient oxygenation secondary to heart defects
- High risk for altered nutrition: less than body requirements related to fatigue and dyspnea
- Altered family processes resulting from knowledge deficit related to the infant's life-threatening illness

PLANNING AND IMPLEMENTATION

The major nursing goals include the improvement of cardiac output and oxygenation, relief of inadequate respirations, adequate nutritional intake, and relief of parental anxiety due to increased knowledge about the infant's condition.

The family's goals include the relief of the infant's symptoms of distress and increased understanding of the condition and its prognosis.

Monitoring Vital Signs. Vital signs must be monitored regularly. If digoxin is ordered, the apical pulse must be counted for a full minute before it is administered. Digoxin should be withheld and the physician notified if the apical rate is lower than the established norms for the child's age and baseline information (90 to 110 beats per minute for infants and 70 to 85 beats per minute for older children). The dosage of digoxin should always be checked with another nurse before it is administered. Evidence of edema, periorbital or peripheral, must be evaluated regularly. Daily weight should be taken early in the morning, before the first feeding of the day, using the same scale with the infant undressed. Careful intake and output measurements should be maintained. If diuretics are administered, serum electrolyte levels should be monitored, especially potassium levels. The infant should be kept at an appropriately warm temperature.

Improving Respiratory Function. The head of the crib mattress should be elevated so that it is at a 30- to 45-degree angle. The infant should not be allowed to shift down in the crib and become "scrunched up," causing decreased expansion room for the chest. Constricting clothing must be avoided. Oxygen is administered as ordered. Respirations should be monitored at least every 4 hours, with close attention paid to breath sounds, dyspnea, tachypnea, retractions, and inspection of the nailbeds for cyanosis. Oxygen saturation levels are monitored with pulse oximetry.

Promoting Energy Conservation. Nursing care should be planned so that the infant has long periods of uninterrupted rest. During the periods when nursing procedures are being carried out, the nurse should talk to the infant softly and soothingly and handle him or her gently, giving loving care. The infant's cries should be responded to quickly so that tiring does not occur.

Maintaining Adequate Nutrition. Feedings should

be given in small, frequent amounts to avoid overtiring the infant. A soft nipple with a large opening may be used to ease the workload of the infant. If adequate nutrition cannot be taken during feedings, gavage feedings may need to be implemented.

Providing Family Teaching. The family of this infant has reason to be apprehensive and anxious. The nurse should be understanding, empathetic, and non-judgmental when communicating with the family members. They need to be given information about CHF in such a way that they can understand it. The nurse should repeat information about signs and symptoms and offer explanations as many times as necessary to help them have good knowledge about the condition. In addition, the nurse should include teaching about medication, feeding, and care techniques, growth and development expectations, and future plans for correction of the defect, if known. The family should be involved in the care of the infant as much as possible within the limitations of the infant's condition.

EVALUATION

- The heart rate is within the normal limits for age; no dysrhythmia or evidence of edema exists.
- The respirations are regular, with no retractions; breath sounds are clear.
- The infant rests quietly.
- The infant feeds with minimal tiring and consumes most of the feeding each time.
- The family verbalizes anxieties, asks appropriate questions, and participates in the care of the infant as able.

Skeletal System Defects

Infants or children with congenital skeletal defects usually receive primary treatment on the general nursery or pediatric unit, and thus the nurse needs to understand the nature and treatment of these anomalies. Children with these conditions and their parents often face long periods of exhausting, costly treatment and therefore need continuing support, encouragement, and education.

The two most common and important skeletal defects are **congenital talipes equinovarus** (clubfoot) and **congenital hip dysplasia** (dislocation of the hip).

Congenital Talipes Equinovarus

Congenital clubfoot is a deformity in which the entire foot is inverted, the heel is drawn up, and the forefoot is adducted. The Latin *talus*, meaning ankle, and *pes*, meaning foot, make up the word *talipes*, which is used in connection with many foot deformities. Equinus, or plantar flexion, and varus, or inversion, denote the kind of foot deformity present in this condition. The equinovarus foot has a clublike appearance, hence the term clubfoot (Figure 7-21).

Congenital talipes equinovarus is the most common congenital foot deformity, occurring in about 7 in 1000 births, appearing as a single anomaly or in connection with other defects, such as myelomeningocele. It may be bilateral (both feet) or unilateral (one foot). The cause is not clear; a hereditary factor occasionally is observed. A hypothesis that receives some acceptance proposes an arrested growth of the germ plasm of the foot during the first trimester of pregnancy.

Diagnosis. Talipes equinovarus is easily detected in a newborn infant but must be differentiated from a persist-

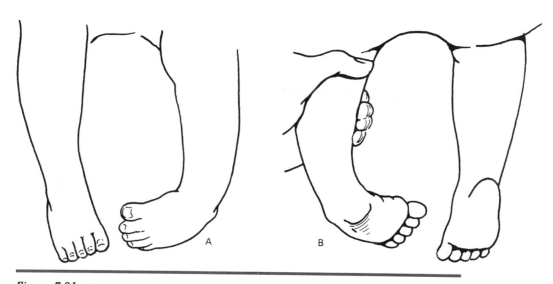

Figure 7-21. Unilateral clubfoot. **A,** Front view. **B,** Back view.

ing fetal "position of comfort" assumed in utero. The positional deformity may be easily corrected by the use of passive exercise, but the true clubfoot deformity is fixed. The positional deformity should be explained to the parents at once to prevent anxiety.

Nonsurgical Treatment. If treatment is started during the neonatal period, correction usually may be accomplished by manipulation and bandaging or by application of a cast. The cast often is applied while the infant is still in the neonatal nursery. While the cast is being applied, the foot is first gently moved into as near-normal position as possible. Force should not be used. If the infant's family caregiver can be present to help hold the infant while the cast is being applied, the caregiver will have the opportunity to understand what is being done. The very young infant gets satisfaction from sucking; therefore, a pacifier helps prevent squirming while the cast is being applied.

The cast is applied over the foot and ankle (and usually to mid-thigh) to hold the knee in right-angle flexion (Figure 7-22). Casts are changed frequently to provide gradual, nontraumatic correction—every few days for the first several weeks, then every week or two. Treatment is continued until complete correction is confirmed by radiograph and clinical observation, usually in a matter of months.

Any cast applied to a child's body should have some type of waterproof material protecting the skin from the sharp plaster edges of the cast. One method is to apply strips of adhesive vertically around the edges of the cast in a manner called petaling. This is done by cutting strips of adhesive 2 or 3 inches long and 1 inch wide. One end is notched and the other end is cut pointed to aid smooth application. Family caregivers must be taught cast care.

Following correction from a cast, a Denis Browne splint with shoes attached is used to maintain correction for another 6 months or longer (Figure 7-23). After overcorrection has been attained, a special clubfoot shoe should be worn, a laced shoe with a turning out of the shoe and the outer wedge of the sole that looks like the shoe is being worn on the wrong foot. The Denis Browne splint still may be worn at night, and passive exercises of the foot should be carried out by the child's caregivers. The older infant may resist wearing the splint, so the family caregivers must be taught the importance of gentle, but firm, insistence that the splint be worn.

Surgical Treatment. Children who do not respond to nonsurgical measures, especially older children, need surgical correction. This approach involves several procedures, depending on the age of the child and the degree of the deformity. It may involve lengthening of the Achilles tendon, capsulotomy of the ankle joint, release of medial strictures, and for the child older than 10 years of age, an operation on the bony structure. Prolonged observation, after correction by either means, should be carried out at least until adolescence; any recurrence is treated promptly.

Congenital Hip Dysplasia

Congenital hip dysplasia results from defective development of the acetabulum with or without dislocation. The malformed acetabulum permits dislocation, the head of the femur becoming displaced upward and backward. The condition is difficult to recognize during early infancy. When there is family history of the defect, increased observation of the young infant is indicated. The condition is approximately seven times more common in girls than in boys and is frequently bilateral.

Diagnosis. Early recognition and treatment, before an infant starts to stand or walk, is extremely important for successful correction. The first examination should be

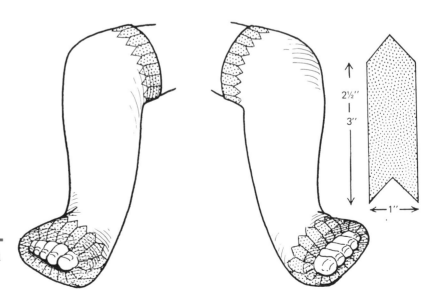

Figure 7-22. Casting for clubfoot in typical overcorrected position showing petaling of cast.

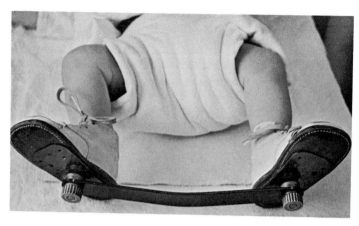

Figure 7-23. A Denis Browne splint with shoes attached.

part of the newborn examination. Experienced examiners may detect an audible "click" when examining the newborn using the Bartow and Ortolani tests. These tests, used together on one hip at a time, involve dislocating and relocating the acetabulum in adduction and abduction and should be conducted only by an experienced practitioner. They are effective only for the first month, after which they disappear. Signs that are useful after this include the following:

1. Asymmetry of the gluteal skin folds (they are higher on the affected side) (Figure 7-24)

2. Limitation of abduction of the affected hip. This is tested by placing the infant in a dorsal recumbent position with his or her knees flexed and then abducting both knees passively until they reach the examination table without resistance. If dislocation is present, the affected side cannot be abducted more than 45 degrees.

3. Apparent shortening of the femur.

Later signs, after the child has started walking, include lordosis, swayback, protruding abdomen, shortened extremity, duck-waddle gait, and a positive Trendel-

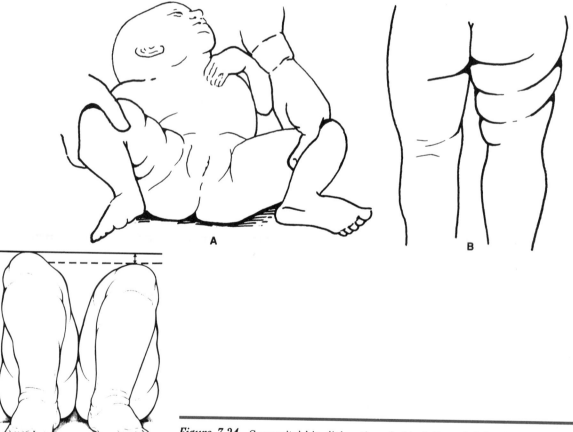

Figure 7-24. Congenital hip dislocation. **A,** Limitation of abduction in the affected leg. **B,** Asymmetry of the gluteal folds of the thighs. **C,** Apparent shortening of the femur.

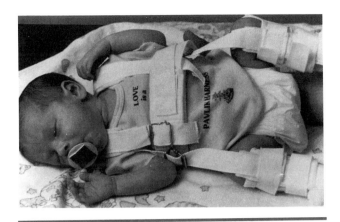

Figure 7-25. Proper positioning of an infant in Pavlik harness. The harness is composed of shoulder straps, stirrups, and a chest strap. It is placed on both legs, even if only one hip is dislocated. (From Jackson DB, Saunders RB. Child Health Nursing. Philadelphia: JB Lippincott, 1993.)

enburg sign. To elicit the sign, the child stands on the affected leg and raises the normal leg. The pelvis tilts downward rather than upward toward the unaffected side.

Roentgen studies usually are made to confirm the diagnosis in the older infant. Uncorrected dislocation causes limping, easy fatigue, hip and low back discomfort, and postural deformities.

Treatment. When the dislocation is discovered during the first few months, treatment consists of manipulation of the femur into position and application of a brace. The most common type of brace in use is the Pavlik harness (Figure 7-25). The physician needs to assess the infant weekly while the infant is in the harness and adjust it to gradually align the femur. In some instances, no further treatment is needed. If treatment is delayed until after the child has commenced to walk or if earlier treatment is not effective, open reduction followed by a spica cast is usually needed. After the cast is removed, a metal or plastic brace is applied to keep the legs in wide abduction.

Nursing Process for the Infant in an Orthopedic Device or Cast

ASSESSMENT

Although the actual hospitalization of the infant is relatively short if there are no other abnormalities that require hospitalization, the nursing responsibility to teach the family cast care or care of the infant in an orthopedic device, such as a Pavlik harness, is of utmost importance. The nurse needs to assess the family's ability to understand and cooperate in the care of the infant. Emotional support of the family is important.

The assessment of the infant varies with the orthopedic device or cast that has been applied. Immediately after the application of a cast, the observations center on

promotion of even drying of the cast. In addition, the toes should be checked for circulation and movement. The skin at the edges of the cast must be checked for signs of pressure or irritation. If an open reduction has been performed, the child should be assessed for signs of shock and bleeding in the immediate postoperative period.

NURSING DIAGNOSES

The nursing diagnoses depend on the defect and the type of treatment. Some diagnoses that may be used are the following:

- Anxiety related to restricted mobility
- High risk for skin impairment related to pressure of the cast on the skin surface
- High risk for altered growth and development related to restricted mobility secondary to orthopedic device or cast
- Family health-seeking behaviors related to the home care of the infant in the orthopedic device or cast

PLANNING AND IMPLEMENTATION

The goals of the family are centered around the desire for correction of the defect with minimal disruption to the growth and development of the infant and care of the infant at home.

Nursing goals include relief of the infant's anxiety, maintenance of skin integrity, nurturance to promote growth and development, and education of the family in the care of the infant at home.

Providing Comfort Measures. The infant may be irritable and fussy because of restriction of movement caused by the device or cast. Methods of soothing the infant that are useful include nonnutritive sucking, stroking, cuddling, and talking or crooning. If irritability seems excessive, the infant should be checked for signs of irritation from the device or cast. The infant in a cast may be held after the cast is completely dry. The harness should not be removed unless specific permission for bathing is granted by the physician. Caretakers must be taught how to reapply the harness correctly. The infant in a Pavlik harness is not difficult to handle.

Promoting Skin Integrity. For the first 24 to 48 hours after application of a cast, the infant should be placed on a firm mattress, and position changes should be supported by firm pillows. When handling the cast, the nurse should use the palms of his or her hands to avoid excessive pressure on the cast. The skin around the cast edges should be carefully inspected for signs of irritation, redness, or edema. The edges of the cast should be petaled around the waist and toes and protected with plastic covering around the perineal area. Great care should be taken to protect the diaper area from becoming soiled and moist. If the covering becomes soiled, it should be removed, washed, dried thoroughly, and reapplied or replaced. With the Pavlik harness, the skin under the straps should be assessed frequently and massaged gently to promote circulation. Extra padding may be placed under the shoulder straps to relieve pressure in that area.

Powders and lotions should be avoided with either the device or cast. "Caking" and "pilling" of the powder or lotion cause areas of irritation. Daily sponge baths are important and must include close attention to the skin under the straps of the device or around the edge of the cast. The infant in a cast should be observed carefully to prevent any restrictions of breathing because of tightness over the abdomen and lower chest area. Also, vomiting after a feeding may be an indication that the cast is too tight over the stomach. Care should be taken to prevent any small particles of food or toys from being pushed down into the cast by the older infant or child.

Diapering can be a challenge for the infant in a cast. Despite environmental concerns, disposable diapers may be the most effective answer in providing good protection of the cast and preventing leakage.

Providing Sensory Stimulation. Because the infant is in the device or cast for an extended period during which much growth and development takes place, efforts should be made to provide the infant with stimulation of a tactile nature. Mobiles, musical toys, and stuffed toys should be provided. The infant should not be permitted to cry for long periods. Feeding times should be relaxed, the infant should be held, if at all possible, and interaction should be encouraged. A pacifier should be provided if the infant desires it. Activities that use the infant's free hands should be encouraged. The older infant may enjoy looking at picture books and interacting with siblings. Diversionary activities should include ways in which the infant may be safely transported to other areas in the home or in the car. Strollers and car seats may be adapted to provide safe transportation. For toddlers, a dolly (a low solid frame on wheels) may provide a movable base to explore the environment and encourage independence.

Providing Family Teaching. The nurse needs to assess the family's knowledge and design a thorough teaching plan because the infant will be cared for at home for most of the time. Complete explanations, written guidelines, demonstrations, and return demonstrations are all useful methods. The family should have a resource person who may be called when a question arises and should be encouraged to feel free to call that person. Definite plans should be made for return visits to have the device or cast checked. The family needs to understand the importance of keeping these appointments. A public health nurse referral may be provided when appropriate (see Nursing Care Plan for the Infant with an Orthopedic Device or Cast).

EVALUATION

- The infant is alert and content with no long periods of fussiness. The skin around the edges of the cast shows no signs of redness or irritation.

- The infant demonstrates evidence of accomplishing appropriate developmental milestones.

- The family demonstrates understanding of the infant's care and asks pertinent questions.

Genitourinary Tract Defects

Most congenital anomalies of the genitourinary tract are not life threatening in a physical sense but may present social problems with lifelong implications for the child and family. Thus, early recognition and supportive, understanding care of these problems are essential.

Hypospadias and Epispadias

Hypospadias is a congenital condition of a male child in which the urethra terminates on the ventral (underside) surface of the penis, instead of at the tip. A cordlike anomaly (called a **chordee**) extends from the scrotum to the penis, pulling the penis downward in an arc. Urination is not interfered with, but the boy is unable to void while standing in the normal male fashion. Surgical repair is desirable between the ages of 6 months and 18 months before body image and castration anxiety become problems. Microscopic surgery makes the early repair possible.

Surgical repair is often accomplished in one stage and is often possible as outpatient surgery. These infants should not be circumcised because the foreskin is used in the repair. Some cases of severe hypospadias may require additional surgical procedures.

In **epispadias**, the opening is on the dorsal (top) surface of the penis. This condition often occurs with exstrophy of the bladder. Surgical repair is indicated.

Exstrophy of the Bladder

This urinary tract malformation occurs in 1 in 30,000 live births in the United States and is usually accompanied by other anomalies, such as epispadias, cleft scrotum, cryptorchidism (undescended testes), a shortened penis in males, and cleft clitoris in females. It is also associated with malformed pelvic musculature, resulting in prolapsed rectum and inguinal hernias. Children with this defect have a widely split symphysis pubis and posterolaterally rotated hip sockets, causing a waddling gait.

In this condition, the anterior surface of the urinary bladder lies open on the lower abdomen (Figure 7-26). The exposed mucosa is red and sensitive to touch and allows direct passage of urine to the outside. This condition makes the area vulnerable to infection and trauma. Surgical closure of the bladder is preferred within the first 48 hours of the infant's life. Final surgical correction is completed before the child goes to school. If repair of the bladder is not done early in the child's life, the family caregivers need to be taught how to care for this condition and how to deal with their own feelings toward this less-than-perfect child. Their emotional reaction may be further complicated if the malformation is so severe that the

Nursing Care Plan
for the Infant with an Orthopedic Device or Cast

Nursing Diagnosis
Anxiety related to restricted mobility

Goal: Reduce infant's anxiety

Nursing Interventions	Rationale	Evaluation
Soothe the infant by stroking, cuddling, talking, crooning, or providing a pacifier.	These are all methods that will help the infant feel safe and loved; they also may provide distraction from the uncomfortable feeling of restriction or irritation from the cast.	The infant is alert and content with no long periods of fussiness.

Nursing Diagnosis
High risk for impaired skin integrity related to pressure of device or cast on skin surface

Goal: Maintain skin integrity

Nursing Interventions	Rationale	Evaluation
For the first 24 to 48 hours after cast application, place infant on a firm mattress and support position changes by firm pillows.	The cast is still wet during this time, and could be pushed out of shape if pressure is too great at any single point.	Cast maintains original shape.
Use palms when handling the cast.	Prevents excessive pressure on wet cast.	
Petal all edges of the cast. Carefully inspect the edges of the cast for signs of irritation, redness or edema.	These are early signs of skin breakdown.	The skin around the edges of the cast show no signs of redness or irritation.
Keep the perineal area of the cast from becoming soiled and wet by protecting with plastic covering. Remove, wash, and thoroughly dry covering if it becomes wet.	Moisture can contribute to skin tissue breakdown.	Perineal covering remains dry and clean.
Frequently assess and gently massage skin under Pavlik harness straps; extra padding may be used under shoulder straps.	The Pavlik harness straps can dig into the infant's shoulders; massaging will improve circulation in that tender area; extra padding also may help to relieve pressure.	Shoulder areas under straps show no signs of redness or irritation.

(continued)

Nursing Care Plan
for the Infant with an Orthopedic Device or Cast (Continued)

Nursing Diagnosis

High risk for altered growth and development related to restricted mobility secondary to orthopedic device or cast

Goal: Provide age-appropriate stimulation

Nursing Interventions	Rationale	Evaluation
Provide infant with mobiles, musical toys, and stuffed toys. Encourage caregiver interaction with the child during feeding time and plan activities that use the infant's free hands.	These toys and activities provide visual, audio, and tactile stimulation to help replace the stimulation an infant without a cast would normally receive through crawling and moving.	The infant demonstrates evidence of accomplishing appropriate developmental milestones.
Plan diversional activities with family caregivers that provide for visual stimulation in different environments.	Because the child cannot move freely, it is important that the environment change visually to provide new sights and sounds.	

Nursing Diagnosis

Family health-seeking behaviors related to the home care of the infant in the orthopedic device or cast

Goal: Provide family teaching

Nursing Interventions	Rationale	Evaluation
Assess the family's knowledge level and design a thorough teaching plan.	It is essential to find out first how much a family understands before beginning any teaching plan.	The family demonstrates understanding of the infant's care and asks pertinent questions.
Choose teaching methods most suited to identified needs and learning style of the family caregivers.	When the appropriate teaching methods are chosen, learning will occur much more quickly.	
Schedule appointments for return visits to have device or cast checked.	Making appointments for return visits before the family leaves will emphasize their importance.	

sex of the child may be determined only by a chromosome test (see the following section on sexual ambiguity).

Nursing care of the infant with exstrophy of the bladder should be directed toward preventing infection, preventing skin irritation around the seeping mucosa, meeting the infant's need for touch and cuddling, and educating and supporting the parents during this crisis.

Sexual Ambiguity

Although rare, the birth of an infant with ambiguous genitalia presents a highly charged emotional climate and has possible long-range social implications. Regardless of the cause, it is important to establish the genetic sex and the sex of rearing as early as possible, so that surgical correction of anomalies may take place before the child begins to function in a sex-related social role. Authorities believe that the infant's anatomic structure, rather than the genetic sex, should determine the sex of rearing. It is possible to surgically construct a functional vagina and to administer hormones to offer an anatomically incomplete female a somewhat normal life. Currently, it is not possible to offer comparable surgical reconstruction to males with an inadequate penis. Par-

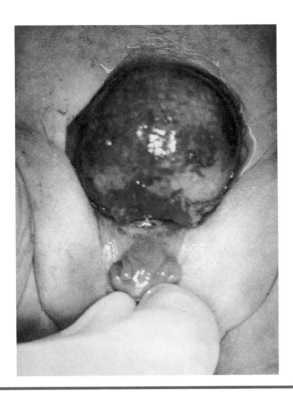

Figure 7-26. Exstrophy of the bladder. (From Avery GB. Neonatalogy, 2nd ed. Philadelphia: JB Lippincott, 1981.)

ents may feel guilt, anxiety, and confusion about their child's condition and need empathic understanding and support to help them cope with this emergency.

Other Congenital Disorders

Infections

Congenital Rubella

The rubella virus infection acquired by the fetus in utero generally persists throughout fetal life and for as long as 18 months after delivery. Persons coming into intimate contact with these babies may develop the disease; therefore, all women of childbearing age who are not immune to rubella should avoid contact with an infected infant.

A large variety of malformations constitute the congenital rubella syndrome, including cataracts and other eye defects, such as glaucoma. Other complications include deafness; cardiac anomalies, especially patent ductus arteriosus, and septal defects; intrauterine growth retardation; subnormal head circumference; and retarded functional development.

Reliance on immunization by presumed attacks of rubella during the person's childhood generally is not dependable because many rashes resemble that of rubella, and symptoms of childhood rubella are mild. Children now receive rubella vaccine as part of their immunizations at 15 months of age. Testing for the presence of

rubella serum antibody is routine in all pregnant women. A positive reaction shows the person to be immune either as a result of the disease itself or from immunization. As a result of these concentrated efforts, neonates are protected from this devastating disease.

Care of the infant is concerned with treating accompanying conditions and giving routine care accorded any newborn infant. Some infants are extremely ill from complications present at birth, and rates of permanent damage are high.

A discussion of maternal immunization for rubella is found in Chapter 4 in the section on maternal infections.

Congenital Syphilis

Syphilis, whether congenital or acquired, is caused by the spirochete *Treponema pallidum*. Fetal infection does not occur much before the fourth month of fetal life, after the fetal organs are formed; therefore, anomalies rarely occur. The infection is contracted through the mother by placental transfer. About one fourth of infected infants are stillborn. Infants born live may not show any clinical symptoms for months or years.

Diagnosis. A VDRL (Venereal Disease Research Laboratory) or Wassermann test on cord blood at delivery is done when congenital syphilis is suspected. Passively acquired antibodies may give false-positive results; therefore, other serologic tests are conducted subsequently. If results are doubtful, treatment usually is instituted to avoid a full-blown infection.

In early congenital syphilis, symptoms may appear before the sixth week of life. Rhinitis, with a profuse, mucopurulent nasal discharge, is usually the first symptom. A maculopapular skin rash appears next, heaviest over the back, buttocks, and backs of the thighs. Bleeding ulcerations and mucous membrane lesions appear around the mouth, the anus, and the genital areas (Figure 7-27). Anemia is present; pseudoparalysis and pathologic fractures may occur. These symptoms usually subside without treatment while the infectious organism lies latent in the child's tissues.

Late symptoms, appearing after infancy, involve the skeletal framework, the eyes, and the central nervous system. The child may acquire a flat bridge of the nose, known as "saddle nose." The permanent teeth are affected in that the incisors are peg shaped (Hutchinson's teeth). A condition of the eyes called **interstitial keratitis** often occurs later in the disease with lacrimation, photophobia, and opacity of the lens that may lead to blindness.

Treatment. Ideally, treatment is preventive, consisting of penicillin therapy for the affected mother early in pregnancy. The physician may order the test to be repeated later in the pregnancy, if infection is suspected, with penicillin therapy instituted at this point if the test is positive. Treatment for the affected infant consists of a

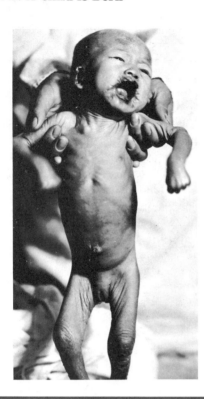

Figure 7-27. Some of the skin manifestations of congenital syphilis. (From Waechter EH, Blake FG. Nursing Care of Children, 9th ed. Philadelphia: JB Lippincott, 1976.)

course of penicillin therapy. Strict isolation of the infant is required.

Early congenital syphilis usually responds to vigorous treatment, and growth and development is not affected. Late congenital syphilis responds well to treatment, but pathologic changes in the bones, eyes, and nervous system are permanent.

Gonorrheal Ophthalmia Neonatorum

Gonorrheal eye infection in the newborn is a serious condition, usually resulting in blindness when prophylactic treatment at birth is omitted. The infectious agent is the gonococcus *Neisseria gonorrhoeae*. The infant becomes infected while passing through the birth canal of an infected mother.

Symptoms are acute redness and swelling of the conjunctiva with a purulent discharge from the eyes, occurring within 36 to 48 hours after birth. The condition is communicable for 24 hours after specific therapy is instituted or when no therapy is used, until discharge from the eyes has ceased.

Prevention and Treatment. In the United States, all states have laws requiring the use of specific preparations instilled into the eyes at birth. States require instillation of 1% silver nitrate or antibiotic drops or ophthalmic ointments, such as tetracycline and erythromycin. Penicillin is the drug of choice for the treatment of gonorrheal

infections, including gonorrheal ophthalmia (see Chapter 5).

Herpes Simplex Virus

Herpes simplex virus, most frequently caused by herpesvirus hominis type 2, is transmitted to the neonate during vaginal delivery of a mother who has an active genital lesion. Cesarean delivery before rupture of membranes is considered a preventive measure, although a small possibility remains that the fetus could have been infected before delivery. The infant usually has no apparent signs of the disease until 6 to 9 days after delivery. In the newborn nursery, those infants who have had possible exposure should be segregated or cared for in the mother's private room.

The infection may be generalized, resembling sepsis. The infant may or may not have lesions. Lesions are highly contagious, if present. The mortality rate is high. Those infants who survive have a high probability for ocular and neurologic damage.

Inborn Errors of Metabolism

Phenylketonuria

Phenylketonuria (PKU) is a recessive hereditary defect of metabolism that, if untreated, causes severe mental retardation in most, but not all, affected children. It is an uncommon trait appearing in about 1 in 10,000 births. In this condition, there is a lack of the enzyme that normally changes the essential amino acid, phenylalanine, into tyrosine.

As soon as the newborn infant with this defect begins to take milk, either breast or cow's milk, phenylalanine is absorbed in the normal manner. However because of the affected infant's inability to metabolize this amino acid, phenylalanine builds up in the blood serum to as much as 20 times the normal level. This build-up takes place at such a rapid pace that increased levels of phenylalanine appear in the blood after 1 or 2 days of ingestion of milk. Phenylpyruvic acid appears in the urine of these infants sometime between the second and the sixth week of life.

Most untreated children with this condition develop severe and progressive mental deficiency, apparently because of the high serum phenylalanine level. The infant appears normal at birth but commences to show signs of mental arrest within a few weeks. It is therefore imperative that these infants be discovered as early in life as possible and placed immediately on a low-phenylalanine formula.

Clinical Manifestations. Untreated infants may show signs of frequent vomiting and aggressive and hyperactive traits. Severe, progressive retardation is characteristic. Convulsions may occur, and eczema, particularly in the perineal area, is common. There is a characteristic musty smell to the urine.

Diagnosis. A blood test is required by most states to detect the phenylalanine level in the newborn. This screening procedure, called the Guthrie inhibition assay test, uses blood from a simple heel prick. The test is most reliable after the infant has ingested some form of protein. Because most infants are discharged early, the accepted practice is to perform the test before the infant is discharged and repeat it again in the third week of life if the first test was done before the infant was 24 hours old. Health practitioners caring for infants not born in a hospital are responsible for the screening of the infant. When screening indicates an increased level of phenylalanine, additional testing is done to make a firm diagnosis.

Treatment. Dietary treatment is required with careful supervision. A formula low in phenylalanine should be started as soon as the condition is detected. (Lofenalac is a low-phenylalanine formula produced by Mead Johnson.) The best results are obtained if the special formula is started before the infant is 3 weeks of age. A low-phenylalanine diet is a very restricted one. Foods to be omitted are breads, meat, fish, dairy products, nuts, and legumes. The diet should be carefully supervised by a nutritionist. The diet should be continued well into the school years. Maintenance of the infant on the restricted diet is relatively simple compared with the problems that arise as the child grows and becomes more independent. Routine blood testing is done to maintain the serum phenylalanine level between 2 and 8 mg/dL. As the child ventures into the world beyond home, more and more dietary temptations are available, and dietary compliance is difficult. The family and child need support and counseling throughout the child's developmental years.

The length of time that the restrictions are necessary is still unclear. Although difficult, the diet seems to be best followed into adolescence.

Galactosemia

Galactosemia is a recessive hereditary metabolic disorder in which the enzyme necessary for converting galactose into glucose is missing. The infants generally appear normal at birth but experience difficulties after the ingestion of milk—whether breast, cow's, or goat's milk—because one of the component monosaccharides of milk lactose is galactose.

Clinical Manifestations and Diagnosis. Early feeding difficulties, with vomiting and diarrhea severe enough to produce dehydration and weight loss, and jaundice are primary manifestations. Unless milk is withheld early, other difficulties include cataracts, liver and spleen damage, and mental retardation, with a high mortality rate early in life. A blood test using the Guthrie inhibition assay method has proved a reliable diagnostic test and is now required by many states as part of routine newborn screening. It may be performed in conjunction with a test for PKU.

Treatment. Galactose must be omitted from the diet, which in the young infant means a substitution for milk. Nutramigen and Pregestimil are formulas that provide galactose-free nutrition for the infant. The diet must continue to be free of lactose when the child moves on to table foods, but the diet does allow for more variety than the phenylalanine-free diet.

Congenital Hypothyroidism

At one time referred to by the now unacceptable term cretinism, congenital hypothyroidism is associated with either a congenital absence of a thyroid gland or with the inability of the infant's thyroid gland to secrete thyroid hormone. The incidence is about 1 in 5000 births, which is approximately twice as frequent as PKU.

Diagnosis. Most states require a routine test for triiodothyronine (T_3) and thyroxine (T_4) levels to determine thyroid function on all newborns before discharge to diagnose congenital hypothyroidism early. This test is done as part of the heel stick screening, which includes the Guthrie screening test for PKU.

Clinical Manifestations. The infant appears normal at birth, but at about 6 weeks of life, clinical signs and symptoms begin to be noticeable. The facial features are typical, with a short forehead, depressed nasal bridge, large tongue, and puffy eyes. The voice (cry) is hoarse, the skin is dry, and there is slow bone development. Two common features are obstinate constipation and umbilical hernia. The infant is a poor feeder, often characterized as a "good" baby by the parent or caretaker because the infant cries very little and sleeps long periods.

Treatment. Replacement of the thyroid hormone is necessary as soon as diagnosis is made. Levothyroxine sodium, a synthetic thyroid replacement, is the drug most commonly used. Blood levels of T_3 and T_4 are monitored to prevent overdosage. Unless therapy is started in early infancy, mental retardation and slow growth occur. The later the therapy is started, the greater the severity of mental retardation. Therapy must be continued for the rest of the person's life.

Summary

Advances in medical technology have improved the outlook for many infants who have sustained damage during intrauterine development or birth, giving them a better chance of an improved quality of life. Nevertheless, many conditions still inflict overwhelming consequences, causing lifelong disabilities. The nurse caring for these infants must use all available resources to deliver quality nursing care to these infants and their families. Many infants injured during the birth process or born with a congenital anomaly have long-term effects from their conditions. Their families may have long-term effects as well. The nurse must be prepared to provide care that stimulates the optimum growth and development of the infant as well as meets the immediate physical problems. The nurse also must include the family, preparing them for home care of the infant and guiding the family to support services that enable them to manage the care for their child for many years. Care of the newborn with special needs is a challenging aspect of nursing.

Review Questions

1. Diane's baby was born with a bilateral cleft lip and cleft palate. When you bring the baby in to her for feeding, she breaks down and sobs uncontrollably. How will you handle this situation?
2. After you talked with her for awhile, Diane is able to get herself under control enough to tell you that she was planning to breastfeed her baby and now she can't because of the cleft lip and palate. What is your response to her? Give her information on feeding as part of your response.
3. You are caring for an infant who has had a cleft lip repair. Describe the care the infant needs concerning elbow restraints.
4. How would you care for the suture line of a cleft lip repair?
5. Why is it important to do a surgical repair on a meningocele?
6. Why is infection control of utmost importance in the care of the infant with myelomeningocele?
7. Your friends have a new baby who has myelomeningocele. The baby is under the care of an well-regarded physician, but your friends still have a lot of questions. What questions will you ask them? What kinds of things will you say to them?
8. How often is the volume of cerebrospinal fluid absorbed and replaced?
9. Tell what happens as fluid builds up in hydrocephalus before the suture lines close; after the sutures line close.
10. What symptoms would an infant display if fluid build-up in the brain is not relieved?
11. What can you do to provide comfort and developmental stimulation to an infant after shunting for hydrocephalus?
12. What are some of the maternal risk factors that may cause congenital heart defects?
13. What is the advantage of using hypothermia during surgery to repair a congenital heart defect?

Reference

1. Alexander MA, Steg NL. Myelomeningocele: Comprehensive treatment. Arch Phys Med Rehabil 70:637–641, 1989.

Bibliography

Aiello DH. Congenital dysplasia of the hip: Diagnosis, treatment, nursing care. AORN J 49(6):1566, 1570, 1574, 1989.

Arn PH, Valle DL, Brusilow SW. Inborn errors of metabolism: Not rare, not hopeless. Contemp Pediatr 5(12):47, 57, 1988.

Byrd LA, Bruton-Maree N. Tetralogy of Fallot. AANA J 57(2): 169–176, 1989.

Carpenito LJ. Handbook of Nursing Diagnosis, 4th ed. Philadelphia: JB Lippincott, 1991.

Castiglia PT, Harbin RE. Child Health Care: Process and Practice. Philadelphia: JB Lippincott, 1992.

Corbett D. Information needs of parents of a child in a Pavlik harness. Orthop Nurs 7(2):20–23, 1988.

Curtin G. The infant with cleft lip or palate: More than a surgical problem. J Perinat Neonat Nurs 3(3):80–89, 1990.

Evans-Berro EA. How to defeat a "tet spell." Am J Nurs 91(7): 46–48, 1991.

Kenner C, Hern MJ. Writing a nursing diagnosis for a complex client: The infant with a congenital heart defect. J Pediatr Nurs 3(4):256–264, 1988.

Peterson PM. Spina bifida: Nursing challenge. RN 55(3):40–46, 1992.

Pillitteri A. Maternal and Child Health Nursing. Philadelphia: JB Lippincott, 1992.

Powell ML, Costanzo JM. Tricuspid atresia: Surgical treatment, pediatric nursing care. AORN J 52(3):567, 570, 1990.

Sampson J, Williams A, McKenna M. The care of children with hydrocephalus. Nursing 3(34):43–48, 1989.

Schaming D, Gorry M, Soroka K, et al. When babies are born with orthopedic problems. RN 53(4):62–67, 1990.

Shaw N. Common surgical problems in the newborn. J Perinat Neonat Nurs 3(3):50–56, 1990.

Steele S. Phenylketonuria: Counseling and teaching functions of the nurse on an interdisciplinarian team. Iss Compr Pediatr Nurs 12(5):395–409, 1989.

Whaley LF, Wong DL. Nursing Care of Infants and Children, 4th ed. St. Louis: Mosby-Year Book, 1991.

A Child Grows

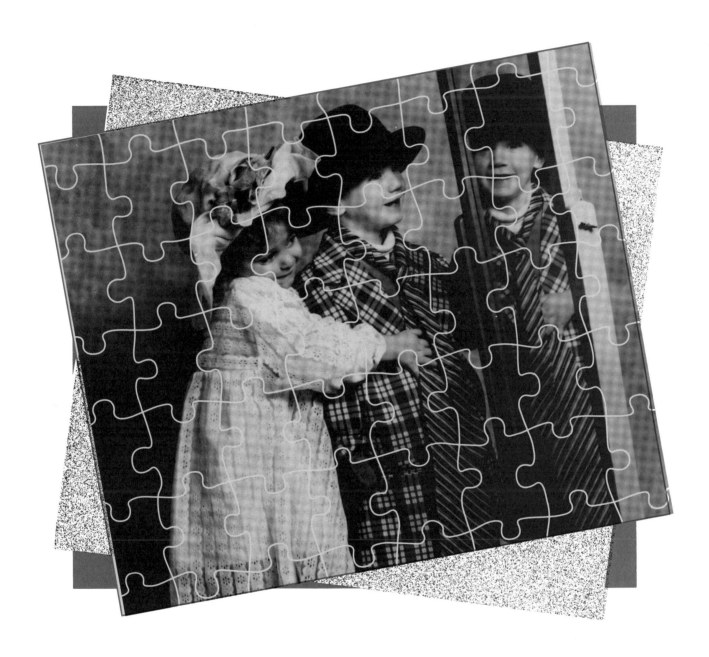

Unit **III**

Growth and Development of the Infant: 28 Days to 1 Year

Chapter 8

Student Objectives

Upon completion of this chapter, the student will be able to:

1. State the ages at which the fontanelles normally close: a.) Anterior fontanelle; b.) Posterior fontanelle.
2. State the ages at which the infant's birth weight: a.) Doubles; b.) Triples.
3. Discuss the eruption of deciduous teeth: a.) Approximate age of the first tooth; b.) First teeth to erupt; c.) Factors that may interfere with eruption; d.) Role of fluoride in dental health.
4. Discuss the appropriate use of developmental tables.
5. State the age at which the child becomes aware of himself or herself as a person.
6. Name the age when the fear of strangers usually appears.
7. State why a baby tends to push food out of his or her mouth with the tongue.
8. State the rationale for introducing new foods one at a time.
9. Discuss "weaning" the infant: a.) Usual age the baby becomes interested in a cup; b.) Criteria to determine the appropriate time.
10. State the cause and prevention of "bottle mouth" caries.
11. List three foods to offer the infant who does not drink enough milk from the cup.
12. List seven communicable diseases against which children are immunized.
13. State at what age immunizations usually begin and which are given in the first year.
14. State one useful purpose of the game "Peek-a-Boo."
15. Discuss the family caregivers' role in the infant's hospital care.

Marks MG: BROADRIBB'S INTRODUCTORY PEDIATRIC NURSING, 4th ed. © 1994 J.B. Lippincott Company.

Key Terms

"bottle mouth" or "nursing bottle" caries

deciduous teeth

extrusion reflex

pedodontist

The infant who has lived through the first month of life has a busy year ahead. During this year the infant grows and develops skills at a rate more rapid than will ever be experienced again. In the brief span of a single year, this tiny, helpless bit of humanity becomes a person with strong emotions of love, fear, jealousy, and anger and gains the ability to rise from a supine to an upright position and move about purposefully.

In the first year, both weight and height increase rapidly. During the first 6 months the infant's birth weight doubles and height increases about 6 inches. Growth slows slightly during the second 6 months but is still rapid. By 1 year of age, the infant's birth weight triples and 10 to 12 inches are added to the height.

Thinking in terms of the "average" child is misleading. To determine whether an infant is reaching acceptable levels of development, birth weight and height must be the standard with which later measurements are compared. A baby weighing 6 lb at birth cannot be expected to weigh as much at 5 or 6 months of age as the baby who weighed 9 lb at birth, but each is expected to double his or her birth weight at about this time. A growth graph is helpful to the nurse, pediatrician, or caregiver for charting a child's progress (Figure 8-1).

Physical Development

Despite the many factors, such as genetic, environmental, health, gender, and race, that affect the growth in the first year of life, the healthy infant progresses in a predictable pattern. By the end of the year, the dependent infant, who at 1 month of age had no teeth and was unable to roll over, sit, or stand, blossoms into an emerging toddler with teeth, the ability to sit alone, stand, and begin to walk alone. The miracle of growth, seen in the prenatal development of the fetus, continues.

Head and Skull

At birth, an infant's head circumference averages about 13 3/4 inches (35 cm) and is usually slightly larger than his or her chest circumference. The chest measures approximately the same as the abdomen at birth.

At about 1 year of age, the head is increased in circumference to approximately 18 inches (47 cm). The chest also grows rapidly, catching up to the head circumference at about 5 to 7 months of age. From then on the chest can be expected to exceed the head in circumference.

Fontanelles and Cranial Sutures
The posterior fontanelle is usually closed by the second or third month of life. The anterior fontanelle may increase slightly in size during the first few months of life. After the 6th month it begins to decrease in size, becoming closed between the 12th and the 18th months. The sutures between the cranial bones do not ossify until later childhood.

Skeletal Growth and Maturation

During fetal life the skeletal system is completely formed in cartilage at the end of 3 months' gestation. Ossification and growth of bones occur during the remainder of fetal life and throughout childhood. The pattern of maturation is so regular that the "bone age" can be determined by radiologic examination. When the bone age matches the child's chronologic age, the skeletal structure is maturing at a normal rate. Radiologic examination is performed *only* if a problem is suspected to avoid unnecessary exposure to radiation.

Eruption of Deciduous Teeth

Calcification of the primary or **deciduous teeth** starts early in fetal life. Shortly before birth, calcification begins in those permanent teeth that are the first to erupt in later childhood. The first deciduous teeth usually erupt between 6 and 8 months of age. The first teeth to erupt are usually the lower central incisors.

Babies in good health who show normal develop-

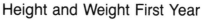

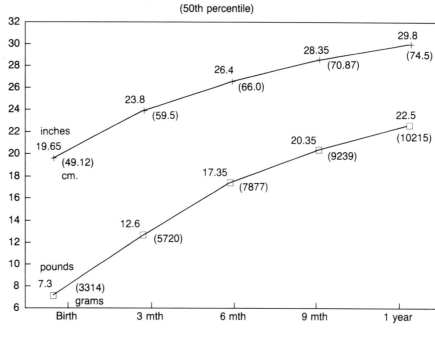

Figure 8-1. Chart of infant growth representing an infant in the mid-range—birthweight 7.3 lb (3314 g) and birth length 19.65 inches (49.12 cm). Infants of different races vary in average size. Asian infants tend to be smaller, African American infants larger.

ment may differ in the timing of tooth eruption. Some families show a tendency toward very early or very late eruption, without other signs of early or late development (Figure 8-2). Some infants may become restless or fussy from swollen, inflamed gums during teething. A cold

teething ring may be helpful in soothing the baby's discomfort. Teething is a normal process of development and does not cause high fever or upper respiratory conditions.

Nutritional deficiency or prolonged illness in infancy may interfere with calcification of both the deciduous and the permanent teeth. The role of fluoride in strengthening calcification of teeth has been well documented. In areas where the fluoride content of drinking water is inadequate or absent, the American Dental Association recommends its administration to infants and children.

Circulatory System

In the first year of life, the circulatory system undergoes several changes. During fetal life high levels of hemoglobin and numbers of red blood cells are necessary for adequate oxygenation. After birth, when oxygen is supplied through the respiratory system, hemoglobin decreases in volume, and red blood cells gradually decrease in number until the third month of life. Thereafter, the count gradually increases until adult levels are reached.

Blood pressure measurement is extremely difficult to obtain with accuracy in an infant. The flush method is sometimes used when a determination of the systolic pressure is desired. Electronic or ultrasonographic monitoring equipment is often used. The average blood pressure during the first year of life is $85/60$ mm Hg. However, variability is expected among children of the same age and body build.

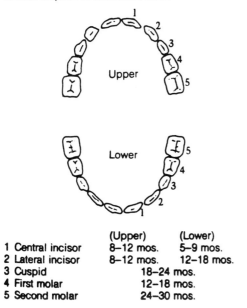

	(Upper)	(Lower)
1 Central incisor	8–12 mos.	5–9 mos.
2 Lateral incisor	8–12 mos.	12–18 mos.
3 Cuspid	18–24 mos.	
4 First molar	12–18 mos.	
5 Second molar	24–30 mos.	

Figure 8-2. Approximate ages for the eruption of deciduous teeth.

An accurate determination of the infant's heart beat requires an apical pulse count. Place a pediatric stethoscope that has a small-diameter diaphragm over the left chest in a position where the heart beat can be clearly heard, and count for 1 full minute. During the first year of life, the average apical rate ranges from 70 (asleep) to 150 (awake) beats per minute and as high as 180 beats per minute while the infant is crying.

Body Temperature and Respiratory Rate

Body temperature follows the average normal range after the initial adjustment to postnatal living. Respirations average 30 breaths per minute, with a wide range (20 to 50 breaths per minute) according to the infant's activity.

Neuromuscular Development

As the infant grows, nerve cells mature, and fine muscles begin to learn to coordinate in an orderly pattern of development. Naturally, the family caregivers are full of pride in the infant who learns to sit or stand before the neighbor's baby does, but accomplishing such milestones early means little. Each child follows a unique rhythm of progress, within reasonable limits.

Average rates of growth and development are useful for purposes of evaluation. There are a few landmarks that call for special attention, even though their absence may indicate the need for additional environmental stimulation. Do not emphasize routine developmental tables with family caregivers; a mild time lag may be insignificant. A large lag may require greater stimulation from the environment or a watchful attitude to discover how overall development is proceeding.

Table 8-1 summarizes the accepted norms in physical, psychosocial, motor, language, and cognitive growth and development in the first year of life (Figure 8-3).

Nutrition

During the first year of life, the infant's rapid growth creates a need for supplies of nutrients greater than at any other time of life. The Academy of Pediatrics Committee on Nutrition has endorsed breastfeeding as the best method of feeding infants. Most of the requirements of the infant for the first 4 to 6 months of life are supplied by either breast milk or commercial infant formulas. Vitamins C and D, iron, and fluoride are the nutrients that may need to be supplemented.

Breastfed infants need supplements of iron as well as vitamin D, which can be supplied as vitamin drops. Most commercial infant formulas are enriched with vitamins C and D. Some infant formulas are iron fortified. Infants who are fed home-prepared formulas (based on evaporated milk) need a supplement of vitamin C and iron;

however, evaporated milk has adequate amounts of vitamin D, which is unaffected by heating in the preparation of formula. Vitamin C can be supplied in orange juice or juices fortified with vitamin C.

Fluoride is needed in small amounts (0.25 mg/day) for strengthening calcification of the teeth and preventing tooth decay. A supplement is recommended for breastfed and commercial formula-fed babies and for those whose home-prepared formulas are made with water that is deficient in fluoride. Vitamin preparations are available combined with fluoride.

Addition of Solid Foods

There is no exact time or order requirement for starting foods. About 4 to 6 months of age, however, the infant's iron supply becomes low and supplements of iron-rich foods are needed. Guidelines for introducing new foods into an infant's diet are provided in Table 8-2.

Infant Feeding

The infant knows only one way to take food and that is to thrust his or her tongue forward as if to suck, which has the effect of pushing the solid food right out of the mouth. This is called the extrusion (protrusion) reflex (Figure 8-4). The process of transferring food from the front of the mouth to the throat for swallowing is a complicated skill that must be learned. The eager, hungry baby is puzzled over this new turn of events and is apt to become frustrated and annoyed, protesting loudly and clearly. It is best, therefore, to take the edge off the very hungry infant's appetite with part of the formula before proceeding with this new experience. If the family caregivers understand that pushing food out with the tongue does not mean rejection, their patience will be rewarded.

The baby's clothing (and the caregiver's as well) needs protection when the baby is being held for a feeding. A small spoon fits the infant's mouth better than a large one and makes it easier to put food further back on the tongue, but not far enough to make the baby gag. The caregiver needs to catch the food if it is pushed out and offer it again, but the baby soon learns how to manipulate the tongue and comes to enjoy this novel way of eating. If the infant is upset and crying for any reason, the caregiver needs to quiet the baby before proceeding with feeding to avoid the danger of aspiration.

Foods are started in small amounts, 1 or 2 tsp daily. Babies like their food smooth, thin, lukewarm, and bland. The choice of mealtime does not matter. It works best, at first, to offer one new food at a time, allowing 4 or 5 days before introducing another so that the baby becomes accustomed to it. This method also helps determine which food is the culprit if the baby has a reaction to a new food.

When teeth start erupting anytime between 4 and 7 months of age, the infant appreciates a piece of zwieback or toast to practice chewing on. At about 9 or 10 months

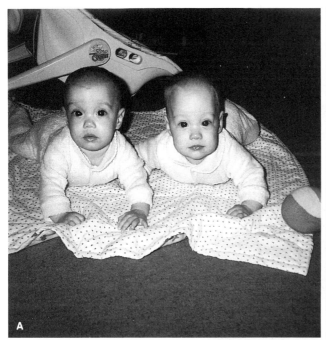

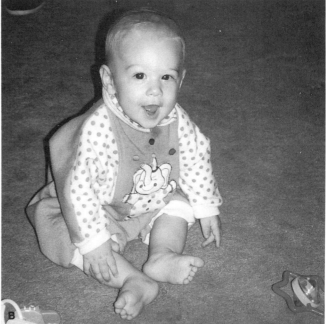

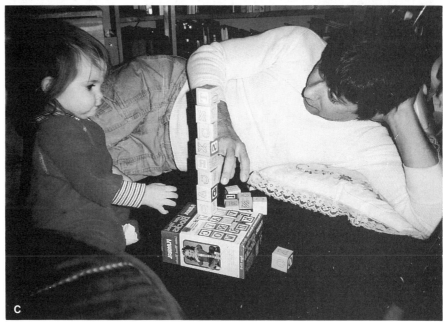

Figure 8-3. Growth and development of the infant: **A**, 10 to 12 weeks, twin girls lifting up their heads from a prone position to look about their world; **B**, 20 weeks, infant tilts forward for balance when sitting; **C**, 11½ months, building a block tower with help.

of age, after a few teeth have erupted, chopped foods can be substituted for pureed foods. Breast milk or formula gradually is replaced with whole milk as the infant learns to drink from the cup. This change takes some time because the infant doubtless continues to derive comfort from sucking at the breast or bottle.

Preparation of Foods

A variety of pureed baby foods, chopped junior foods, and prepared milk formulas are available on the market, and these products certainly relieve caregivers of much preparation time. However, using prepared foods can be an expense that many families cannot afford. Family caregivers must learn that no matter which type of food they are feeding the infant, it is important to carefully read food labels to avoid any foods that have undesirable additives.

The nurse can point out that vegetables and fruits can be cooked and strained or pureed in a blender and are just as acceptable to the baby. Baby foods prepared at home should be made from freshly prepared foods, not canned, to avoid any commercial additives. Labels of frozen foods that are used should be checked for added sugar, salt, or

(text continued on page 174)

Table 8-1. Growth and Development Chart: Birth to 1 Year.

Age	Physical	Psychosocial	Fine Motor	Gross Motor	Language	Cognition
Birth–4 wk	Weight gain of 5–7 oz (150–270 g) per wk Height gain of 1 inch per mo first 6 mo Head circumference increases ½ inch per mo Moro, Babinski, rooting, and tonic neck reflexes present	Some smiling Begins Erikson's stage of "trust vs. mistrust"	Grasp reflex very strong Hands flexed	Catches and holds objects in sight that cross visual field Can turn head from side to side when lying in a prone position When prone, body in a flexed position When prone, moves extremities in a crawling fashion	Cries when upset Makes enjoyment sounds during mealtimes	At 1 mo, sucking activity associated with pleasurable sensations
6 wk	Tears appear	Smiling in response to familiar stimuli	Hands open Less flexion noted	Tries to raise shoulders and arms when stimulated Holds head up when prone Less flexion of entire body when prone	Cooing predominant Smiles to familiar voices Babbling	**Primary Circular Reactions** Begins to repeat actions
10–12 wk	Posterior fontanelle closes	Aware of new environment Less crying Smiles at significant others	No longer has grasp reflex Pulls on clothes, blanket, but does not reach for them	No longer has Moro reflex Symmetric body positioning Pumps arms, shoulders, and head from prone position (Figure 8-3A)	Makes noises when spoken to	Beginning of coordinated responses to different kinds of stimuli
16 wk	Moro, rooting, and tonic neck reflexes disappear; drooling begins	Responses to stimulus Sees bottle, squeals, laughs Aware of new environment and shows interest	Grasps objects with two hands Grasps objects in crib voluntarily and brings them to mouth Eye–hand coordination beginning	Plays with hands Brings objects to mouth Balances head and body for short periods in sitting position	Laughs aloud Sounds "n," "k," "g," and "b"	Likes social situations Defiant, bored if unattended

Age	Physical	Social/Emotional	Fine Motor	Gross Motor	Language	Cognitive
20 wk	May show signs of teething	Smiles at self in mirror; Cries when limits are set or when objects are taken away	Holds one object while looking for another one; Grasps objects wanted	Able to sit up (Figure 8-3B); Can roll over; Can bear weight on legs when held in a standing position; Able to control head movements	Cooing noises; Squeals with delight	Visually looks for an object that has fallen
24 wk	Birth weight doubles; weight gain slows to 3–5 oz (90–150 g) per wk; Height slows to ½ inch per mo; Teething begins with lower central incisors	Likes to be picked up; Knows family from strangers; Plays "Peek-a-Boo"; Knows likes and dislikes; Fear of strangers	Holds a bottle fairly well; Tries to retrieve a dropped article	Tonic neck reflex disappears; Sits alone in high chair, back erect; Rolls over and back to abdomen	Makes sounds "guh," "bah"; Sounds "p," "m," "b," and "t" are pronounced; Bubbling sounds	**Secondary Circular Reactions** Repeats actions that affect an object; Beginning of object permanence
28 wk	Lower lateral incisors are followed in the next month by upper central incisors	Imitates simple acts; Responds to "no"; Shows preferences and dislikes for food	Holds cup; Transfers objects from one hand to the other	Reaches without visual guidance; Can lift head up when in a supine position	Babbling decreases; Duplicates "ma-ma" and "pa-pa" sounds	
32 wk	Teething continues	Dislikes diaper and clothing change; Afraid of strangers; Fear of separating from mother	Adjusts body position to be able to reach for an object; May stand up while holding on	Crawls around; Pulls toy toward self	Combines syllables but has trouble attributing meaning to them	
36 wk	Bladder and bowel patterns more stable; upper lateral incisors erupt	Imitates waving "bye-bye"; Repeats facial expressions; cries when yelled at	Releases objects with flexed wrist; Good finger and thumb grasp (pincer grasp)	Creeps around, stands when holding onto furniture; Pulls self to stand; Sits up; Recovers balance when falls over	Imitates sounds; Knows what "no" means	Now aware that objects are separate from self; **Secondary Circular Reactions** Actions memorized
40 wk–1 yr	Birth weight tripled; has six teeth; Babinski reflex disappears; Anterior fontanelle closes between now and 18 mo	Does things to attract attention; Tries to follow when being read to; Imitates parents; Looks for objects not in sight	Holds tool with one hand and works on it with another; Puts toy in box after demonstration; Stacks blocks (Figure 8-3C); Holds crayon to scribble on paper	Stands alone, begins to walk alone; Can change self from prone to sitting to standing position	Words emerge; Says "da-da" and "ma-ma" with meaning	Coordination of secondary schemes; masters barrier to reach goal, symbolic meaning

other unnecessary ingredients. Excess blended food can be stored in the freezer in ice cube trays for future use. Cereals may be cooked and formulas may be prepared at home as well. Preparation of baby food at home demands careful sanitary practices for preparation and storage. All equipment used in the preparation of the infant's food must be carefully cleaned with hot, soapy water and rinsed thoroughly. Instead of purchasing junior foods, the parent can substitute well-cooked, unseasoned table foods that have been mashed or ground. Some families prefer to spend more money for convenience and economize elsewhere, but no one should be made to feel that a baby's health or well-being depends on commercially prepared foods.

The well baby's appetite is the best index of the proper amount of food. Healthy babies enjoy eating and accept most foods, but they do not like strong-flavored or bitter foods. If the baby shows a definite dislike for any particular food, there is no reason to force it because this may develop into a battle of will power. However, a dislike for a certain food does not need to be permanent, and the rejected food may be offered again at a later date. The important point is to avoid making an issue of likes or dislikes. The caregiver also should avoid introducing any personal attitudes about food preferences.

Self-Feeding

The infant has an overpowering urge to investigate and to learn. At around 7 or 8 months of age, the baby may grab the spoon from the caregiver, examine it, and mouth it. The baby also sticks his or her fingers in the food to feel the texture and to bring it to the mouth for tasting (Figure

Table 8-2. Suggested Feeding Schedule: Birth to 1 Year

Age	Food Items	Amounts*		Rationale
Birth–6 mo	Human milk or iron-fortified formula	0–1 mo 1–2 mo 2–3 mo 3–4 mo 4–5 mo 5–6 mo	18–24 oz 22–28 oz 25–32 oz 28–32 oz 27–39 oz 27–45 oz	Infants' well-developed sucking and rooting reflexes allow them to take in milk and formula Infants do not accept semisolids because their tongues protrude when a spoon is put in their mouths (extrusion reflex) Infants are unable to transfer food to the back of their mouths Human milk requires supplementation
	Water	Not routinely recommended		Small amounts may be offered under special circumstances, such as hot weather, elevated bilirubin levels, or diarrhea
4–6 mo	Iron-fortified instant cereal†; begin with rice cereal (delay adding barley, oats, and wheat until the sixth mo)	4–8 tbsp (after mixing)		At this age, the extrusion reflex decreases. The infant is able to depress the tongue and transfer semisolid food from a spoon to the back of the pharynx to swallow it
	Unsweetened fruit juices†: plain, vitamin C–fortified; dilute juices with equal parts of water	2–4 oz		Cereal adds a source of iron and vitamins A, B, and E. Fruit juices introduce a source of vitamin C Withhold orange, pineapple, grapefruit, or tomato juice until the sixth mo
7–8 mo	Fruits, plain strained†; avoid fruit desserts Yogurt†	1–2 tbsp		Teething is beginning; thus, there is an increased ability to bite and chew
	Vegetables, plain strained†; avoid combination meat and vegetable dinners	5–7 tbsp		Vegetables introduce new flavors and textures
	Meats, plain strained†; avoid combination or high-protein dinners	1–2 tbsp		Meat provides additional iron, protein, and B vitamins
	Zwieback, toast, crackers†	1 small serving		
	Iron-fortified infant cereal or enriched cream of wheat	4–6 tbsp		
	Fruit juices	4 oz		
	Human milk or iron-fortified formula	24–32 oz		Iron-fortified formula or iron supplementation with human milk continues to be needed, because the infant is not consuming significant amounts of meat
	Water	As desired		May introduce a cup to the infant

(continued)

Table 8-2. Suggested Feeding Schedule: Birth to 1 Year *(Continued)*

Age	Food Items	Amounts*	Rationale
9–10 mo	Finger foods—well-cooked, mashed, soft, bite-sized pieces of meat and vegetables	In small servings	Rhythmic biting movements begin; enhance this development with foods that require chewing Decrease amounts of mashed foods as amounts of finger foods increase
	Iron fortified infant cereal or enriched cream of wheat	4–6 tbsp	
	Fruit juices	4 oz	
	Fruits	6–8 tbsp	
	Vegetables	6–8 tbsp	
	Meats, fish, poultry, yogurt, cottage cheese	4–6 tbsp	Formula consumption may begin to decrease; thus, begin other sources of calcium, riboflavin, and protein (such as cheese, yogurt, and cottage cheese)
	Human milk or iron-fortified formula	24–32 oz	
	Water	As desired	
11–12 mo	Soft table foods† as follows: Cereal: iron-fortified infant cereal; may introduce dry, unsweetened cereal as a finger food	4–6 tbsp	Motor skills are developing; enhance this with more finger foods
	Breads: zwieback, toast, crackers	1–2 small servings	Rotary chewing motion develops; thus, child is able to handle whole foods, which require more chewing.
	Fruit: soft canned fruits or ripe banana, cut up; peeled raw fruit as infant approaches 12 mo	½ cup	Infant is relying less on breast milk or formula for nutrients. A proper selection of a variety of solid foods (fruits, vegetables, starches, protein sources, and dairy products) will continue to meet the young child's needs
	Vegetables—soft cooked, cut up	½ cup	
	Meats: strips of tender, lean meat	2 oz or ½ cup chopped	
	Cheese strips, peanut butter Mashed potatoes, noodles		Delay peanut butter until the 12th mo
	Fruit juices	4 oz	
	Human milk or iron-fortified infant formula	24–30 oz	
	Water	As desired	

* Amounts listed are daily totals.
† New food item for that age group.
Adapted from Eschleman MM. Introductory Nutrition and Diet Therapy, 2nd ed. Philadelphia: JB Lippincott, 1991.

8-5). All this is an essential, although messy, part of the learning experience. After preliminary testing, the infant's next task is to try self-feeding. The baby soon finds that the motions involved in getting a spoon right side up into the mouth are too complex, thus fingers become favored over the spoon. However, the infant returns to the spoon again, until eventually succeeding to get some food from spoon to mouth at least part of the time. The nurse can help family caregivers understand that all this is not deliberate messing, to be forbidden, but rather a necessary part of the infant's learning.

Weaning the Infant

Weaning, either from the breast or bottle, needs to be attempted gradually, without fuss or strain. The infant is still testing the environment, and an abrupt removal of a main source of satisfaction—sucking—before basic distrust of the environment has been conquered may prove detrimental to normal development. The speed with which weaning is accomplished should be suited to each infant's readiness to give up this form of pleasure for a more mature way of life.

At the age of 5 or 6 months, the infant who has watched others drink from a cup usually is ready to try a sip when it is offered. The infant seldom is ready at this point, however, to give up the pleasures of sucking altogether. Forcing the child to give up sucking creates resistance and suspicion. It is better to let the infant set the pace. An infant who takes food from a dish and milk from a cup during the day may still be reluctant to give up a bedtime bottle. However, the infant should never be permitted to take a bottle along to bed. **Pedodontists** (dentists who specialize in the care and treatment of children's teeth) discourage the bedtime bottle because the sugar from formula or sweetened juice coats the infant's teeth for long periods and causes erosion of the enamel on the deciduous teeth, resulting in a condition known as **"bottle mouth"** or **"nursing bottle" caries**. This condition can also occur in infants who sleep with their mother and nurse intermittently throughout the night. In addition to the caries, liquid from milk, formula, or juice can pool in the mouth and flow into the eustachian tube, causing otitis media, if the infant falls asleep with the bottle. A bottle of plain water or a pacifier can be substituted for the infant who needs the comfort of sucking at bedtime.

A few babies resist drinking from a cup. Milk needs (calcium, vitamin D) may be met by offering yogurt, custards, cottage cheese, and other milk dishes until the infant becomes accustomed to the cup. The caregiver should be cautioned not to use honey or corn syrup to sweeten milk because of the danger of botulism in these products, which the infant's system is not strong enough to combat.

During the second half of the first year, the infant's milk consumption alone is not likely to be sufficient to meet caloric, protein, mineral, and vitamin needs.

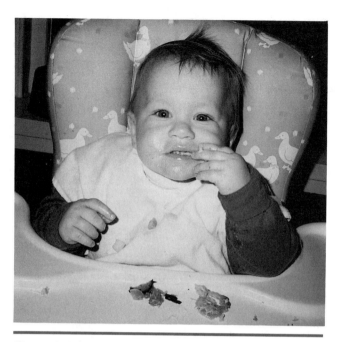

Figure 8-5. Eating by yourself is a messy business but so much fun!

Women, Infants, Children Food Program

Women, Infants, Children (WIC) is a special supplemental food program for pregnant, breastfeeding, or postpartum women and infants and children as old as 5 years of age. This federal program is available to those people who are eligible based on financial and nutritional needs and who live in a WIC service area. The program provides nutritious supplemental foods, nutrition information, and health care referrals. There is no cost to any people who are determined to be eligible, and the family's food stamp benefits or school children's breakfast and lunch program benefits are not affected. The foods prescribed by the program that may be purchased with vouchers or distributed through clinics include iron-fortified infant formula and cereal, infant juices, milk, dry beans or peas, peanut butter, cheese, cereal, juice, and eggs. Many health care facilities give WIC information to eligible mothers who are there for prenatal visits or at the time of delivery to encourage the use of WIC services.

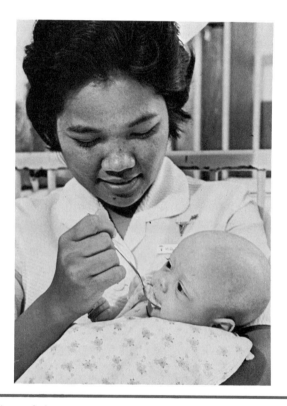

Figure 8-4. A baby tends to push his or her first solids out of the mouth with the tongue.

Health Maintenance

Every infant is entitled to the best possible protection against disease. Because of immaturity, the infants are not able to take proper precautions, therefore family caregivers and health professionals must be responsible for them. This care extends beyond the daily needs for food, sleep, cleanliness, love, and security to a concern for the infant's future health and well-being (Table 8-3).

Medical science has discovered measures that provide immunity for a number of serious or disabling diseases. Protection is available for conditions such as diphtheria, smallpox, tetanus, hepatitis, polio, mumps, measles, German measles (rubella), and *Hemophilus influenzae* meningitis, making it unnecessary to take chances with children's health owing to inadequate immunization.

Immunization Schedule

The Academy of Pediatrics, through its committee on the control of infectious diseases, has recommended a schedule of immunizations for healthy children living in normal conditions (Table 8-4). Immunizations should be given within the prescribed timetable, unless physical conditions of the child make this impossible. The common cold

is not a reason for postponement, but acute febrile conditions, conditions causing immunosuppression, and administration of corticosteroids and radiation or antimetabolites are all reasons for postponement.

Some side effects from the immunizations may occur, varying with the type of immunization. The most common side effect is a fever within the first 24 to 48 hours and possibly a local reaction at the site of injection. These reactions are treated symptomatically with acetaminophen for the fever and warm compresses to the injection site.

Many children do not get the initial immunizations in infancy and may not get them until they reach school age, when the immunizations are required for school entrance. Health care personnel should make every effort to encourage parents to have their children immunized in infancy to avoid the danger of possible epidemic outbreaks. For instance, measles outbreaks, resulting in the deaths of children, have been increasing at an alarming

Table 8-3. Recommended Health Maintenance Age: 2 Weeks to 1 Year

Procedure	2 Weeks	2 Months	4 Months	6 Months	9 Months	12 Months
Health history	Take prenatal and birth history; family and social history; discuss events in first 2 weeks, family concerns	Update history including eating, sleeping, and elimination patterns Discuss family concerns and infant's reaction to immunizations	Update history; discuss family concerns and infant's reactions to immunizations	Same as earlier	Same as earlier	Same as earlier
Physical examination	Measure height, weight, and head circumference; take infant's temperature; perform a complete physical examination and vision evaluation	Same as for 2 weeks, except include hearing and vision evaluation Development and behavior assessment by history and physical. If questionable, perform appropriate developmental test	Same as at 2 weeks, with vision examination	Same as at 2 weeks, except include hearing and vision evaluation	Same as at 2 weeks, except add dental examination and vision evaluation	Same as at 2 weeks, except include dental examination
Laboratory Procedures	PKU test repeated if done before 2 days old				Hematocrit, hemoglobin and blood cell count; sickle cell screening	Lead screening; urinalysis

(continued)

Table 8-3. Recommended Health Maintenance Age: 2 Weeks to 1 Year *(Continued)*

Procedure	Age					
	2 Weeks	2 Months	4 Months	6 Months	9 Months	12 Months
Immunizations	HBV (recommended before discharge from newborn nursery)	DPT, OPV, HBV, HbCV	DPT, OPV, HbCV	DPT, HbCV,* OPV,* HBV		Tuberculin test
Feeding	See Table 8-2 for suggested guidelines					
Teaching and counseling†	Discuss normal variations of newborn (*eg,* skin color, head shape); need for tactile and visual stimulation; prevention of infection; hygiene; differences in infant temperament; attachment behaviors; and need for consistency (basic trust)	Discuss immunizations and possible reactions, sleep patterns; accident prevention; differences in temperament; visual, tactile, and auditory stimulation; repetition of infant sounds and vocal stimulation; family needs for rest, privacy, and break from routine; need for consistency; and attachment behaviors	Discuss immunizations and possible reactions; sleep and wake patterns; need for activities to strengthen head (*eg,* infant swing); stimulation of all senses; moving baby around in home; and opportunity for movement on floor	Discuss immunizations and possible reactions; accident prevention; care of minor infections such as colds, diarrhea, and vomiting; teething; family interactions; continued need for stimulation, including roughhouse play; need for room to crawl, scoot, and roll over; and fear of strangers	Discuss accident prevention, including possibility of walking; care of teeth; separation anxiety; surprise toys like jack-in-the-box and separation games like "Peek-a-Boo"; sound and language stimulation; and childrearing practices	Discuss accident prevention (the toddler years are here!); dental care and care of minor accidents (falls, cuts); developing sense of autonomy; satisfaction of curiosity needs; language stimulation; putting-in and taking-out activities; and developing independence and start of temper tantrums

* Optional doses at this time.
† Suggested teachings to be personalized for each child.
DPT, diptheria, pertussis, tetanus; *OPV,* trivalent oral polio vaccine; *HBV,* hepatitis B vaccine; *HbCV, Hemophilus influenzae* type B conjugate vaccine.
Adapted from Wieczorek R, Natapoff J. A Conceptual Approach to the Nursing of Children: Health Care from Birth Through Adolescence. Philadelphia: JB Lippincott, 1981.

rate because of inadequate immunization. Serious illnesses, permanent disability, and deaths from inadequate immunizations are senseless and tragic.

Psychosocial Development

The give-and-take of life is experienced by the infant who actively seeks food to fulfill feelings of hunger. The infant begins to develop a sense of trust when fed on demand. However, the infant eventually learns that every need is not always met immediately when demanded. Slowly, the infant becomes aware that one's needs are fulfilled by something or someone separate from one's self. Gradually, as a result of the loving care of family caregivers, the infant learns that the environment responds to desires expressed through one's own efforts and signals. The infant is now aware that the environment is separate from self.

The caregivers who expect too much too soon from the infant are not encouraging optimal development. Rather than teaching the rules of life before the infant has learned to trust the environment, the caregivers are actually teaching that nothing is gained by one's own activity and that the world does not respond to one's needs.

Conversely, the caregivers who rush to anticipate every need give the infant no opportunity to test the environment. The opportunity to discover that through one's own actions the environment may be manipulated to suit one's own desires is withheld from the infant by

Table 8-4. Immunization Schedules: Recommended Schedule for Active Immunization of Normal Infants and Children

Age	Immunization			
0–2 wk	HBV			
2 mo	DPT	OPV	HBV	HbCV
4 mo	DPT	OPV		HbCV
6 mo	DPT	OPV*	HBV	HbCV*
15 mo	MMR			
18 mo	DTaP	OPV		
4–6 yr	DTaP	OPV	MMR†	
10–12 yr	MMR†			
14 yr	dT			

*Depends on type of vaccine used.
†MMR second dose can be administered at either of these ages.
HBV, hepatitis B vaccine; *DPT*, diphtheria, tetanus toxoids with pertussis vaccine; *OPV*, oral polio vaccine; *HbCV*, *Haemophilus influenzae* type b conjugate vaccine; *MMR*, measles, mumps, and rubella vaccine; *DTaP*, diphtheria, tetanus toxoids with attenuated pertussis vaccine; *dT*, reduced dose of diphtheria, full adult dose of tetanus toxoid; to be repeated every 10 yr throughout life.

Parent Teaching

Tips for Infants from Birth to 1 Year

First 6 weeks of life includes frequent holding of infant, gives infant feeling of being loved and cared for. Rocking and soothing baby important.

6 weeks to 3 1/2 months: continue to give infant feeling of being loved and cared for; respond to cries; provide visual stimulation with toys, pictures, and mobiles; auditory stimulation by talking and singing to baby.

3 1/2 to 5 months: play regularly with child; give child variety of things to look at; talk to the child; offer a variety of items to touch—soft, fuzzy, smooth, and rough, to provide tactile stimulation; continue to respond to infant's cries.

5 to 8 months: continue to give infant feeling of being loved and cared for by holding, cuddling, and responding to needs; talk to infant; put infant on floor more to roll and move about.

8 to 12 months: time to accident-proof the house; give infant maximum access to living area; supply infant with playthings; stay close by to support infant in difficult situation; continue to talk to infant to provide language stimulation.

these "smothering" caregivers. The display on parent teaching tips for infants in the first year of life suggests healthy childrearing patterns during infancy.

No one is perfect, and every family caregiver misinterprets the infant's signals at times. The caregiver may be tired, preoccupied, and responding momentarily to needs of self. The caregiver may not be able to ease the pain or soothe the restlessness, but this also is a learning experience for the baby.

As mentioned earlier, the infant's development depends on a mutual relationship, with a give-and-take, between the infant and the environment, of which the family caregivers play the most important role. Table 8-5 summarizes significant caregiver–infant interactions indicating positive and negative behaviors.

During the first few weeks of life, actions such as kicking and sucking are simple reflex activities. In the next sequential stage, reflexes are coordinated and elaborated. For example, the eyes follow random hand movements (Figure 8-6). The infant finds that repetition of chance movements brings interesting changes, and in the latter part of the first year these acts become clearly intentional actions (Figure 8-7). The infant expects that certain results follow certain actions.

The smiling face looking down is soon connected by the infant with the pleasure of being picked up, fed, or bathed. Anyone who smiles and talks softly to the infant may make that small face light up and cause squirming of anticipation. In only a few weeks, however, the infant

learns that one particular person is the main source of comfort and pleasure.

An infant cannot apply abstract reasoning but understands only through the five senses. As the infant matures enough to recognize the mother or primary family caregiver, the infant becomes fearful when this person disappears. Out of sight has always meant, to the infant, out of existence, and the infant cannot tolerate this. Thus, to the infant, self-assurance is necessary to confirm that objects and people do not cease to exist when out of sight. This is a learning experience on which the infant's entire attitude toward life depends.

The ancient game of "Peek-a-Boo" is a universal example of this learning technique. It is also one of the joys of infancy, as the child affirms the ability to control the disappearance and reappearance of self. In the same manner by which the infant affirms self-existence, the existence of others is confirmed even when temporarily out of sight.

Implications for Hospital Care

Hospitalization, however brief, hampers the infant's normal pattern of living. Disruption occurs even when a family caregiver can stay with the infant during hospitali-

Table 8-5. Criteria of Positive Caregiver–Infant Interactions

Area of Interaction	Positive Caregiver Response
Feeding of infant	Offers infant adequate amounts and appropriate types of food and prepares food appropriately Hold infant in comfortable, secure position during feeding Burps infant during and/or after feeding Offers food at a comfortable pace for the infant
Stimulation of infant	Provides appropriate nonaggressive verbal stimulation to infant Provides a variety of tactile experiences and touches infant in caring ways other than during feeding times or when moving infant away from danger Provides appropriate toys and interacts with infant in way that is satisfying to infant
Rest and sleep for infant	Provides a quiet, relaxed environment, and a regular, scheduled sleep time for infant Makes certain infant is adequately fed and is warm and dry before putting him or her down to sleep
Understanding of infant	Has realistic expectations of infant and recognizes infant's developing skills and behavior Has realistic view of one's own parenting skills View of infant's health condition corresponds to the view of medical and/or nursing diagnosis
Problem-solving initiative	Motivated to manage infant's problems; diligently seeks information about infant; follows through on plans involving infant
Interaction with other children	Demonstrates positive interaction with other children in home without aggression and hostility
Caregiver's recreation	Seeks positive outlets for own recreation and relaxation
Parenting role	Expresses satisfaction with parenting role; positive attitudes expressed

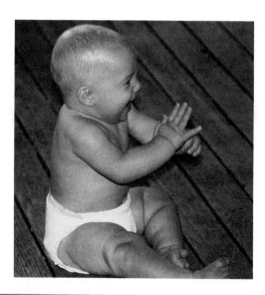

Figure 8-6. Infant looking at hands. (From Castiglia PT, Harbin R. Child Health Care. Philadelphia: JB Lippincott, 1992.)

zation. All or most of the sick infant's energies may be needed to cope with the illness. However, if given sufficient affection and loving care and if promptly restored to the family, the infant is not likely to suffer any serious psychological problems. Long-term hospitalization, however, may present serious problems, even with the best of care.

Illness in itself is frustrating, causing pain and discomfort and limiting normal activity, none of which the infant can understand. In the situations in which the hospital setting may be an emotionally unresponsive, unfamiliar atmosphere, providing little, if any, cuddling or rocking, an infant may fail to respond to treatment, despite cleanliness and proper hygiene. When this happens, it becomes readily apparent that touching, rocking, and cuddling a child are essential elements of nursing care (Figure 8-8).

Hospitalization may have other adverse effects. The small infant matures largely as a result of physical development. If hindered from reaching out and responding to the environment, the infant becomes apathetic and ceases

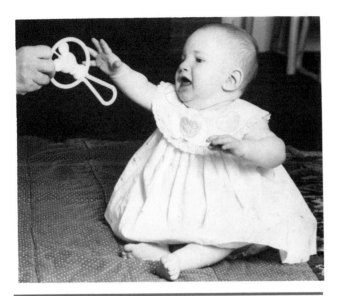

Figure 8-7. A 6-month-old girl reaching for a toy. (From Castiglia PT, Harbin RE. Child Health Care: Process and Practice. Philadelphia: JB Lippincott, 1992.)

to learn. This situation is particularly apparent when restraints are necessary to keep the child from undoing surgical procedures or dressings or to prevent injury. The child in restraints needs an extra measure of love and attention from nurses and family caregivers and the use of every possible method available to provide comfort.

Parent–Nurse Relationship

The nurse's relationship with family caregivers is extremely important. The hospitalized infant needs continuity of the stimulation, empathic care, and loving attention

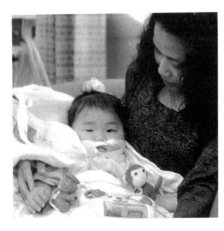

Figure 8-8. Holding and cuddling can ease the discomfort and fear of the hospital experience. (From Jackson DB; Saunders RB. Child Health Nursing: A Comprehensive Approach to the Care of Children and Their Families. Philadelphia: JB Lippincott, 1993.)

from family caregivers. These caregivers need encouragement and support from the nurses to feed, hold, diaper, and participate in the care of their infant as much as they are capable of doing. Through conscientious use of the nursing process, the nurse may evaluate the needs of the caregivers and the infant and may plan care with these needs in mind. The caregivers' apprehensions should be identified and acknowledged, and plans must be developed to resolve or eliminate them. Arrangements for rooming-in for the family caregiver should be made, if possible. Family caregivers often are sensitive to those changes in their infant that may help to identify discomfort, pain, or fears. Caregivers may sometimes assist during treatments and other procedures by stroking, talking to, and looking directly at the infant, thus helping to provide comfort during the time of stress. After the procedure, the infant may benefit from rocking, cuddling, singing, stroking, and other comfort measures that the family caregivers may provide. In situations in which the family caregivers are unavailable or are limited in being with the infant, the nursing staff must meet these emotional needs.

Physical Care

Children enter the hospital to become physically stable. They cannot thrive physically if they are emotionally disturbed or allowed to stagnate mentally. All the child's needs—physical, psychosocial, and cognitive—must be met as completely as possible.

Bathing the Infant

A daily bath is desirable if the infant's condition permits. Placing the baby into a small tub for a bath rather than giving a sponge bath may have a soothing and comforting effect, as long as there are no contraindications.

Tub Bath. Wash hands, put on protective cover, and assemble the following equipment before starting:

- Large basin or small tub
- Mild soap
- Nonsterile protective gloves
- Clean cotton balls
- Soft washcloth
- Large, soft towel or small cotton blanket
- Clean diaper and shirt

The room should be a comfortable temperature and draft free. The bath water should be about 95° to 100°F (35.2° to 37.8°C), measured with a bath thermometer or comfortably warm to the elbow. Small babies squirm and move about much more than an inexperienced person might expect. (An absolute rule is *never* to turn one's back on an infant when the crib side is down, and *always* keep a hand on the infant). A sensible precaution when bathing a baby is to put the bath basin into the crib and thus eliminate the need for turning from the baby. Crib mattresses are plastic covered and sheets may be changed, so that splashed water is no problem.

Before undressing the baby, wash the baby's face with clean water, using the washcloth or cotton balls. Do not use soap on the baby's face. A clean, moist cotton ball is used to wash each eye, wiping from the inner to the outer canthus and discarding the cotton ball after use. A clean, moist cotton ball also is used for each ear, taking care to clean any discharge, if present. If dried mucus is present in the anterior nares, a wisp of cotton may be twisted, dipped in clear water, and used for cleaning the nose. This cleaning may cause the baby to sneeze and bring down more mucus, which may be wiped away.

Applicators should *not* be used in the ordinary cleaning of a baby's eyes, ears, or nose. Injury to the mucous membranes may easily occur if the baby squirms. Any material in the ears or nose that is too deep to remove without probing should be removed, if necessary, only by the use of appropriate instruments in the hands of a trained person.

Next, the baby's scalp may be soaped; then the baby may be picked up and held in a securely in a "football" hold, with the head over the basin to rinse the soap away.

After drying the head, undress the baby and examine the skin for rashes or excoriations. If the baby's diaper is soiled, the feces should be wiped from the buttocks before placing the infant into the basin. Protective, non-sterile gloves are worn when cleaning the infant's diaper area. Soap the infant's body all over, and lift him or her into the basin, holding securely while supporting the head and shoulders on your arm. Some nurses prefer to soap the infant with their free hands while holding the infant in the tub because a soapy baby is slippery and difficult to pick up. Use the technique that feels most secure to you. If the baby's skin is dry, soap may be omitted or used only in the perineal area. A prescribed soap substitute also may be used.

If the baby is enjoying this experience, make it a leisurely one, engaging the infant in talk, paddling in the water, and playing for a few extra minutes (Figure 8-9). When finished, lift the infant out and pat dry, paying attention to creases (especially under the arms, chin, and perineal area).

After the bath, the labia of female infants should be separated and gently cleansed with moist cotton balls and clean water. Wipe from *front to back* to avoid introducing any bacteria from the anal region into the vagina or urethra. Male infants who have been circumcised need only to be inspected for cleanliness. An uncircumcised male infant may have the foreskin gently retracted and any accumulation of smegma or debris washed off and the foreskin returned in place. If the foreskin does not easily retract, it must not be forced, but this must be documented and reported appropriately.

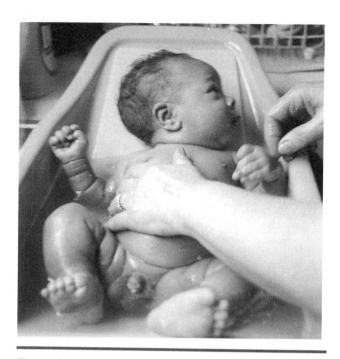

Figure 8-9. Bath time can be an enjoyable experience for the infant. (From Jackson DB, Saunders RB. Child Health Nursing: A Comprehensive Approach to the Care of Children and Their Families. Philadelphia: JB Lippincott, 1993.)

The use of scented or talcum powder is discouraged. Powders tend to cake in the creases, causing irritation, and also may be inhaled by the infant, causing respiratory problems. Scented powders and lotions may cause allergic reactions in some babies. In any case, a clean baby has a sweet smell without the use of additional fragrances.

Excessively dry skin may benefit from the application of lanolin or A & D ointment, but oils are believed to block pores and cause infection. Various medicated ointments are available for excoriated skin areas.

A baby's fingernails need to be inspected and cut if they are long because the baby may scratch his or her face during random arm movements. The nails should be cut straight across with great care, holding the arm securely and the hand firmly while cutting.

The bathing procedure is essentially the same for the older infant. When old enough to sit and move about freely, the infant may enjoy the regular bathtub, but usually this is frightening to him or her. Splashing about in a small tub may be more fun, especially with the addition of a floating toy. Always keep a secure hold on any infant in a tub. Try to schedule your time so that this is a leisurely process, a time for the nurse and baby to enjoy, and an excellent time to teach the family caregivers. For the procedure on the sponge bath, see Chapter 5.

Dressing the Infant

Hospitalized infants wear cotton shirts, gowns, or one-piece sleeper sets and diapers, except in hot weather if there is no air conditioning, when a diaper alone is sufficient. The easiest way to put an infant's arm into a sleeve is to work the sleeve so that the arm hole and the opening are held together, then to reach through the armhole and pull the arm through the opening. If gowns that tie in back are used, care must be taken to see that they fit properly—not too tight around the neck or too loose—to avoid the danger of the baby becoming entangled.

Diapers come in various sizes and shapes. Debate surrounds the issue of cloth versus disposable diapers. The issue of the environmental impact of disposable diapers concerns health care personnel. Whatever the type, size, and folding method used, there should be no bunched material between the thighs. Two popular cloth diaper styles are either the oblong strip pinned at the sides or the square diaper folded "kite" fashion. The latter kind has the advantage of being useful for different ages and sizes. When folding the cloth diaper for a male infant, the excess material is folded in the front; for the female, the excess fabric is folded to the back. A word of caution is necessary. If cloth diapers are used and fastened with safety pins, the safety pins must always be closed when they are fastening the diaper. When removed, safety pins must be closed and placed out of the reach of the infant.

The older infant needs the diaper fastened snugly at the hips and legs to prevent feces from running out at the open spaces. Cleaning a soiled crib and a smeared baby once or twice serves as an effective reminder for the nurse.

Weighing the Infant

The hospitalized infant often needs to be weighed daily to assess growth or fluid balance. Weights should be taken every day at the same time, with the same scale.

1. Prepare the scale by covering it with paper, cloth diaper, or sheet and by balancing it.
2. Place the naked infant on the scale, and weigh the infant. *Always* hold your hand within an inch or so of the infant to be ready to take hold if necessary.
3. Pick up the infant and discard the scale cover.
4. Read the weight and record it on the work sheet or scrap paper.
5. Clean the scale according to hospital policy.

If the baby's weight varies significantly from the previous weight, have another person check it with you. Document and report the weight as appropriate.

Hospital Safety

All safety factors that are age appropriate apply when the infant is hospitalized. A few rules are specific to the hospital environment. The crib sides must always be kept fully raised, except when someone is directly working with the baby. Never turn your back to an infant while the

Parent Teaching

Tips for Infant Safety

1. The infant should always be placed in an approved infant car carrier when in the car.
2. Crib and playpen bars should be spaced less than 2½ inches apart.
3. Never leave infant unattended on a high surface.
4. Always close safety pins and keep out of infant's reach.
5. Choose toys carefully:
   a. Watch for loose or sharp parts.
   b. Avoid small buttons or parts that can come off and choke infant.
   c. Check for nontoxic material.
5. Never leave the infant unattended in a car, absolutely not in warm weather.
6. Baby-proof your home:
   a. Cover unused plugs with plastic covers.
   b. Keep electrical cords out of sight.
   c. Move all toxic substances (cleaning fluids, detergents, insecticides) out of reach and keep locked.
   d. Keep small articles (such as buttons and marbles) off the floor and out of the infant's reach.
   e. Remove table cloths or dresser scarfs that the infant might grasp and pull.
   f. Remove any house plants that may be poisonous.
   g. Pad sharp corners of low furniture (or remove from infant's living area).
7. Never leave the infant alone in the bath.
8. Turn household hot water to a safe temperature—120°F (48.8°C)—to avoid burns.
9. Protect infant from inhaling lead paint dust (from remodeling) or chewing on surfaces painted with lead paint.
10. Place medicines in locked cupboards; remind family and friends (especially those with grown children or no children) to do the same.
11. Be "one step ahead" of the baby's development, prepared for the next stage.

side rails are down. (Safety jackets and restraints are discussed in detail in Chapter 2.) Never leave any equipment within the reach of an infant. Be alert to the family caregivers' safety practices, and reinforce good safety rules at every opportunity (see Parent Teaching Tips for Infant Safety.) Remind the caregivers that the infant is rapidly developing and that safety precautions should stay one step ahead of the infant's developmental capabilities.

Summary

The growth and development in the first year of life is truly remarkable. The infant progresses from a totally dependent being to one who is ready to "take off and cruise solo." The infant who finds a secure world with loving caregivers learns to trust and is able to progress comfortably to the next developmental stage. Family caregivers need support and guidance from health care personnel throughout this time of rapid change. During this year, teeth have erupted, and the infant's diet has progressed from breast or formula to milk and table food, with many messes along the way. Weight has tripled, and the infant has grown 10 to 12 inches in length. Much socialization has taken place, as shown in Table 8-1. The infant has gone through the first stage of stranger anxiety and now has learned how to "charm" caregivers and admirers. The infant's social circle consists of parents, caregivers, siblings, grandparents, aunts, uncles, and baby-sitters. Safety, important in all stages of life, becomes even more critical as the infant moves on to autonomy, the next stage of development.

Review Questions

1. Tony Ricardo brings 6-month-old Essie for a routine checkup. Describe the information you will gather, the extent of the physical examination, any immunizations (assuming that she is up to date), review of feeding, and other teachings that you will perform.
2. Tony R. tells you that Essie loves her bedtime bottle. What teaching will you stress to him?
3. Describe a 9-month-old infant, including psychosocial, fine motor, gross motor, language, and cognitive development.
4. Kathy Kelly brings 9-month-old Sean to the clinic. She tells you she is worried because he has only two teeth. How would you answer her?
5. Sue Sankey, an unmarried 17-year-old mother of 4-month-old Samantha, is not employed. She says she has no money for baby food. What guidance will you give her?
6. Find out how an eligible mother in your area can get assistance from WIC.
7. If Sue Sankey later tells you that Samantha does not like her food because she spits it out, what will be your reply?
8. Demonstrate how to hold an infant in a football hold. Why is this a good way to hold a baby?
9. Kathy Kelly lives in an apartment with her baby. The rooms are a living room, kitchen, bathroom, bedroom, and nursery (baby's bedroom). Going room to room, make a list of all the safety precautions that Kathy should take to protect Sean as he becomes mobile.

Bibliography

Brazelton TB. To Listen to a Child. Reading, MA: Addison-Wesley, 1985.

Brazelton TB. What Every Baby Knows. New York: Ballantine Books, 1987.

Castiglia PT, Harbin RE. Child Health Care: Process and Practice. Philadelphia: JB Lippincott, 1992.

Coryell J, Provost B. Stability of Bayley Motor Scale scores in the first year of life [Abstr]. Phys Ther 69(10):834–841, 1989.

Eschleman MM. Introductory Nutrition and Diet Therapy, 2nd ed. Philadelphia: JB Lippincott, 1991.

Pillitteri A. Maternal and Child Health Nursing. Philadelphia: JB Lippincott, 1992.

Premomo J, Bruck AM, Greenstreet PK, et al. The high environmental cost of disposable diapers. MCN 15(5):279; 282; 284, 1990.

Schuster CS, Ashburn SS. The Process of Human Development, 3rd ed. Philadelphia: JB Lippincott, 1992.

Spock B, Rothenberg MB. Dr. Spock's Baby and Child Care. New York: Pocket Books, 1992.

Whaley LF, Wong DL. Nursing Care of Infants and Children, 4th ed. St. Louis: Mosby-Year Book, 1991.

Health Problems of the Infant

Student Objectives

Upon successful completion of this chapter, the student will be able to:

1. Identify seven ways the infant's respiratory system differs from the adult's.
2. Describe the characteristics of the child with nonorganic failure to thrive.
3. Differentiate between mild diarrhea and severe diarrhea.
4. Identify the symptoms of pyloric stenosis.
5. State another name for congenital megacolon, and list the common symptoms.
6. Describe the diagnosis and treatment of intussusception.
7. Identify the common causes of iron deficiency anemia.
8. Explain how sickle cell disease is inherited: a.) Sickle cell trait; b.) Sickle cell anemia.
9. Describe the behavior of the infant with acute otitis media.
10. Describe the effect sudden infant death syndrome has on the infant's family.
11. Describe the nursing care specific to a child at high risk for seizures.
12. List four complications of *Hemophilus influenzae* meningitis.
13. Identify the causative organism of thrush.

Marks MG: BROADRIBB'S INTRODUCTORY PEDIATRIC
NURSING, 4th ed. © 1994 J.B. Lippincott Company.

Key Terms

colic

craniotabes

currant jelly stools

enteric precautions

febrile seizure

gastroenteritis

invagination

kwashiorkor

lactose

lactose intolerance

marasmus

urticaria

myringotomy

nuchal rigidity

opisthotonos

orchiopexy

pruritus

purpuric rash

rumination

teratogenicity

*I*nfancy is a period of continuing adjustment for the child and the family. The infant is adjusting to physical life outside the uterus and social life within the family. Family members are adjusting to their new roles as parents or siblings and to the presence of this new person in their midst. Although the adjustment is more gradual than the abrupt transition required at birth, it can still involve sufficient physiologic and psychosocial stresses to create health problems during the first year of life.

Three factors that help determine how health problems are manifested in the infant are the following:

1. The pathogenic agent—how virulent the organism or how great the stress.

2. The environment—how favorable or unfavorable external conditions are, including nutrition and hygiene.

3. The individual infant—the infant's resistance to stress and ability to adapt to it, and body responses to biologic, chemical, and physical injuries.

All three factors need to be considered when planning nursing care for the infant and family, remembering that even a minor health problem can create great anxiety for concerned parents.

Infants can rapidly become very ill, often with a high fever (102° to 104°F [38.9° to 40°C] or more). Fortunately, with prompt intervention, they usually recover just as quickly. Diagnosis of an infant's health problem is no simple matter, partly because the infant cannot "tell you where it hurts," and partly because the clinical manifestations are similar for many different disorders, some minor, some serious.

Most acute health problems result from a respiratory or gastrointestinal infection, or from an uncorrected, or perhaps even undetected, congenital deviation. Respiratory problems occur more often and with greater severity in infants because of their immature body defenses and small and undeveloped anatomic structures (Figure 9-1). Sometimes these problems require hospitalization, interrupting development of the infant–family relationship and the infant's patterns of sleeping, eating, and stimulation. Although the illness may be acute, if the recovery is rapid and the hospitalization brief, the infant probably will experience few if any long-term effects. If, however, the condition is chronic or so serious that it requires a long hospitalization, both infant and family may suffer serious consequences.

Psychological Problems

Failure to Thrive

Infants who fail to gain weight and show signs of delayed development are classified as failure-to-thrive infants. Failure to thrive can be divided into two classifications: organic failure to thrive, which is a result of a disease condition, and nonorganic failure to thrive (NFTT), which has no apparent physical cause. Often when the NFTT infants are hospitalized, they show a rapid weight gain.

Four principal factors are necessary for human growth: food, rest and activity, adequate secretions of hormones, and a satisfactory relationship with a parent (or nurturing person), who provides consistent, loving, human contact, and stimulation. When any of these four factors are missing, or when the infant has a major birth defect, such as congenital heart disease or a metabolic disorder, growth is disturbed and development can be delayed.

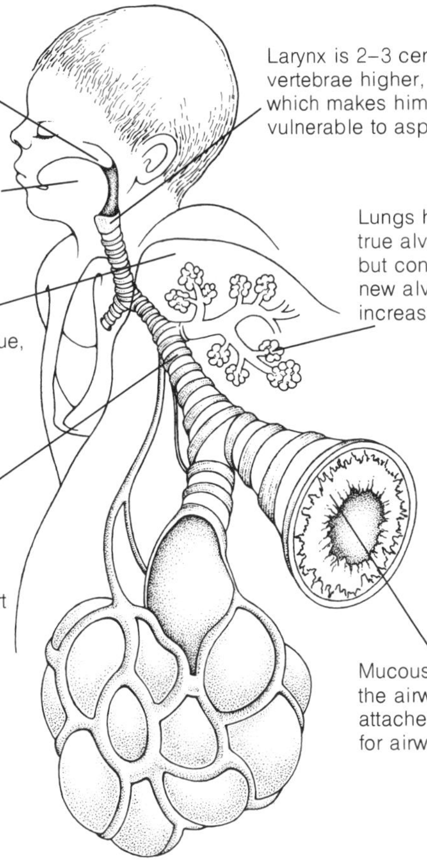

The infant's respiratory system differs from the adult's in that the infant's:

Soft palate is much greater

Larynx is 2–3 cervical vertebrae higher, which makes him more vulnerable to aspiration

Tongue is larger in proportion to mouth, so potential for airway obstruction is greater

Lungs have fewer true alveoli at birth, but continue to gain new alveoli and existing ones increase in size

Airway has larger proportion of soft tissue, so potential for edema is greater

Cricoid cartilage encircles airway, so support is less; cartilaginous support increases in late school-age

Mucous membranes lining the airway are more loosely attached, so potential for airway edema is greater

Figure 9-1. The infant or young child is at greater risk than the adult for airway obstruction due to anatomic differences in the respiratory tract. Alveolar damage in infancy is often not permanent, but airway damage remains throughout life. (Redrawn from Simkims R. The crises of bronchiolitis. Am Nurs 81:514–516, 1981.)

Clinical Manifestations

Infants with NFTT are often listless, seriously below average weight and height, immobile for long periods, and may be unresponsive to (or actually try to avoid) cuddling and vocalization. Examination of the infant is likely to reveal no organic cause for this condition. Examination of the family relationship, particularly the mother–infant relationship, however, can often provide important insight into the problem.

The family relationships of these infants are often so disrupted that there is no warm, close relationship with a parent or family caregiver. For some reason or reasons, proper attachment has not occurred. Often the father is absent or emotionally unavailable, adding to the mother's feelings of isolation and inadequacy, leading to an atmosphere of additional stress and conflict.

It is important that the nurse understand that the problem is not with the parent alone, nor with the infant, but instead with their interaction and mutual lack of responsiveness. They are not in harmony. The parent does not stimulate the infant; therefore, the infant has no one to respond to and fails to do the "cute baby" things that would gain attention and stimulation. The infant is unable to accomplish the developmental task of establishing basic trust, which Erikson identifies as the primary task of infancy.

NFTT infants often fall into the classification of "difficult" or irritable babies, but others may be listless, passive, and seem to not care about feedings. A frequent characteristic is **rumination** (voluntary regurgitation), perhaps as a means of self-satisfaction when the desired response is not received from the caregiver. When rumination occurs, a series of events are activated that further strains the parent–infant relationship. The infant loses weight, sometimes becoming severely emaciated, grows increasingly listless and irritable, and because of the frequent vomiting, smells "sour" from a strong odor of vomitus. None of this makes for an attractive baby to love, cuddle, and "show off."

Diagnosis

The infant needs to be thoroughly evaluated by the physician to rule out any possible systemic or congenital disorder. Signs of deprivation are important elements in the diagnosis. When the infant begins to improve in a nurturing atmosphere, the diagnosis is confirmed.

Treatment

Treatment initially depends almost entirely on good nursing care. By teaching child care skills, acting as a role model, and supporting parent–infant interactions, the nurse can play a critical role in helping reverse the infant's growth failure and begin an improved parent–infant relationship. Prognosis of the NFTT infant is uncertain. Much depends on the support and counseling the family receives. Long-term care is almost certainly necessary and may require involvement of several members of the health care team, such as the family therapist, clergy, social worker, and public health nurse. The nurse must guard against judgmental and stereotypical feelings about the family of these infants. The nurse's positive and nonjudgmental attitude can have a direct and lasting effect on the family's interaction with these infants.

Nursing Process for the NFTT Infant

ASSESSMENT

The nurse must conduct a careful physical assessment of the infant, including evaluation of skin turgor, assessment of the anterior fontanelle, signs of emaciation, weight, temperature, apical pulse, respirations, responsiveness, listlessness, and irritability. The nurse observes for rumination or odor of vomitus.

When interviewing the family caregiver, the nurse must observe carefully the interaction between the caregiver and the infant and note the caregiver's responsiveness to the infant's needs and the infant's response to the caregiver. The nurse listens carefully for underlying problems while talking with the family caregivers. The nurse notes if other supportive, involved people are present or if the caregiver is a single parent with no support system. The nurse takes a careful history of feeding and sleeping patterns or problems, assessing the caregiver's confidence in handling the infant and noting any apparent indication of feelings of inadequacy or stress.

NURSING DIAGNOSES

The nursing diagnoses for the infant with failure to thrive must include as much interaction with the family caregiver as possible. Careful assessment, diagnosis, and planning provide for sensory stimulation, adequate food (140 cal/kg) for weight gain, and tender loving care. As the infant becomes less fretful, more responsive, and gains weight, the caregiver will find the infant much more appealing. Some nursing diagnoses might include the following:

- Sensory–perceptual deprivation related to deficient nurturing
- Altered nutrition: less than body requirements and fluid volume deficit related to inadequate intake
- Constipation and altered urinary elimination related to dehydration
- Altered parenting related to lack of knowledge and confidence in parenting skills
- Altered growth and development related to inadequate environmental stimulation
- High risk for injury related to uninvolved caregiver and infant's developmental age
- High risk for infection related to malnourishment
- High risk for impaired skin integrity related to malnourishment

PLANNING AND IMPLEMENTATION

Based on the interview with the parent (or family caregiver), observation, and the physical assessment of the infant, the nursing care plan is formulated. The parent's participation in the infant's care is important. The major nursing goals are to improve the interaction between the infant and the parent, improve the infant's nutritional state, and initiate improvement in developmental tasks that can be continued by the parent.

Providing Sensory Stimulation. The nurse can play a critical role in reversing the infant's growth failure and improving the mother–infant relationship. Providing sensory stimulation plays an important part in the care of the infant. The infant needs to be cuddled, cooed to, played with (such as "Peek-a-Boo," and "Patty-Cake"), talked to in warm and soft tones, and provided opportunities to fulfill sucking needs and with toys that stimulate interest and responsiveness.

Maintaining Adequate Nutrition and Fluid Intake. The infant must be fed slowly and carefully in a quiet environment. The nurse might snuggle the infant closely and rock gently while feeding the infant. Feedings may need to be given every 2 or 3 hours initially. The infant is burped frequently during and at the end of each feeding, then placed on his or her abdomen with the head slightly elevated or held in a chest to chest position. A family caregiver who is present can become involved in the infant's feedings. The child who is older can sit at a low table facing the nurse while eating. The nurse should feed the infant until good eating habits are established. Extra fluids of unsweetened juices are encouraged. The nurse can demonstrate to the caregiver the importance of talking encouragingly as the baby eats. The feeding time should be made pleasant and comforting. Food intake must be carefully documented with caloric intake and strict intake and output measurement records.

Monitoring Elimination Patterns. As food and fluids are gradually increased and the infant becomes hydrated, bowel and urine production return to normal. Careful documentation of urine and stool output is essential.

Providing Family Teaching. While caring for the infant, the nurse can point out the infant's development and responsiveness, noting and praising any positive parenting behaviors that the family caregiver displays. The caregiver who has felt the absence of a close, warm childhood relationship may not understand the infant's needs for cuddling and stimulation. Teaching about these needs must be done carefully, so as not to further damage the caregiver's self-esteem. Many of these family caregivers are sometimes overly concerned about "spoiling" the infant. The nurse can do much to dispel these fears, explaining the need for the development of trust and introducing the caregiver to the developmental tasks appropriate for the infant. Long-term care of these infants and their families may require counseling that involves several members of the health care team—family therapist, clergy, social worker, and public health nurse.

Promoting Safety Practices. Safety considerations must be conscientiously followed, and the nurse should review and reinforce these safety practices with the family caregivers. Side rails must be kept up completely; infant seats are recommended instead of high chairs; restraints should be used with extreme caution and only if necessary to keep the child from interfering with treatments.

Preventing Infection. The infant may be especially susceptible to infectious diseases because of his or her malnourished condition. The child's immune system can be weakened and become a host to any opportune disease. To protect the infant, caretakers should screen anyone who will come in contact with the infant for respiratory conditions or any other bacterial or viral illness.

Promoting Skin Integrity. The infant's skin needs to be protected to prevent irritation. Lanolin or A&D ointment can be used to lubricate areas of dry skin. The ointment should be applied at least once each shift. The infant should be turned at least every 2 hours.

EVALUATION

- The infant is less fretful and more responsive. The infant appears more alert and visually follows the caregiver around the room.
- The infant increases his or her oral intake. The baby's weight increases at a predetermined goal of 1 or more ounces per day.
- Intake and output is within normal limits. Daily stools are of a soft consistency and the urine is not concentrated, as indicated by color or odor.
- The family caregivers demonstrate positive signs of good parenting: they feed the infant successfully, exhibiting an appropriate response to the child. Referrals to support agencies are made before discharge.
- The infant remains uninjured.
- The infant remains free of respiratory or other types of infection.

- The infant's skin remains intact and shows no signs of redness or irritation.

Gastrointestinal Disorders

The gastrointestinal system is responsible for taking in and processing nutrients that nourish all parts of the body. As a result, any problem of the gastrointestinal system, whether it is a lack of nutrients, an infectious disease, or a congenital disorder, can quickly affect other parts of the body and ultimately affect general health and growth and development.

Malnutrition

The World Health Organization has abundantly publicized the malnutrition and hunger that affect more than half the world's population. In the United States, malnutrition contributes to the high death rate of the children of migrant workers and Native Americans. Malnourished children grow at a slower rate, have a higher rate of illness and infection, and have more difficulty concentrating and achieving in school. Table 9-1 lists foods that provide the essential nutrients that a child needs for healthy growth.

Protein Malnutrition

Protein malnutrition results from an insufficient intake of high-quality protein or from conditions in which protein absorption is impaired or there is an increased loss of protein. Clinical evidence of protein malnutrition may not be apparent until the condition is well advanced.

Kwashiorkor results from severe deficiency of protein with an adequate caloric intake and is a condition that accounts for most of the malnutrition in the world's children today. Its highest incidence is among children ages 4 months to 5 years.

An affected child develops a swollen abdomen; retarded growth with muscle wasting; edema; gastrointestinal changes; thin, dry hair with patchy alopecia; apathy; and irritability. In untreated patients, mortality rates are 30% or higher. Although strenuous efforts are being made around the world to prevent this condition, its causes are complex.

Traditionally, these babies have been breast-fed until the age of 2 or 3 years. The child is weaned abruptly when the next child is born and is given the regular family diet, which consists mostly of starchy foods with little meat or vegetable protein. Cow's milk generally is not available, and in many places where goats are kept, their milk is not considered fit for human consumption.

In fact, the name *kwashiorkor* in African dialect means "the sickness the older baby gets when the new baby comes" (Figure 9-2).

Marasmus is a deficiency in calories as well as protein. The child with marasmus is seriously ill. The

Table 9-1. Good Sources of Essential Nutrients

Protein	Vitamin A	Vitamin B			Vitamin C	Vitamin D	Minerals		
		Thiamine	Riboflavin	Niacin			Calcium	Iron	Iodine
Meat, poultry, fish, milk products and eggs. Whole wheat grains, nuts, peanut butter, legumes are also good sources of protein, but need to be supplemented by some animal protein, such as meat, eggs, milk, cheese, cottage cheese or yogurt.	Green leafy vegetables, deep yellow vegetables and fruits, whole milk or whole milk products, egg yolk.	Meat, fish, poultry, eggs, whole grain, legumes, potatoes, green leafy vegetables.	Milk (best source), meat, egg yolk, green vegetables.	Meat, fish, poultry, peanut butter, wheat germ, brewer's yeast. Although the amount in milk is small, children whose intake of milk is adequate do not develop pellagra.	Citrus fruits and tomatoes, fresh or frozen citrus fruit juices, strawberries, cantaloupe. Breast milk is an adequate source of vitamin C for young infants only if the mother's diet contains sufficient vitamin C.	Sunlight, fish liver oils, fortified milk and synthetic vitamin D.	Milk and milk products, squash, sweet potatoes, raisins, rhubarb, well-cooked dried beans, turnip greens, Swiss chard, mustard greens.	Green leafy vegetables, liver, meats and eggs, dried fruits, whole grain or enriched bread and cereals.	Seafoods, plants grown on soil near the sea, iodized salt.

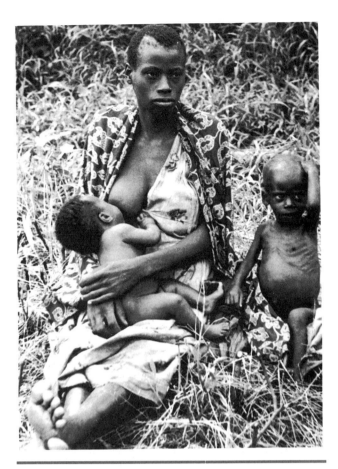

Figure 9-2. The older child in this picture shows the protein-calorie deprivation and the malnutrition that occurred when he was disposessed or replaced at his mother's breast by the new baby. (From Eschleman MM. Introductory Nutrition and Diet Therapy, 2 ed. Philadelphia: JB Lippincott, 1991, p. 139.)

condition is common among children of Third World countries because of severe drought conditions. There is not enough food to supply everyone in these countries, and the children are not fed until adults are fed. The child is severely malnourished and highly susceptible to disease. This syndrome may be seen in the child with NFTT.

Vitamin Deficiency Diseases

Rickets is caused by a lack of vitamin D. Rickets is a disease affecting the growth and calcification of bones. The absorption of calcium and phosphorus is diminished owing to the lack of vitamin D, the function of which is to regulate the use of these minerals. Early manifestations include **craniotabes** (a softening of the occipital bones) and delayed closure of the fontanelle. There is delayed dentition, with defects in tooth enamel and a tendency to develop caries. As the disease advances, thoracic deformities, softening of the shafts of long bones, and spinal and pelvic bone deformities develop. The muscles are poorly developed and lacking in tone, thus delaying standing and walking. Deformities occur during periods of rapid growth, and although rickets itself is not a fatal disease, complications such as tetany, pneumonia, and enteritis are more likely to cause death in rachitic children (children with rickets) than in healthy children.

Infants and children require an estimated 400 U of vitamin D daily for the prevention of rickets. Because of the uncertainty of a small child receiving sufficient exposure to ultraviolet light in temperate climates, it is administered orally in the form of fish liver oil or synthetic vitamin. Whole milk and evaporated milk, fortified with 400 U of vitamin D per quart, are available throughout the United States. Breast-fed infants should receive vitamin D supplements, especially if the mother's intake of vitamin D is poor.

Scurvy is caused by inadequate vitamin C (ascorbic acid) available in the diet. Early inclusion of vitamin C in the form of orange or tomato juice or in a vitamin preparation prevents the development of this disease. Febrile diseases seem to increase the need for vitamin C. A variety of fresh vegetables and fruits supply vitamin C for the older infant and child. Because a considerable proportion of vitamin C content is destroyed by boiling or by exposure to air for long periods, the person who prepares the family's food should be taught to cook vegetables with minimal water in a covered pot and to store juices in a tightly covered opaque container. Vegetables that are cooked in a microwave oven retain more vitamin C because little water is added in the cooking process.

Early clinical manifestations of scurvy are irritability, loss of appetite, and digestive disturbances. A general tenderness in the legs severe enough to cause a "pseudoparalysis" develops. The infant is apprehensive about being handled and assumes a "frog" position, with hips and knees semiflexed and the feet rotated outward. The gums become red and swollen, and hemorrhages occur in various tissues. Characteristic hemorrhages in the long bones are subperiosteal, especially at the ends of the femur and tibia.

Recovery is rapid with adequate treatment, but death may occur from malnutrition or exhaustion in untreated cases. Treatment consists of therapeutic daily doses of ascorbic acid.

Thiamine is one of the major components of the vitamin B complex. Children whose diets are deficient in thiamine exhibit irritability, listlessness, loss of appetite, and vomiting. A severe lack of thiamine in the diet causes the disease called beriberi, characterized by cardiac and neurologic symptoms. Beriberi does not occur when balanced diets are eaten that include whole grains.

Riboflavin deficiency usually occurs in association with thiamine and niacin deficiencies. It is manifested mainly by skin lesions. The primary source of riboflavin is milk. It is destroyed by ultraviolet light; thus, opaque milk cartons are best for storage. Whole grains are also a good source of riboflavin.

Niacin insufficiency in the diet causes a disease known as **pellagra**, which has gastrointestinal and neurologic symptoms. Pellagra does not occur in children whose intake of whole milk is adequate or in those whose diet is well balanced.

Mineral Insufficiency

Iron deficiency results in anemia. The condition is the most common cause of nutritional deficiency among children older than 4 to 6 months whose diets lack iron-rich foods. Anemia is often found in poor children younger than 6 years of age in the United States. Iron deficiency anemia is discussed more fully later in this chapter in the section on circulatory system disorders.

Calcium is necessary for bone and tooth formation. It also is needed for proper nerve and muscle functioning. Hypocalcemia (insufficient calcium) causes neurologic damage, including mental retardation. Rich sources of calcium include milk and milk products. Observe for hypocalcemia in children with milk allergies.

Food Allergies

Children with food allergies exhibit symptoms that vary from one child to another. Common symptoms are **urticaria** (hives), **pruritus**, (itching), stomach pains, and respiratory symptoms. Some of the symptoms may appear quickly after the child has eaten the offending food, but others may have a delayed reaction, thus the investigation needed to find the cause can be frustrating.

Milk

Milk allergy is the most common food allergy in the young child. Symptoms that may indicate an allergy to milk are diarrhea, vomiting, colic, irritability, respiratory symptoms, or eczema. Infants who are breast-fed for the first 6 months or more may avoid developing milk allergies entirely unless there is a strong family history of allergies. Infants with severe allergic reactions to milk are given commercial formulas that are soybean or meat based and formulated to be similar in nutrients to other infant formulas. If the infant has a severe milk allergy, the parent needs to learn to read prepared food labels carefully to avoid lactose or lactic acid ingredients.

Other Food Allergies

Foods should be introduced to the infant one food at a time, with an interval of 4 or 5 days between each new food (Table 9-2). If any gastrointestinal or respiratory reaction occurs, the food should be eliminated. Foods that are among those most likely to cause allergic reactions are eggs, wheat, corn, legumes (including peanuts and soybeans), oranges, strawberries, and chocolate. Suspected foods are eliminated and reintroduced one at

Table 9-2. Some Foods That May Cause Allergies and Possible Sources

Food	Sources
Milk	Yogurt, cheese, ice cream, puddings, hot dogs, foods made with nonfat dry milk, lunch meat, chocolate candies
Eggs	Baked goods, ice cream, puddings, meringues, candies, mayonnaise, salad dressings, custards
Wheat	Breads, baked goods, hot dogs, lunch meats, cereals, cream soups. Oat, rye, and corn-meal products may have wheat added.
Corn	Products made with cornstarch, corn syrup, or vegetable starch; many children's juices, popcorn, cornbreads or muffins, tortillas
Legumes	Soybean products, peanut butter and peanut products
Citrus fruits	Oranges, lemons, limes, grapefruit, gelatins, children's juices, some pediatric suspensions
Strawberries	Gelatins, some pediatric suspensions
Chocolate	Cocoa, candies, chocolate drinks or desserts, colas

a time in small amounts to test for reaction. This testing should be done in a carefully controlled situation to avoid serious or life-threatening reactions. Many allergies disappear as the child's gastrointestinal tract matures.

Nursing Process for the Nutritionally Deprived Infant

ASSESSMENT

The family caregiver interview must be carefully conducted to determine the underlying cause. If the difficulty lies in the caregiver's inability to give proper care, the nurse must try to determine if this can be attributed to lack of information, financial problems, indifference, or other reasons. Do not make assumptions until the interview is completed. Several cases of malnutrition have been reported in infants of families who believed it was better for their infants to eat vegetables only and, in the process, severely limited needed fat intake. If food allergies are suspected as the cause of malnourishment, a careful history of food intake should be included. In addition, a history of stools and voiding should be obtained from the parent.

The physical assessment of the infant includes an evaluation of skin turgor and skin condition, assessment of the anterior fontanelle, signs of emaciation, weight, temperature, apical pulse, respirations, responsiveness, listlessness, and irritability.

NURSING DIAGNOSES

The infant who is admitted to the hospital with the diagnosis of malnourishment often is seriously ill. The nursing diagnoses depend in part on the physical as well as the sociocultural causes of the condition. The nurse needs to reevaluate the nursing diagnoses as the infant improves. Nursing diagnoses that may be used include the following:

- Altered nutrition: less than body requirements related to inadequate intake of nutrients secondary to poor sucking ability, lack of interest in food, lack of adequate food sources, or the caregiver's lack of knowledge of infant requirements
- Fluid volume deficit related to inadequate intake
- Constipation and altered urinary elimination related to insufficient fluid intake
- High risk for infection, impaired skin integrity, and altered growth and development related to malnourishment

PLANNING AND IMPLEMENTATION

Developing a plan of care for the malnourished infant may be challenging. The nurse may need to try a variety of tactics to successfully feed the child. Including the family caregiver in the plan of care is in the best interest of both the infant and the caregiver. The major nursing goals include improvement in the infant's dietary intake and teaching the caregivers methods to avoid nutritional deficiencies within their economic means.

Maintaining Adequate Nutrition
One of the primary nursing care problems may be persuading the infant to take more nourishment than he or she wants. Inexperienced nurses may find it difficult to persuade an uninterested infant to take his or her formula, and it can become frustrating. Perhaps the nurse's insecurity and uncertainty communicate themselves to the child in the way he or she handles the child. An experienced nurse may succeed in feeding an infant 3 or 4 oz in a short period, whereas the inexperienced nurse who seems to be going through the same motions persuades the infant to take only 1 oz or less. As the nurse and the infant become accustomed to each other, however, they both relax, and feeding becomes easier.

The baby who is held snugly in the nurse's arms, wrapped closely and rocked gently, finds it easier to relax and take in a little more feeding. An impatient, hurried nurse nearly always communicates tension to the child. If the nurse is tense because of other feedings that must be attended to, he or she should ask for help. The bottle should never be propped in the crib.

Gavage feedings or intravenous fluids may be needed to improve the nutritional status of the infant, but it is important for the infant to develop an interest in food and in the process of sucking. A hard or small-holed nipple may completely discourage the infant. The nipple should be soft, with holes large enough to allow the formula to drip without pressure but not so soft that it offers no resistance and collapses when it is sucked on or with holes so large that milk pours out, causing him or her to choke. This situation can frustrate a weak infant, who then no longer attempts to nurse. Scheduling feedings every 2 or 3 hours is best because most weak babies are able to handle frequent, small feedings better than every-4-hour feedings. With more frequent feedings, promptness is important. Feedings should be limited to no more than 20 to 30 minutes so that the infant does not tire. Demand schedules are not wise with the malnourished infant because he or she has probably lost the power to regulate the supply and demand schedule.

If malnutrition is related to economic factors or inadequate caregiver knowledge of the infant's needs, teaching the family caregivers the essential facts of infant and child nutrition and making referrals for social services may be necessary. In teaching the caregivers, the nurse must be alert to the possibility that the caregiver is not able to read or understand English and should be certain that the teaching materials used are understood. Simply asking the family caregivers if they have questions is not adequate in determining whether the material has been understood.

Family caregivers may need information regarding assistance in obtaining sound nutritional food for the infant. Infant formulas and baby food can be expensive, and economic factors can be the actual cause of the infant's state of malnutrition. The Women, Infant, Children (WIC) program should be recommended to them (see Chapter 8).

Improving Fluid Intake. In addition to a lack of interest, the infant is weak and debilitated, with little strength to suck. Intravenous fluids may be needed initially to build enough energy in the infant to take more oral nourishment and correct his or her fluid and electrolyte balance. Accurate intake and output measurements are essential along with checking fontanelles and daily weighing in the early morning. Intravenous infusion placement, patency, and site must be monitored every 2 hours.

Monitoring Elimination Patterns. Careful documentation of intake and output, as well as character, frequency, and amount of stools is essential. Any unusual characteristics of the stools or urine should be reported at once.

Preventing Infection and Promoting Skin Integrity and Sensory Stimulation. Infection is always a concern when a child is in a debilitated state. Good aseptic technique must be followed. The family caregivers should be taught good handwashing technique. Care in keeping other people with infectious diseases away from the infant is necessary. Close observation of skin condition, with careful attention to mucous membranes, use of vitamin A & D ointment or lanolin for dry or reddened skin, and prompt changing of soiled diapers are necessary to prevent skin breakdown in weakened infants.

While caring for the infant, the nurse should create an atmosphere in which the infant can respond as he or she gets stronger. The nurse should use every opportunity to reinforce to the caregivers the appropriate developmental tasks that the infant accomplishes and to suggest ways the family caregivers can stimulate additional responses from the infant.

EVALUATION

- The infant gains a prescribed number of ounces in weight per day. Evidence of improved nutritional status is noted by assessing improved signs of hydration.
- The infant shows evidence of adequate sucking by increasing oral intake daily. The infant displays interest in feedings and extending the amount of time nursing without showing signs of tiring.

- If parenteral fluids are administered, the site remains intact. No signs of redness or induration are evidenced at the intravenous infusion site. Restraints are adequate but kept to a minimum.
- Bowel and urine output is sufficient and of normal character and is documented accurately.
- The family caregivers demonstrate, through discussion, questions, and verbal responses, a beginning knowledge of appropriate nutrition for a growing infant. The caregivers follow through with the referrals that have been made to assist them.
- The skin and mucous membranes of the infant show evidence of improved hydration; redness and skin breakdown are improved. The infant is more alert, smiling, and responsive to sensory stimulation.

Diarrhea and Gastroenteritis

Diarrhea in infants is a fairly common symptom of a variety of conditions. It may be mild with a small amount of dehydration, or it may be extremely severe, requiring prompt and effective treatment (Figure 9-3).

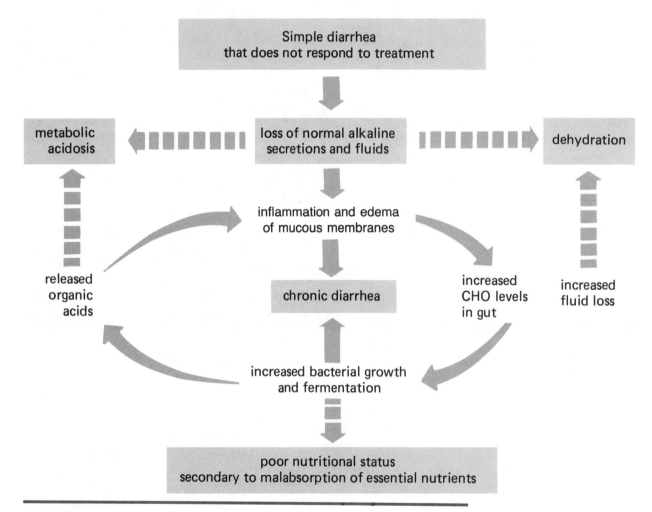

Figure 9-3. The vicious cycle of infant diarrhea. (Redrawn from Copeland L. Chronic diarrhea in infancy. Am J Nurs 77:461–463, 1977. Copyright © 1977, American Journal of Nursing Company. Reproduced with permission.)

Chronically malnourished infants with diarrheal symptoms constitute a common problem in many areas of the world. This condition is prevalent in areas where clean water and sanitary facilities are lacking or inadequate. Certain metabolic diseases, such as cystic fibrosis, have diarrhea as a symptom. Diarrhea also may be caused by antibiotic therapy.

Some conditions that cause diarrhea may require readjustment of the infant's diet. Allergic reactions to food are not uncommon and can be controlled by avoidance of the offending food. Congenital lactose intolerance is seen in some infants of African American, Native American, Eskimo, Asian, and Mediterranean heritage. Infants with **lactose intolerance** are unable to digest **lactose**, the primary carbohydrate in milk, because of an inborn deficiency of the enzyme lactase. Symptoms include cramping, abdominal distention, flatus, and diarrhea after ingesting milk. Formulas such as Isomil, Nursoy, Nutramigen, and Prosobee are commercially available that are made from soybean, meat-based, or protein mixtures and have no lactose. Overfeeding as well as underfeeding or an unbalanced diet may be the cause of diarrhea in an infant. Adjusting the infant's diet, cutting down on the amount of sugar added to formula, or reducing bulk or fat in the diet may be necessary.

Many diarrheal disturbances in infants may be caused by contaminated food or from human or animal fecal waste through the oral fecal route. Infectious diarrhea is commonly referred to as **gastroenteritis**. The infectious organisms may be salmonella, *Escherichia coli*, dysentery bacilli, and various viruses, most notably rotaviruses. It is difficult to determine the causative factor in most patients. Because of the seriousness of infectious diarrhea among infants and the danger of spreading diarrhea throughout a pediatric unit, most hospitals isolate the child with moderate or severe diarrhea until the causative factor definitely has been proved to be noninfectious.

Clinical Manifestations

Mild diarrhea may show little more than loose stools, which may number from 2 to 4 to as many as 10 to 12 per day. There may be irritability and loss of appetite. Vomiting and gastric distention are not significant factors, and dehydration is minimal.

Mild or moderate diarrhea can convert rather quickly to severe diarrhea in an infant. Vomiting usually accompanies the diarrhea; together, they cause large losses of body water and electrolytes. The infant becomes severely dehydrated and is gravely ill. The skin becomes extremely dry and loses its turgor. The fontanelle becomes sunken, and the pulse is weak and rapid. The stools become greenish liquid and may be blood tinged.

Diagnosis

Treatment to stop the diarrhea must be initiated immediately; however, stool specimens may be collected to be tested for culture and sensitivities. This test determines the causative infectious organism, if there is one, and effective antibiotics can be prescribed as indicated.

Treatment

Establishing normal fluid and electrolyte balance is the primary concern in treating gastroenteritis. The infant with mild dehydration may be given oral feedings of commercial electrolyte solutions, such as Pedialyte and Lytren. As the diarrhea clears, gradual additions can be made. The BRAT diet, which consists of ripe *b*anana, *r*ice cereal, *a*pplesauce (preferably canned), and *t*oast is often ordered by the physician because it is nonirritating to the gastrointestinal tract. Salty broths should be avoided. Foods can be gradually added as the condition of the infant improves, with milk products last on the list.

In severe diarrhea, oral feedings are discontinued completely. Fluids to be given intravenously must be carefully calculated to replace the lost electrolytes. Frequent laboratory determination of the infant's blood chemistries are necessary to guide the physician in this replacement therapy. After a serious bout of diarrhea, the physician may prescribe soybean formula for a few weeks to avoid possible reaction to milk proteins.

Nursing Process for the Infant with Diarrhea and Gastroenteritis

ASSESSMENT

In addition to basic information on the infant, the interview with the family caregiver must include specific information about the history of bowel patterns and questions concerning the onset of diarrheal stools, with details on number and type of stools per day. The caregiver may need help in describing the color and odor of stools, and the nurse can assist with suggested terms. The nurse also should inquire about recent feeding patterns, nausea, and vomiting. The caregiver also should be asked about fever and other signs of illness and signs of illness in any other family members.

The physical assessment of the infant involves evaluation of skin turgor and condition, including excoriated diaper area, temperature, anterior fontanelle (depressed, normal, or bulging), apical pulse rate (observing for weak pulse), stools (character, amount, and color and presence of blood), irritability, lethargy, vomiting, urine (amount and concentration), lips and mucous membranes of the mouth (dry, cracked), eyes (bright, glassy, sunken, dark circles), and any other notable physical signs.

NURSING DIAGNOSES

A primary nursing diagnosis is "Diarrhea related to . . . [whatever cause exists]." Other nursing diagnoses vary with the intensity of the diarrhea (mild or severe) as determined by the physical assessment and parent interview. Some nursing diagnoses are the following:

- High risk for infection transmission related to gastro-intestinal infection
- Altered skin integrity related to the constant presence of diarrheal stools
- Altered elimination related to dehydration
- Parental anxiety and infant diversional activity deficit related to the seriousness of infant's illness
- Altered nutrition: less than body requirements related to diarrhea
- Increased sucking needs related to NPO status
- High risk for hyperthermia related to dehydration
- High risk for infection related to weakened state
- High risk for injury related to developmental age
- Parental health-seeking behaviors related to therapy for diarrhea

PLANNING AND IMPLEMENTATION

The major goals of the nurse include the elimination of any danger of infecting other patients, stopping the diarrhea, and maintaining good skin condition in the infant.

Preventing Infection. To prevent the spread of possibly infectious organisms to other pediatric patients, it is necessary for the nurse to follow **enteric precautions** of the Centers for Disease Control. Gowns and gloves are worn when handling articles contaminated with feces. Masks are not necessary. Contaminated linens and clothing are placed in specially marked containers to be processed according to hospital policy. Disposable diapers and other disposable items are placed in specially marked bags and disposed of according to hospital policy. Visitors are limited to family only.

The nurse must teach the family caregivers the principles of aseptic technique and observe them to ensure understanding and compliance. Good handwashing must be carried out, and it also must be taught to the caregivers. The nurse should stress that gloves are needed for added protection, but careful handwashing is also absolutely necessary.

Promoting Skin Integrity. To reduce irritation and excoriation of the buttocks and genital area, the nurse should cleanse those areas frequently and apply a soothing protective preparation such as lanolin or A&D ointment. Diapers should be changed as quickly as possible after soiling. Some infants' skin may be sensitive to cloth diapers, and others may be sensitive to disposable diapers, so it may be necessary to try either type. It is often helpful to leave the diaper off, exposing the buttocks and genital area to the air. Disposable pads under the infant can facilitate easy and frequent changing. Caregivers should be taught that waterproof diaper covers hold moisture in and do not allow circulation of air, increasing irritation and excoriation of the diaper area.

Preventing Dehydration. An infant can dehydrate quickly and can get into serious trouble after only 3 days or less of diarrhea. Careful counting of diapers is required, and even weighing diapers may be necessary to determine the infant's output more accurately. Careful observation of all stools is essential. Documenting the number and character of the stools, as well as the amount and character of any vomitus, is important.

Providing Comfort Measures. Being the family caregiver of an infant who has become so ill in such a short time is frightening. Meeting the emotional needs of the infant is difficult but of great importance. The caregiver benefits from suggestions of ways that the infant might be consoled without interfering with the infant's care. Soothing, gentle stroking of the head and speaking softly help the infant bear the frustrations of the illness and its treatment. The infant can be picked up and rocked, as long as this can be done without jeopardizing the intravenous infusion site. If the intravenous infusion is in a position that may be displaced, this is not permitted. Threading a needle into the small veins of a dehydrated infant is difficult, and replacement may be nearly impossible, but the infant's life may depend on the proper parenteral fluids. The nurse needs to help fill the emotional needs of the infant and also encourage the family caregiver to have some time away from the infant's hospital room without feeling guilty about leaving the infant.

Maintaining Adequate Nutrition. Daily weights on the same scale are necessary, taken in early morning before the morning feeding, if infant is on oral feedings. Isolation precautions are maintained while the infant is weighed. Strict intake and output determinations are maintained.

Intravenous fluids are administered in severe dehydration to rest the gastrointestinal tract and restore the hydration status. Placement, patency, and site of the intravenous infusion should be monitored at least every 2 hours. Restraints with relevant nursing interventions may be necessary. Good mouth care is essential while the infant is NPO.

When oral fluids are administered, the infant is given oral pediatric electrolyte replacement fluids, such as Pedialyte and Lytren. After the infant tolerates the oral electrolyte fluids, half-strength formula may be introduced, then several days later full-strength formula (possibly lactose-free or soy formula to avoid disaccharide intolerance or reaction to milk proteins). The mother of a breast-fed infant should be given access to a breast pump if her infant is NPO.

Satisfying Sucking Needs. The infant who is NPO needs to have his or her sucking needs fulfilled. This can be accomplished by offering a pacifier.

Maintaining Body Temperature. Monitor vital signs (at least every 2 hours if there is fever). *Do not take the temperature rectally.* Insertion of a thermometer into the rectum can cause stimulation of stools as well as trauma and tissue injury to sensitive mucosa. Follow the appro-

Parent Teaching

Tips on Diarrhea

The danger in diarrhea is dehydration (drying out). If the child becomes dehydrated, he or she can become very sick. Increasing the amount of liquid the child drinks is helpful. Solid foods may need to be decreased so the child will drink more.

Suggestions

1. Give liquids in small amounts (2 to 4 tbsp) about every half hour. If this goes well, increase the amount a little each half hour. Don't force the child to drink because he or she may vomit.

2. Give solid foods in small amounts. Do not give milk for a day or two because this can make diarrhea worse.

3. Give only soups or broths that are nonsalty.

4. Liquids recommended for vomiting may be given for diarrhea also.

4. Soft foods to give (small amounts): applesauce, fine chopped or scraped apple without peel, bananas, toast, rice cereal, plain unsalted crackers or cookies, any meats

Call the Physician if

1. Child develops sudden high fever.

2. Stomach pain becomes severe.

3. Diarrhea becomes bloody (more than a streak of blood).

4. Diarrhea becomes more frequent or severe.

5. Child becomes dehydrated (dried out).

Signs of Dehydration

1. Child has not urinated for 6 hours or more.

2. Child has no tears when crying.

3. Child's mouth is dry or sticky to touch.

4. Child's eyes are sunken.

5. Child is less active than usual.

6. Child has dark circles under eyes.

Warning

Do not use medicines to stop diarrhea for children younger than 6 years of age unless specifically directed to by the physician. These medicines can be dangerous if not used properly.

Diaper Area Skin Care

1. Change diaper as soon as it is soiled.

2. Wash area with mild soap, dry, and rinse well.

3. Use soothing, protective lotion recommended by your physician or hospital.

4. Do not use waterproof diaper covers—they increase diaper area irritation.

5. Wash hands with soap and water after changing diapers or wiping the child.

priate procedures for fever reduction, and administer anti-pyretics and antibiotics as prescribed. The infant's temperature should be taken with a thermometer that can be left in the isolation room.

Preventing Infection. The infant is susceptible to the invasion of bacteria because of a weakened immune system. Careful observation of vital and neurologic signs, careful aseptic technique, and prompt reporting of any signs of systemic infection are necessary.

Promoting Safety Practices. Safety measures should be maintained at all times. The nurse must be constantly aware of the infant's increasing developmental skills.

Promoting Family Teaching. The nurse should explain to the family caregivers the importance of gastrointestinal rest for the infant. The family caregivers (especially if young or poorly educated) may not understand the necessity for NPO status. Cooperation of the parent is improved with increased understanding (see Parent Teaching Tips on Diarrhea and Vomiting).

EVALUATION

- Infection control is maintained as evidenced by careful handwashing, gowning, and gloving
- The infant's diaper area shows no evidence of redness or excoriation
- The infant's urine and stool output are accurately documented
- The infant rests quietly; caregivers console infant effectively
- The infant is well hydrated as evidenced by good turgor, moist mucous membranes, and clear eyes
- The infant uses a pacifier to satisfy nonnutritive sucking needs
- The infant is afebrile
- The infant shows no signs of a secondary infection
- Safety measures are maintained; the infant is free from injury
- The family demonstrates understanding of infant's treatment through cooperation and appropriate questions

Colic

Colic is the recurrent paroxysmal bouts of abdominal pain that are fairly common among young infants. The fact that it often disappears around the age of 3 months gives small comfort to the parent vainly trying to soothe a colicky infant. Although many theories have been proposed, none has been accepted as the causative factor.

Clinical Manifestations and Diagnosis
Attacks occur suddenly, usually late in the day or evening. The infant cries loudly and continuously. The infant appears to be in considerable pain, but otherwise seems healthy, nurses or takes formula well, and gains weight as

expected. The baby may be momentarily soothed only by rocking or holding but eventually falls asleep, exhausted from crying. The infant with colic is often classified as a "difficult" baby.

Differential diagnosis should be made to rule out allergic reaction to milk or certain foods. If the baby is breast-fed, the mother's diet should be studied to determine if anything she is eating may be affecting the baby. Intestinal obstruction or infection also must be ruled out.

Treatment
No single treatment is consistently successful. Changing to a nonallergenic formula helps determine if there is an allergic factor or perhaps if the infant has lactose intolerance. Otherwise, a number of measures may be employed, one or more of which might work. The point the family must remember is that the condition will pass, even though at the time it seems as though it will last forever. Medications such as sedatives, antispasmodics, and antiflatulents are sometimes prescribed, but their effectiveness is not consistent. Family caregivers need to be reassured that their parenting skills are not inadequate (see Parent Teaching Tips for Colic).

Pyloric Stenosis

Pyloric stenosis is rarely symptomatic during the first days of life. It has occasionally been recognized shortly after birth, but the average affected infant does not show symptoms until about the third week of life. Symptoms rarely appear after the second month. Although symptoms appear late, pyloric stenosis is classified as a congenital defect. Its cause is not known.

The pylorus is the muscle that controls the flow of food from the stomach to the duodenum. Pyloric stenosis is characterized by hypertrophy of the circular muscle fibers of the pylorus, with a severe narrowing of its lumen. The pylorus is thickened to as much as twice its size, is elongated, and has a consistency resembling cartilage. As a result of this obstruction at the distal end of the stomach, the stomach becomes dilated (Figure 9-4).

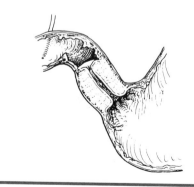

Figure 9-4. Pyloric stenosis. (narrowed lumen of the pylorus).

Parent Teaching

Tips for Vomiting

Vomiting will usually stop in a couple of days and can be treated at home as long as the child is getting some fluids.

Warning

Some medications used to stop vomiting in older children or adults are dangerous in children. DO NOT use any medicines unless your physician has told you to use it for *this child*.

Give child clear liquids to drink in small amounts.

Suggestions

1. Flat soda (no fizz). Use caffeine-free type; do not use diet soda.
2. Jello water—double the amount of water, let stand to room temperature.
3. Ice popsicles
4. Gatorade
5. Pedialyte, Lytren (buy at the drugstore, no prescription needed)
6. Tea
7. Solid Jello
8. Broth (not salty)

How to Give

Give small amounts often. One tbsp every 20 minutes for the first few hours is a good rule of thumb. If this is kept down without vomiting, increase to 2 tbsp every 20 minutes for the next couple of hours. If there is no vomiting, increase the amount the child may have. If child vomits, wait for 1 hour before offering more liquids.

Clinical Manifestations

During the first weeks of life, the infant with pyloric stenosis often eats well and gains weight, but then he or she starts vomiting occasionally after meals. Within a few days, the vomiting episodes increase in frequency and force, becoming projectile. The vomited material is sour, undigested food, which may contain mucus, but never bile, because it has not progressed beyond the stomach.

Because the obstruction is a mechanical one, the baby does not feel ill, is ravenously hungry, and is eager to try again and again, but the food invariably comes back. As the condition progresses the baby becomes irritable, loses weight rapidly, and becomes dehydrated. A condition of alkalosis develops from the loss of potassium and hydrochloric acid, and the baby becomes seriously ill.

Constipation becomes progressive because little food gets into the intestine and the urine is scanty. Gastric peristaltic waves passing from left to right across the abdomen usually can be seen during or after the feedings.

Diagnosis

Diagnosis is usually made on the clinical evidence. The nature, type, and times of vomiting, observation of gastric peristaltic waves, and a history of weight loss with hunger and irritability point in this direction. The olive-sized pyloric tumor often can be felt through deep palpation by an experienced physician. Ultrasonographic or radiographic studies with barium swallow show an abnormal retention of barium in the stomach and increased peristalsis. Pyloric stenosis occurs more frequently in white males and has a familial tendency.

Treatment

Surgery is the treatment of choice in this condition. The surgical procedure is called a pyloromyotomy (also known as Fredet-Ramstedt operation). This procedure simply splits the hypertrophic pyloric muscle down to the submucosa, allowing the pylorus to expand so that food may pass. Prognosis is excellent if surgery is performed before the infant is severely dehydrated.

Nursing Process for the Infant with Pyloric Stenosis

ASSESSMENT

When the infant of 1 or 2 months of age is admitted to the hospital with a history of projectile vomiting, pyloric ste-

Parent Teaching

Tips for Colic

1. Pick up and rock the baby, in a rocker, or tummy down across your knees, swinging legs side to side. (Be sure head is supported.)
2. Walk around the room while rocking baby in your arms (hum or sing to baby).
3. Try a bottle, but don't overfeed. Give a pacifier if baby has eaten well within 2 hours.
4. Baby may like rhythmic movements of baby swing.
5. Try taking baby for a drive.
6. When feeding baby, try methods to decrease gas formation: frequent burping, smaller feedings more frequently; position baby in infant seat after eating.
7. Try doing something to entertain but not overexcite baby.
8. Gently rub baby's abdomen if it is rigid.
9. Sit with baby resting on your lap, with legs toward you; gently move baby's legs in pumping motion.
10. Try putting baby down to sleep in a darkened room.
11. Keep remembering it's temporary. Try to stay as calm and relaxed as possible.

nosis is suspected. A careful interview with the family caregiver should include questions concerning when the vomiting started, the character of the vomitus (undigested formula with no bile), hunger, and vomitus progressively more projectile. The caregiver will relate a story of a baby who is an eager eater but who cannot retain food. The caregiver should be asked about constipation and scanty urine. Physical assessment of the infant reveals an infant who may show signs of dehydration. Weight, evaluation of skin turgor and skin condition (including excoriated diaper area), anterior fontanelle (depressed, normal, bulging), temperature, apical pulse rate (observing for weak pulse, tachycardia), irritability, lethargy, urine (amount and concentration), lips and mucous membranes of the mouth (dry, cracked), eyes (bright, glassy, sunken, dark circles), and observation of visible gastric peristalsis when infant is eating are all important assessments. Documenting and reporting signs of severe dehydration assists in the determination of the need for fluid and electrolyte replacement.

NURSING DIAGNOSES

The severity of the state of dehydration and malnutrition determines to some extent the appropriate nursing diag-

noses for this infant. Some preoperative diagnoses that may be used are the following:

- Altered nutrition: less than body requirements related to inability to retain food
- Fluid volume deficit related to frequent vomiting
- Parental anxiety related to seriousness of illness and impending surgery
- Altered oral mucous membranes and increased sucking needs related to NPO status
- High risk for infection related to malnutrition
- High risk for impaired skin integrity related to dehydration
- High risk for altered growth and development related to prolonged illness

Postoperative nursing diagnoses may include:

- High risk for aspiration related to postoperative condition
- Parental anxiety related to postoperative condition
- High risk for impaired skin integrity related to surgery
- Pain related to surgical trauma

PLANNING AND IMPLEMENTATION: PREOPERATIVE

Preoperatively, the major nursing goals include rehydration of the infant, relieving the family's anxiety, and preparing the infant for surgery.

Maintaining Adequate Nutrition and Fluid Intake. The pylorus is hypertrophied, and food (breast milk or formula) cannot pass through because of the narrow passage from the stomach into the duodenum. As a result, the child is unable to retain any feedings, and projectile vomiting occurs with greater frequency. The vomitus is characteristically undigested food with perhaps some shreds of mucus and streaking of blood. This causes the baby to become irritable, lose weight, and become dehydrated. If the infant is severely dehydrated and malnourished, intravenous fluids and electrolytes are necessary for rehydration to prepare for surgery and correct hypokalemia and alkalosis.

Feedings of formula thickened with infant cereal and fed through a large-holed nipple may be given to improve nutrition before surgery. A smooth muscle relaxant may be ordered to be administered before feedings. The infant should be fed slowly while sitting in an infant seat or being held in an upright position. During the feeding, the infant should be burped frequently to avoid gastric distention. Accurate documentation of the feeding given and the approximate amount retained is required. The frequency and type of emesis also must be recorded. Oral fluids are omitted for a specified time before surgery. To empty the stomach after the barium swallow to prepare for the surgery, the physician may order a nasogastric tube with saline lavage. The nasogastric tube is left in place when the infant goes to surgery.

Reducing Family Anxiety and Providing Family Teaching. The family caregivers are anxious because their infant is obviously seriously ill, and when they learn that their young infant is to undergo surgery, their apprehensions increase. The nurse must include the caregivers in the preparation for surgery, explaining the following:

1. The importance of added intravenous fluids preoperatively to improve electrolyte balance and rehydrate the infant

2. The reason for ultrasonographic or barium swallow examination

3. The function of the nasogastric tube and saline lavage

4. The location of the pylorus at the distal end of the stomach, and what happens when the circular muscle fibers hypertrophy. (You can liken it to a doughnut, which gets thicker, so that the opening closes and very little food gets through.)

5. The surgery is called pyloromyotomy (or Fredet-Remstedt). The muscle is simply split down to, but not through, the submucosa, allowing it to balloon and let food pass through.

The family caregivers are directed to the appropriate waiting area during surgery, so that the surgeon can find them and communicate with them immediately after surgery. The nurse can tell the caregivers what to expect and approximately how long the surgery will be. In addition, the procedure for the postanesthesia care unit (PACU) should be explained to the caregivers so that they know that the infant will be under close observation postoperatively until fully recovered.

Providing Mouth Care and Nonnutritive Sucking. Mucous membranes of the mouth may be dry because of dehydration, and oral fluids are omitted before surgery, therefore the infant needs good mouth care. In addition, a pacifier can satisfy the sucking needs that the baby has because of the interruption in normal feeding and sucking habits.

Preventing Infection. Malnutrition and dehydration can compromise the infant's ability to fight off infection. Aseptic technique must be followed carefully. Good handwashing procedures are essential. The nurse should teach the family that visitors must be free of any kind of respiratory or viral infection.

Promoting Skin Integrity. Depending on the severity of the infant's dehydration, the skin may easily break down and become irritated. The infant should be turned, diapers changed, and lanolin or A&D ointment applied to dry skin areas. Close observation of skin condition and documentation are important.

Providing Sensory Stimulation. In the first few weeks and months of life, the infant is developing at a fast pace. Illness can slow the developmental process. The nurse must remember that the major task of infancy according to Erikson is the development of trust. In light of this, the nurse must encourage the family caregivers to soothe and cuddle the infant as much as possible within the limits of treatments that must be carried out. Stroking, cuddling, and talking to the baby are all important aspects of the care, and the caregivers can help fulfill these needs. This approach also helps the caregiver to feel needed and useful.

PLANNING AND IMPLEMENTATION: POSTOPERATIVE

Postoperatively, the major nursing goals include prevention of aspiration, maintenance of fluid balance, and relief of parental anxiety.

Preventing Aspiration. Postoperatively, the infant should be positioned on the side and watched carefully to prevent aspiration of mucus or vomitus, particularly during the anesthesia recovery period. After fully awaking from surgery, the infant may be held by a family caregiver. The nurse can assist the caregiver to find a position that does not interfere with intravenous infusions and that is comforting to both caregiver and child.

The first feeding, given 4 to 6 hours postoperatively, is usually an electrolyte replacement, such as Lytren and Pedialyte. Feedings should be given in small amounts, slowly, with frequent burping. Intravenous fluid administration is necessary until the infant is taking sufficient oral feedings. The nurse continues to use all nursing measures that relate to intravenous care that were followed preoperatively. Accurate intake and output and daily weight determinations are required.

Reducing Family Anxiety. The family caregivers will be anxious if the infant vomits after the surgery, but they need to be reassured that this is not uncommon. The nurse can reassure the caregivers that this most likely will occur only once or twice. The caregivers should be involved in the infant's postoperative care. Caregivers need reassurance that the care they gave the infant at home did not cause the condition. The nurse must give the caregivers support and understanding and encourage them in feeding and providing for the infant's needs. They can be told that the likelihood of a satisfactory recovery in a few weeks with steady progression to complete recovery is excellent. The operative fatality rate under these conditions has become less than 1%.

Promoting Skin Integrity. The surgical site needs to be observed closely for blood, drainage, and secretions. Observations should be made at least every 4 hours. Any odor should be recorded and reported. The incision and dressings are cared for as ordered by the physician.

Relieving Pain. The infant's behavior is observed to evaluate discomfort and pain. Excessive crying, restlessness, listlessness, resistance to being held and cuddled, rigidity, and increased pulse and respiratory rates can indicate pain. Analgesics should be administered to provide comfort. Nursing interventions that may provide comfort include rocking, holding, cuddling, and offering a pacifier. The family caregivers can be included in helping provide comfort to the infant.

EVALUATION

- Preoperatively, the infant's hydration is improved, with improved skin turgor, increased weight gain, correction of hypokalemia and alkalosis, adequate intake of fluids, and no evidence of gastric distention.

- The intravenous infusion site remains intact with no signs of redness or induration. The infant's stomach is clear of barium following gastric lavage.

- The family caregivers verbalize an understanding of the procedures and treatments, cooperate with the nursing staff, ask appropriate questions, and express confidence in the surgeon.

- The mucous membranes of the mouth are not coated. Saliva is sufficient as evidenced by typical drooling. The infant has a pacifier to satisfy sucking needs.

- No evidence of infection is noted in the infant as evidenced by elevated temperature, nasal or respiratory congestion, redness, or irritation.

- Skin integrity is maintained with no signs of irritation or breakdown.

- The infant responds positively to the sensory stimulation of the nursing personnel and family.

- Postoperatively, the infant does not aspirate vomitus or mucus and is comforted by caregivers and family caregivers.

- Postoperatively, intravenous infusions do not infiltrate as evidenced by absence of redness, edema, pain, or leakage. The infant retains oral fluids with minimal vomiting.

- The family caregivers are involved in the postoperative feeding of the infant and demonstrate an understanding of feeding technique.

- The surgical site shows no signs of infection as evidenced by absence of redness, foul odor, or drainage.

- The infant shows no signs of discomfort as evidenced by sleeping and resting in a relaxed manner, cuddling with caregivers and nurses, and lack of excessive crying.

Congenital Aganglionic Megacolon

Congenital aganglionic megacolon, also called Hirschsprung disease, is characterized by obstinate constipation resulting from partial or complete intestinal obstruction of mechanical origin. The condition may be severe

enough to be recognized during the neonatal period, but in other patients it may not be diagnosed until later infancy or early childhood.

Parasympathetic nerve cells regulate peristalsis in the intestine. The name *aganglionic megacolon* actually describes the condition because there is an absence of parasympathetic ganglion cells within the muscular wall of the distal colon and the rectum. As a result, the affected portion of the lower bowel has no peristaltic action, thus it narrows, and the portion directly *proximal to* (above) the affected area becomes greatly dilated and filled with feces and gas (Figure 9-5).

Clinical Manifestations

Accurate reporting of the first meconium stool in the *newborn* is vitally important. Failure of the newborn to have a stool in the first 24 hours may indicate a number of conditions. One of the conditions that must be considered is megacolon. Other neonatal symptoms are suggestive of complete or partial intestinal obstruction, such as bile-stained emesis and generalized abdominal distention. Gastroenteritis with diarrheal stools may be present, and ulceration of the colon may occur.

Symptoms in the *older infant* or *young child* are obstinate, severe constipation dating back to early infancy. Stools are ribbonlike or consist of hard pellets. Formed bowel movements do not occur except with the use of enemas, and soiling does not occur. The rectum is usually empty because the impaction occurs above the aganglionic segment.

As the child grows older, the abdomen becomes progressively enlarged and hard (Figure 9-6). General debilitation and chronic anemia are usually present. Differentiation must be made between this condition and psychogenic megacolon owing to coercive toileting or other emotional problems. In aganglionic megacolon there is an absence of withholding of stool, defecating in inappropriate places, and soiling.

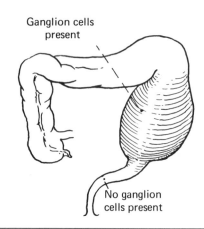

Figure 9-5. Dilated colon in Hirschsprung disease.

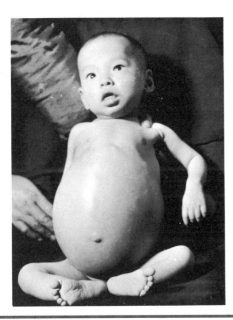

Figure 9-6. A baby with Hirschsprung disease. (From Waechter EH, Blake FG. Nursing Care of Children, 9th ed. Philadelphia: JB Lippincott, 1976.)

Diagnosis

In the newborn, the absence of a meconium stool within the first 24 hours, and in the older infant or young child, a history of obstinate, severe constipation may indicate the need for further testing. Definitive diagnosis is made through barium studies and must be confirmed by rectal biopsy.

Treatment

Treatment involves surgery with the ultimate resection of the aganglionic portion of the bowel. Frequently, a colostomy is performed to relieve the obstruction. This allows the infant to regain any weight lost; the colostomy also gives the bowel a period of rest to return to a more normal state. Resection is deferred until later in infancy.

⌐⌐ Nursing Process for the Infant Undergoing Surgery for Congenital Megacolon

ASSESSMENT

A careful history gathered from the family caregivers is useful, noting especially the history of stooling. If the child is not a young infant, onset of constipation, character and odor of stools, and frequency of bowel movements, poor feeding habits or lack of appetite (anorexia), and irritability are significant.

Physical assessment of the child must include observation for a distended abdomen, signs of poor nutrition (*review signs listed in assessment of the malnourished*

infant), and recording of weight and vital signs. Assessment of developmental milestones is included.

NURSING DIAGNOSES

Many of the nursing diagnoses for pyloric stenosis also may be appropriate for congenital megacolon, with some adjustment. The following are some of the diagnoses that may apply:

- Preoperative diagnoses:
  - Constipation related to intestinal obstruction
  - Altered nutrition and fluid volume deficit: less than body requirements related to anorexia
  - Parental anxiety and knowledge deficit related to the serious condition of the infant and lack of knowledge about impending surgery
  - High risk for infection related to debilitated state
  - High risk for injury related to developmental age
  - High risk for altered growth and development related to illness and hospitalization
  - Fear (in the older child) related to impending surgery
- Postoperative diagnoses:
  - High risk for impaired skin integrity related to irritation from the colostomy
  - Pain related to the surgical procedure
  - High risk for infection related to surgery
  - Fluid volume deficit related to postoperative condition after colostomy
  - Altered oral and nasal mucous membranes related to NPO status and irritation from nasogastric tube
  - Parental health-seeking behaviors related to postoperative care of the colostomy

PLANNING AND IMPLEMENTATION: PREOPERATIVE CARE

The major nursing goals preoperatively include cleaning of the intestinal tract, fluid balance, and relief of parental anxiety.

Relieving Constipation. The colon must be emptied of fecal material before diagnostic and surgical procedures are performed. Colonic irrigations with isotonic saline solution and neomycin or other antibiotics are administered to cleanse the bowel and prepare the gastrointestinal tract. Soapsuds or tap water enemas are never administered because the lack of peristaltic action causes the enemas to be retained and absorbed into the tissues, causing water intoxication. This could cause syncope, shock, or even death after only one or two irrigations.

Maintaining Adequate Nutrition and Fluid Intake. Parenteral fluids may be needed to improve the infant's state of hydration because the constipation and distended abdomen cause loss of appetite; thus, the infant is in a poor nutritional state. All the precautions used with parenteral fluid administration are appropriate.

Providing Family Teaching. Family caregivers are apprehensive about the preliminary procedures as well as the impending surgery. The nurse must explain to the caregivers all aspects of the preoperative care, including examinations, colonic irrigations, and intravenous fluid therapy. As with other surgerical procedures, the nurse should inform the caregivers about the waiting area, the PACU, and the approximate length of the surgery and answer any other questions they may have. Building good rapport preoperatively is an essential aspect of good nursing care. The family caregivers need to have their questions answered about the later resection of the aganglionic portion. With successful surgery, these children grow and develop normally.

Preventing Infection. Any infant or child undergoing surgery is at risk for infection. Aseptic technique, good handwashing practices by health care personnel and family caregivers, and monitoring staff, family, and other visitors for respiratory or viral infections are necessary.

Promoting Safety Practices. The infant is growing, and safety measures are vital. The nurse must be alert to changing developmental abilities. Family caregivers also must be made aware of these changes so that they can be alert to safety hazards. Safety measures must be conscientiously implemented.

Providing Sensory Stimulation. The growth and development of this infant may have been slowed because of poor nutrition and dehydration. Sensory stimulation should be integrated into the nursing care, and the nurse should teach the family caregivers methods of encouraging developmental tasks in the infant.

Reducing Anxiety. Children who are preschool and older are more aware of the approaching surgery and have a number of fears as a result of their developmental stage. Preschoolers are still in the age of magical thinking. They may overhear a word or two that they misinterpret and exaggerate, imagining pain and danger. Careful explanation must be provided for the preschooler to reduce any fears about mutilation. The nurse can talk about the surgery, reassuring the child that the "insides won't come out," and answer questions seriously and with sincerity. Family caregivers are encouraged to stay with the young child if possible to increase the child's feelings of security.

The older school-age child may have a more realistic view of what is going to happen but may be upset by a disruption in peer relationships. Efforts should be made to provide contact with the school-age child's peers through telephone contact or by letter writing. A school teacher can be encouraged to have the child's class write letters as a class project. At all times, for any child, the nurse must remember to treat the child as a person and respect the feelings that are being expressed.

PLANNING AND IMPLEMENTATION: POSTOPERATIVE CARE

The major nursing goals include reduction of the family caregivers' anxiety and preparation for home care of the infant, care of the colostomy and surgical site, maintenance of fluid and nutrition, and prevention of skin breakdown and mucous membrane irritation.

Promoting Skin Integrity. When routine colostomy care is performed, careful attention should be given to the area around the colostomy. Observations of redness, irritation, and rashy appearance should be recorded and reported. The skin should be prepared with skin-toughening preparations that strengthen the skin and provide better adhesion of the appliance.

Relieving Pain. The child may have abdominal pain postoperatively. Assess for signs of pain, such as crying, pulse and respiration rate increase, restlessness, and guarding of abdomen or drawing up the legs. Analgesics must be administered as ordered. Additional nursing measures that can be used are changing the child's position, holding the child when possible, stroking, cuddling, and engaging in age-appropriate activities. The child must be observed carefully for signs of pain, and analgesic administration should not be delayed. The child is observed for abdominal distention, which must be reported and documented promptly.

Preventing Infection. Preoperative procedures for infection control and administration of antibiotics are continued postoperatively. Observe the dressings for drainage, odor, and bleeding, and change them using sterile technique.

Maintaining Fluid Intake. A nasogastric tube is left in place after surgery, and intravenous feedings are given until bowel function is established. Accurate intake and output determinations and reporting of the character, amount, and consistency of stools help determine when the child may have oral feedings. The drainage from the nasogastric tube should be recorded and reported every 8 hours. Any unusual drainage (eg, bright bleeding) must be reported immediately.

Providing Oral and Nasal Care. Good mouth care must be performed at least every 4 hours. At the same time, the nares should be gently cleaned to relieve any irritation from the nasogastric tube. If the infant is young, sucking needs can be satisfied with a pacifier.

Providing Family Teaching. The family caregiver must be shown how to care for the colostomy at home. If available, an ostomy nurse may be consulted to assist in teaching the family caregivers. Devices and their use, daily irrigation, and skin care are topics that should be discussed. The caregivers should demonstrate their understanding by caring for the colostomy under the supervision of nursing personnel several days before discharge. Family caregivers also need referrals to support personnel.

EVALUATION

Preoperative:

- The colon is cleaned and well prepared for surgery.
- The child is well hydrated preoperatively.
- Family caregivers demonstrate an understanding of preoperative procedures by cooperating and asking relevant questions. When asked to repeat information, caregivers are able to do so and indicate their comprehension.
- The child is infection free.
- The child receives no injuries.
- Family caregivers and staff involve the infant in age-appropriate activities within the limitations of the preparations for surgery. Postoperatively, activities continue as the infant's condition permits.
- The older child displays minimum fear of bodily injury; the older child continues contact with peers and interacts with the nursing staff in a positive manner.

Postoperative:

- Colostomy care is performed, and no skin breakdown or infection occurs around the site. No incisional infection is evidenced.
- The child rests quietly and shows no signs of restlessness; he or she verbalizes comfort if old enough to communicate.
- Accurate intake and output determinations are documented. Nasogastric drainage is recorded and reported. Stools are described and documented.
- Oral and mucous membranes are moist and nonirritated. The infant uses a pacifier to meet sucking needs.
- Family caregivers demonstrate skill and knowledge in caring for the colostomy. Caregivers receive information about appropriate referrals.

Intussusception

Intussusception is the **invagination**, or telescoping, of one portion of the bowel into a distal portion. It occurs most frequently at the juncture of the ileum and the colon, although it can appear elsewhere in the intestinal tract. The invagination is from above downward, the upper portion slipping over the lower portion, pulling the mesentery along with it (Figure 9-7).

The condition occurs more often in boys than in girls and is the most frequent cause of intestinal obstruction in childhood. The highest incidence occurs in infants between the ages of 4 and 10 months.

The condition usually appears in healthy babies without any demonstrable cause. Possible contributing factors may be the hyperperistalsis and the unusual mobility of the cecum and ileum normally present in early life. Occasionally, a lesion such as Meckel's diverticulum or a polyp may be present.

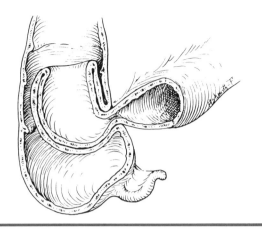

Figure 9-7. In this drawing of intussusception, note the telescoping of a portion of the bowel into the distal portion.

Clinical Manifestations

The infant who has previously appeared healthy and happy suddenly becomes pale, cries out sharply, and draws up his or her legs in a severe colicky spasm of pain. This spasm may last for several minutes, after which the infant relaxes and appears well until the next episode, which may be 5, 10, or 20 minutes later.

Most of these infants start vomiting early, a vomiting that becomes progressively more severe and eventually is bile stained. The infant strains with each paroxysm, emptying his or her bowels of fecal contents. The stools consist of blood and mucus, thereby earning the name of **currant jelly stools**.

Symptoms of shock appear quickly and characteristically include a rapid, weak pulse; increased temperature; shallow, grunting respirations; pallor; and marked sweating. Shock, vomiting, and currant jelly stools are the cardinal symptoms of this condition. These symptoms, coupled with the paroxysmal pain, are severe enough to bring the child into the hospital early.

The nurse, who is often consulted by neighbors, friends, and relatives if things go wrong, needs to be informed and alert; therefore, a word of caution is needed. On rare occasions a more chronic form appears, particularly during an episode of severe diarrheal disturbance. The onset is more gradual and may not show all the classic symptoms, but the danger of a sudden, complete strangulation is present. Such an infant should already be in the care of a physician because of the diarrhea.

Diagnosis

Diagnosis usually can be made by the physician from the clinical symptoms, rectal examination, and palpation of the abdomen during a calm internal when it is soft. A baby is often unwilling to tolerate this palpation, and sedation may be ordered. In many patients, a sausage-shaped mass can be felt through the abdominal wall.

Treatment

Unlike pyloric stenosis, this condition is an emergency in the sense that prolonged delay is dangerous. The telescoped bowel rapidly becomes gangrenous, thus markedly reducing the possibility of a simple reduction. Adequate treatment during the first 12 to 24 hours should have a good outcome, with complete recovery. The outcome becomes more uncertain as the bowel deteriorates, making resection necessary.

Immediate treatment consists of intravenous fluids, NPO status, and a diagnostic barium enema. The barium enema often can reduce the invagination simply by the pressure of the barium fluid pushing against the telescoped portion. The barium enema should not be done if signs of bowel perforation or peritonitis are evident. Abdominal surgery is performed if the barium enema does not correct the problem. Surgery may consist of manual reduction of the invagination or resection with anastomosis or possible colostomy if the intestine is gangrenous.

Nursing Process for the Infant with Intussusception

ASSESSMENT

Because this is an emergency situation, the initial assessment is brief. Collecting information from the parent needs to be limited to information about the immediate episode. Information about sudden acute abdominal pain evidenced by shrieking screams and drawn-up knees, vomiting, and currant jelly stools is essential.

Physical assessment of the infant includes the vital signs, assessment of abdomen for pain and tenderness, irritability, and pallor. This should be completed before the infant is sent to the radiology department for the barium enema.

NURSING DIAGNOSES

The nursing diagnoses depend on the outcome of the barium enema. If the invagination was reduced, the infant is returned to normal feedings within 24 hours and discharged in about 48 hours. Careful observation for recurrence is important during this period. If surgery is necessary, the nurse can implement many of the same diagnoses that are recommended for congenital aganglionic megacolon, including the following:

- Parental anxiety related to the serious condition of the infant and impending surgery
- High risk for infection related to surgery
- High risk for injury related to developmental age
- Pain on admission related to intussusception and postoperatively related to surgical procedure
- Fluid volume deficit and altered nutrition: less than body requirements related to preoperative status and postoperative recovery period

PLANNING AND IMPLEMENTATION

As previously stated, much depends on the results of the barium enema. The major preoperative nursing goals include preparing the infant and his or her parents for the barium enema, monitoring the infant's condition, observing for possible shock, and helping the parents deal with their anxiety. Postoperatively, major nursing goals include fluid and electrolyte balance, relief of abdominal pain in the infant, monitoring of vital signs and bowel sounds, prevention of infection at the surgical site, and if gastric suction is used, monitoring of the gastric contents, maintenance of the airway, and prevention of respiratory complications. Refer to the section on congenital aganglionic megacolon for suggested implementation of postoperative nursing goals.

Reducing Family Anxiety. The family caregivers' anxiety level is high, and the nurse must make every effort to keep them informed as the infant is cared for and procedures are done. The nurse must maintain a calm, reassuring, but concerned manner throughout this time of urgency. If surgery is indicated, the caregivers need a complete explanation of the problem and information regarding the procedure, where they can wait, when the surgeon will talk to them postoperatively, and the PACU routine. The caregivers also should be reassured that they have not done anything that has caused this condition.

EVALUATION

- The family caregivers demonstrate confidence in the care that the infant is receiving, evidenced by their cooperation and appropriate questions.
- The surgical site is free of foul drainage, redness, or other signs of infection. The infant's lungs and upper respiratory tract remain free of signs of infection.
- The infant receives no injuries.
- Postoperative pain is alleviated by the administration of analgesics and palliative nursing measures.
- The parents gain an accurate understanding of the disease process and relate this understanding to nursing personnel when questioned.
- Adequate hydration is evidenced by skin turgor, moist mucous membranes, and other signs of hydration. Bowel sounds are promptly recorded and reported so that oral nutrition may be restarted.

Circulatory System Disorders

Anemia is a common childhood blood disorder. It may be the result of an inadequate production of red blood cells or hemoglobin, or from an excessive loss of either red cells or hemoglobin. The following are examples of the more common types of anemia found in childhood; there are many others.

1. Inadequate production of erythrocytes or of hemoglobin, as in iron deficiency anemia and in anemia of chronic infection.
2. Excessive loss of red cells, as in hemorrhage.
3. Hemolytic anemia associated with congenital abnormalities of erythrocytes or hemoglobin, as in thalassemia or sickle cell disease.
4. Hemolytic anemia associated with acquired abnormalities of erythrocytes or hemoglobin, from drugs, chemicals, or bacterial reaction.

Iron Deficiency Anemia

Iron deficiency anemia is a common nutritional deficiency among young children. It is a hypochromatic, microcytic anemia (ie, the blood cells are smaller than normal and deficient in hemoglobin) common between the ages of 9 and 24 months. The full-term newborn has a high hemoglobin level (needed during fetal life to provide adequate oxygenation) that decreases during the first 2 or 3 months of life. However, considerable iron is reclaimed and stored, usually in sufficient quantity to last for 4 to 9 months of life.

A child needs to absorb 0.8 to 1.5 mg of iron per day. Because only 10% of dietary iron is absorbed, a diet containing 8 to 10 mg of iron is needed for good health. During the first years of life, it is often difficult for a child to obtain this quantity of iron from food. If the diet is inadequate, anemia quickly results.

Babies with an inordinate fondness for milk can take in an astonishing amount and, with their appetites satisfied, show little interest in solid foods. These babies are prime candidates for iron deficiency anemia. Infants and toddlers have come into the hospital with a history of taking 2 or 3 quarts of milk daily and accepting no other foods, or at best, only foods with a high carbohydrate content. Many parents believe, incorrectly, that milk is a perfect food, so why not let the baby have all the milk desired? These infants are commonly known as milk babies. They have pale, almost translucent (porcelainlike) skin and are chubby and susceptible to infections.

Many children with iron deficiency anemia, however, are undernourished because of the family's economic problems. Along with the economic factor, a parental knowledge deficit about nutrition is frequently present. The WIC program, discussed in Chapter 8, does much to alleviate this problem.

Clinical Manifestations

The signs of iron deficiency anemia include underweight, anorexia, growth retardation, and listlessness in addition to the characteristics of milk babies described earlier.

Diagnosis

In blood tests that measure hemoglobin, a level lower than 11 g/dL or a hematocrit lower than 33% is highly suspect.

Treatment

Treatment consists of improved nutrition, with ferrous sulfate administered between meals with juice, preferably orange juice for better absorption. The family caregivers need to be taught to brush the child's teeth after administration of ferrous sulfate to prevent staining. For best results, iron should not be given with meals. Caregivers also should be told that ferrous sulfate can cause constipation or turn the child's stools black. A few children have a hemoglobin level so low or anorexia so acute that they need additional therapy. An iron dextran mixture for intramuscular use (Imferon) is administered. This medication should be administered in the vastus lateralis by the Z-track method to avoid leakage into the subcutaneous tissues because of its irritating nature.

For those infants who are ill enough to be admitted to the hospital, the nurse should refer to the nursing process for the nutritionally deprived infant. For most infants with iron deficiency anemia, teaching for home care is needed. When teaching caregivers, the nurse should keep in mind that attitudes and food choices are often influenced by cultural differences (see Parent Teaching Tips for Iron Deficiency Anemia).

Sickle Cell Disease

Sickle cell disease is a hereditary trait occurring most commonly in blacks that is characterized by the production of an abnormal hemoglobin that results in the red blood cells taking on a "sickle" shape. It appears as an asymptomatic trait when the sickling trait is inherited from one parent alone (heterozygous state). When inherited from both parents (homozygous state), the child has sickle cell disease and anemia develops (Figure 9-8A). A rapid breakdown of red blood cells carrying hemoglobin S, the abnormal hemoglobin, causes a severe hemolytic anemia. The sickling trait occurs in about 10% of African Americans; there is a much higher incidence in parts of Africa. In African Americans, the disease itself, sickle cell anemia, has an incidence of 0.3% to 1.3%. The tendency to sickle can be demonstrated by a laboratory test. In those people who carry one gene for the sickle cell trait, the hemoglobin level and red blood cell count are normal, and the child is asymptomatic. However, there is a 50% probability that each child born to one parent carrying the sickle cell trait will inherit the trait from that parent (Figure 9-8B).

Clinical Manifestations

Clinical symptoms of the disease itself do not usually appear before the latter half of the first year of life because

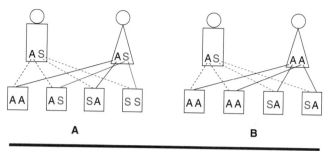

Parent Teaching

Tips for Iron Deficiency Anemia

Figure 9-8. Inheritance patterns. **A**, Homozygous type. Each parent is carrying one hemoglobin A gene and one hemoglobin S gene. One child is free of the gene (AA), two are carriers (AS), and one has sickle cell diseases (SS). **B**, Heterozygous type. One parent carriers a hemoglobin S gene, and one does not. Two children will be free of the gene (AA), and two will be carriers (AS).

Foods High in Iron

1. One of the most important things you can do for your baby and family is to learn about the foods that will help them stay healthy.

2. Milk is good for your baby, but no more than a quart a day (3 8-oz bottles).

3. Shop for baby cereals fortified with iron.

4. Some baby formulas are iron fortified.

5. Egg yolks are rich in iron. Avoid egg white for young babies because of allergies.

6. Green vegetables such as peas, green beans, lettuce, and spinach are good sources.

7. Dried beans, dried peas, canned refried beans, and peanut butter provide good sources for toddlers and older children.

8. Fruits that are iron rich include peaches, prune juice, raisins (don't give to child younger than 3 years of age because of danger of choking).

9. For older children fortified instant oatmeal and cream of wheat are good sources of iron.

10. Read labels to check for iron content of processed foods.

11. Organ meat, poultry, and fish are good iron sources.

12. Orange juice helps iron to absorb in the body.

13. Liquid iron preparations should be taken through a straw to prevent staining of teeth.

---

sufficient fetal hemoglobin is still present to prevent sickling. Sickle cell disease causes a chronic anemia with hemoglobin levels of 6 to 9 g/dL. (Normal levels in infants are between 11 and 15 g/dL.) The chronic anemia causes the child to be tired and have a poor appetite and pale mucous membranes.

The sickle cell crisis is the most severe manifestation of the condition. Normal red blood cells, which carry oxygen to the tissues, are disc shaped and normally move through the blood vessels, bending and flexing to flow through smoothly. The smooth, uniform shape of the red blood cells and the low viscosity (thickness) of the blood is such that these cells split relatively easily at Y-intersections and go single file through the capillaries with little or no clustering. The affected red blood cells (hemoglobin S) do much the same thing until there is an episode that causes sickling. These episodes (sickle cell crises) can

be precipitated by low oxygen levels (which can be caused by respiratory infection or extreme strenuous exercise), dehydration, acidosis, or stress. When sickling occurs, the affected red blood cells become crescent-shaped and therefore do not slip through as easily as do the disk-shaped cells. The viscosity of the blood increases (becomes thicker), causing slowdown and sludging of the red blood cells. The impaired circulation results in tissue damage and infarction. A sickle cell crisis may be the first clinical manifestation of the disease and may recur frequently during early childhood. This disturbance presents a variety of symptoms. The most common symptom is severe, acute, abdominal pain (caused by sludging in the spleen causing enlargement), together with muscle spasm, fever, and severe leg pain that may be muscular, osseous (bony), or localized in the joints, which become hot and swollen. The abdomen becomes boardlike, with an absence of bowel sounds, making it extremely difficult to distinguish the condition from an abdominal condition requiring surgery. Several days after a crisis, the child will be jaundiced, evidenced by yellow sclera, as a result of the hemolysis that has occurred. The crisis may have a fatal outcome caused by cerebral, cardiac, or hemolytic complications.

Diagnosis

Screening for the presence of hemoglobin S may be done with a test called Sickledex (fingerstick screening test that gives results in 3 minutes). Definite diagnosis is made through hemoglobin electrophoresis ("fingerprinting"). This can be done after the Sickledex screening results are positive.

Treatment

Prevention of crises is the goal between episodes. Adequate hydration is vital; fluid intake of 1500 to 2000 mL daily is desirable for a child weighing 20 kg, and this should be increased to 3000 mL during the crisis. Extremely strenuous activities that may cause oxygen depletion are to be avoided, and these children should avoid visiting areas of high altitude. Small blood transfusions help bring the hemoglobin to a near normal level temporarily. Iron preparations have no effect in sickle cell disease. Treatment for a crisis is supportive and symptomatic, and bed rest is indicated. Oxygen may be administered. Analgesics are given for pain. Dehydration and acidosis are vigorously treated. Prognosis is guarded, depending on the severity of the disease.

Nursing Process for the Child with Sickle Cell Crisis

ASSESSMENT

The parents who have a child with sickle cell disease may suffer a great deal of guilt for having passed the disease to their child. Care must be taken not to increase this guilt but to help them cope with it. The interview with the parent includes questions concerning activities or events that lead to this crisis, a history of the child's health and any previous episodes, and an evaluation of the parents' knowledge about the condition.

Assessment of the child varies somewhat with the age of the infant or child. Vital signs are recorded, particularly noting fever, abdominal pain observed, presence of bowel sounds, pain or swelling and warmth in the joints, and muscle spasms. The young child is observed for dactylitis (hand–foot syndrome) resulting from soft-tissue swelling caused by interference with circulation. This swelling then further impairs circulation.

NURSING DIAGNOSES

Nursing diagnosis varies somewhat with the age of the child and the stage of advancement of the disease. Some diagnoses that may be used are the following:

- Activity intolerance related to oxygen depletion
- Parental anxiety related to child's condition
- Parental health-seeking behaviors related to the disorder and appropriate care measures
- Hyperthermia related to the disease process
- Fluid volume deficit related to low fluid intake, impaired renal function, or both
- Altered growth and development related to chronic condition
- High risk for infection related to decreased hemoglobin level
- High risk for injury related to developmental age
- Impaired physical mobility related to muscle and joint involvement

- Pain related to disease condition affecting abdominal organs or joints and muscles
- High risk for impaired skin integrity related to altered circulation

PLANNING AND IMPLEMENTATION

The major nursing goals are to relieve pain, increase fluid intake, improve gas exchange, relieve parents' and child's anxiety, and decrease the number of future episodes by improving the parents' knowledge of the causes of crisis episodes.

Promoting Energy Conservation. The child may become dyspneic on any kind of activity. Nursing activities must be planned so that the child is disturbed as little as possible and is able to rest. Bed rest is necessary to decrease the demands on oxygen supply. Oxygen may be administered by mask or nasal cannula to improve tissue perfusion.

Reducing Family Anxiety and Providing Family Teaching. Guilt plays an important part in the anxiety that the family caregivers experience. Explaining procedures and planned treatments and care helps the caregivers feel that they are being included in the care. Involving the caregivers in learning measures that may help alleviate pain, encouraging fluid intake, and emphasizing the importance of protecting the child from situations that will cause overexhaustion or otherwise deplete the child's oxygen supplies help them feel they have some control over the disease. In addition, they may need more information concerning the disorder. If the child has been previously diagnosed, the caregivers should already have had information presented to them. In this instance, the nurse should assess their knowledge base and supplement and reinforce that information.

Maintaining Body Temperature. Vital signs are taken at least every 4 hours, and if fever is noted, every 2 hours. Measures to control fever, such as sponging, increased fluid intake, and antipyretics, are implemented as needed.

Maintaining Fluid Intake. The child is prone to dehydration because of the inability of the kidneys to concentrate urine. Signs of dehydration to observe are dry mucous membranes, weight loss, or in the case of infants, sunken fontanelles. Strict intake and output measurements and daily weights are necessary. The nurse should teach the family caregivers that fluid intake is important in caring for the child and intake should be maintained between 1500 and 2000 mL when the child is not in crisis. The child can be offered appealing fluids, such as juices, popsicles, noncaffeinated soda, and favorite flavored gelatins.

Providing Sensory and Cognitive Stimulation. Chronic illness affects the growth and development of a child. Family caregivers need information about normal developmental activities appropriate for the child and should be encouraged to provide sensory and cognitive stimulation in the young child. As the child gets older, the caregivers should encourage educational, recreational, and vocational goals that are suitable.

Preventing Infection. In any child with anemia or with other debilitating conditions, infection is a constant concern. Careful handwashing practices and aseptic technique are fundamental to good nursing care. Any family and visitors with an infectious or viral disease should not be permitted in the child's room. This rule also applies to the nursing staff. The child must be observed for signs of infection, which must be recorded and reported. Antibiotic therapy may be ordered if required.

Promoting Safety Practices. Safety precautions must be maintained, and family caregivers and visitors should be made aware of the safety needs of the child. These precautions vary with the age of the child.

Improving Physical Mobility. Sickling that affects the muscles and joints causes a great deal of pain for the child. The child needs careful handling and should be moved slowly, and gently. Joints can be supported with pillows. Warm soaks and massages may help relieve some of the discomfort. Analgesics also should be administered as needed. Passive exercises help prevent contractures and wasting of muscles.

Relieving Pain. The child in sickle cell crisis often has severe pain. The enlargement of the spleen (splenomegaly) causes severe abdominal pain. Joint and muscle pain are also common owing to poor perfusion of the tissues. Assessment of pain, nursing measures to relieve pain, and prompt administration of analgesics are essential. The family caregivers can be involved, if they wish, in helping administer comfort measures to the child. Sometimes diversional activities can help alleviate perceived pain but be assured that these children are in pain and need analgesics promptly.

Promoting Skin Integrity. Increased fluid intake and improved nutrition are important. The child's skin is regularly observed each shift, and good skin care, consisting of lotion, massage, and skin-toughening agents, especially over bony prominences, is necessary. Additional padding in the form of foam protectors and egg crate–type pads or mattresses may be helpful where there is irritation from bedding.

EVALUATION

- The child rests with minimum disturbance from nursing activities.
- The family caregivers appear more confident and demonstrate increased knowledge of the condition by cooperation and verbal confirmation.
- The child's temperature remains within normal limits.
- The intake of the child is at least 3000 mL/day.

- The family caregivers verbalize an understanding of normal growth and development goals.
- The child remains free of infection.
- Safety precautions appropriate for developmental stage are implemented.
- Passive exercises keep the child's muscles flexible.
- Pain is reduced or eliminated as evidenced by the child's relaxation and resting or the child's report.
- The child's skin shows no signs of redness, irritation, or breakdown.

Respiratory System Disorders

Acute Nasopharyngitis (Common Cold)

The common cold is one of the most common infectious conditions of childhood. The young infant is as susceptible as the older child but is generally not as frequently exposed.

The illness is of viral origin, rhinoviruses being the principal agents. Bacterial invasion of the tissues may cause complications such as ear, mastoid, and lung infections. The young child appears to be more susceptible to complications than an adult.

Clinical Manifestations

The infant older than the age of 3 months usually develops fever early in the course of the infection, often as high as 102° to 104°F (38.9° to 40°C). Younger infants usually are afebrile. The infant sneezes and becomes irritable and restless. The congested nasal passages interfere with nursing, increasing the infant's irritability. The infant may have accompanying vomiting or diarrhea that may be caused by mucous drainage into the digestive system. The infant should be protected from people who have colds because complications in the infant can be serious.

Diagnosis

This nasopharyngeal condition may appear as the first symptom of many childhood contagious diseases, such as measles, and needs to be observed carefully. The common cold also needs to be differentiated from allergic rhinitis.

Treatment

The child with an uncomplicated cold may not need any treatment in addition to rest, increased fluids and nutrition, normal saline nose drops, suction with a bulb syringe, and a humidified environment. In the older child, acetaminophen can be administered as an analgesic and antipyretic. Aspirin is best avoided. If the nares or upper lip become irritated, cold cream or petrolatum (Vaseline) can be used. The infant needs to be comforted by holding, rocking, and soothing.

It the symptoms persist for several days, the child needs to be seen by a physician to rule out complications such as otitis media.

Otitis Media

Otitis media is one of the most common infectious diseases of childhood. Two out of three children have at least one episode of otitis media by their third birthday.[1] The eustachian tube in an infant is shorter and wider than in the older child or adult (Figure 9-9). The tube is also straighter, thereby allowing nasopharyngeal secretions to enter the middle ear more easily. *Hemophilus influenzae* is an important causative agent of otitis media in infants.

Clinical Manifestations

A restless infant who repeatedly shakes his or her head and rubs or pulls at one ear should be checked for ear

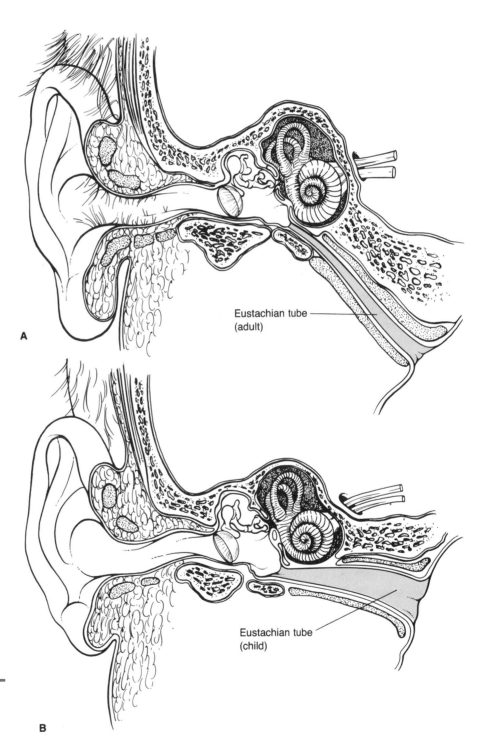

Figure 9-9. Comparison of the eustachian tube in the adult (**A**) and the infant (**B**).

infection. Symptoms include fever and irritability. There may be vomiting or diarrhea.

Diagnosis

Examination of the ear with an otoscope reveals a bulging eardrum. Spontaneous rupture of the eardrum may occur, in which case there will be purulent drainage, and the pain caused by the pressure built up in the ear will be relieved.

Treatment

Antibiotics are used during the period of infection and for several days following to prevent mastoiditis or chronic infection. A 10-day course of amoxicillin is a common treatment. Most infants respond well to antibiotics.

Some infants and young children have repeated episodes of otitis media. Children with chronic otitis media may be put on a prophylactic course of an oral penicillin or sulfonamide drug. **Myringotomy** (incision of the eardrum) may be performed to establish drainage and to insert tiny tubes into the tympanic membrane to facilitate drainage. The tubes eventually fall out spontaneously. Attention to chronic otitis media is essential because permanent hearing loss can result from frequent occurrences with scarring. Mastoiditis (infection of the mastoid sinus) is a possible complication of acute otitis media that is not treated. The occurrence of mastoiditis was much more frequent before the advent of antibiotics. Currently, it is seen only in children who have an untreated ruptured eardrum or inadequate treatment (through noncompliance of parents or improper care) of an acute episode.

Most infants and young children with otitis media are cared for at home, therefore a primary responsibility of the nurse is to teach the family caregivers about prevention and the care of the child (see Parent Teaching Tips for Otitis Media).

Acute Bronchiolitis

Acute bronchiolitis (acute interstitial pneumonia) occurs with the greatest frequency during the first 6 months of life and is rarely seen after the age of 2 years. Most cases occur in infants who have been in contact with older children or adults with upper respiratory viral infections.

Acute bronchiolitis is caused by a viral infection. The causative agent in more than 50% of cases has been shown to be the respiratory syncytial virus (RSV). Additional viruses associated with the disease are parainfluenza virus, adenoviruses, and other viruses not always identified.

The bronchi and bronchioles become plugged with a thick, viscid mucus, causing air to be trapped in the lungs. The infant can breathe air in but has difficulty expelling it. This result hinders the exchange of gases, and cyanosis appears.

Clinical Manifestations

Seen in the winter and early spring months, the onset of dyspnea is abrupt, sometimes preceded by a cough or a nasal discharge. There is a dry, persistent cough, extremely shallow respirations, air hunger, and cyanosis, which is frequently marked. Suprasternal and subcostal retractions are present (see Figure 3-3). The chest becomes barrel shaped from the trapped air. Respirations are 60 to 80 breaths per minute.

Body temperature elevation is not extreme, seldom increasing higher than 101° to 102°F (38.3° to 38.9°C). Dehydration may become a serious factor if competent care is not given. The infant appears apprehensive, irritable, and restless.

Diagnosis

Diagnosis is made from clinical findings and can be confirmed by laboratory testing (enzyme-linked immunosorbent assay) of the mucus obtained by direct nasal aspiration or nasopharyngeal washing.

Treatment

The infant is usually hospitalized and treated with high humidity by mist tent, rest, and increased fluids (Figure 9-10). Oxygen may be administered in addition to the mist tent. Monitoring of oxygenation may be done by means of capillary gases or pulse oximetry. Antibiotics are not prescribed because the causative organism is a virus. Intravenous fluids often are administered to ensure an adequate intake and to permit the infant to rest. The hospitalized infant is placed on respiratory isolation to prevent spread.

Ribavirin (Virazole), is an antiviral drug that may be used to treat certain infants with RSV. It is administered as an inhalant by hood, mask, or tent. The American Academy of Pediatrics states that the use of ribavirin must be limited to infants at high risk for severe or complicated RSV, such as infants with chronic lung disease, premature infants, transplant recipients, and those infants receiving chemotherapy. Ribavirin is classified as a category X drug, signifying a high risk for potential **teratogenicity** (causing damage to a fetus) from inhalation of mist that may escape into the room atmosphere and be inhaled by health care personnel and others. Women who might be pregnant should be advised to stay out of the room where ribavirin is being administered.

Bacterial Pneumonia

Pneumococcal pneumonia is the most common form of bacterial pneumonia found among infants and children. Its incidence has decreased during the last several years. This disease occurs mainly during the late winter and early spring months, principally in children younger than 4 years of age.

In the infant, pneumococcal pneumonia is generally

Parent Teaching

Tips for Otitis Media

The eustachian tube is a connection between the nasal passages and the middle ear. The eustachian tube is wider, shorter, and straighter in the infant, allowing organisms from respiratory infections to travel into the middle ear to cause infection (otitis media).

Prevention

1. Hold infant in an upright position, or position with head slightly elevated while feeding to prevent formula from draining into the middle ear through the wide eustachian tube of infant.
2. Never prop a bottle.
3. Do not give infant a bottle in bed. This allows fluid to "pool" in the middle ear, encouraging organisms to grow.
4. Protect infant from exposure to others with upper respiratory infections.
5. Protect infant from passive smoke; don't permit smoking by others in baby's presence.
6. Remove sources of allergies from home.
7. Observe for clues of ear infection: shaking head, rubbing or pulling at ears, fever, combined with restlessness or screaming and crying.
8. Be alert to signs of hearing difficulty in toddlers and preschoolers. This may be the first signs of an ear infection.
9. Teach toddler or preschooler gentle nose blowing.

Care of Child with Otitis Media

1. Have child with upper respiratory infection who shows symptoms of ear discomfort checked by a health care professional.
2. Be sure to complete the entire amount of antibiotic prescribed, even though the child seems better.
3. Heat (such as a heating pad on low setting) may provide comfort, but an adult must stay with a child.
4. Soothe, rock, and comfort child to help relieve discomfort. The child is more comfortable sleeping on side of infected ear.
5. Give pain medications (such as acetaminophen) as directed.
6. Provide liquid or soft foods; chewing causes pain.
7. Hearing loss may last up to 6 months after infection.
8. Follow-up with hearing tests should be scheduled as advised.

of the bronchial rather than the lobar type seen in older children. It is usually secondary to an upper respiratory viral infection. The most common finding in infants is a patchy infiltration of one or several lobes of the lung. Pleural effusion is frequently present.

H. influenzae pneumonia also occurs in infants and young children. Its clinical manifestations are similar to those of pneumococcal pneumonia. Its onset is more insidious, its clinical course longer and less acute, and it is usually lobar in distribution. Complications in the young infant are frequent, usually bacteremia, pericarditis, and

empyema (pus in lungs). The treatment is the same. Immunization with *H. influenzae* type B conjugate vaccine (HbCV) is currently recommended beginning at 2 months of age.

Clinical Manifestations

The onset of the pneumonic process is usually abrupt, following a mild upper respiratory illness. Temperature increases rapidly to 103° to 105°F (39.4° to 40.6°C). Respiratory distress is marked, with obvious air hunger, flaring of the nostrils, circumoral cyanosis, and chest retrac-

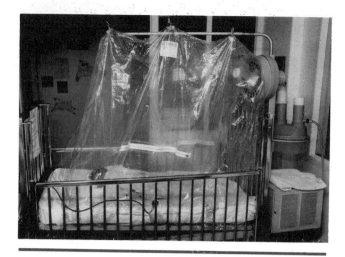

Figure 9-10. Mist tent. The side rails are down for photographic purposes only. (From Skale N. Manual of Pediatric Nursing Procedures. Philadelphia: JB Lippincott, p. 1981.)

tions. Tachycardia and tachypnea are present, with a pulse rate frequently as high as 140 to 180 beats per minute, and respirations as high as 80 breaths per minute.

Generalized convulsions may occur during the period of high fever. Cough may not be noticeable at the onset but may appear later. Abdominal distention due to swallowed air or paralytic ileus commonly occurs.

Diagnosis

Diagnosis is made based on clinical symptoms, chest radiograph, and culture of the organism from secretions.

Treatment

The use of antibiotics early in the disease gives a prompt and favorable response. Penicillin or ampicillin has proved to be the most effective treatment and is generally used unless the infant has a penicillin allergy. Oxygen started early in the disease process is important. Infants are sometimes placed in a Croupette or mist tent. Currently, there is some controversy concerning the safety of mist tents unless constant observation can be provided. Children have become cyanotic in mist tents with subsequent arrest owing to difficulty in seeing the child; therefore, a mask or hood is thought to be the better choice.

Intravenous fluids are often necessary to supply the needed amount of fluids. Prognosis for recovery is excellent.

◪ Nursing Process for the Infant with a Respiratory Disorder

ASSESSMENT

A thorough parent interview is conducted, which includes the standard information needed as well as specific information, such as when the family caregiver first noticed

the symptoms; the course of the fever thus far; the caregiver's description of respiratory difficulties; how well the infant was taking nourishment and fluids; nausea; vomiting; urinary and bowel output; and history of exposure to other family members with respiratory infections.

The nurse needs to conduct a physical assessment of temperature, apical pulse, respirations (rate, respiratory effort, retractions [costal, intercostal, sternal, suprasternal, substernal], and flaring of nares), breath sounds (crackles, wheezing), cough (dry, productive, hacking), irritability, restlessness, skin color (pallor, cyanosis), circumoral (around the mouth) cyanosis, skin turgor, anterior fontanelle (depressed or bulging), nasal passage congestion (color, consistency), mucous membranes (mouth dry, lips dry or cracked), and eyes (bright, glassy, sunken, moist, crusted).

NURSING DIAGNOSES

Nursing diagnoses are based on the interview with the family caregivers and the specific physical findings and should be reasonable and realistic. Some nursing diagnoses that may be used for the infant with a respiratory condition are the following:

- Ineffective airway clearance related to nasal and chest congestion and obstructed airway
- Altered nutrition: less than body requirements and fluid volume deficit related to inability to nurse, suck, or swallow adequately with congested nasal passages
- Hyperthermia related to infection process
- High risk for otitis media related to current respiratory illness and the size and location of the eustachian tubes
- High risk for injury related to maturational level
- Altered growth and development related to hospitalization
- Parental anxiety related to child's illness
- Activity intolerance related to inadequate gas exchange

PLANNING AND IMPLEMENTATION

The major nursing goals depend on the infant's status. The infant may need to be placed in respiratory isolation. Many infants hospitalized with a respiratory condition need to be placed in a Croupette or mist tent. Additional nursing interventions are required for the infant in a mist tent. If intravenous fluids are ordered, nursing diagnoses are necessary that focus on tissue and skin integrity and appropriate restraints to ensure that the infant does not interfere with the intravenous infusion site. Intravenous administration and the use of restraints are discussed in Chapter 3.

Monitoring Respiratory Function. Respirations are monitored, with observations for tachypnea and retractions and assessment of breath sounds made at least every 4 hours. If deep retractions are noted, observations should be made more frequently. A moisturized atmosphere is provided with an ice-cooled mist tent or cool vaporizer. The moisturized air helps thin the mucus in the respiratory tract to ease respirations. Oxygen can be added if the physician desires, especially in cases of pneumococcal pneumonia.

Maintaining Adequate Nutrition and Fluid Intake. The infant's nasal passages are cleared using a bulb syringe, being certain to clear the passages immediately before feeding. Normal saline nose drops to thin secretions are administered approximately 10 to 15 minutes before feedings and at bedtime. The infant is fed slowly, allowing frequent stops, with suctioning during feeding as needed. Overtiring the infant during feeding must be avoided. Juices and water appropriate for the infants' age are offered between meals. A relatively small-holed nipple should be used so that the infant does not choke, but caution should be used to avoid making the infant work too hard. Accurate intake and output measurements are maintained. The infant must be observed for dehydration. Skin turgor, anterior fontanelle, and urine output are good indicators. Diaper counts should be kept, and if necessary, diapers can be weighed to determine the amount of urine output.

The infant may be so exhausted by respiratory effort that intravenous fluids are necessary. Observation of patency, placement, site integrity, and flow rate must be made at least hourly.

Maintaining Body Temperature. Monitor the infant's temperature frequently (at least every 2 hours if it is higher than 38.5°C). If the infant has an elevated temperature, remove excess clothing and covering. Antipyretic medications may be ordered. A tepid sponge bath may be administered in accordance with hospital policy. Tepid water is used, and the infant is sponged for approximately 20 minutes, after which the nurse should redress the infant lightly. Thirty minutes after completing the sponge bath, the temperature is taken, recorded, and reported.

Preventing Otitis Media. The infant's position is changed, turning from side to side every hour so that mucus is less likely to drain into the eustachian tubes. Maintaining the infant in an infant seat facilitates breathing and helps prevent the complication of otitis media as well. The infant is observed for irritability, shaking of his or her head, or pulling at the ears. The infant must not be given a bottle while he or she is lying in bed. The best position for feeding is upright to avoid excessive drainage into the eustachian tubes.

Promoting Safety Practices. Side rails must be kept up full at all times. Pad the side of the crib as necessary to protect the infant. Toys must be chosen with safety in mind, and have no sharp edges, small parts, strings, or ropes in which the infant can become entangled. Stuffed toys are not recommended in a mist tent

because they become saturated and provide an environment in which organisms flourish.

Providing Sensory Stimulation. Age-appropriate sensory stimulation should be provided within the constraints of the infant's condition. The nurse talks to the infant during care, encouraging response but being careful not to overtire the infant. The use of a soothing, reassuring voice is comforting to the infant. As the infant responds with smiles and coos, the nurse offers encouragement. Toys should be introduced that are safe for use in a moist atmosphere and that are age-appropriate for the infant. Balloons are not safe if they are within the infant's reach.

Reducing Family Anxiety. Family caregivers need teaching and reassurance. The nurse must talk to the parents while working with the infant, explaining what is happening and why. Equipment and treatments must be explained to caregivers so that their questions (both spoken and unspoken) are answered. The nurse must actively listen to caregivers and use communication skills to respond to their worries. The family caregivers should be taught the following:

1. How to clear nasal passage with bulb syringe
2. How to feed infant slowly and allow the infant a chance to nurse without tiring, burping frequently to expel swallowed air
3. The importance of a croup tent and the necessity to leave the infant in it except for feedings and bathing (unless otherwise indicated)
4. Ways to soothe infant while he or she remains in the tent
5. The need for respiratory precautions and good handwashing technique
6. The importance of extra fluids for the infant
7. The desirability of using a humidifier at home after discharge
8. Proper cleaning techniques of a humidifier
9. That the infant should not be in contact with people who have infections during hospitalization or after discharge

Promoting Energy Conservation. During an acute stage, the infant is allowed to rest as much as possible. Work is planned so that rest and sleep are not interrupted more than absolutely necessary (see Nursing Care Plan for the Infant with Respiratory Dysfunction).

EVALUATION

■ The respiratory accessory muscles are no longer used. Breath sounds are clear. The infant rests and sleeps quietly. Respirations are regular and even. Mucous secretions are thinned and diminished. The infant is not chilled from wet clothing.

(text continued on page 218)

Nursing Care Plan
for the Infant with Respiratory Dysfunction

Nursing Diagnosis
Ineffective airway clearance related to infectious process

Goal: Improve respiratory function

Nursing Interventions	Rationale	Evaluation
Monitor respiratory function: observe for tachypnea and retractions; assess breath sounds at least every 4 hours. If deep retractions are noted, assess more frequently.	Changes in the infant's breathing may be early indication of respiratory distress.	Infant's respirations are regular and even, and the infant no longer uses accessory muscles in breathing.
Provide a moisturized atmosphere with ice cooled mist tent or cool vaporizer; oxygen can be added if physician desires.	The high moisture content of the air in a mist tent helps to liquify secretions for easier removal by coughing, expectoration, or suctioning.	Infant rests and sleeps quietly. Mucous secretions are thinned and diminished.

Nursing Diagnosis
Altered nutrition: less than body requirements related to inability to nurse/suck/swallow with congested nasal passages or fatigue from difficulty with breathing

Goal: Maintain adequate food and fluid intake

Nursing Intervention	Rationale	Evaluation
Keep nasal passages clear using a bulb syringe. Clear nasal passages immediately before feeding.	Infants are obligatory nasal breathers. Clearing eases infant's breathing to permit adequate feeding.	Infant takes in adequate nutrition as evidenced by no loss of weight or some weight gain.
Administer normal saline nose drops before feedings and at bedtime.	Normal saline nose drops help to thin mucous secretions.	Infant sucks adequately without excessive tiring.

Nursing Diagnosis
Activity intolerance related to inadequate gas exchange

Goal: Promote energy conservation

Nursing Interventions	Rationale	Evaluation
Plan procedures so that rest and sleep is not interrupted more than absolutely necessary.	The infant in respiratory distress needs as much rest as possible in order to meet minimum energy requirements.	Infant has extended periods of uninterrupted rest.

(continued)

Nursing Care Plan
for the Infant with Respiratory Dysfunction (Continued)

Nursing Diagnosis
Hyperthermia related to infectious process

Goal: Maintain normal body temperature

Nursing Interventions	Rationale	Evaluation
Monitor temperature frequently (at least q2h if over 38.5°C (101.3°F).	Temperature can fluctuate rapidly in the infant with a respiratory infection.	Temperature documented q2h or more frequently when elevated.
Remove excess clothing and covering; administer antipyretic medications as ordered; administer tepid sponge bath in accordance with hospital policy; redress lightly; record temperature before and after bath.	Lowering the infant's temperature is of vital importance since a fever depletes fluids rapidly and the infant may become dehydrated.	Temperature returns to within a normal range (between 37° and 37.8°C or 98.6 and 100.1°F).

Nursing Diagnosis
High risk for otitis media related to current respiratory infection and size and location of the eustachian tube

Goal: Prevent otitis media

Nursing Interventions	Rationale	Evaluation
Change infant's position, turning from side to side every hour; feed infant in upright position.	Turning infant prevents mucous from pooling into the eustachian tubes; keeping the infant upright during feeding improves drainage.	Chart indicates that infant has been turned regularly. Infant remains free of complication of otitis media with no evidence of ear pain or discomfort.
Observe for irritability, shaking of head, or pulling at ears.	Early recognition of signs of otitis media promotes early diagnosis and treatment.	Signs and symptoms of otitis media are documented and reported promptly.

Nursing Diagnosis
High risk for injury related to age and maturational level

Goal: Prevent injury to infant during hospitalization

Nursing Intervention	Rationale	Evaluation
Maintain side rails up full at all times; pad side of crib as necessary; explain to family caregivers the need for maintaining such precautions.	The infant may be more mobile than nurses or family caregivers expect.	Safety precautions are maintained and the child experiences no injury.

(continued)

Nursing Care Plan
for the Infant with Respiratory Dysfunction (Continued)

Nursing Diagnosis
Parental anxiety related to child's illness

Goal: Reduce family anxiety

Nursing Interventions	Rationale	Evaluation
Actively listen to family caregivers' concerns regarding child and child's illness.	Caregivers are reassured when encouraged to express their concerns about their child.	Caregivers express feelings and apprehensions about child and child's illness. Nurses respond fully to caregivers' questions.
Provide reassurance and explain what is happening when working with infant.	Understanding both the disease and treatment methods helps family to feel that child's illness is under control.	Caregivers demonstrate understanding of child's illness and treatment through appropriate questions and responses when discussing child's illness.
Involve family caregivers in caring for child. Teach caregivers techniques of care for infant after discharge.	Family caregivers benefit from security of practicing techniques under guidance of nursing staff.	Caregivers describe specific care measures they will follow at home.

Nursing Diagnosis
Altered growth and development related to hospitalization

Goal: Provide sensory stimulation

Nursing Intervention	Rationale	Evaluation
Provide age-appropriate stimulation within the constraints of the infant's condition; talk and sing to the infant while giving care, encouraging response.	The infant needs tactile, visual, and auditory stimulation; caregiving activities provide a wonderful opportunity for both physical and verbal play.	Infant responds to various types of stimulation with coos, smiles, age-appropriate verbalization, and activity.

- The infant has an adequate intake. Skin turgor is improved, and nasal passages are clear.
- The temperature ranges between 37° and 37.8°C.
- The child is free of complication of otitis media.
- The child is not injured.
- The infant responds appropriately to sensory stimulation.
- The family caregivers demonstrate understanding and reflect confidence in the staff evidenced by cooperation and appropriate questions.
- The infant has extended periods of uninterrupted rest.

Sudden Infant Death Syndrome

Sudden infant death syndrome (SIDS) has caused much grief and anxiety among many families for centuries. SIDS, one of the leading causes of infant mortality worldwide, claims an estimated 7000 to 8000 lives annually in the United States alone.

Throughout history, this syndrome has presented a most exasperating problem. Commonly called "crib death," it is the sudden unexpected death of an apparently healthy infant in whom the postmortem fails to reveal an adequate cause. SIDS is not a diagnosis but a description of a syndrome. It is the leading cause of death in infants older than 1 month of age.[2]

Varying theories have been suggested about the cause of SIDS. In ancient writings, it was attributed to "overlaying" by the infant's mother or nurse. The adult supposedly rolled over onto the infant during sleep. This cause was eventually ruled out, particularly because many affected infants were alone in their cribs when they ceased breathing. Over the years much investigation and research has been done, but no single cause has been identified, and physicians can neither prevent nor predict the event.

A closely related syndrome is apparent life-threatening events (ALTE). These are episodes in which the infant is found in distress but, when quickly stimulated, recovers with no lasting problems. These were formerly called "near-miss SIDS." These infants are placed on home apnea monitors. The apnea monitor is set to alarm if the infant has not taken a breath within a given number of seconds. Family caregivers are taught infant cardiopulmonary resuscitation so that they can respond quickly if the alarm sounds (Figure 9-11). Infants who have had an episode of ALTE are at risk for additional episodes and may be at risk for SIDS. Infants are usually kept on home apnea monitors until they are 1 year old. This is a stressful time for the family because someone who is trained in infant cardiopulmonary resuscitation must be with the infant at all times.

Infants affected with SIDS are most frequently between the ages of 2 and 3 months, although some deaths have occurred during the first and second weeks of life. Few infants older than 6 months of age die of SIDS. SIDS is a greater threat to low-birth-weight infants than to term infants. It occurs more often in winter and affects more male infants than female infants as well as infants from minority and lower socioeconomic groups. Babies born to mothers younger than 20 years of age, infants who are not firstborn, and those whose mothers smoked during pregnancy also have been found to be at greater risk. Research has revealed that a greater number of infants with SIDS have been sleeping in a prone position than in a supine position. As a result of these studies, the American Academy of Pediatrics recommends that infants must *not* be placed in a prone position to sleep. Infants must be placed only in a supine or side-lying position until they are 6 months old.

SIDS is rapid and silent. Previous studies had suggested nighttime as the peak time of death, but the time of day is apparently not clear because recent studies reveal that about half of the attacks may occur during the day. The history reveals that no outcry has been heard, nor is there any evidence of a struggle. People who have been sleeping nearby claim to have heard nothing unusual before the death was discovered. It is not uncommon for the infant to have been recently examined by a physician and found to be in excellent health. Autopsies frequently reveal a mild respiratory disorder but nothing considered serious enough to have caused the death. Emergency personnel need to be observant for possible clues that may indicate that this is a case of child abuse, but they must be cautious not to cast any suspicion on the family caregivers. The guilt feelings of the caregivers are over-

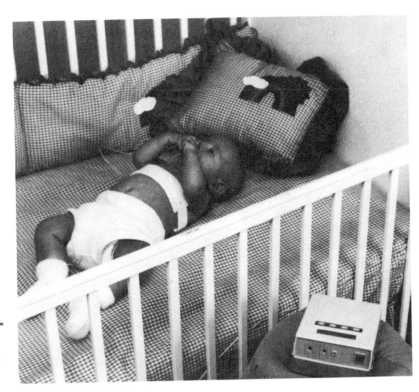

Figure 9-11. An apnea monitor for home monitoring. (Courtesy of Life Watch Systems, 1050 17th St. Suite 900, Denver, CO 80265.)

whelming, and any suggestion from medical personnel that the cause of death is questionable is inexcusable and may be more than the caregivers can handle.

Emotional Support for Parents and Families

The effects of SIDS on caregivers and families are devastating. Grief is coupled with guilt, even though it is known that SIDS cannot be predicted or prevented. Disbelief, hostility, and anger are common reactions that families exhibit. An autopsy must be done and the results promptly made known to the family. Even though the family caregivers are told that they are not to blame for the infant's death, it is difficult for most caregivers not to keep searching for evidence of some possible neglect on their part. Prolonged depression usually follows the initial shock and anguish over the infant's death. The immediate response of the emergency department staff should be one of allowing them to express their grief, encouraging them to say "good bye" to their baby and providing a quiet private place for them to do so. Compassionate care of the family caregivers includes helping to find someone to accompany them home or to meet them there. Referrals should be made to the local chapters of the National SIDS Foundation immediately. In some states, specially trained community health nurses who are knowledgeable about SIDS are available. These nurses are prepared to help families and can provide written materials as well as information, guidance, and support in the family's home. In addition, they maintain contact with the family as long as necessary and will provide support in a subsequent pregnancy.

A concern of the parents is how to tell other children in the family. A booklet written by Jacques Bell and Linda Esterling, "What Will I Tell the Children?" provides sound advice with guidance at each age level.[3]

Parents are particularly concerned about subsequent infants. Data previously had suggested that these infants were at greater risk, but more recent studies have indicated that this risk is no greater than in the general population. However, many physicians continue to recommend monitoring these infants for the first few months of life to help reduce the stress of the family. This is a decision that each physician and family must make together after looking at all the pros and cons. Monitoring is usually maintained until the new infant is past the age of the SIDS infant's death.

Grief waxes and wanes for months and years for these parents. Having another child is by no means going to cause them to forget the one they lost. Mothers often relate that they think they are healing, only to have some small incident set them off again. Friends and acquaintances need to be sensitive to their needs. Comments such as "You are young, you can always have more children," "God must have needed a little angel," and "Well, you have the other children" are inappropriate. The best way to interact with these parents is by actively listening and showing compassionate concern.

Genitourinary System Disorders

There are a few conditions that may affect the genitourinary system of the infant in the first year of life. Structurally, two defects, hydrocele (fluid in the saclike cavity around the testes) and cryptorchidism (undescended testes) occur in a small percentage of male infants. Urinary tract infections may occur when poor hygiene exists in infants wearing diapers, and the most common type of renal cancer, Wilms' tumor (nephroblastoma), may first be seen in infancy. Each of these conditions is briefly discussed in this section.

Hydrocele

Hydrocele is a collection of peritoneal fluid that accumulates in the scrotum through a small passage called the processus vaginalis. This processus is a fingerlike projection in the inguinal canal through which the testes descend. Usually the processus closes soon after birth, but if it does not close, fluid from the peritoneal cavity passes through, causing hydrocele. This is the same passage through which intestines may slip, causing an inguinal hernia. If the hydrocele remains by the end of the first year, corrective surgery is performed.

Cryptorchidism

Shortly before or soon after birth, the male gonads (testes) descend from the abdominal cavity into their normal position in the scrotum. Occasionally, one or both of the testes do not descend, a condition called cryptorchidism (Figure 9-12). The testes are usually normal in size; the cause for nondescent is not clearly understood.

In most male infants with cryptorchidism, the testes descend by the time the infant is 1 year old. If one or both testes have not descended by this age, treatment is recommended. If both testes remain undescended, the male will be sterile.

A surgical procedure called **orchiopexy** is used to bring the testis down into the scrotum and anchor it there. Some physicians prefer to try medical treatment before doing surgery. This treatment consists of injections of human chorionic gonadotropic hormone. If this is not successful in bringing the testis down, orchiopexy is performed. Surgery usually is performed when the child is between 1 and 2 years of age. The prognosis for a normal functioning testicle is good when the surgery is performed at this young age and no degenerative action has taken place before treatment.

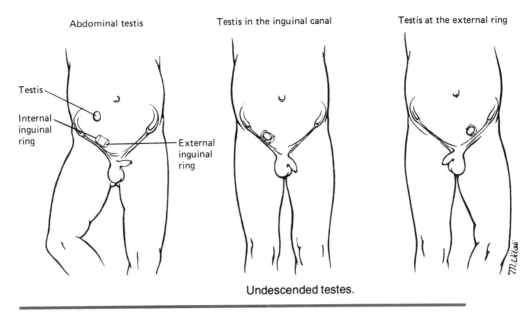

Abdominal testis   Testis in the inguinal canal   Testis at the external ring

Testis

Internal
inguinal
ring

External
inguinal
ring

Undescended testes.

Figure 9-12. Undescended testes. (From Wieczorek RR, Natapoff J. A Conceptual Approach to the Nursing of Children: Health Care from Birth Through Adolescence. Philadelphia: JB Lippincott, 1981.)

Urinary Tract Infections

Infections of the urinary tract are fairly common in the "diaper age," in infancy, and again between the ages of 2 and 6 years. The condition occurs more commonly in girls than in boys, except in the first 4 months of life, when it appears more commonly in boys. Although many different bacteria may infect the urinary tract, intestinal bacteria, particularly *E. coli*, account for the infection in about 80% of acute episodes. The female urethra is shorter and straighter than the male urethra; thus, it is more easily contaminated with feces. Inflammation may extend into the bladder, ureters, and kidney.

Clinical Manifestations

In infants the symptoms may be fever, nausea, vomiting, foul-smelling urine, weight loss, and increased urination. Occasionally, there is little or no fever. Vomiting is common, and diarrhea may occur. The infant is irritable. In acute pyelonephritis (inflammation of the kidney and renal pelvis), the onset is abrupt with a high fever for 1 or 2 days. Convulsions may occur during the period of high fever.

Diagnosis

Diagnosis is based on the finding of pus in the urine under microscopic examination. It is important that the urine specimen be fresh and uncontaminated. A "clean catch" voided urine, properly performed, is essential for microscopic examination. If a culture is needed, the infant must be catheterized, but this is usually avoided if possible. In

the cooperative, toilet-trained child, a clean midstream urine may be used successfully.

Treatment

Simple urinary tract infections may be treated with antibiotics at home. The child with acute pyelonephritis is hospitalized. Fluids are given freely. The symptoms usually subside within a few days after antibiotic therapy (usually sulfisoxazole or ampicillin) has been initiated, but this is not an indication that the infection is completely cleared. Medication must be continued after symptoms disappear. An intravenous pyelogram or ultrasonographic study may be performed to assess the possibilities of structural defects if the child has problems with recurring infections

Nursing Process for the Child with a Urinary Tract Infection

ASSESSMENT

The interview with the family caregiver includes basic information about the child, such as feeding and sleeping patterns, and history of other illnesses. Information regarding the present illness includes when the fever started and its course thus far, signs of pain or discomfort on voiding, recent change in feeding pattern, if the child had vomiting or diarrhea, irritability, lethargy, abdominal pain, unusual odor to urine, chronic diaper rash, and signs of febrile convulsions. If the child is toilet trained, questions about toileting habits are important (how does the child wipe? does the child wash his or her hands when toileting?). The caregiver also should be questioned about the use of bubble baths and the type of soap used, especially for girls.

Physical assessment of the child includes temperature; pulse (alert for tachycardia) and respiration rates; weight; height; observation of wet diaper, or urine in an older child; the perineal area for rash; signs of irritability and lethargy; and general skin condition, color, and turgor. A urine specimen is needed on admission. A midstream urine collection method is desirable, and catheterization is avoided, if possible. Any indications of urinary burning, frequency, urgency, or pain are recorded and reported.

In the child who has repeated urinary tract infections, the nurse should observe the interaction between the child and the family caregivers to detect any indications that the infection may be caused by sexual abuse. The alert nurse looks for possible indications of sexual abuse, such as bruising, bleeding, and lacerations of the external genitalia in the child who is extremely shy and frightened.

NURSING DIAGNOSES

Nursing diagnoses vary with the age and condition of the child. Some nursing diagnoses that may be used are the following:

- Altered urinary elimination related to pain and burning on urination
- High risk for injury related to developmental stage
- Parental anxiety and health-seeking behaviors related to the child's urinary tract infection

PLANNING AND IMPLEMENTATION

The major nursing goals are to relieve pain, increase the child's fluid intake, and teach family caregivers methods for prevention of recurrent infections.

Maintaining Normal Elimination. Because of pain and burning on urination, the toilet-trained child may try to hold urine and not void. The child is encouraged to void every 3 or 4 hours, so that recurrences of infection do not occur. The child is assessed for burning, pain, and frequency. If possible, the voiding pattern is observed to note trickling or other signs that the bladder is not being emptied completely. Urine output is carefully monitored and measured. An infant's diaper can be weighed for accuracy. Accurate intake and output measurements are important.

Antibiotics are administered as ordered. The infant or child is observed for signs of any reactions to the antibiotics. The family caregivers and the child are prepared for any other procedures that may be ordered, including appropriate explanations. Increasing the child's fluid intake is necessary to help dilute the urine and flush the bladder. An increase in fluid intake also helps decrease

the pain experienced on urination. Frequent, small amounts of fluids, such as glucose water and liquid gelatin, for the infant are usually well accepted. Persistence on the part of the nurse may be necessary. Enlisting the help of the family caregivers may be useful, but if they are not successful, the nurse must persevere. Most infants and children like apple juice that helps acidify the urine. Cranberry juice is a good choice for the older child, if he or she tolerates it. Analgesics and antispasmodics are administered as ordered.

Promoting Safety Practices. Safety factors appropriate to child's age are carefully followed. Family caregivers' involvement in keeping the environment safe for the child is desirable.

Reducing Family Anxiety and Providing Family Teaching. The family caregivers are the key people in helping prevent recurring infections (see Parent Teaching Tips for Urinary Tract Infection).

EVALUATION

- The child's urine culture is negative.
- The child voids normally, emptying the bladder each time.
- The child is pain free.
- The child is safe and uninjured.
- Family caregivers demonstrate an understanding of the genitourinary system and good hygiene habits as evidenced by the ability to discuss information and ask appropriate questions.

Parent Teaching

Tips for Urinary Tract Infection

1. Change infants diaper when soiled, and clean with mild soap and water. Dry completely.
2. Girls should *always* wipe from front to back.
3. Teach your child to wash hands before and after going to the toilet.
4. Bubble baths create a climate that encourages bacteria to grow, especially in young girls.
5. Teach young girls to learn to take showers. Avoid water softeners in tub baths.
6. Encourage your child to try to urinate every 3 or 4 hours and to empty her bladder.
7. Girls should wear cotton underpants to provide air circulation to perineal area.
8. Encourage child to drink fluids, especially cranberry juice.
9. Older girls should avoid whirlpools or hot tubs.

Wilms' Tumor (Nephroblastoma)

Wilms' tumor is an adenosarcoma in the kidney region and is one of the most common of the abdominal neoplasms found in early childhood. The tumor arises from bits of embryonic tissue remaining after birth. This tissue has the capacity to begin rapid cancerous growth in the area of the kidney.

The tumor is rarely discovered until it has reached a size large enough to be palpated through the abdominal wall. As the tumor grows, it invades the kidney or the renal vein and disseminates to other parts of the body. When the child is admitted for evaluation and treatment, a sign must be posted on the head of the bed stating that abdominal palpation should be avoided because cells may break loose and spread the tumor. Treatment consists of surgical removal as soon as possible after the growth is discovered combined with radiation and chemotherapy.

Prognosis is best for the child younger than 2 years of age but has improved markedly for others with improved chemotherapy. Follow-up consists of regular evaluation for metastasis to the lungs or other sites. All implications for long-term chemotherapy apply to this child.

Nervous System Disorders

Acute or Nonrecurrent Seizures

A seizure (convulsion) may be a symptom of a wide variety of disorders. In infants and children between the age of 6 months and 3 years, febrile seizures are the most common. These seizures occur in association with a high fever, frequently one of the initial symptoms of an acute infection somewhere in the body. Less frequent causes of convulsions are intracranial infections, such as meningitis, toxic reactions to certain drugs or minerals, such as lead, metabolic disorders, and a variety of brain disorders.

Clinical Manifestations

A seizure may occur suddenly without warning; however, restlessness and irritability may precede an episode. The body stiffens, and the infant loses consciousness. In a few seconds, clonic movements occur. These movements are quick, jerking movements of the arms, legs, and facial muscles. Breathing is irregular, and there is an inability to swallow saliva.

Febrile seizures usually occur in the form of a generalized seizure early in the course of a fever. Although commonly associated with high fever, 102° to 106°F (38.9° to 41.1°C), some children appear to have a low seizure threshold and convulse when a fever of 100° to 102°F (37.8° to 38.9°C) is present.

Diagnosis

Immediate treatment is based on presenting symptoms. Further evaluation is made after the urgency of the seizure has passed.

Treatment

Emergency care to protect the child during the seizure is the primary concern. Diazepam (Valium) is the drug of choice, usually administered intravenously, if necessary.

Nursing Process for the Child at Risk for Seizures

ASSESSMENT

The family caregiver interview should include questions about any history of seizure activity. The caregivers are asked to describe any previous episodes, including the infant's temperature, how the infant behaved immediately before the seizure, movements during the seizure, and any other information they believe to be related. Ask about the presence of any fever during this present illness and any indications of seizure activity before admission for this illness. Seizure precautions should be instituted if the child has a history of a previous febrile seizure.

An infant or child whose fever or other symptoms indicate that a seizure may be anticipated should be placed where constant observation is possible. The physical assessment includes careful evaluation of temperature, neurologic assessment, and other assessments appropriate for the present illness.

NURSING DIAGNOSES

In addition to nursing diagnoses related to the presenting symptoms, those specific to anticipated seizure activity are suggested in this section. If the seizure is preceded by fever, nursing diagnoses and measures for fever reduction also would be included. Some of the diagnoses specific to possible seizure activity are the following:

- Ineffective airway clearance during seizure episode related to loss of consciousness
- High risk for injury related to uncontrolled muscular activity during seizure
- Parental anxiety related to the child's seizure activity
- Parental health-seeking behaviors related to prevention of and precautions during seizures

PLANNING AND IMPLEMENTATION

The immediate nursing goal is to maintain an unobstructed airway and protect the child from injury. Additional nursing goals include relieving parental anxiety and helping the parents understand what is occurring.

Preventing Aspiration. When an infant starts to convulse, the nurse should turn the infant to one side to prevent aspiration of saliva or vomitus. Nothing is put into the child's mouth. Blankets, pillow, or other items that may keep the child from having a clear airway are removed. Oxygen and suction equipment must be readily available for emergency use.

Promoting Safety Practices. The child who has a history of previous seizures must be kept under close observation. The crib sides are padded, and sharp or hard items are kept out of the crib. Care must be taken to avoid making the child feel isolated by completely hiding the view of the surroundings outside the crib. During the seizure, the nurse stays with the child, protecting but not restraining. If clothing is tight, it should be loosened. The child should be moved to a flat surface if not in bed when the seizure starts.

The nurse documents the seizure completely after the episode. The type of movements, (rigidity, jerking, twitching), parts of the body that were involved, duration of the seizure, pulse and respirations, the child's color, and any deviant eye movements or other notable signs are documented.

Reducing Family Anxiety. A convulsion, or seizure, is a frightening occurrence to family caregivers. A calm, confident attitude on the part of the nurse reassures caregivers that the child is in good hands. Explanations are needed to reassure them that febrile seizures are not uncommon in small children. Parents need to be reassured that the physician will evaluate the child to determine if the seizure has any cause other than nervous system irritation resulting from the high fever.

Providing Family Teaching. Family caregivers must be taught seizure precautions so that they can handle a seizure that occurs at home. They also are instructed on what observations to make during a seizure, so that they can report these to the physician to assist in evaluating the child. Methods to control fever in the child should be included in teaching. When teaching the family caregivers about tepid sponge baths, the nurse explains to them that when the child shivers, the body is working to conserve its temperature, and sponging should be stopped until shivering stops because this could increase temperature (see Parent Teaching Tips to Reduce a Fever).

EVALUATION

- The child's airway remains patent, with no aspiration of saliva or vomitus.
- The child is uninjured during the seizure.
- The family caregivers verbalize their concerns.
- The family caregivers demonstrate an understanding of the methods to reduce fever and safe handling of seizures at home by verbal interaction with the nurse.

Hemophilus Influenzae *Meningitis*

Purulent meningitis in infancy and childhood is caused by a variety of agents. Among these are the meningococ-

Parent Teaching

Tip on Ways to Reduce Fever

If temperature is above 103°F (39.4°C) or child "acts sick," call the physician.

1. Use infant tub for baby or regular tub for child.
2. Use clean washcloths and towels.
3. Use about 2 inches of water, lukewarm to your wrist.
4. Place child in tub or on padded surface.
5. Sponge child's body with wet washcloth, using long, soothing strokes, rubbing lightly. Start with face, neck, arms, and chest. Be sure to get underarms well.
6. Sponge abdomen, back, and legs. Be sure to include groin and diaper area.
7. Sponge 20 minutes, remove child and cover lightly.
8. Take temperature after 30 minutes. Repeat until temperature is below 101°F (38.3°C).

Note:

If child shivers, stop sponging. When shivering stops, begin sponging again. Encourage child to drink as much water or juice as much as possible. Ice popsicles are good, too. Check with doctor about giving child acetaminophen (Tylenol).

DO NOT USE alcohol or ice water to sponge your child.

cus, tubercle bacillus, and the *H. influenzae* type B bacillus. The most common form is the *H. influenzae* meningitis. Meningococcal meningitis is spread by means of droplet infection from an infected person, all other forms are contracted by invasion of the meninges via the blood stream from an infection elsewhere.

Peak occurrence of *H. influenzae* meningitis is between the ages of 6 and 12 months. It is rare during the first 2 months of life and is seldom seen after the fourth year. Purulent meningitis is an infectious disease. Respiratory isolation techniques should be carried out for 24 hours after the start of effective antimicrobial therapy or until pathogens can no longer be cultured from nasopharyngeal secretions. Current immunizations include the HbCV, which is given at 2 months and repeated at 4, 6, and 15 months (see Table 8-4 in Chapter 8).

Clinical Manifestations

The onset may be either gradual or abrupt following an upper respiratory infection. Young infants with meningitis may have a characteristic high-pitched cry, fever, and irritability. Other symptoms include headache, **nuchal rigidity** (stiff neck) that may progress to **opisthotonos** (arching of the back), and delirium. Projectile vomiting may be present. Generalized convulsions are common in infants. Coma may occur early, particularly in the older child. Meningococcal meningitis, which tends to occur as epidemics in older children, exhibits a **purpuric rash** (caused by bleeding under the skin) in addition to the other symptoms.

Diagnosis

Early diagnosis and treatment are essential for uncomplicated recovery. A spinal tap is performed promptly whenever symptoms raise a suspicion that the disease may be present. The spinal tap is done before any antibiotics are administered to have accurate results. The nurse assists by holding the infant during the spinal tap procedure (Figure 9-13).

The spinal fluid will be under increased pressure. Laboratory examination of the fluid will reveal increased protein and decreased glucose content. Early in the disease, the spinal fluid may be clear, but it rapidly becomes purulent. The causative organism usually can be determined from stained smears of the spinal fluid, enabling specific medication to be started early, without waiting for growths of organisms on culture media.

Treatment

Treatment consists initially of intravenous administration of antibiotics in an effective dose. Third-generation cephalosporins, such as ceftazidime (Fortaz) or ceftriaxone (Rocephin), usually are used. Later in the disease, medications may be given orally. Treatment depends on the progress of the condition and continues as long as there is fever or signs of subdural effusion or otitis media. The administration of intravenous steroids early in the course has decreased the occurrence of deafness as a complication.

Subdural effusion may complicate the condition among infants during the course of the disease. Fluid accumulates in the subdural space between the dura and the brain. Needle aspirations through the infant's open suture lines or burr holes (in the skull of the older child) are used to remove the fluid. Repeated aspiration may be required.

Complications of *H. influenzae* meningitis with long-term implications are hydrocephalus, nerve deafness, mental retardation, and paralysis. The risk of complications is lessened when appropriate medication is started early in the disease.

Nursing Process for the Child with Meningitis

ASSESSMENT

The infant or child with meningitis is obviously extremely sick, and the anxiety level of the family caregivers is understandably high. The nurse needs to be patient and sensitive to their feelings when doing the assessment interview. A complete history is obtained with particular emphasis on the present illness, including any recent

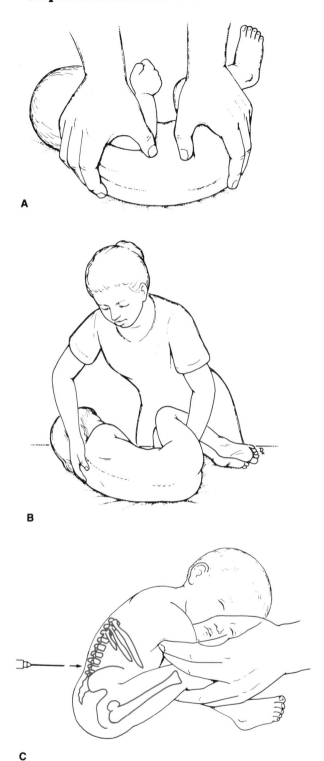

Figure 9-13. Three positions for a spinal tap. **A,** Knee-chest position for young infant. The nurse can hold the infant securely. **B,** Recumbent position. The nurse places one arm under flexed knees and grasps the child's hands; the other arm is placed around the neck and shoulders. **C,** Sitting position. Small infant is held in a sitting position, the knees flexed on the abdomen, and the nurse holds the elbow and knee in each hand, flexing the spine. (From Skale N. Manual of Pediatric Nursing Procedures. Philadelphia: JB Lippincott, p. 301.)

upper respiratory infection or middle ear infection. Information on other children in the family and their ages is also important.

The physical assessment of the infant includes temperature, pulse, and respirations, neurologic evaluation, which includes the level of consciousness (see section on neurologic evaluation). The young infant is examined for a bulging fontanelle, and the head circumference is measured for a baseline. This assessment needs to be performed after the spinal tap and starting of the intravenous fluids are completed because these procedures take precedence over everything else.

NURSING DIAGNOSES

The following nursing diagnoses are some of those that may be used in planning the care of the child with meningitis:

- Altered cerebral tissue perfusion related to cerebral edema
- Parental anxiety related to the child's condition and prognosis
- High risk fluid volume deficit related to vomiting, fever, and fluid restrictions
- High risk for ineffective airway clearance related to level of consciousness
- Fluid volume excess related to syndrome of inappropriate antidiuretic hormone
- High risk for infection transmitted to others

PLANNING AND IMPLEMENTATION

The major nursing goals are maintaining a patent airway, maintaining isolation for 24 hours after antibiotics have been started, monitoring neurologic status and vital signs, administering antibiotics, maintaining strict fluid intake and output measurements, and observing for signs of increased intracranial pressure (increased head size, headache, bulging fontanelle, decreased pulse, seizures, high-pitched cry, increased blood pressure, change in level of consciousness, and irritability or other behavioral changes). An additional nursing goal includes the relief of the caregivers' and child's anxiety.

Monitoring Vital Signs and Neurologic Status. The child may have signs of cerebral edema (see planning and implementation section). The child must be observed for seizure activity, temperature, blood pressure, pulse, respirations, neurologic changes, and change in level of consciousness every 2 hours. An increase in blood pressure, decrease in pulse, change in neurologic signs, or signs of respiratory distress are all signs that must be reported at once. The child's head circumference is measured at least every 4 hours. The child's room should be quiet and darkened to decrease stimulation that may cause seizures. The nurse must speak softly, move quietly, and raise and lower side rails carefully. The head of the bed can be elevated.

Reducing Family Anxiety. The parents are taught isolation techniques and good handwashing technique and are encouraged to stay with their child, if possible. Family caregivers need to be supported through every step of the process. Their anxiety about procedures, the child's seizures and condition, and the possible complications are all serious concerns. Family caregivers need to be included and to feel useful. If they are not too apprehensive, the nurse can help them to find small things that they can do for their child. They must be kept advised about the child's progress at all times.

Maintaining Fluid Intake. Fluid balance is an important aspect in the care of the child. Strict intake and output measurements are critical. Methods of reducing fever may be used as needed. Intravenous fluids are administered, with observation and monitoring of the intravenous infusion site and safety precautions to maintain the site.

Preventing Aspiration. The child should be positioned in a side-lying position with the neck supported for comfort and the head elevated. Pillows, blankets, and soft toys that might obstruct the airway are removed. Excessive mucus is watched for and removed as much as possible. Suction is used sparingly.

Monitoring Fluid Volume. Secretion of the antidiuretic hormone that is produced by the posterior pituitary gland may be increased by the infectious process. The child may not excrete urine adequately, and a body fluid excess will occur. Strict intake and output measurements are necessary; daily weight and electrolytes are monitored. Signs for concern that must be reported immediately are decreased urinary output, hyponatremia, increased weight, nausea, and irritability. The child is placed on fluid restrictions if signs occur.

Preventing Infection. *H. influenzae* is a highly contagious organism that may spread to other people by means of droplet transmission. Isolation precautions must be adhered to for the first 24 hours after the antibiotic is administered. Staff members and family caregivers must follow proper isolation procedures. Other children in the family may need to be assessed to determine if they should receive prophylactic antibiotics.

EVALUATION

- The child has no seizure activity.
- The parents' anxiety is decreased as evidenced by their cooperation.
- The child's temperature remains normal. Strict intake and output measurements are maintained. Intravenous fluids flow at the correct rate and are not infiltrated.
- The child's airway is clear.
- The child's fluid and electrolyte balance is adequate.
- Isolation precautions are maintained. Children in the home are assessed for prophylaxis.

Skin and Mucous Membrane Disorders

Miliaria Rubra

Miliaria rubra, often called prickly heat, is common in infants who are exposed to summer heat or are overdressed. It also may appear in febrile illnesses and may be mistaken for the rash of one of the communicable diseases. The rash appears as pinhead-sized erythematous (reddened) papules. It is most noticeable in areas where sweat glands are concentrated, such as folds of the skin, the chest, and about the neck. It usually causes itching, making the infant uncomfortable and fretful.

Treatment primarily should be preventive. Family caregivers should be taught to avoid bundling their infants in layers of clothing in hot weather. A diaper may be all that the child needs. Tepid baths without soap help control the itching. A thin sprinkling of cornstarch at diaper changes help relieve the infant's discomfort. The cornstarch should be carefully applied and brushed off so that it does not cake in the folds, but simply makes a smooth, soothing surface on the skin. Cornstarch is preferred over talc because talc may contain asbestos fibers that can cause aspiration pneumonia in the infant or young child if inhaled. Cornstarch has been associated with the promotion of growth of *Candida albicans*, but a study by Leyden in 1984 found that neither talc nor cornstarch supported growth of *C. albicans* under the conditions normally found in the diaper area.[4]

Diaper Rash

Diaper rash is a common occurrence in infancy, causing the baby discomfort and fretfulness. Bacterial decomposition of urine produces ammonia that is irritating to an infant's tender skin. Diarrheal stools also produce a burning erythematous area in the anal region. Some infants seem to be more susceptible than others, possibly owing to inherited sensitive skin. Prolonged exposure to wet or soiled diapers, use of plastic or rubber pants, infrequently changed disposable diapers, inadequate cleansing of the diaper area, especially after bowel movements, sensitivity to some soaps or disposable diaper perfumes, and the use of strong laundry detergents without thorough rinsing are considered to be causes. Yeast infections, notably candidiasis, are also causative factors.

Treatment

The primary treatment is one of prevention. Diapers need to be changed frequently, without waiting for obvious leaking. Regular checking is necessary. Manufacturers of disposable diapers are constantly trying to improve the ability of disposable diapers to take the wetness away from the infant's skin. Diapers washed at commercial laundries are sterilized, preventing the growth of ammonia-forming bacteria. Although convenient, disposable diapers and commercial diaper service can be an expense that the young parent may not be able to afford. Diapers washed at home should be presoaked (good commercial products are available, such as Diaperene), washed in hot water with a mild soap, rinsed thoroughly, and have an antiseptic added to the final rinse. Drying diapers in the sun, or in a heated dryer, also helps destroy bacteria.

Exposure of the diaper area to the air helps clear up the dermatitis. It is important to discourage the use of baby powder when diapering. Caked powder helps create an environment in which organisms love to grow. Teaching the caregiver to clean the diaper area from front to back with warm water and drying thoroughly with each diaper change helps improve or prevent the condition. If soap is necessary when cleaning stool from the infant's buttocks and rectal area, the caregiver must be certain that the soap is completely rinsed before diapering. Caregivers should be alerted that the use of commercial wet wipes may aggravate the condition. If the area becomes excoriated and sore, the health care provider may prescribe an ointment to be used (See Parent Teaching Tips for Diaper Rash).

Candidiasis

C. albicans is the causative agent for thrush and some cases of diaper rash. Newborns can be exposed to a candidiasis vaginal infection in the mother during delivery. Thrush appears in the infant's mouth as a white coating that looks like milk curds. Poor handwashing practices and inadequate washing of bottles and nipples are contributing factors. In addition, infants and toddlers may experience episodes of thrush or diaper rash after antibiotic therapy caused by the upset of the normal intestinal flora that allows an overgrowth of *Candida*.

Treatment for a diaper rash caused by *Candida* is the application of nystatin ointment or cream to the affected area. Application of nystatin (Mycostatin, Nilstat) to the oral lesions every 6 hours is an effective treatment. A reliable treatment for thrush is painting the infant's mouth with 1% gentian violet 3 times a day. This is effective but unsightly. Except in cases caused by antibiotic therapy, good hygiene practices should be reinforced.

Seborrheic Dermatitis

Generally, seborrheic dermatitis (cradle cap) can be prevented by daily washing of the infant's hair and scalp. Characterized by yellowish, scaly, or crusted patches on the scalp, it occurs in newborns and in older infants possibly as a result of excessive sebaceous gland activity. Family caregivers may be afraid to wash vigorously over the "soft spot." They need to understand that this is where cradle cap often begins and that careful but vigorous washing of the area with a washcloth can prevent this disorder. Using a fine-toothed baby comb after shampoo-

Parent Teaching

Tips for Diaper Rash

1. Rinse all baby's clothes thoroughly to eliminate soap or detergent residue that may irritate baby's skin.

2. Rinse diapers two times in clear water. Do not use fabric softeners because these can cause a skin reaction.

3. Use plastic or rubber diaper covers only when absolutely necessary. They hold moisture, which makes rash worse.

4. Change diapers as soon as wet or soiled. Disposable diapers hold moisture the same as plastic or rubber covers.

5. Avoid fastening diaper too tight, irritating baby's skin.

6. Expose baby's bottom to air without diapers as much as possible to help rash heal.

7. Do not overdress or overcover baby. Sweating makes rash worse.

8. Wash baby's bottom only with lukewarm water, using wet cotton balls or pouring over in bath basin or sink. Pat dry with soft cloth. Do not use commercial baby wipes. Do not rub rash.

9. A cool, wet cloth placed over red diaper rash is very soothing. Try this for 5 minutes three or four times a day.

10. Use ointment only as recommended by health care provider. Apply very thin layer only. Wash off at each diaper change.

11. Dry baby's diaper area thoroughly before rediapering. A hair dryer on low warm setting used after patting dry may help.

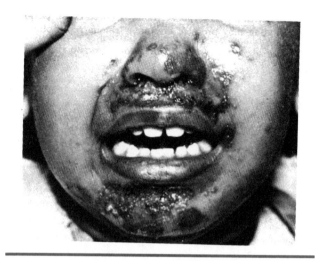

Figure 9-14. Typical lesion of impetigo. (From Pillitteri A. Maternal and Child Health Nursing. Philadelphia: JB Lippincott, 1992, p. 1353.)

ing is also a helpful preventive measure. These principles are stressed as part of care of the newborn teaching in maternal–newborn care.

Once the condition exists, daily application of mineral oil helps loosen the crust. No attempt should be made to loosen it all at once, however, as the delicate skin on the scalp may break and bleed and easily become infected.

Impetigo

Impetigo is a superficial bacterial skin infection. In the newborn infant, the primary causative organism is *Staphylococcus aureus*. In the older child, the most frequent causative organism is group A beta-hemolytic *Streptococcus* (Figure 9-14). Impetigo in the newborn is usually bullous (blisterlike), and in the older child the lesions are nonbullous.

Impetigo in the newborn nursery is cause for immediate concern. The condition is highly contagious and can spread through a nursery quickly. The nurse caring for an infant who has impetigo must follow contact (skin and wound) precautions, including wearing a cover gown and gloves. The infant should be segregated from other infants in the nursery to deter spread of the disease. Crusts can be soaked off with warm water followed by application of topical antibiotics, such as bacitracin and neosporin. The infant's hands must be covered or elbow restraints applied to prevent scratching of lesions. Careful handwashing by nursing personnel and family members is essential.

The older child with impetigo is treated at home. The family caregivers must be taught hygiene practices to prevent the spread of impetigo to other children in the household or other contacts of the child in the day care center, nursery school, or elementary school. Lesions occur primarily on the face but may spread to any part of the body. The crusts and drainage are contagious. Because the lesions are *pruritic* (itchy), the child must learn to keep his or her fingers and hands away from the lesions. Nails should be trimmed to prevent scratching of lesions. Further teaching of the family includes not sharing towels and washcloths. Medical treatment includes oral penicillin or erythromycin for 10 days. Daily washing of the crusts helps speed the healing process. Mupirocin (Bactroban) ointment may be used.

Because this is commonly a streptococcal infection in the older child, rheumatic fever or acute glomerulonephritis may follow, and family caregivers should be alerted to this possibility, but the occurrence of either of these complications is rare.

Acute Infantile Eczema

Infantile eczema is an atopic dermatitis considered to be at least in part an allergic reaction to some irritant or irritants. It is fairly common during the first year of life after the age of 3 months. It is uncommon in breast-fed babies before they are given additional foods.

Infantile eczema is characterized by (1) hereditary disposition; (2) hypersensitivity of the deeper layers of the skin to protein or proteinlike allergens; and (3) allergens to which the child is sensitive that may be inhaled, ingested, or absorbed through direct contact, such as house dust, egg white, and wool. Those infants who have eczema tend to have hay fever or asthma later in life.

Clinical Manifestations

Eczema usually starts on the cheeks and spreads to the extensor surfaces of the arms and legs. Eventually the entire trunk may become involved. The initial reddening of the skin is quickly followed by papule and vesicle formation. Itching is intense, and the scratching the infant does makes the skin weep and crust. The areas easily become infected by hemolytic streptococci or by staphylococci.

Diagnosis

The most common allergens concerned in the manifestation of eczema are the following:

- Foods: egg white, cow's milk, wheat products, and orange and tomato juice
- Inhalants: house dust, pollens, and animal dander
- Materials: wool, nylon, and plastic

However, diagnosis is not simple. Often, trial by elimination is as effective as any other diagnostic tool. Skin testing on a young infant generally is not considered to be valid; thus, it is discouraged as a means of diagnosis.

Diagnostic Diet. An elimination diet may be helpful in ruling out offending foods. A hypoallergenic diet consisting of a milk substitute such as soy formula, vitamin supplement, and other foods known to be hypoallergenic is given. If the child's skin condition shows improvement, other foods are added one at a time, with an interval of approximately 1 week, noting effects and eliminating any foods that cause a reaction. The protein of egg white is such a common offender that most pediatricians advise against feeding whole eggs to any infant until late into the first year of life (see Table 9-2).

Great care must be taken not to allow the child to become undernourished. An elimination program must always be initiated under the supervision of a competent pediatric nurse practitioner, dietitian, or physician.

Treatment

Smallpox vaccination is definitely contraindicated for the child with eczema. In fact, such a child must be kept away from anyone who has recently been vaccinated. A serious condition called *eczema vaccinatum* results when an infant with eczema is vaccinated or is exposed to the vaccination of another person. The infant becomes seriously ill, and mortality rates have been high. Fortunately because smallpox vaccination is no longer required, this is not a major concern but could occur if the child is exposed to someone preparing to go overseas. Of greater current concern is protecting the child from any person who has a herpes simplex infection. If the lesions become infected with herpes simplex (cold sore), a generalized reaction may occur. In the child with severe eczema with a large number of lesions, body fluid loss from oozing through the lesions can be serious. The infant may have severe pain and be gravely ill with this complication.

Oral antibiotics may be ordered for a coexistent infection, such as *Staphylococcus*, *Streptococcus*, or viral infections. Oral antihistamines and sedatives may help relieve the itching and provide for rest. If no infection exists, topical hydrocortisone ointments may be used to relieve inflammation. Wet soaks or colloidal baths also may be prescribed. Both are used for their soothing effects. Water should be tepid for further soothing, and soap may not be used because of its drying effect. Some physicians recommend the use of a mild soap, such as Dove, or a soap substitute. Lubrication is essential to retain moisture and prevent evaporation after the baths. Emollients containing lanolin or petrolatum, such as Eucerin, may be prescribed.

Inhalant and contact allergens should be avoided as far as possible. In the infant's sleeping room, window drapes or curtains, dresser scarfs, and rugs should be removed or made of washable fabric that can be frequently laundered. Furniture should be washed off frequently. The mattress of the crib should have a nonallergenic covering and be washed frequently, cleaning carefully along the binding. Feather pillows must be eliminated, and stuffed toys should be washable. It may be necessary to provide new homes for household pets. However, dander from the pets can remain in carpets, crevices, and overstuffed furniture for a long time. Carpets and area rugs may need to be removed. A home, especially an older one with a damp basement, may be harboring molds that shed allergenic spores. Bathrooms are also places for molds and mildews to hide, especially in warm, humid climates.

Nursing Process for the Child with Infantile Eczema

ASSESSMENT

The family caregivers of the child with infantile eczema are often frustrated and exhausted. Although the caregiver can be assured that most cases of infant eczema clear up by the age of 2, this does little to relieve the present situation. Hospitalization is avoided whenever possible because these infants are highly susceptible to infections. Sometimes, however, hospitalization seems to be the only answer to provide more intensive therapy or relieve an exhausted caregiver. The interview with the family caregivers must cover the history of the condition, including those treatments that have been tried already and those foods that have been ruled out as allergens. A thorough review of the home environment must be included. An evaluation of the caregivers' knowledge of the condition is an important part of the assessment.

The assessment of the infant includes vital signs, general nutritional state, and a complete examination of all body parts with careful documentation of the eruptions, location, and size. Areas that are weeping and crusted should be indicated, as well as those areas that are not affected.

NURSING DIAGNOSES

Regardless of the severity of the eczema, the nursing diagnoses are much the same. Nursing diagnoses that may be used are the following:

- Sleep pattern disturbance related to itching and discomfort
- High risk for altered nutrition: less than body requirements related to elimination diet
- High risk for infection related to skin lesions
- Altered growth and development related to chronic condition and confining treatments
- Parental health-seeking behaviors related to disease condition and treatment

PLANNING AND IMPLEMENTATION

The major nursing goals are to provide the infant with treatments that are soothing and relieve pruritus, to maintain skin integrity with no infected lesions, to provide good nutrition within the constraints of allergens, and to provide sensory stimulation and diversional activities that contribute to the developmental needs of the infant.

Providing Comfort Measures. Soothing baths, such as the colloidal bath (Aveeno), should be planned just before naptime or bedtime. Medications such as sedatives or antihistamines should be timed so that they will be effective immediately after the bath, when the infant is most relaxed.

Maintaining Adequate Nutrition. The child is weighed on admission and daily thereafter. This procedure gives some indication regarding weight gain. If an elimination diet is being used, the diet should be carefully balanced, within the framework of the foods permitted, and supplemented with vitamin and mineral preparations as needed. Fluids are encouraged to prevent dehydration.

Preventing Infection. As stated earlier, usually these children are kept out of the hospital because of the con-

cern about infection. However, they also can become infected at home. If hospitalized, the infant should be placed in a room alone or in a room where there is no other child with any type of infection.

The infant's lesions can be covered with light clothing. Especially appropriate are the one-piece loose-fitting, terry pajamas or one-piece cotton underwear known as "onesies." This type of clothing helps keep the infant from scratching. In addition, the nails must be kept closely cut, and mittenlike hand coverings can be worn. Restraints are used only if absolutely necessary, but sometimes elbow restraints must be used. Restraints are removed at least every 4 hours and more often, if feasible. Care should be taken to avoid allowing the child to rub or scratch while restraints are off. If ointments or wet dressings need to be kept in place on the infant's face, a mask may be made by cutting holes into a cotton stockinette-type material to correspond to eyes, nose, and mouth. Wet dressings on the rest of the body can be kept in place by wrapping the infant "mummy" fashion. Dressings may be left on for an extended period but should not be allowed to become dry because that can create open areas when they are removed. Antibiotics should be administered as ordered.

Providing Sensory Stimulation. Every effort should be made to provide sensory stimulation by involving the infant in age- and developmentally appropriate activities. Singing songs, looking at picture books, reading stories, engaging in rhymes, cuddling, "Peek-a-Boo," a pacifier, safe toys, and other activities are strongly recommended. Such activities also serve as a diversion to prevent complications. The infant who is old enough to self-feed should be permitted to do so with restraints removed under supervision.

Providing Family Teaching. The family caregivers need help in understanding the condition, possible food, contact, and inhalant allergens, and ways to soothe the infant. They also need assistance in determining ways to encourage normal growth and development. Caregivers need instruction on reading labels of prepared foods, watching carefully for "hidden" allergens. Family caregivers may feel apprehensive of or repulsed by this unsightly infant. They need support to be able to express their feelings and to view this as a distressing, but temporary, skin condition.

Infants and children with eczema are frequently active, "behaviorally itchy" children, so caregivers need support in handling challenging behavior. Family caregivers also need guidance in ways to promote development of a strong self-image in the child to protect against strangers' openly negative reactions.

EVALUATION

- The child rests an adequate amount for his or her age.
- The child's nutrition meets the needs for growth and development as evidenced by desirable weight gain.
- The child's skin lesions are not infected.

- The child engages in activities appropriate to age and developmental stage within the confines of the treatment.
- Family caregivers verbalize an understanding of the disease and its treatment. Caregivers demonstrate an acceptance of the infant and the condition by interacting in a positive fashion with the child

Summary

The first year of life is one in which many rapid changes take place. Small and immature anatomic structures make the infant vulnerable to many health problems. Adequate nutrition is essential to the development of a healthy infant. Infants who are nutritionally deprived are especially defenseless against opportunistic organisms. The infant's digestive system is easily upset. Vomiting and diarrhea are frequent signs of distress in the infant. The immaturity of the respiratory system creates hazards for the typical infant and is especially hard on the child with other problems. *H. influenzae* is a common bacteria that causes serious respiratory infections to which the infant is vulnerable and is also the most common cause of meningitis in this age group. New immunizations promise to change this. Infants become feverish quickly and must be observed for febrile seizures and protected from injury. Urinary tract infections are frequent in infant girls older than 2 months because of the short urethra. The infant's skin is sensitive, and rashes, infections, and eczema are relatively common. Nonirritating and moisturizing soaps should be used. All these conditions can occur in the infant with good nutrition and a warm family relationship. When the further insult of socioeconomic and emotional deprivation is added to all of this, the minor problems become serious and major problems are life threatening. Nurses need to use all the skills of the nursing process to plan and administer optimum nursing care.

Review Questions

1. You are caring for Jimmy, a 6-month-old boy with the diagnosis of NFTT. What observations will you make? What might you expect to find? What are some nurturing practices you can incorporate into your nursing care? Tell how you will work with his 16-year-old mother, Jill, to set positive parenting behaviors for her.
2. Discuss the reasons infection control practices must be implemented when caring for the debilitated infant. Identify those practices that you would implement when caring for an 8-month-old infant with malnutrition.
3. Nine-month-old Mandy has severe diarrhea. What symptoms would you look for in Mandy? What documenting is especially important in her care?
4. Mandy has progressed to a BRAT diet. Describe it, and tell how you might fix it and serve it to Mandy.
5. Jane Brown is your neighbor. Two-month-old Kevin, her only child, has colic. Jane is overwhelmed and almost frantic. Discuss what you can say to her and the suggestions you can make.
6. Ten-month-old Sarah is chubby and pale, with skin like a china doll. The family lives on a small farm and keep a milk cow. Sarah's grandmother brings her in for a regular checkup. What concerns would you have, and what teaching would you give Sarah's grandmother?
7. Review the inheritance of sickle cell disease. Explain how the disease is passed from generation to generation.
8. Eddie, age 4 months, is admitted with bronchiolitis, suspected to be caused by RSV. What observations must you make when assessing him? He is placed in a mist tent. Discuss nursing care, and include any measure that may help ease his breathing.
9. Describe the emergency care of a child during a seizure.
10. Tell how you would instruct family caregivers about isolation precautions when caring for a child with meningitis.
11. What teaching might you give a father whose infant has miliaria rubra?
12. Tell what the relationship *Candida albicans* has to some cases of diaper rash. What might you teach the mother about treating diaper rash?
13. Billy Joe has impetigo. He goes to a day care center. Make a teaching plan for the family and the day care workers.

References

1. Kline MK. Otitis media. In Oski FA (ed). Principles and Practices of Pediatrics. Philadelphia: JB Lippincott, 1990.
2. Loughlin GM, Carroll JL. Sudden unexplained death and apparent life-threatening events. In Oski FA (ed). Principles and Practices of Pediatrics. Philadelphia: JB Lippincott, 1990.
3. Bell J, Esterling LS. What Will I Tell the Children? Omaha: University of Nebraska Medical Center Child Life Department and Meyer Children's Rehabilitation Institute, 1986.
4. Leyden JJ. Cornstarch, *Candida albicans*, and diaper rash. Pediatr Dermatol 1(4):322–325, 1984.

Bibliography

Bell J, Esterling LS. What Will I Tell the Children? University of Nebraska Medical Center Child Life Department and Meyer Children's Rehabilitation Institute, 1986.

Carpenito LJ. Handbook of Nursing Diagnosis, 4th ed. Philadelphia: JB Lippincott, 1991.

Castiglia PT, Harbin RE. Child Health Care: Process and Practice. Philadelphia: JB Lippincott, 1992.

Demmler GJ. Rotaviruses. In Oski FA (ed). Principles and Practices of Pediatrics. Philadelphia: JB Lippincott, 1990.

Engel NS. Phenobarbital for pediatric febrile seizures: Risk-benefit update. MCN 15(4):257, 1990.

Eschleman MM. Introductory Nutrition and Diet Therapy, 2nd ed. Philadelphia: JB Lippincott, 1991.

Facione N. Otitis media: An overview of acute and chronic disease. Nurse Pract 15(10):11–20, 1990.

Gino C. SIDS research that causes pain. Am J Nurs 88(10): 1353–1354, 1988.

Janai H, Stutman HR, Marks MI. Invasive *Hemophilus influenzae* type B infections: A continuing challenge. Am J Infect Control 18(3):160–166, 1990.

Jurgrau A. Why aren't we protecting our children? RN 53(11): 30–35, 1990.

Klein MJA. The home health nurse clinician's role in the prevention of nonorganic failure to thrive. J Pediatr Nurs 5(2):129–135, 1990.

Loughlin GM, Carroll JL. Sudden unexplained death and apparent life-threatening events. In Oski FA (ed). Principles and Practices of Pediatrics. Philadelphia: JB Lippincott, 1990.

Pillitteri A. Maternal and Child Health Nursing. Philadelphia: JB Lippincott, 1992.

Reeves-Swift R. Rational management of a child's acute fever. MCN 15(3):82–85, 1990.

Rivers R, Williamson N. Sickle cell anemia complex disease—nursing challenge. RN 53(6):24–28, 1990.

Sperhac AM. Abdominal pain in pediatric patients: Assessment and management update. J Emerg Nurs 15(2):93–100, 1989.

Whaley LF, Wong DL. Nursing Care of Infants and Children, 4th ed. St. Louis: Mosby-Year Book, 1991.

Wilson D, Killion D. Urinary tract infections in the pediatric patient. Nurse Pract 14(7):38–40, 1989.

Woolsey SF. Support after sudden infant death. Am J Nurs 88(10):1348–1352, 1988.

Growth and Development of the Toddler: 1 to 3 Years

Chapter 10

Student Objectives

Upon completion of this chapter, the student will be able to:

1. State the age group identified as toddler.
2. State why parenting a toddler is often frustrating for caregivers.
3. Describe physical growth that occurs during toddlerhood.
4. List three reasons why eating problems often appear in this age group.
5. Describe the progression of the toddler's self-feeding skills.
6. State why accident prevention is a primary concern when caring for a toddler.
7. State the four leading causes of accidental death of toddlers, and list preventive measures for each.
8. List eight types of medications most frequently involved in childhood poisonings.
9. State the age at which a child should be taught toothbrushing, and discuss why this is an appropriate age.
10. Describe the relationship of sweet foods and plaque formation on the teeth.
11. Discuss the purpose of the toddler's first dental visit and the ideal age for it.
12. Describe the elements in timing of the beginning of toilet training.
13. Identify six suggestions to aid in bowel training.
14. State when complete bowel and bladder control might be achieved.
15. Define the following terms as they relate to the psychosocial development of the toddler: a) Negativism; b) Ritualism; c) Dawdling.
16. List desirable information to be gathered in a social assessment when a toddler is admitted to the hospital.

Marks MG: BROADRIBB'S INTRODUCTORY PEDIATRIC NURSING, 4th ed. © 1994 J.B. Lippincott Company.

Key Terms

autonomy	parallel play
dawdling	punishment
discipline	ritualism
negativism	temper tantrum

*S*oon after a child's first birthday, important, sometimes dramatic changes take place. Physical growth slows considerably, mobility and communication skills improve rapidly, and a determined, often stubborn little person begins to create a new set of challenges for the parents. "No" and "want" are favorite words. Temper tantrums appear.

During this transition from infancy to early childhood, the child learns many new physical and social skills. With additional teeth and better motor skills, the toddler's self-feeding abilities improve and include the addition of a new assortment of foods. Left unsupervised, the toddler also may taste many nonfood items that may be harmful, even fatal.

This transition is a time of unpredictability: one moment, the toddler insists on "me do it"; the next moment, the child reverts to dependence on his or her mother or other caregiver. As the toddler seeks to assert independence and achieve autonomy, fear of separation develops. The toddler's curiosity about the world increases, as does his or her ability to explore (Figure 10-1). Family caregivers soon discover that this exploration can wreak havoc on orderly routine and a well-kept house and that the toddler requires close supervision to prevent injury to self or objects in the environment. The toddler justly earns the title of "explorer."

Toddlerhood can be a difficult time for family caregivers. Just as they are beginning to feel confident in their ability to care for and understand their infant, the toddler changes into a walking, talking person whose attitudes and behaviors disrupt the entire family. Accident-proofing safety measures and firm but gentle discipline are primary tasks for parents of toddlers. Learning to discipline with patience and understanding is difficult but eventually rewarding. At the end of the toddlerhood stage, the child's behavior generally becomes more acceptable and predictable.

Erikson's psychosocial developmental task for this age group is **autonomy** while overcoming doubt and shame. As the infant's task was one of building trust, the toddler seeks independence, wavering between dependence and freedom, gaining self-awareness. This behavior is so common that the stage is commonly referred to as the "terrible twos," but it is just as often referred to as the "terrific twos" because of the toddler's exciting language development, the exuberance with which the toddler greets the world, and a newfound sense of accomplishment. Both aspects of being 2 years of age are essential to the child's development, and caregivers must learn how to manage the fast-paced switches between anxiety and enthusiasm.

Physical Development

Toddlerhood is a time of slowed growth and rapid development. Each year the toddler gains 5 to 10 lb in weight and about 3 inches in height. Continued eruption of teeth, particularly the molars, help the toddler learn to chew food. The toddler learns to stand alone (Figure 10-2) and to walk between the ages of 1 and 2 years. During this time, most children say their first words and continue to improve and refine their language skills. By the end of this period, the toddler may have learned partial or total toilet training.

The rate of development varies with each child, depending on the individual personality and the opportunities available to test, explore, and learn. Significant landmarks in growth and development of the toddler are summarized in (Table 10-1).

Nutrition

Between the ages of 1 and 3 years, eating problems frequently appear. These problems occur for a number of reasons, such as the following:

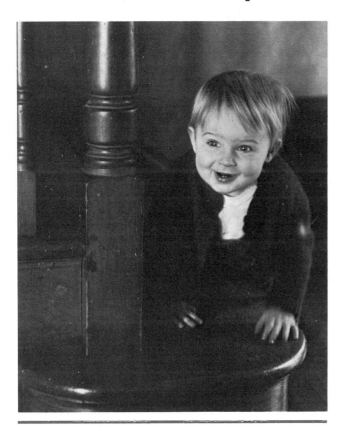

Figure 10-1. The toddler explores the stairs independently. (Photo by Carol Baldwin.)

1. Growth rate has slowed; therefore, the toddler may want and need less food than before. Family caregivers need to know that this is normal.

2. The child's strong drive for independence and autonomy compels an assertion of will to prove to himself or herself and others the fact of individuality.

3. A child's appetite varies according to the kind of foods offered, and "food jags" are common, with a desire for only one kind of food for awhile.

To minimize these eating problems and ensure that the child gets a balanced diet with all the proteins, carbohydrates, minerals, and vitamins essential for health and well-being, meals should be planned with an understanding of the toddler's developing feeding skills (Table 10-2). Messiness is to be expected and prepared for when learning begins but gradually improves as the child gains skill in self-feeding. The following suggestions also may be helpful to caregivers in the home and in the hospital:

1. Serve small portions, and provide second servings when the first has been eaten. Remember, 1 or 2 tbsp is an adequate serving for the toddler. Do not overwhelm the child with too much food on the dish.

2. Remember that there is no *one* food positively essential to health. Allow substitution for a dis-

liked food. Food jags in which toddlers prefer one food for days on end are common and not harmful. If the child refuses a particular food, such as milk, use appropriate substitutes like puddings, cheeses, yogurt, and cottage cheese. Do not let eating become a battle of wills.

3. Toddlers like simply prepared foods, served warm or cool, *not* hot or cold.

4. Provide a social atmosphere at mealtimes, allowing the toddler to eat with others in the family. They learn by imitating the acceptance or rejection of foods by other family members.

5. Children prefer foods they can pick up with their fingers; however, they should be allowed to use a spoon or fork when they want to try.

6. Try to plan regular mealtimes with small nutritious snacks planned between meals. Do not attach too much importance to food by urging the child to choose what to eat.

7. Dawdling at mealtime is common with this age group and can be ignored unless it stretches on to unreasonable lengths or becomes a play for power.

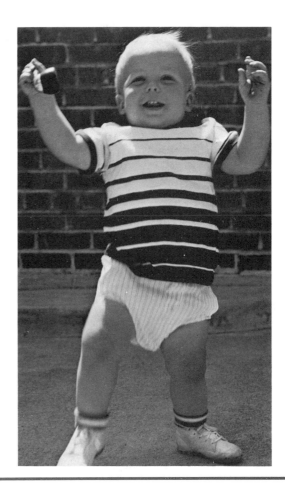

Figure 10-2. The toddler is proud of his ability to stand alone. (Photo by Carol Baldwin.)

Table 10-1. Growth and Development: The Toddler

Age (months)	Personal–Social	Fine Motor	Gross Motor	Language	Cognition
12–15	Begins Erikson's stage of "autonomy vs shame and doubt" Seeks novel ways to pursue new experiences Imitations of people are more advanced	Builds with blocks, finger paints Able to reach out with the hands and bring food to the mouth Holds a spoon Drinks from a cup	Movements become more voluntary Postural control improves; able to stand and may take few independent steps	First words are not generally classified as true language. They are generally associated with the concrete and are usually activity-oriented	Begins to accommodate to the environment, and the adaptive process evolves
18	Extremely curious Becomes a communicative social being Parallel play Fleeting contacts with other children "Make-believe" play begins	Better control of spoon; good control when drinking from cup Turns pages of a book Places objects in holes or slots	Walks alone; gait may still be a bit unsteady Begins to walk sideward and backward	Begins to use language in a symbolic form to represent images or ideas that reflect the thinking process Uses some meaningful words such as "hi," "bye-bye," and "all gone" Comprehension is significantly greater	Demonstrates foresight and can discover solutions to problems without excessive trial-and-error procedures Is able to imitate without the presence of a model (deferred imitation)
24	Language facilitates autonomy Sense of power from saying "no" and "mine" Increased independence from mother	Turns pages of a book singly Adept at building a tower of 6–7 cubes When drawing, attempts are made to enclose a space	Runs well with little falling Throws and kicks a ball Walks up and down stairs—one step at a time	Beings to use words to explain past events or to discuss objects not observably present Rapidly expands vocabulary to approximately 300 words; uses plurals	Enters preconceptual phase of cognitive development State of continuous investigation Primary focus is egocentric
36	Basic concepts of sexuality are established Separates from mother more easily Attends to toilet needs	Copies a circle and a straight line Grasps spoon between thumb and index finger Holds cup by handle	Balances on one foot; jumps in place; pedals tricycle	Quest for information furthered by questions like "why," "when," "where," and "how" Has acquired the language that will be used in the course of simple conversation during the adult years	Preconceptual phase continues; can think of only one idea at a time; unable to think of all parts in terms of the whole

From Wieczorek RR, Natapoff JN: A Conceptual Approach to the Nursing Care of Children: Health Care from Birth Through Adolescence. Philadelphia: JB Lippincott, 1981.

Then the food can be calmly removed without comment. Mealtime for the toddler should not exceed 20 minutes.

8. Making desserts a reward for good eating habits is not appropriate. It gives unfair value to the dessert and makes vegetables or other foods seem less desirable.

9. Offer regularly planned nutritious snacks, such as milk, crackers and peanut butter, cheese cubes, and pieces of fruit. Plan snacks midway between meals and at bedtime.

10. Remember that the total amount eaten each day is more important than the amount eaten at a specific meal.

A sample daily food plan is provided in Table 10-3.

Table 10-2. Feeding Skills of the Toddler

Age	Skills
1 year	May need a toy to hold attention while sitting for meals (enjoys holding cup—tilts head backward to drain last drop; enjoys finger feeding
15 months	Better gross motor control; able to sit through meals; finger feeding is preferred method; increased desire to use spoon, however, has difficulty "scooping up" foods (much spilling); grasps cup more with thumb and forefingers; now tilts cup with fingers rather than tilting head; child more insistent about feeding self
18 months	Appetite decreasing; refusals and preferences not clearly defined; better control of spoon; replaces spilled food back on spoon; holds cup with both hands; has good control with fingers and spills very little; often throws cup when finished if no one is there to take it
21 months	Easily distracted; enjoys pouring things from one container to another; rituals/patterns prevalent (eg, same spoon, cup)
2 years	Appetite fair to moderate; "finicky" or "fussy" (definite likes and dislikes); food jags; spoon grasped between thumb and index finger; able to place food on spoon without assistance of other hand; still considerable spilling; accepts no help ("Me do!")
30 months	Appetite fluctuates between very good and very poor; usually takes in *one* good meal (noon or evening); refusals and preferences still prevalent; rituals persist
3 years	Refusals and preferences less evident; spoon held between thumb and index finger (some hold it in adult fashion with palm turned inward); cup held by the handle in adult fashion; once again head tilts back to secure last drop

From Wieczorek RR, Natapoff JN: A Conceptual Approach to the Nursing of Children: Health Care From Birth Through Adolescence. Philadelphia: JB Lippincott, 1981.

Health Maintenance

Activities that protect the health of the toddler and help ensure continuing growth and development include prevention of accidents and infection, current immunizations (see Table 8-4 in Chapter 8), formation of good oral health habits, toilet training, and provision of a stimulating environment and the opportunity to explore it. Nurses assist families with toddlers in these activities by health teaching, support of positive parenting behaviors, and reinforcement of the toddler's achievements (Table 10-4).

Sleep Needs

The toddler's sleep needs change gradually between the ages of 1 and 3 years. A total need for 12 to 14 hours of sleep is to be expected in the first year of toddlerhood, decreasing to 10 to 12 hours by 3 years. The toddler soon gives up a morning nap, but most continue to need an afternoon nap until sometime toward the third birthday. Rituals are a common part of bedtime procedures. A bedtime ritual provides structure and a feeling of security because the toddler knows what to expect and what is expected of him or her. The separation anxiety that is common in the toddler may contribute to some of the toddler's reluctance to go to bed. Family caregivers must be careful that the toddler does not use this to manipulate them and delay bedtime. The gentle, firm consistency of caregivers is ultimately reassuring to the toddler. Regular schedules, with set bedtimes with a story time, or quiet time beforehand often helps the toddler settle for the night. There are many wonderful stories to be read to the toddler that can provide a calming end to a busy day.

Accident Prevention

Toddlers are explorers who require constant supervision in a controlled environment to encourage autonomy and prevent injury. When supervision is inadequate, or the environment unsafe, tragedy often results, making accidents the leading cause of death for children between the ages of 1 and 4 years. Accidents involving motor vehicles, drowning, burns, poisoning, and falls are the most frequent causes of death. Burns and drownings are similar in numbers of deaths that occurred, but motor vehicle deaths for this age group are more than 3 times greater than either of these causes.

Motor Vehicle Accidents

Many childhood deaths or injuries resulting from motor vehicle accidents can be prevented by proper use of restraints when toddlers are passengers in moving vehicles. Federally approved child safety seats are designed to give the child maximum protection if used correctly. Children need to be taught that they must be securely fastened in the car seat before the car starts. Adults must be responsible for teaching the child that seat belts are required for safe car travel. Many other toddlers are killed or injured by moving vehicles while playing in their own driveways or garages. Caregivers need to be aware that these tragedies can occur and take proper precautions at all times. Adults in the car with a child should set the example by also using seat belts (see Parent Teaching: Parent Tips to Prevent Motor Vehicle Accidents).

Drowning

Although drowning of young children is often associated with bathtubs, the increased number of home-owned

Table 10-3. Suggested Daily Food Guidelines for the Toddler

Food Items	Daily Amounts*	Comments/Rationale
Cooked eggs†	3–5/wk	Good source of protein; moderate use is recommended because of high cholesterol content in egg yolk
Breads, grains, and cereals: whole-grain or enriched	4 or more servings (eg, ½ slice bread, ¼ cup cereal, 2 crackers, ¼ cup noodles)	Provides thiamine, niacin, and, if enriched, riboflavin and iron Encourage the child to identify and appreciate a wide variety of foods
Fruit juices; fruit—canned or small pieces	3–4 child-sized servings (eg, ½ cup juice, ¼–½ cup fruit pieces)	Use those rich in vitamins A and C; also source of iron and calcium Self-feeding enhances the child's sense of independence
Vegetables	1–2 child-sized servings (eg, ¼–½ cup)	Include at least 1 dark green or yellow vegetable every other day for vitamin A
Meat, fish, chicken, casseroles, cottage cheese, peanut butter, dried peas and beans	2 child-sized servings (eg, 1 oz meat, 1 egg, ½ cup casserole, ¼ cup cottage cheese, 1–2 tbsp peanut butter)	Source of complete protein, iron, thiamine, riboflavin, niacin, and vitamin B_{12} Nuts and seeds should not be offered until after age 3 when the risk of choking is minimal
Milk, yogurt, cheese	4–6 child-sized servings (eg, 4–6 oz milk, ½ cup yogurt, 1 oz cheese)	Cheese, cottage cheese, and yogurt are good calcium and riboflavin sources; also sources of calcium, phosphorus, complete protein, riboflavin, and niacin; also vitamin D if fortified milk used
Fats and sweets	In moderation	May interfere with consumption of nutrient-rich foods. Chocolate should be delayed until the child is 1 year old
Salt and other seasonings	In moderation	Children's taste buds are more sensitive than those of adults. Salt is a learned taste, and high intakes are related to hypertension

* Amounts are daily totals and goals to be achieved gradually.
†New food item for the age group.
Adapted from Eschleman MM: Introductory Nutrition and Diet Therapy, 2nd ed. Philadelphia: JB Lippincott, 1991, pp. 286–287.

swimming pools has added significantly to the number of accidental drownings. Often, these pools are fenced on three sides to keep out nonresidents but are bordered on one side by the family home, making the pool accessible to infants and toddlers. These and small plastic wading pools hold enough water to drown an unsupervised toddler. Any family living near even a small body of water must be cautioned not to leave a mobile infant or toddler unattended, even for a moment, to avoid potential tragedy. Even a small amount of water such as that in a bucket may be enough water to drown a small child.

Burns
Burn accidents occur most often as scalds from immersions and spills and from exposure to uninsulated electrical wires or live extension cord plugs. Children also are burned while playing with matches or while left unattended in a home where a fire breaks out. Whether the fire results from a child's mischief, an adult's carelessness, or some unforeseeable event, the injuries, even if not fatal, can have long-term or permanent effects. Many burns can be prevented by following simple safety practices also the display on Parent Teaching: Tips to Prevent Burns).

Ingestion of Toxic Substances
The curious toddler wants to touch and taste everything. Left unsupervised, the toddler may sample household cleaners, parents' prescriptions, children's or regular aspirin, kerosene, gasoline, or peeling lead-based paint chips or dust particles. Poisoning is still the most common medical emergency in children, with the highest incidence occurring between the ages of 1 and 4 years.

Table 10-4. Guidelines for Health Promotion in the Toddler

Developmental Characteristics of Toddler (2–3 yr)	Possible Deviations from Health	Nursing Measures to Ensure Optimal Health Practices
Self-feeding (foods/objects more accessible for mouthing, handling, and eating)	Inadequate nutritional intake Accidental poisoning Gastrointestinal disturbances: Instability of gastrointestinal tract Infection from parasites (pinworm)	Diet teaching Childproofing the home Careful handwashing (before meals, after toileting) Avoidance of rich foods Observe for perianal itching (Scotch tape test, administer anthelmintic)
Toilet training	Constipation (if too rigid training procedures initiated) Urinary tract infection (especially prevalent in girls owing to anatomic structure and poor toilet habits)	Teaching regarding toileting procedures Urinalysis when indicated (eg, burning) Teaching hygiene (at the onset of training instruct girls to wipe from front to back, hand-wash—to prevent cross-infection)
Increased socialization	Increase prevalence of upper respiratory infections (immune levels still at immature levels)	Hygienic practices (eg, use of tissue or handkerchief, not drinking from same glass) Immunizations for passive immunity against communicable disease (MMR; boosters of HbCV, DPT, OPV)
Primary dentition	Caries with resultant infection or loss of primary as well as beginning permanent teeth	Initiation or oral hygiene, regular teeth brushing, dental examination at 21½ months–3 year Proper nutrition to ensure dentition
Sleep disturbances	Lack of sleep may cause irritability, lethargy, decreased resistance to infection	Teaching regarding recommended amounts of sleep (12–14 h in first year, decreasing to 10–12 h by age 3); need for rituals to enhance the transition process to bedtime; possibility of need for nap; setting bedtime limits

MMR, measles, mumps, rubella; *HbCV*, hepatitis B conjugate vaccine; *DPT*, diptheria, pertussis, tetanus; *OPV*, oral polio vaccine.
Adapted From Wieczorek RR, Natapoff JN: A Conceptual Approach to the Nursing of Children: Health Care From Birth Through Adolescence. Philadelphia: JB Lippincott, 1981.

Parents need continual cautioning about the possibility of childhood poisoning. Even with precautionary labeling and packaging of medication and household cleaning supplies, children display amazing ingenuity in opening bottles and packages that catch their curiosity. Mr. Yuk labels are available from the nearest poison control center. The child can be taught that products are harmful if they have the Mr. Yuk label on them. However, labeling is not sufficient. All items that are in any way toxic to the child must be placed under lock and key or totally out of the child's reach.

The preventive measures should be observed by all caregivers of small children (see Parent Teaching: Tips for Prevention of Poisoning).

The following medications are most frequently involved in cases of childhood poisoning:

- Acetaminophen
- Salicylates—aspirin
- Laxatives
- Sedatives
- Tranquilizers
- Analgesics
- Antihistamines
- Cold medicines
- Birth control pills

The importance of careful, continuous supervision of toddlers and other young children cannot be overemphasized.

Teaching Oral Hygiene

Dental caries (cavities) constitute a major health problem among children and young adults. Although sound teeth depend in part on sound nutrition, the process of dental caries is linked to the effect of diet on the oral environment. Tooth decay is caused by bacteria that act in the

Parent Teaching

Parent Tips to Prevent Motor Vehicle Accidents

1. Never start the car until the child is securely in the car seat.

2. If the child manages to get out of the car seat or unfasten it, pull over to the curb or side of the road as soon as possible, turn off the car, and tell the child the car will not go until the child is safely in the seat. Children love to go in the car, and if they learn that they cannot go unless in the car seat, they will comply.

3. Never permit a child to stand in a car while it is in motion.

4. Teach the toddler to stop at a curb and wait for an adult escort to cross the street. An older child should be taught to look both ways for traffic. Start this as a game with toddlers, and continually reinforce it.

5. Teach the child to cross only at corners.

6. Begin in toddlerhood to teach awareness of traffic signals and the meaning. As soon as color recognition is achieved, the child can tell you when it is all right to cross.

7. Never let a child run into a street after a ball.

8. Teach child to never walk between parked cars to cross.

9. As a driver, always be on the alert for children running into the street when in a residential area.

presence of sugar and form a film, or dental **plaque**, on the teeth. People who eat sweet foods frequently accumulate plaque easily and are prone to dental caries. Sugars eaten at mealtime appear to be neutralized by the presence of other foods and therefore are not as damaging as between-meal sweets and bedtime bottles. Foods consisting of hard or sticky sugars, such as lollipops and caramels, that remain in the mouth for longer periods tend to cause more dental caries than those that are eaten quickly. Sugarless gum or candies are not as harmful.

When the child is about 2 years of age, he or she should be taught tooth brushing, or if brushing is not possible, to rinse the mouth after each meal or snack. Because this is the period in which the toddler likes to imitate others, the child is best taught by example. Plain water should be used until the child has learned how to spit out toothpaste or toothpowder. The caretaker should also brush the toddler's teeth until the child becomes experienced. One good method is to stand behind the child in front of a mirror and brush the child's teeth. In addition to cleaning adequately, this also helps the child learn how it feels to have the teeth thoroughly brushed.

In communities where the water is not fluoridated, the use of a fluoride toothpaste strengthens tooth enamel and helps prevent tooth decay. Supervision in using fluoride toothpaste is desirable, keeping the amount of toothpaste used to a small pea-sized amount. Supplemental fluoride may be recommended by the physician; however, this can be an added cost to those on limited incomes. A fluoride supplement is a medication and should be treated and stored as such. Fluoride also can be applied during regular visits to the dentist, but the greatest benefit to the tooth enamel occurs before the eruption of the teeth.

The first visit to the dentist should occur at about this same time, just to get acquainted with the dentist, including the staff and office. A second visit might be a good time for a preliminary examination, and subsequent visits twice a year for checkups are recommended. If there are older siblings, the toddler can go along on a visit with them to help overcome the fears of a strange setting. Some clinics are recommending earlier visits to check the child and give dietary guidance. Children of low-income families often have poor dental hygiene and care, both because of the cost of care and parental lack of knowledge about proper care and nutrition. Some families may believe it is not necessary to take proper care of baby teeth because "they just fall out anyway." Nurses have a great responsibility to teach and guide these families.

Parent Teaching

Tips to Prevent Burns

1. Do not let electrical cords dangle over a counter or table. Repair cords if frayed. Newer small appliances have shorter cords to prevent dangling.

2. Cover electrical wall outlets with safety caps.

3. Turn handles of pans on the stove toward the back of the stove. If possible, place pans on back burners out of the toddler's reach.

4. Place cups of hot liquid out of reach. Do not use overhanging tablecloths that toddlers can pull.

5. Use caution when serving foods heated in the microwave—they can be hotter than apparent.

6. Supervise small children at all times while in the bathtub, so they cannot turn on the hot water tap.

7. Turn thermostat on home water heater down so that water temperature is no higher than 120°F.

8. Place matches in metal containers, out of reach of small children. Keep lighters out of reach of children.

9. Never leave small children unattended by an adult or responsible teenager.

Parent Teaching

Tips for Prevention of Poisoning

1. Keep medicines in original containers in a locked cupboard. Do not rely on a high shelf being out of a child's reach.

2. Never refer to medicines as candy.

3. Discard unused medicines by a method that eliminates any possibility of access by children, other persons, or animals (eg, flush them down the toilet).

4. Replace safety caps properly, but do not depend on them to be childproof. Children can sometimes open them easier than adults.

5. Keep a bottle of syrup of ipecac in a locked cupboard to induce vomiting if needed.

6. Keep the telephone number of the nearest poison control center posted near the telephone.

7. Keep a chart with emergency treatment for poisoning in a handy permanent spot.

8. Store household cleaning and laundry products out of reach of children.

9. Never put kerosene or other household fluids in soda bottles or other drink containers.

Toilet Training

Learning control of the bowel and bladder is an important part of the socialization process. In Western culture, a great sense of shame and disgust has been associated with body waste products. To function successfully in this culture, one must learn to dispose of body waste products in a place considered proper by society.

The toddler has been operating on the pleasure principle, simply emptying the bowel and bladder when the urge is present without any thought of anything but personal comfort. During toilet training, the child, who is just learning about control of the personal environment, finds that some of that control must be given up to please those most important people, the parent or family caregivers. The toddler must now learn to conform not only to please those special loved ones but, to preserve self-integrity, must persuade himself or herself that this acceptance of the dictates of society is voluntary. These new routines make little sense to the child.

Timing

To be able to cooperate in toilet training, the child's sphincter muscles must have developed to the stage at which the child can control them. Control of the rectal sphincter develops first. The child also must be able to postpone the urge to defecate until reaching the toilet or potty and must be able to signal the need *before* the event. This level of maturation seldom takes place before the age of 18 to 24 months.

At the start of training, the child has no understanding of the uses of the potty chair but, to please the parent, the child will sit there for a short time. If the child's bowel movements occur at approximately the same time every day, one day a bowel movement will occur while sitting on the potty. Although there is no sense of special achievement as yet, the child does like the praise and approval. Eventually, connection of this approval with the bowel movement in the potty occurs and the child will be happy that the parent is pleased.

Suggestions for Bowel Training

1. A potty chair in which a child can comfortably sit with his or her feet on the floor is preferable. Most small children are afraid of a flush toilet.

2. The child should be left on the potty chair for only a short time. The caregiver should be readily available but should not hover anxiously over the child. If a bowel movement occurs, approval is in order; if not, no comment is necessary.

3. During the beginning stages of training, the child is likely to have a movement soon after leaving the potty. This is not willful defiance and need not be mentioned.

4. The potty should be emptied unobtrusively after the child has resumed playing. The child has cooperated and produced the product desired. If it is immediately thrown away, the child may be confused and not so eager to please the next time.

5. The ability to feel shame and self-doubt appears at this age. Therefore, the child should not be teased about reluctance or inability to conform. This teasing can shake the child's confidence and cause feelings of doubt in self-worth.

6. The caregiver should not expect perfection, even after control has been achieved. Lapses inevitably occur, perhaps because the child is completely absorbed in play (Figure 10-3) or because of a temporary episode of loose stools. Occasionally, a child feels aggression, frustration, or anger and may use this method to "get even." As long as the lapses are occasional, they should be ignored. If the lapses are frequent and persistent, the cause should be sought.

Bladder Training

Generally, the first indication of readiness for bladder training is when the child makes a connection between

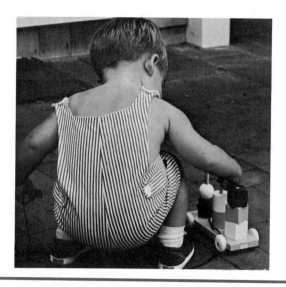

Figure 10-3. The 2-year-old child is capable of complete absorption in play and may forget or ignore the signals of a full bowel or bladder. (Photo by Carol Baldwin.)

the puddle on the floor with something he or she did. In the next stage, the child runs to the parent or caretaker and indicates a need to urinate but only after it has happened.

Not until there is sufficient maturity to control the bladder sphincter and reach the desired place is there much benefit to be gained from a serious program of training. When the child stays dry for about 2 hours at a time during the day, sufficient maturity may be indicated.

Each child follows an individual pattern of development. No parent needs to feel embarrassed or ashamed because the child is still having accidents. No one should expect the child to accomplish self-training, and family caregivers should be alert to the signs of readiness. Patience and understanding by the caregivers are essential. Complete control, especially at night, may not be achieved until the fourth or fifth year of age. Each child should be taught a term or phrase to use for toileting that is recognizable to others, clearly understood, and socially acceptable. This is especially true for children who are cared for outside the home.

Psychosocial Development

The toddler develops a growing awareness of self as a being, separate from other people or objects. Intoxicated with newly discovered powers and lacking experience, the child tends to test personal independence to the limit. This age has been called an age of **negativism**. Certainly the toddler's response to nearly everything is a firm "no," but this is more an assertion of individuality than of an intention to disobey. Ritualism, dawdling, and temper tantrums also characterize this age.

Ritualism is a practice employed by the young child to help develop security. A certain routine must be followed, making rituals of simple tasks. At bedtime, all toys must be in accustomed places, and the caregiver must follow a habitual practice. This passion for a set routine is not found in every child to the same degree, but it does provide a comfortable base from which to step out into new and potentially dangerous paths. These practices often become more evident when a sitter is in the home, especially at bedtime. This gives the child some measure of security when the primary caregiver is absent.

Dawdling serves much the same purpose. The young child has to decide between following the wishes and routines of the parent or caregiver and asserting independence by following personal desires. Being incapable of making such a choice, the toddler compromises and tries both. If the matter is of any importance, the caregiver should help the child to follow along the way to go, in a firm and friendly manner, otherwise dawdling can be ignored within reasonable limits.

Temper tantrums spring from frustrations. The child's urge to be independent naturally results in many frustrations. Add to this the fact that the child is reluctant to leave the scene for necessary rest, and one can see that frequently the frustrations become too great. Even the best of parents or caregivers may lose patience, showing a temporary lack of understanding. The child reacts with enthusiastic rebellion, but this, too, is a phase that must be lived through while working toward becoming a person.

Reasoning with the child, scolding, or punishing during the tantrum is useless. A trusted person needs to be nearby who remains calm and patient until the child gains self-control. After the tantrum is over, it is best to help the child relax by diverting attention with a toy or some other interesting distraction but not yielding the point or giving in to the child's whim. That would tell the child that to get whatever one wants, one needs only to throw oneself on the floor and scream. The child would have to learn, painfully, later in life that one cannot control others in this manner.

Admittedly it is not easy to handle a small child who drops to the floor screaming and kicking in rage in the middle of the supermarket or the sidewalk nor are comments from onlookers at all helpful. The best a caregiver can do is pick up the out-of-control child as calmly as possible and carry the child to a quiet, neutral place to regain self-control. These tantrums can be accompanied by head-banging and breath-holding. Breath-holding can be frightening to the caregiver, but the child will shortly lose consciousness and begin breathing. Head-banging can cause injury to the child, so the caregiver needs to provide protection. Calmness should be employed by the caregiver of a toddler having a tantrum. The child is out of control and needs help to regain control; the adult must maintain self-control to reassure the child and provide security.

Play

The play of the toddler moves from the solitary play of the infant to **parallel play** in which the toddler plays alongside other children but not with them (Figure 10-4). Much of the play time is filled with imitation of those people the child sees as role models: adults around him or her, siblings, and other children. Toys, such as push-pull toys, rocking horses, large blocks, and balls, that involve the new gross motor skills of the toddler are popular. Fine motor skills are developed by use of thick crayons, play dough, finger paints, wooden puzzles with large pieces, toys that fit pieces into shaped holes, and cloth books. The toddler enjoys "talking" on a play telephone and likes pots, pans, and toys such as brooms, dishes, and lawnmowers that help in imitating the adults in the child's environment, promoting socialization. The toddler is not able to share toys until the later stage of toddlerhood. Adults should not make an issue of sharing at this early stage.

Toys should be carefully checked for loose pieces and sharp edges to ensure the toddler's safety. Toddlers still put a lot of things into their mouths, therefore small pieces that may come loose, such as small beads and buttons, must be avoided.

For an adult, just staying quietly on the sidelines, observing and listening to the toddler play, can be a fascinating revelation of what is going on in the child's world.

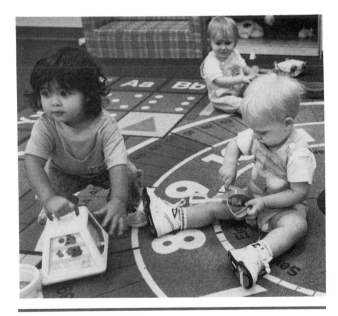

Figure 10-4. Toddlers engaged in parallel play. (From Castiglia PT, Harbin RE. Child Health Care: Process and Practice. Philadelphia: JB Lippincott, 1992.)

Discipline

The word discipline has come to mean punishment to many people. The concepts are not the same. **Discipline** means to train or instruct to produce a particular behavior pattern, especially moral or mental improvement, and self-control. **Punishment** means to penalize for wrongdoing. Although all small children need discipline, the need for punishment occurs much less frequently.

The toddler learns self-control gradually. The development from an egotistic being, whose world exists only to give self-satisfaction, into a person who understands and respects the rights of others is a long, involved process. The child cannot do this alone but must be taught.

Two-year-old children begin to show some signs of accepting responsibility for their own actions, but because of their egocentricity, they lack inner controls. The toddler still wants the forbidden thing but may repeat "no, no, mustn't" while reaching for a desired treasure, recognizing the act is not approved. Although the child understands the act is not approved, the desire is too strong to resist. Even at this age, children want and need limits. With no limits set, the child develops a feeling of insecurity and fear. With proper guidance, the child gradually absorbs the restraints and develops self-control or conscience.

Consistency and timing are important in the approach that the caregiver uses when disciplining the child. Those people caring for the child should agree on the methods of discipline and should be consistent. This need for consistency can cause disagreement for family caregivers who have experienced different types of childrearing themselves. The toddler needs a lot of help during this time. The caregivers may be confused by this child who had been a sweet, loving baby that has now turned into a belligerent little being who throws tantrums at will. This period can be challenging to adults. The child needs to learn that the adults are in control and will help the child gain self-control while learning to be independent. When the toddler hits or bites another child, the offender should be calmly removed from the situation. Negative messages, such as "You are a bad boy for hitting Mario" or "Bad girl—you don't bite people," are not helpful. Instead, messages that do not label the child as bad but label the act as unacceptable should be used (eg, "Biting hurts—be gentle"). Another method that can be used with a child who is not cooperating or who is out of control is to send the child to a "time out" chair. This should be a place where the child can be alone, but observed, without other distractions. The duration of the isolation should be limited—1 minute per year of age is usually adequate. The child should be warned in advance of this possibility, but only one warning per event is necessary. Children should be praised for good behavior and, when possible, the negative behavior can be ignored.

One of the most important points to remember is that the adults should all operate by the same rules, so that the child knows what is expected. Spanking or other physical punishment usually does not work well because the child is merely taught that hitting or other physical violence is acceptable, and the child who is spanked frequently becomes immune to it.

Sharing with a Sibling

The first child has the parents' undivided attention until a new baby arrives, frequently in the first child's toddlerhood. It is difficult to prepare a child just emerging from babyhood for this arrival. Although the toddler can feel the mother's abdomen and understand that this is where the new baby lives, it does not give adequate preparation for the baby's arrival. This real baby represents a rival for the mother's affection.

As in many stressful situations, the toddler frequently regresses to more infantile behavior. The toddler who no longer takes milk from a bottle may need or want a bottle when the new baby is being fed. Toilet-training, which may have been moving along well, may regress, with the toddler having episodes of soiling and wetting.

The new infant creates considerable change in the home, whether he or she is the first child or the fifth. In homes in which the previous baby is being displaced by the newcomer, however, some preparation is necessary. Moving the older child to a larger bed some time before the new baby appears lets the toddler take pride in being "grown up" now. Preparation of the toddler for a new brother or sister is helpful but should not be intense until just before the expected birth. Many hospitals have sibling classes for new siblings-to-be planned to occur shortly before the anticipated delivery. These classes geared to the young child give the child some tasks to do for the new baby and talk about the way the new baby will be, including negative as well as positive aspects of having a new baby in the home. Many books are available for the parent to use to help prepare the young child for birth and that also talk about sibling rivalry.

Probably the greatest help in preparing the child of any age to accept the new baby is to help the child feel that this is "our baby," not just "mommy's" baby (Figure 10-5). Helping to care for the baby according to the child's ability contributes to a feeling of continuing importance and self-worth.

The displaced toddler almost certainly will feel some jealousy. With careful planning, however, the mother can reserve some time for cuddling and playing with the toddler just as before. Perhaps the toddler may profit from a little extra parental attention for a time. The toddler needs to feel that parental love is just as great as ever and there is plenty of room in their lives for both children.

The child should not be made to grow up too soon. The parents should not shame or reprove the toddler for

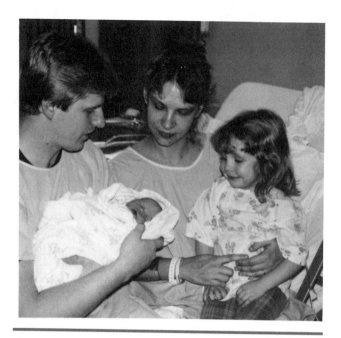

Figure 10-5. This toddler is meeting her new baby sister.

reverting to babyish behavior but try to be understanding and give the sibling a bit more love and attention. Perhaps the father or other family member can occasionally take over the care of the new baby while the mother devotes herself to the toddler. The mother also may plan special times with the toddler when the new infant is sleeping and she has no interruptions. This approach helps the toddler feel special.

Implications for Hospital Care

Although hospitalization is difficult and frightening for a child of any age, the developmental stage of the toddler intensifies these problems. The nurse caring for the toddler must keep in mind the developmental tasks and needs of the toddler when planning care. The toddler, engaged in trying to establish self-control and autonomy, finds that strangers seem to have total control, eliminating any control on the part of the child. Add these fears to the inability to communicate well, discomfort from pain, separation from family, unfamiliar people and surroundings, physical restraint, and uncomfortable or frightening procedures and the reaction of the toddler is clearly understood.

As part of the admission procedure for the child, a social assessment survey should be completed by interviewing the family caregiver who has accompanied the child to the hospital. Usually part of the standard pediatric nursing assessment form, the social assessment covers eating habits and food preferences, toileting habits and terms used for toileting, family members and the names the child calls them, the name the child is called by family members, pets and their names, favorite toys, sleeping or napping patterns and rituals, and other significant data and helps the staff better plan care for the toddler (see Figure 2-3 in Chapter 2). This information should become an indispensable part of the nursing care plan. Using this information, the nurse should develop a nursing care plan that provides opportunities for independence for the toddler whenever possible.

Separation anxiety is high during the toddler age. As discussed in detail in Chapter 2, the stages of protest and despair are commonplace. The nurse must acknowledge these stages and communicate to the child that feeling angry and anxious at the separation from the person (parent or primary family caregiver) foremost in the child's life is accepted. The nurse must *never* interpret the toddler's angry protest as a personal attack. Many hospitals encourage family involvement in the care of the child to minimize the separation anxiety. The mother is frequently the family member who stays with the child, but in many families other members who are close to the child may take turns staying. Having a parent or family caregiver with the toddler can be extremely helpful. Nurses must be cautious, however, not to neglect caring for the toddler who has a loved one present. In addition, many children come from families in which a family caregiver is not able to stay with the child for any of a number of reasons. These children need extra attention and care. All children should be assigned a constant caregiver while in the hospital, but this is especially important for the toddler who is alone.

The nurse assigned to the toddler will become a surrogate parent while caring for the child. Maintaining, as much as possible, the pattern, schedule, and rituals that the toddler is used to helps provide some measure of security to the child. This is a time when the toddler needs the security of a beloved thumb, or other "lovey." The nurse needs to recognize that importance of this means that the toddler uses to provide self-comfort. The lovey, a favorite stuffed animal or blanket, may be well worn and dirty, but the toddler finds great reassurance in having it to snuggle or cuddle. No one should ridicule the child for its unkempt appearance. Every effort should be made to allow the toddler to have it whenever desired. When the family caregiver has to leave the toddler, it may be helpful for the adult to give the child some personal item to keep until the adult returns and tell the child they will return "when the cartoons come on TV" or "when your lunch comes." These are concrete times that the toddler will most likely understand.

Toilet Training

The toddler just learning sphincter control is still dependent on familiar surroundings and the family caregiver's support. For this reason, some pediatric personnel automatically put toddlers back in diapers when they are admitted; this practice should be discouraged. Under the right circumstances, and especially with the caregiver's help, many of these children can maintain control. They at least should be given a chance to try. Potty chairs can be provided for the child when appropriate. The nursing staff needs to understand the method and times of accomplishing toilet training that had been used in the home and try to comply with them as closely as possible in the hospital setting.

Communication

Communicating with the toddler requires the nurse to talk in terms that the child understands. Giving one direction or request at a time is necessary. The request or direction should be made as a positive statement and in a firm but friendly, matter-of-fact way. Rather than towering over the small child, the nurse should approach the child at the child's level. That is, the nurse should stoop, sit, or squat to get down to the toddler's eye level. Helping the toddler learn new words and praising for the use of new words are important ways to encourage development. The nurse also communicates with the toddler through nonverbal communications. Displaying a pleasant, soothing presence more likely communicates friendliness to the toddler than abrupt or quick actions do. Never ask a toddler a yes/no question if you are not willing to live with the answer. Toddlers should be given an opportunity to make choices, however. For example, instead of saying, "Do you want to eat now?" say "Would you like to eat in your room or in the playroom?"

Discipline

Discipline in the hospital setting can be perplexing at times. Children come to the hospital from many backgrounds with a great variety in the types of control (or lack of control) to which they are accustomed. The nurse must set some limits for the toddler but must be careful in doing so. This can be a time when the family caregiver and nursing personnel can share their expertise and knowledge about the child and normal growth and development. The toddler, as do children of any age, needs to feel that someone is in control and needs limits, but these limits must be set with love and understanding. A child who has been overindulged for a long time may need firm, calm statements of limits, delivered in a no-nonsense but kind manner. Explaining what is going to be done, what is expected of the toddler, and what the toddler can expect from the nurse may be helpful. Sometimes the nurse may have to give some tactful guidance to the family caregiver to help set some limits for the toddler. This is an area in which experience helps the nursing personnel solve difficult problems.

Eating Concerns

A toddler's eating habits may loom large in the nurse's mind as a potential problem. In the hospital, as at home, food can assume an importance out of all proportion to its value and create an unnecessary problem.

Eating Is a Social Activity

In some hospitals, the staff may tend to forget that in our culture, eating is a social activity. Many a toddler who sits in a crib playing with food would eat with gusto if placed in a high chair or at the table with peers. The way that meals are served depends partially on the physical set-up of the individual pediatric unit, but the nurse often can provide opportunities for company while eating even under limited circumstances. Some suggestions for avoiding eating problems are offered earlier in this chapter. Other approaches are as follows:

1. Some calculated neglect at mealtime often works wonders. Self-feeding should be encouraged. Hovering over the child, urging just one more bite, makes it irresistible for the toddler to say "no." If it appears to the toddler that eating or not makes no difference, there is no need to resist. The toddler can be influenced by the attractiveness of the food and the behavior of peers. An adult nearby eating in a businesslike manner also offers a helpful example. Permitting guest trays for the family caregiver may provide this opportunity. The nurse must remember, however, that caregivers may take a break only when going out for their own meal, therefore this solution may not always be best.

2. Serve the dessert along with the rest of the meal. It does not matter whether the child eats it first or last because hospital desserts for children are usually as nourishing as other foods.

3. If the child is accustomed to cultural foods, such as Mexican tortillas or Italian spaghetti, find out if the hospital will allow the mother or family caregiver to bring in these foods. A small child finds it particularly difficult to eat strange foods, especially when illness takes the appetite away. Family members need to be reminded that they must let the nursing staff know if they bring food into the hospital for the child so that the child's intake can be recorded.

Fluids

"Push fluids" is an order that is frequently difficult to carry out with a toddler. A small child cannot take much fluid at any one time, so persistence seems to be the answer. Fluids should be offered in a small cup or glass. Providing fluids such as juices and ices that are appealing to the child within the limitations of the diet can be helpful.

A tea party with small cups and a pot to pour from provides entertainment as well as fluid. Taking turns pouring prolongs the party until everyone has had a turn, including a favorite doll or teddy bear. The pot may need many fillings, but the fluid chart is going to look much better. Often a little imagination helps solve the problems of young children. The cooperation of the family caregiver may be helpful, but the caregiver should not have cause to feel that this is work that the nursing staff should be doing.

Safety

All activities must be approached with safety in mind. The toys that are provided for the toddler should be assessed for safety. Restraints should not be used to substitute for good nursing care but must be used when the toddler's safety is in question. When restraints are used, extra emotional care should be given and frequent observation of the restraints should be carried out. An area safe for the child to be permitted to move around freely is desirable. Safety in the hospital setting is discussed in detail in Chapter 2.

Summary

"It was the best of times, it was the worst of times" may well be a quote from a family caregiver of a toddler rather than a quote from Dickens' *A Tale of Two Cities*. Toddlers are delightful in their continuous exploring and adventuring into a new world. However, the drive for independence can be so intense and frustrating to all involved that the toddler and the family can seem to be at opposite ends of the world. The toddler is no longer a baby but is not very "grown up" either, extremely difficult 1 minute and totally lovable and loving the next. The ability to communicate, imitate, and imagine makes this a fascinating stage for parents and caregivers to observe. The ability to walk, run, and climb makes this stage potentially dangerous for the toddler, demanding continuous supervision by a responsible person. If family caregivers can summon sufficient patience and understanding to deal with the toddler's search for autonomy and the resulting frustration that leads into displays of temper that accompany that search, this time can be an especially close one for the family. Once the child begins to interact with people outside the family, in a nursery school or day care center, family influence is never again as strong.

The toddler's search for independence, with the need to frequently touch base to gain reassurance and security, causes traumatic reactions to hospitalization. The toddler's language skills are not developed enough for him or her to fully understand what is going on and so the toddler's feelings of anxiety increase. Nursing personnel must be acutely aware of the toddler's needs and plan care to provide for developmental progress. The toddler is truly an explorer in all aspects of life and must be encouraged, and at the same time he or she must be protected from harm.

Review Questions

1. Jeff is the father of 2½-year-old Shane. Shane likes to go to his daddy's workshop with him. What will you teach Jeff to help him make this a safe experience for Shane?
2. Marti complains to you that 2-year-old Sasha is very difficult to put to bed at night. Give Marti some tips that might help her make bedtime easier.
3. You are caring for 18-month-old Kyle. What information do you need to know from his family caregiver to help you plan nursing care for him? How will you gain this information?
4. You are at the supermarket with your 2-year-old niece, Deanna. Deanna has a temper tantrum because you have refused to buy her some cookies she wants. You are embarrassed by the scene she is making. What are you going to do?
5. Describe a typical bedtime routine for a toddler. In a class discussion, list as many bedtime rituals as you can.
6. Why is the toddler called an "explorer?"
7. Why do eating problems frequently occur during toddlerhood?
8. Give Holly, the teen mother of toddler Chris, some tips to help her solve her worries about Chris' eating habits.
9. You hear Mike, the father of 2-year-old Jed, complain that "Jed just stands there and wets himself instead of going to the pot." What guidance can you give him about toilet training a toddler that will help him?
10. Eighteen-month-old Jodi's grandparents are getting ready to keep her for a week. What guidance will you give them about making their house safe for her visit?
11. What do you consider good dental care for a toddler? What would you teach a family with a toddler about oral hygiene?
12. Why is a toddler exciting and fun to be around?

Bibliography

Brazelton TB. To Listen to a Child. New York: Addison-Wesley, 1984.

Brazelton TB. What Every Baby Knows. New York: Ballentine Books, 1987.

Castiglia PT, Harbin RE. Child Health Care: Process and Practice. Philadelphia: JB Lippincott, 1992.

Eschlemann MM. Introductory Nutrition and Diet Therapy, 2nd ed. Philadelphia: JB Lippincott, 1991.

Greenspan SI. Development and behavior: The very young child. Pediatr Clin North Am 38(6):1370–1383, 1991.

Pillitteri A. Maternal and Child Health Nursing. Philadelphia: JB Lippincott, 1992.

Schuster CS, Ashburn SS. The Process of Human Development, 3rd ed. Philadelphia: JB Lippincott, 1992.

Spock B, Rothenberg MB. Dr. Spock's Baby and Child Care. New York: Pocket Books, 1992.

Whaley LF, Wong DL. Nursing Care of Infants and Children, 4th ed. St. Louis: Mosby-Year Book, 1991.

Health Problems of the Toddler

Student Objectives

Upon completion of this chapter, the student will be able to:

1. Describe four characteristics of infantile autism.
2. Identify four goals of treatment of infantile autism.
3. Describe treatment for bacterial conjunctivitis.
4. Describe the diagnosis of celiac disease.
5. Describe the usual treatment for spasmodic laryngitis.
6. Discuss acute laryngotracheobronchitis, including the symptoms and treatment.
7. Identify the basic defect in cystic fibrosis.
8. State the major organs affected by cystic fibrosis.
9. Name the most frequent type of complication in cystic fibrosis.
10. List the diagnostic procedures used to diagnose cystic fibrosis.
11. Describe the dietary and pulmonary treatment of cystic fibrosis.
12. State the most common cause of poisoning that occurs in the toddler-age group.
13. List five common substances children ingest.
14. List seven sources of lead that may cause chronic lead poisoning.
15. Describe lead poisoning a.) Symptoms; b.) Diagnosis; c.) Treatment; d.) Prognosis.
16. Discuss the incidence of burns in small children.
17. State the three major causes of burns in small children.
18. Differentiate between first-, second-, and third-degree burns.
19. Describe emergency treatment of a a.) Minor burn. b.) Moderate or severe burn.
20. State why hypovolemic shock occurs in the first 48 hours after a burn.
21. Describe the treatment of a child who has swallowed a foreign object.

Marks MG: BROADRIBB'S INTRODUCTORY PEDIATRIC NURSING, 4th ed. © 1994 J.B. Lippincott Company.

Key Terms

achylia

allograft

amblyopia

autistic

autograft

binocular vision

cataract

celiac syndrome

chelating agent

conjunctivitis

contractures

coryza

croup

débridement

diplopia

dysphagia

echolalia

emetic

encephalopathy

eschar

esotropia

exotropia

external hordeolum

goniotomy

heterograft

homograft

hydrotherapy

hyperpnea

hypochylia

hypovolemia

lacrimation

orthoptics

photophobia

pica

steatorrhea

strabismus

stridor

sympathetic ophthalmia

*C*hildren from ages 1 to 3 years are likely to have a number of minor health problems, many of them caused by infection or environmental hazards. Most of these health problems can be managed at home after a visit to the pediatrician's office or clinic. Some of the problems, however, are serious enough to require hospitalization, thus separating the toddler from his or her family caregivers. This separation increases the seriousness of the health problem and the need for loving and understanding attention to the child's emotional needs as well as physical condition.

Psychological Problems

Infantile Autism

Although called *infantile* because it is thought to be present from birth, autism usually is not conclusively diagnosed until after 12 months of age. The word *autism* comes from the Greek word *auto* meaning "self" and was first used by Dr. Leo Kanner in 1943 to describe a group of behavioral symptoms in children. The term *pervasive developmental disorder* was introduced in 1980 when the terminology was revised by the American Psychiatric Association. Disorders in this category are characterized by severe behavioral disturbance that affects the practical use of language as a means of communication, interpersonal interaction, attention, perception, and motor activity. **Autistic** children are totally self-centered and unable to relate to others, often exhibit bizarre behaviors, and often are destructive to themselves and others.

Autism occurs in 1 in 2500 births and twice as often in males as in females. Several theories exist about its cause as well as its treatment or management. Originally thought to result from an unsatisfactory early mother–child relationship (emotionally cold, detached mothers, sometimes described as "refrigerator mothers"), autism now appears to have organic, and perhaps genetic, causes instead. Researchers suggest that autism may result from a disturbance in language comprehension, a biochemical problem involving neurotransmitters, or from abnormalities in the central nervous system, probably brain metabolism. These children score poorly on intelligence tests but have good memories and good intellectual potential.

Because the cause of autism is not understood, treatment attempts have met with limited success. These children experience the normal health problems of childhood in addition to those that result from their behaviors. Therefore, it is important that nurses understand this unexplained disorder and how it affects children and families.

Characteristics

The American Psychiatric Association lists 16 characteristics of autism divided into the following three categories:

1. Qualitative impairment in reciprocal social interaction (inability to relate to others)
2. Qualitative impairment in verbal and nonverbal communication and imagination (inability to communicate with others)
3. Markedly restricted repertoire of activities and interests.[1]

To diagnose infantile autism, eight characteristics must be identified, and all three categories must be represented.

Children with autism do not develop a smiling response to others or an interest in being touched or cuddled. In fact, they can react violently at attempts to hold them. Their blank expressions and lack of response to verbal stimulation can suggest deafness. They do not show the normal fear of separation from parents that most toddlers exhibit. Often they seem not to notice when family caregivers are present.

During their second year, autistic children become completely absorbed in strange repetitive behaviors, such as spinning an object, flipping an electrical switch on and off, or walking around the room feeling the walls. Their bodily movements are bizarre: rocking, twirling, flapping arms and hands, walking on tip-toe, twisting and turning fingers. If these movements are interrupted, or if objects in the environment are moved, a violent temper tantrum may result. These tantrums may include self-destructive acts such as hand biting and head banging.

Although infants and toddlers normally are self-centered, ritualistic, and prone to displays of temper, autistic children show these characteristics to an extreme degree, coupled with an almost total lack of response to other people.

The autistic child is slow to develop speech, and any that does develop is primitive and ineffective in its ability to communicate. **Echolalia** ("parrot speech") is typical of autistic children; they echo words they have heard, such as a television commercial, but offer no indication that they understand the words. Although autistic children are self-centered, their speech indicates that they seem to have no sense of self because they never use the pronouns "I" or "me."

Standard intelligence tests that count on verbal ability usually indicate that these children are mentally deficient. However, many of these children also demonstrate unusual memory and mathematic, artistic, and musical abilities.

Diagnosis

The symptoms of autism can suggest other disorders such as lead poisoning, phenylketonuria, congenital rubella, and measles encephalitis. Therefore, a complete pediatric physical and neurologic examination is necessary, including vision and hearing testing, electroencephalography, radiographic studies of the skull, urine screening, and other laboratory studies. In addition, the nurse usually takes a complete prenatal, natal, and postnatal history, including development, nutrition, and family dynamics. Other members of the health team may be involved in the evaluation and treatment of the autistic child, including audiologists, psychiatrists, psychologists, special education teachers, speech and language therapists, and social workers.

Treatment

The treatment of an autistic child is extremely challenging. The child is mentally retarded but may demonstrate exceptional talent in areas such as factual memory and art or music. Four goals toward which treatment is geared are:

- Promotion of normal development
- Specific language development
- Social interaction
- Learning

The treatment must be individually planned and is highly structured. Behavioral modification techniques are often used. The family needs therapy to help relieve guilt and help them understand this puzzling child. The overall long-term prognosis for these children is not optimistic, but the earlier treatment is started, the better the long-term outlook is. Researchers are working with language development of autistic children by aiding them to express themselves in language through use of a computer keyboard. This method needs further study to determine its validity.

Nursing Care

Caring for the autistic child means recognizing that autism creates great stresses for the entire family. The problems that cause family caregivers to seek diagnosis are difficult to live with; diagnosis itself is usually a lengthy and expensive process, and the hope for successful treatment is slight. Most caregivers of autistic children feel guilty, despite the fact that current theories accept organic rather than psychological causes for this disorder. The possibility of genetic factors adds to this guilt. Often, there are other children in the family who are normal but who suffer from a lack of attention because the caregivers' energies are almost totally directed to solving the problems of the autistic youngster.

Nurses who care for these children in a hospital setting should consider the family caregivers their most valuable source of information about the child's habits and communication skills. A private or semiprivate room is generally preferred; visual and auditory stimulation should be minimized. Familiar toys or other valued objects from home reduce the child's anxiety about the strange environment. The nurse needs to learn what techniques have been used by the caregivers to communicate with the child and gain his or her cooperation. Establishing a relationship of trust between the child and the nurse is essential. This child should be cared for by a constant primary nurse to provide consistency.

Sensory Disorders

Eye Conditions

Cataracts

A **cataract** is a development of opacity in the crystalline lens that prevents light rays from entering the eye. Congenital cataracts may be hereditary, or they may be complications of maternal rubella during the first trimester of pregnancy. Cataracts also may develop later in infancy or childhood from eye injury or from metabolic disturbances, such as galactosemia and diabetes.

Surgical extraction of the cataracts is performed at an early age. With early removal, the prognosis for good vision is improved. The infant or child is fitted with contact lens, and if only one eye is affected, the "good" eye is patched to prevent amblyopia (see discussion in the section on strabismus). Numerous lens changes will be needed to change the strength as the child gets older.

Glaucoma

Glaucoma may be of the congenital infantile type, occurring in children younger than 3 years of age; juvenile glaucoma, showing clinical manifestations after the age of 3; or secondary glaucoma, resulting from injury or disease. Increased intraocular pressure due to overproduction of aqueous fluid causes the eyeball to enlarge and the cornea to become large, thin, and sometimes cloudy. Untreated, the disease slowly progresses to blindness. Pain may be present. **Goniotomy** (surgical opening into Schlemm's canal), which provides drainage of the aqueous humor, is effective in relieving intraocular pressure in many instances. Goniotomy may need to be performed multiple times to control intraocular pressure. Surgery is performed as early as possible to prevent permanent damage.

Strabismus

Strabismus is the failure of the two eyes to direct their gaze at the same object simultaneously, commonly called "squint" or "crossed eyes." **Binocular** (normal) **vision** is maintained through the muscular coordination of eye movements, so that a simple vision results. In strabismus, the visual axes are not parallel, and **diplopia** (double vision) results. In an effort to avoid seeing two images, the child's central nervous system suppresses vision in the deviant eye, causing a condition of **amblyopia** (dimness of vision from disuse of the eye), sometimes called "lazy eye."

A wide variation in the manifestation of strabismus exists; there are lateral, vertical, and mixed lateral and vertical types. There may be monocular strabismus, in which one eye deviates while the other eye is used, or alternating strabismus, in which deviation alternates from one eye to the other. The term **esotropia** is used when the eye deviates toward the other eye; **exotropia** denotes a turning away from the other eye (Figure 11-1).

Treatment depends on the type of strabismus present. In monocular strabismus, occlusion of the better eye by patching to force the use of the deviating eye should be initiated at an early age. Patching will be continued for weeks or months. The younger the child, the more rapid the improvement. The patching may be for set periods or continuous, depending on the age of the child. The older child needs continuous periods of patching, whereas the younger one may respond quickly to short periods of patching. The child should be stimulated to use the unpatched eye by occupations such as puzzles, drawing, sewing, and similar activities.

Glasses can correct a refractive error if amblyopia is not present. **Orthoptics** (therapeutic ocular muscle exercises) to improve the quality of vision may be prescribed to supplement the use of glasses or surgery.

Surgery on the eye muscle to correct the defect is necessary for those children who do not respond to glasses and exercises. Many children need surgery after amblyopia has been corrected. Early detection and treatment of strabismus is essential for a successful outcome. The correction is believed to be necessary before the child reaches 6 years of age, or the visual damage may be

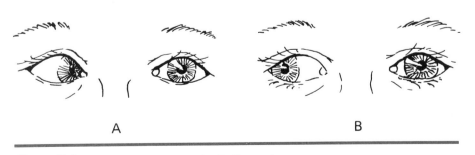

A   B

Figure 11-1. Strabismus. **A**, Esotropia. **B**, Exotropia.

permanent; however, some authorities believe that correction can be successful even up to the age of 10 years.[2]

Eye Injury and Foreign Objects in the Eye

Eye injuries are fairly common, particularly in older children. Ecchymosis of the eye (black eye) is of no great importance unless the eyeball is involved. A penetrating wound of the eyeball is potentially serious—BB shots in particular are dangerous—and requires the attention of an ophthalmologist. With any history of an injury, a thorough examination of the entire eye is necessary.

Sympathetic ophthalmia may follow perforation wounds of the globe, even if the perforations are small. **Sympathetic ophthalmia** is an inflammatory reaction of the uninjured eye, which often includes **photophobia** (intolerance of light), **lacrimation** (secretion of tears), pain, and some dimness of vision. The retina may finally become detached, and atrophy of the eyeball may occur. Prompt and skillful treatment at the time of the injury is essential to avoid involvement of the other eye.

Small foreign objects, such as specks of dust, that have lodged inside the eyelid may be removed by rolling the lid back and exposing the object. Cotton-tipped applicators should not be used for this purpose because of the danger of sudden movement and of possible perforation of the eye. If the object cannot be easily removed with a small piece of moistened cotton or soft clean cloth, or flushed out with a saline solution, the child should be taken to the physician.

Eye Infections

A condition called properly **external hordeolum**, but known commonly as a sty, is a purulent infection of the follicle of an eyelash, generally caused by *Staphylococcus aureus*. Localized swelling, tenderness, and pain are present, with a reddened lid edge. The maximum tenderness is over the infected site. The lesion progresses to suppuration, with eventual discharge of the purulent material. Warm saline compresses applied for about 15 minutes three or four times daily give some relief and hasten resolution, but recurrence is common. The sty should never be squeezed. Antibiotic ointment may help prevent accompanying conjunctivitis and recurrence.

Conjunctivitis is an acute inflammation of the conjunctiva. In children, conjunctivitis may be caused by a virus, bacteria, allergy, or foreign body. Conjunctivitis caused by bacteria is the most common type. The purulent drainage, a common characteristic, can be cultured to determine the causative organism. Bacterial conjunctivitis is treated with ophthalmic antibacterial agents such as erythromycin, bacitracin, sulfacetamide, and polymyxin because of the danger of contagion. Ointments blur vision, therefore drops usually are used during the day and ointments at night. Before applying medication, warm moist compresses can be used to remove the crusts that form on the eyes. The child who has bacterial conjunctivitis should be kept separate from other young children until the condition has been treated. Precautions, such as a separate wash cloth and towel and disposable tissues, are important to prevent spread of infection among family members.

Hospital Care for the Child Undergoing Eye Surgery

A person experiencing any kind of sensory deprivation may find it difficult to stay in touch with reality. A child whose eyes must be covered is particularly vulnerable. The implications of not being able to see are not always appreciated by nurses who have not themselves experienced this. A young child who wakens from surgery to total darkness may well go into a state of panic. Observation of the child returning from surgery may reveal the panic and anxiety as evidenced by trembling and nervousness. The child needs a family caregiver or close loved one to stay during the time when vision is restricted.

Preparation for the event should, of course, be carried out as well as it is possible to do so, but the small child has no experience to help in understanding what actually is going to happen. The darkness, pain, and total strangeness of the situation can be overwhelming.

Restraints should not be used indiscriminately, but most small children do need some reminder to keep their hands away from the sore eye, unless someone is beside them to prevent them from rubbing or from removing eye dressings. Elbow restraints are useful, although they do not prevent rubbing the eye with the arm. Flannel strips applied to the wrists in clove-hitch fashion can be tied to the cribsides in such a manner as to allow freedom of arm movement but to prevent the child from causing damage to the operative site.

To alert the child, the nurse should speak when approaching. The child does need tactile stimulation; therefore, after speaking, the nurse would do well to stroke or pat the child. If permitted, the nurse may hold the child for additional reassurance.

Gastrointestinal System Disorders

Celiac Syndrome

Intestinal malabsorption with **steatorrhea** (fatty stools) is a condition brought about by various causes, the most common being cystic fibrosis (CF) and gluten-induced enteropathy, the so-called idiopathic celiac disease. The term **celiac syndrome** is used to designate the complex of malabsorptive disorders.

Gluten-Induced Enteropathy

The idiopathic celiac disease is a basic defect of metabolism precipitated by the ingestion of wheat gluten or rye gluten, leading to impaired fat absorption. The exact cause is not known; the most acceptable theory is that of an inborn error of metabolism with an allergic reaction to the gliadin fraction of gluten (a protein factor in wheat) as a contributing or, possibly, the sole factor.

Severe manifestations of the disorder have become rare in the United States and in western Europe, but mild disturbances in intestinal absorption of rye, wheat, and sometimes oat gluten are common, occurring in about 1 in 2000 children.

Clinical Manifestations. Signs generally do not appear before the age of 6 months and may be delayed until the age of 1 year or later. Manifestations include chronic diarrhea with foul, bulky, greasy stools and progressive malnutrition. Anorexia and a fretful, unhappy disposition are typical. The onset is generally insidious, with failure to thrive, bouts of diarrhea, and frequent respiratory infections. If the condition becomes severe, the effects of malnutrition are prominent. Retarded growth and development, a distended abdomen, and thin, wasted buttocks and legs are characteristic symptoms (Figure 11-2).

The chronic course of this disease may be interrupted by a celiac crisis, an emergency situation. This frequently is triggered by an upper respiratory infection. The child commences to vomit copiously, has large, watery stools, and becomes severely dehydrated. As the child becomes drowsy and prostrate, an acute medical emergency develops. Parenteral fluid therapy is essential to combat acidosis and to achieve normal fluid balance.

Diagnosis and Treatment. Currently, the only way to determine if a small child's failure to thrive is caused by celiac disease is to initiate a trial gluten-free diet and to evaluate the results. Improvement in the nature of the stools and general well-being with a gain in weight should follow, although several weeks may elapse before clear-cut manifestations can be confirmed.

Response to a diet from which rye, wheat, and oats are excluded is generally good, although probably no cure can be expected, and dietary indiscretions or respiratory infections may bring relapses. The omission of wheat products, in particular, should continue through adolescence because the ingestion of wheat appears to inhibit growth in sensitive people.

Dietary Program. The young child is usually started on a starch-free, low-fat diet. If the condition is severe, this consists of skim milk, glucose, and banana flakes. Bananas contain invert sugar and are usually well tolerated. Additions to the diet of lean meats, pureed vegetables, and fruits are made gradually. Eventually, fats may be added, and the child can be maintained on a regular diet with the exception of all wheat and rye products.

Commercially canned creamed soups, cold cuts, frankfurters, and pudding mixes generally contain wheat products. The forbidden list also includes malted milk drinks, some candies, many baby foods, and of course, breads, cakes, pastries, and biscuits, unless the latter are made from corn flour or corn meal. It is important for

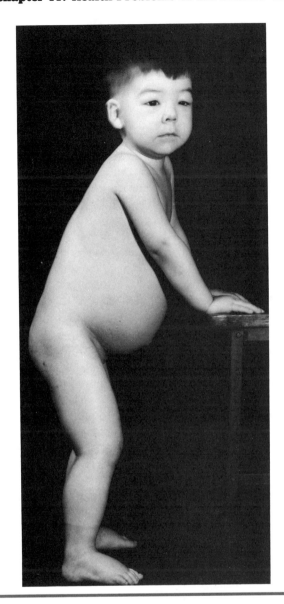

Figure 11-2. A child with celiac disease. Notice the protruding abdomen.

caregivers to read the list of ingredients on packaged foods carefully before purchasing anything. Vitamins A and D in water-miscible solutions are needed in double amounts to supplement the deficient diet.

Respiratory System Disorders

Croup

Croup is not a disease but a general term that typically exhibits symptoms of a barking cough, hoarseness, and inspiratory **stridor** (shrill, harsh respiratory sound). The disorders are named for the respiratory structures that are involved. For instance, acute laryngotracheobronchitis affects the larynx, trachea, and major bronchi.

Spasmodic Laryngitis

Spasmodic laryngitis occurs in children between the ages of 1 and 3 years. The cause is undetermined; it may be of infectious or of allergic origin, but certain children seem to develop severe laryngospasm with little, if any, apparent cause. The attack may be preceded by **coryza** (runny nose) and hoarseness or by no apparent signs of respiratory irregularity during the evening. The child awakens after a few hours of sleep with a barklike cough, increasing respiratory difficulty, and stridor. The child becomes anxious and restless, and there is marked hoarseness. There may be a low-grade fever and mild upper respiratory infection.

This condition is not serious but is frightening, both to the child and the family. The episode subsides after a few hours; little evidence remains the next day when an anxious caregiver takes the child to the physician. Attacks frequently occur two or three nights in succession.

Treatment. Humidified air is helpful in reducing the laryngospasm. Taking the child into the bathroom and opening the hot water taps, with the door closed, is a quick method for providing moist air—provided that the water runs hot enough. The physician may prescribe an **emetic** (an agent that causes vomiting), such as syrup of ipecac, in a dosage less than that needed to produce vomiting, which usually gives relief by helping to reduce spasms of the larynx. Humidifiers may be used in the child's bedroom to provide high humidity. Cool humidifiers are recommended, but vaporizers may be used. If a vaporizer is used, caution must be taken to place it away from the child's reach to protect the child from danger of being burned. Cool-mist humidifiers can be purchased and provide safe humidity. Humidifiers and vaporizers need to be cleaned regularly to prevent growth of undesirable organisms. Sometimes the spasm is relieved by exposure to cold air, for instance, when the child is taken out into the night to go to the emergency department or to see the physician.

Acute Laryngotracheobronchitis

Laryngeal infections are common in small children, and they often involve tracheobronchial areas as well. Acute laryngotracheobronchitis (bacterial tracheitis or laryngotracheobronchitis) may progress rapidly and become a serious problem within a matter of hours. The toddler is the most frequently affected member of the 1- to 4-year age group. This condition is usually of viral origin, but bacterial invasion, most frequently staphylococcal, follows the original infection. It generally occurs after an upper respiratory infection with fairly mild rhinitis and pharyngitis.

The child develops hoarseness and a barking cough, with a fever that may reach 104°F (40°C) or 105°F (40.6°C). As the disease progresses, marked laryngeal edema occurs, and the child's breathing becomes difficult; the pulse is rapid, and cyanosis may appear. Congestive heart failure and acute respiratory embarrassment can result.

Treatment. The major goal of treatment for acute laryngotracheobronchitis is to maintain an airway and adequate air exchange followed by antimicrobial therapy. The child is placed in a supersaturated atmosphere, such as that obtained in a croupette or some other kind of mist tent that also can include the administration of oxygen. Racemic epinephrine (Vaponefrin) may be administered by means of a nebulizer to effect bronchodilation, usually by a respiratory therapist. Rapid improvement may be seen because of vasoconstriction, but the child must be carefully watched for reappearance of symptoms. Nebulization is usually administered every 3 or 4 hours. The use of nebulization frequently produces relief, but if necessary, intubation with a nasotracheal tube may be performed for a child with severe distress unrelieved by other measures. Tracheostomies, once performed frequently, are rarely performed because intubation is preferred. Antibiotics are administered parenterally initially and continued after the fever has returned to a more normal range.

Close and careful observation of the child is important. Observation includes checking the pulse, respirations, color, listening for hoarseness and stridor, and noting any state of restlessness that indicates an impending respiratory crisis. Pulse oximetry is used to determine the degree of hypoxia.

Epiglottitis

Epiglottitis is acute inflammation of the epiglottis (the cartilaginous flap that protects the opening of the larynx). Commonly caused by the *Hemophilus influenzae* type B, it most often affects children between 2 and 7 years of age. The epiglottis becomes inflamed and swollen with edema. The edema decreases the ability of the epiglottis to move freely, which results in blockage of the airway, creating an emergency.

The child may have been well or may have had a mild upper respiratory infection before the development of a sore throat, **dysphagia** (difficulty swallowing), and a high fever of 39°C to 40°C (102.2 to 104°F). The dysphagia may cause drooling. *A tongue blade should never be used to initiate a gag reflex because complete obstruction may occur.* The child is very anxious, preferring to sit up, leaning forward to breathe. Immediate emergency attention is necessary.

The child may need endotracheal intubation or a tracheostomy if the epiglottis is so swollen that intubation cannot be performed. Moist air is necessary to help reduce the inflammation of the epiglottis. Pulse oximetry is required to evaluate oxygen requirements. Antibiotics are administered intravenously. After 24 to 48 hours of antibiotic therapy, the child may be extubated. Antibiotics are continued for the customary 10 days. Although this condition does not occur frequently, it is an extremely frightening condition for the child and the family.

Nursing Process of the Young Child with an Upper Respiratory Disorder

ASSESSMENT

A thorough interview is conducted with the caregiver, which includes the standard information needed as well as specific information, such as when the symptoms were first noticed, if the child has had fever, a description of respiratory difficulties, signs of hoarseness, the character of any cough, and any other information that can be determined about the condition.

The nurse must conduct a physical assessment of temperature, pulse, observing respiratory effort that includes a visual examination of the accessory muscles, lung sounds, signs of impending respiratory obstruction, observing circumoral pallor, cyanotic nail beds, irritability, or mental confusion. If the child is old enough to communicate verbally, the nurse should ask the child questions to determine how the child feels.

NURSING DIAGNOSES

The nursing diagnoses depend on the assessment of the child and the severity of the respiratory distress. The following nursing diagnoses are among those that may be appropriate:

- High risk for ineffective airway clearance related to obstruction associated with edema and mucus secretions of the upper airway
- High risk for fluid volume deficit related to respiratory fluid loss, fever, and difficulty swallowing
- Anxiety related to dyspnea, invasive procedures, and separation from caregiver
- Parental anxiety related to child's respiratory symptoms
- Parental health-seeking behaviors related to child's condition and home care

PLANNING AND IMPLEMENTATION

The major nursing goals for the young child with an upper respiratory disorder are to observe closely for respiratory or cardiac changes. The need for immediate intubation is always a possibility; thus, close vigilance is essential. The child's energy must be conserved to reduce oxygen requirements.

Monitoring Respiratory Function. The nurse must be on the alert continuously for warning signs of airway obstruction. The child should be monitored at least every hour. The nurse should uncover the child's chest and make observations of the child's breathing efforts, noting the amount of chest movement, shallow breathing, and retractions. The nurse should listen with a stethoscope for breath sounds, particularly noting the amount of stridor, which indicates difficult breathing. Increasing hoarse-

ness should be reported. In addition, pallor, listlessness, circumoral cyanosis, cyanotic nail beds, and restlessness are indications of impaired oxygenation and should be reported at once. The heart rate should be evaluated for rate, strength, and regularity. A rapid, weak pulse may indicate impending cardiac problems. Cool, high humidity provides relief. Oxygen may be administered. Pulse oximetry may be used to evaluate oxygen requirements.

Monitoring Adequate Fluid Intake. Maintaining adequate fluid intake may be a problem. Adequate hydration helps to reduce thick mucus. The child may be too ill to want to eat, but warm, clear oral fluids may be tolerated. However, in the case of severe respiratory distress, aspiration is a constant danger. The child may need to be NPO to prevent this threat. Parenteral fluids are administered to replace those lost through respiratory loss, fever, and anorexia. Fluid needs are determined by the amount needed to maintain body weight with sufficient amounts added to replace the additional losses. Daily weights and accurate intake and output records are essential. Serum electrolyte levels are monitored to maintain them within normal limits. Observation of skin turgor and mucous membranes are necessary and should be recorded at least once per shift.

Reducing the Child's Anxiety. When frightened or upset and crying, the child with croup or a related upper respiratory condition may hyperventilate, and additional respiratory distress occurs. For this reason, maintaining a calm, soothing manner while caring for the child is essential. When possible, the child should be cared for by a constant caregiver with whom a trusting relationship has been achieved. Avoiding any nonessential invasive procedures helps decrease the child's reasons for anxiety. The family can provide the child with a favorite blanket or toy. The parent or caregiver should be encouraged to stay with the child, if at all possible, to provide reassurance and avoid separation anxiety in the child. Care should be planned so that the child has minimal interruptions of much-needed rest. Age-appropriate explanations of treatment and procedures should be given to the child. As the child improves, age-appropriate diversional activities can be provided to aid in relieving anxiety and boredom. For the child in respiratory isolation, the nurse must make extra efforts to relieve the child's feelings of loneliness.

Reducing Parental Anxiety. For the parent or family caregiver, watching a child who has severe respiratory symptoms is a frightening experience. The parent or caregiver may feel helpless, and these feelings of anxiety and helplessness may be exhibited in a variety of ways. To alleviate these feelings, the nurse can encourage discussion of these feelings. The nurse should explain procedures, treatments, the illness, and the prognosis to the parent, making certain to use terminology that can be understood. The parent or caregiver should be included in the care of the child as much as possible and encouraged to soothe and comfort the child.

Providing Family Teaching. The parent or caregiver needs thorough explanations of the signs and symptoms of the condition. The nurse should explain the symptoms that can be handled at home (hoarseness, croupy cough, and inspiratory stridor when disturbed) and those that indicate the child needs to be seen by the physician (continuous stridor, use of accessory muscles, labored breathing, lower rib retractions, restlessness, pallor, and rapid respirations). The family needs to be aware that recurrence of these conditions is common. Use of cool humidifiers or vaporizers should be explained, including cleaning methods and safety in the use of a steam vaporizer to avoid burns. Explanations of medications are necessary. The nurse, who needs to be certain that the information was understood, can have the parent relate back specific facts. Information should be written also but must be done in a simple way so that it can be clearly understood. The nurse must determine that the parent can actually read and understand the written material. When appropriate, the parent can demonstrate care of equipment and any treatments to be done at home.

EVALUATION

- Airway is clear, no evidence of retractions, stridor, hoarseness, or cyanosis
- Fluid intake is adequate for age and weight; good skin turgor and moist mucous membranes
- Rests quietly, no evidence of dyspnea on exertion, cooperates with care, smiles, and plays contentedly
- Parent or caregiver cooperates with and participates in care, appears more relaxed, states feelings, and accurately describes facts about child's condition
- Parent or caregiver demonstrates understanding of child's home care, asks appropriate questions, and verbally relates signs and symptoms to observe

Cystic Fibrosis

When first described, cystic fibrosis (CF) was called fibrocystic disease of the pancreas. Further research has revealed that this disorder represents a major dysfunction of all exocrine glands. The major organs affected are the lungs, the pancreas, and the liver. Because about half of all children with CF experience pulmonary complications, this disorder is discussed here with other respiratory conditions.

CF is hereditary and is transmitted as an autosomal recessive trait. Both parents must be carriers of the gene for CF to appear. With each pregnancy, the chance is one in four that the child will have the disease. The incidence is about 1 in 2000 in white children in the United States. The incidence in African Americans is 1 in 17,000.

Although the cause of CF is unknown, the basic defect is related to abnormal secretions of the exocrine (mucus-producing) glands, which produce thick, tenacious mucus rather than the thin, free-flowing secretion normally produced. This abnormal mucus leads to obstruction of the secretory ducts of the pancreas, liver, and reproductive organs. Thick mucus obstructs the respiratory passages, causing air trapping and overinflation of the lungs. In addition, the sweat and salivary glands excrete excessive electrolytes, specifically sodium and chloride (Figure 11-3).

Clinical Manifestations

Meconium ileus is the presenting symptom of CF in 5% to 10% of the newborns who later develop additional manifestations. Depletion or absence of pancreatic enzymes before birth results in impaired digestive activity, and the meconium becomes *viscid* (thick) and *mucilaginous* (sticky). The *inspissated* (thickened) meconium fills the small intestine, causing complete obstruction. Clinical manifestations are bile-stained emesis, a distended abdomen, and an absence of stool. Intestinal perforation with symptoms of shock may occur. These newborns taste salty when kissed because of the high sodium chloride concentrations in their sweat.

Symptoms of CF may occur at varying ages during infancy, childhood, or adolescence. A hard, nonproductive chronic cough may be the first sign. Later, bronchial infections become frequent. Development of a barrel chest and clubbing of fingers indicates chronic lack of oxygen. Despite an excellent appetite, malnutrition is apparent and becomes increasingly severe. The abdomen becomes distended, and body muscles become flabby.

Pancreatic Involvement. Thick, tenacious mucus obstructs the pancreatic ducts, causing **hypochylia** (diminished flow of pancreatic enzymes) or **achylia** (absence of pancreatic enzymes). This achylia or hypochylia leads to intestinal malabsorption and severe malnutrition. The pancreatic enzymes that are deficient are lipase, trypsin, and amylase. Malabsorption of fats causes frequent steatorrhea (bulky and greasy stools, with a distinctively foul odor). Anemia or rectal prolapse frequently occurs if the pancreatic condition remains untreated. The incidence of diabetes is greater in these children than in the general population, possibly owing to changes in the pancreas. The incidence of diabetes in patients with CF is expected to increase because of the increasing life expectancy of these patients.

Pulmonary Involvement. The degree of lung involvement determines the prognosis for survival. The severity of pulmonary involvement differs in individual children, a few showing only minor involvement. More than half of the children with CF can now be expected to live beyond age 18, with increasing numbers living into their late 20s and even 30s.

Respiratory complications pose the greatest threat to children with CF. Abnormal amounts of thick, viscid mucus

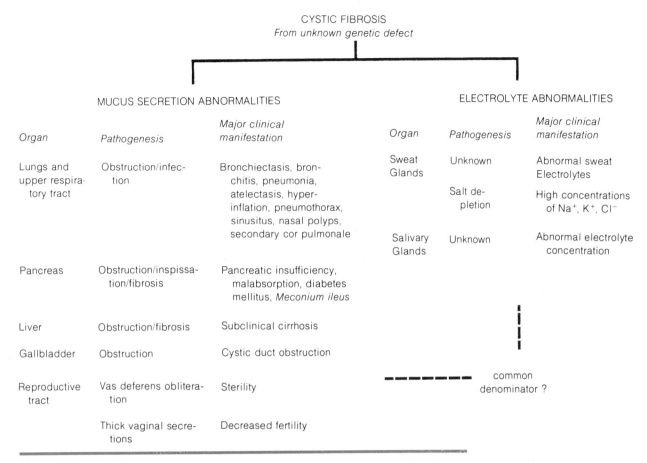

CYSTIC FIBROSIS
From unknown genetic defect

MUCUS SECRETION ABNORMALITIES

Organ	Pathogenesis	Major clinical manifestation
Lungs and upper respiratory tract	Obstruction/infection	Bronchiectasis, bronchitis, pneumonia, atelectasis, hyperinflation, pneumothorax, sinusitus, nasal polyps, secondary cor pulmonale
Pancreas	Obstruction/inspissation/fibrosis	Pancreatic insufficiency, malabsorption, diabetes mellitus, *Meconium ileus*
Liver	Obstruction/fibrosis	Subclinical cirrhosis
Gallbladder	Obstruction	Cystic duct obstruction
Reproductive tract	Vas deferens obliteration	Sterility
	Thick vaginal secretions	Decreased fertility

ELECTROLYTE ABNORMALITIES

Organ	Pathogenesis	Major clinical manifestation
Sweat Glands	Unknown	Abnormal sweat Electrolytes
	Salt depletion	High concentrations of Na^+, K^+, Cl^-
Salivary Glands	Unknown	Abnormal electrolyte concentration

common denominator ?

Figure 11-3. CF defects and manifestations. (From Larter N. Cystic fibrosis. Am J Nurs 81:527–532, 1981.)

clog the bronchioles and provide an ideal medium for bacterial growth. *S. aureus coagulase* can be cultured from the nasopharynx and sputum of most patients. *Pseudomonas aeruginosa* and *H. influenzae* also are found frequently. The basic infection, however, appears most often to be caused by *S. aureus*.

Numerous complications arise from severe respiratory infections. Atelectasis and small lung abscesses are common early complications. Bronchiectasis and emphysema develop, with pulmonary fibrosis and pneumonitis, eventually leading to severe ventilatory insufficiency. These children often have barrel chests and clubbing of the fingers. In advanced disease, pneumothorax, right ventricular hypertrophy, and cor pulmonale are common complications. Cor pulmonale is a frequent cause of death.

Other Affected Organs. The tears, saliva, and sweat of children with CF contain abnormally high concentrations of electrolytes, and the submaxillary salivary glands are enlarged in most of these children. In hot weather, the loss of sodium chloride and fluid through sweating produces frequent heat prostration. Additional fluid and salt in the diet should be given as a preventive measure.

Diagnosis

Diagnosis is based on family history, elevated sodium chloride levels in the sweat, analysis of duodenal secretions via a nasogastric tube for trypsin content, a history of failure to thrive, chronic or recurrent respiratory infections, and radiologic findings of hyperinflation and bronchial wall thickening. In the event of a positive sodium chloride sweat test, at least one other criterion must be met to make a conclusive diagnosis.

The principal diagnostic test to confirm CF is a sweat chloride test using the pilocarpine iontophoresis method. This method induces sweating by using a small electric current that carries topically applied pilocarpine into a localized area of the skin. Elevations of 60 mEq/L or above are diagnostic, with values between 50 and 60 mEq/L highly suspect. Although the test itself is fairly simple, false positive results do occur, and conducting the test on a young infant is difficult.

Treatment

In the newborn, meconium ileus is treated nonoperatively with hyperosmolar enemas administered gently. In the patients in whom this does not resolve the blockage of thick, gummy meconium, surgery is necessary. During surgery, a mucolytic such as Mucomyst may be used to liquefy the meconium. If this procedure is successful, resection may not be necessary. Most of these infants develop CF of varying degrees of severity.

In the older child, treatment is aimed at correcting pancreatic deficiency, improving pulmonary function, and preventing respiratory infections. If bowel obstruction does occur (meconium ileus equivalent), the preferred management includes hyperosmolar enemas and oral or nasogastric administration of mucolytics.[2]

The overall treatment goals are to improve the child's quality of life and to provide for long-term survival. A health care team is needed, including a physician, a nurse, a respiratory therapist, a dietitian, and a social worker, to work together with the child and family. CF treatment centers with a staff of specialists are becoming more available, particularly in the larger medical centers.

Dietary Treatment. Commercially prepared pancreatic enzymes given during meals or snacks aid digestion and absorption of fat and protein. Because pancreatic enzymes are inactivated in the acidic environment of the stomach, microencapsulated capsules that deliver the enzymes to the duodenum, where they are needed, are preferred. These enzymes are administered either as capsules to be swallowed or can be opened and sprinkled on the child's food.

The child's diet should be high in carbohydrates and protein, with no restriction of fats. The child may need $1\frac{1}{2}$ to 2 times the normal caloric intake to promote growth. Unless acutely ill, these children have large appetites, but they can receive little nourishment without a pancreatic supplement. With proper diet and enzyme supplements, these children show evidence of improved nutrition, and their stools become relatively normal. Enteric-coated pancreatic enzymes now essentially eliminate the need for dietary restriction of fat.

Because of the increased loss of sodium chloride, these children are allowed to use as much salt as they wish, even though onlookers may think it is too much. During hot weather, additional salt may be provided with pretzels, salt bread sticks, and saltines.

Supplements of fat-soluble vitamins A, D, E, and K are necessary because of the poor digestion of fats. Water-miscible (the ability to be mixed with water) preparations can be given to provided the needed supplement.

Pulmonary Treatment. The goal of treatment is to prevent and treat respiratory infections. Respiratory drainage is provided by thinning the secretions and by mechanical means, such as postural drainage and clapping, to loosen and drain the secretions from the lungs. Antibacterial drugs for the treatment of infection are necessary as indicated. Some physicians may prescribe a prophylactic antibiotic therapy when the child is diagnosed. Antibiotics may be administered orally or parenterally, even in the home. In the event of home parenteral administration of antibiotic therapy, a central venous access device is used. Immuni-

zation against childhood communicable diseases is extremely important for these chronically ill children. All immunization measures may be used and should be maintained at appropriate intervals. Physical activity is essential because it improves mucus secretion. In addition, exercise helps the child to "feel good," and the child can be encouraged to participate in any aerobic activity he or she enjoys. Activity, along with physical therapy, should be limited only by the child's endurance.

Inhalation therapy can be preventive or therapeutic for the child with CF. Hand-held nebulizers are easy to use and convenient for the ambulatory child. In some instances, a bronchodilator drug, such as theophylline or beta-adrenergic agonists (metaproterenol, terbutaline, and albuterol, may be administered either orally or through nebulization. The addition of a mucolytic agent, such as Mucomyst, may be prescribed during periods of acute infection.

A humidified atmosphere can be provided with humidifiers. The use of mist tents at night is no longer recommended. In summer, a room air conditioner can help provide comfort and controlled humidity to the child.

Chest physical therapy (*CPT*) is performed routinely at least every morning and evening, even if little drainage is apparent (Figure 11-4). CPT is a combination of postural drainage and chest percussion. Chest percussion, which is clapping and vibrating of the affected areas, if performed correctly, helps loosen and move the secretions out of the lungs. The physical therapist usually performs this procedure in the hospital and demonstrates it to the family because this will be an essential part of home care.

Home Care

The home care for children with CF places a tremendous burden on the concerned families. This is not one-time hospital treatment, nor is there a prospect of cure to brighten the horizon. Each day, much time is spent in the performance of treatments. Family caregivers must learn to perform CPT and how to operate any respiratory equipment and administer intravenous antibiotics when necessary. The child's diet must be planned, with the regulation of additional enzymes according to need. Great care is needed to prevent exposure to infections.

In addition, the family caregivers must guard against overprotection and against undue limitation of their child's physical activity. Somehow, a good family relationship must be preserved, with time allowed for attention to other members of the family.

Physical activity is an important adjunct to the child's well-being and is a necessary help in getting rid of secretions. Capacity for exercise is soon learned, and the child can be trusted to become self-limiting as necessary, especially if given an opportunity to learn the nature of the disease. The child may find postural drainage fun when a caregiver raises the child's feet in the air and walks the

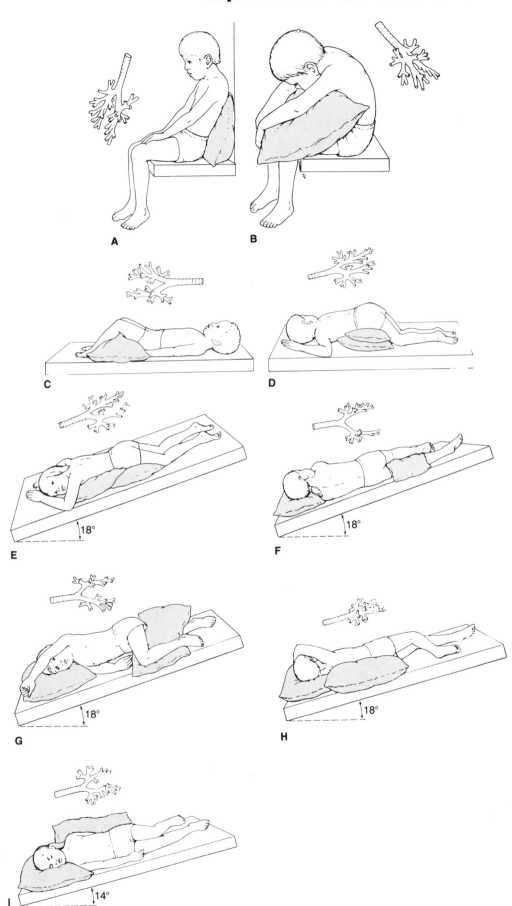

Figure 11-4. Bronchial drainage positions for the main segments of all lobes in children. **A**, Apical segment of right upper lobe and apical subsegment of apical-posterior segment of left upper lobe. **B**, Posterior segment of right upper lobe and posterior subsegment of apical-posterior segment of left upper lobe. **C**, Anterior segments of both upper lobes. **D**, Superior segments of both lower lobes. **E**, Posterior basal segments of both lower lobes. **F**, Lateral basal segment of right lower lobe. **G**, Anterior basal segment of left lower lobe. **H**, Right middle lobe. **I**, Lingular segments of left upper lobe. (From Skale N. Manual of Pediatric Nursing Procedures. Philadelphia: JB Lippincott, 1992.)

child around "wheelbarrow" fashion, or the older child can learn to hang from a monkey bar by the knees. Providing as much normalcy as possible is always desirable.

Hot weather activity should be watched a little more closely, with additional attention directed toward increased salt and fluid intake during periods of exercise.

Caring for a child with CF places great stress on a family's financial resources. The expense of daily medications, frequent clinic or office visits, and sometimes lengthy hospitalizations can be devastating to an ordinary family budget, even with hospital-medical insurance coverage. The Cystic Fibrosis Foundation, with chapters throughout the United States, is helpful in providing education and services. Some assistance may be available through local agencies or community groups.

Nursing Process for the Child with Cystic Fibrosis

ASSESSMENT

The assessment of the child with CF varies with the age of the child and the circumstances of the admission. A complete parent interview is conducted that includes the standard information as well as questions concerning respiratory infections, the child's appetite and eating habits, stools, noticeable salty perspiration, history of bowel obstruction as an infant, and family history for CF, if known. The parent's or caregiver's knowledge of the condition also must be assessed.

The assessment of the child includes routine vital signs; observation of respirations, including cough, breath sounds, and barrel chest; respiratory effort, such as retractions and nasal flaring; clubbing of the fingers; and signs of pancreatic involvement, such as failure to thrive and steatorrhea. The skin around the rectum should be examined for irritation and breakdown from the frequent foul stools. The nurse should ask the child age-appropriate questions, involve the child in the assessment, and determine the child's own perception of the disease and this current illness.

NURSING DIAGNOSES

The nursing diagnoses for CF may be many and varied. The reason for the present admission, the age of the child, the progression of the condition, the level of understanding that the child and the caregiver have about the condition, and the current illness all merge to determine the pertinent nursing diagnoses for this admission. For the child who has just been diagnosed, the nursing diagnoses may be much more complex than for one who has been admitted for complications of a longstanding condition. The family caregiver and the child, as suitable for age, should be included in the determination of current nursing diagnoses. Some of the diagnoses that may be appropriate include the following:

- Ineffective airway clearance related to thick, tenacious mucus production
- High risk for infection related to bacterial growth medium provided by pulmonary mucus and impaired body defenses
- High risk for altered nutrition: less than body requirements related to impaired absorption of nutrients
- Activity intolerance related to dyspnea secondary to mucopurulent secretions
- Anxiety of child related to hospitalization
- Altered family processes related to child's chronic illness and its demands on the caregivers

PLANNING AND IMPLEMENTATION

Nursing diagnoses need to be developed and prioritized before planning and implementation can begin. As stated earlier, much depends on the reason for the specific admission and other factors discussed under Nursing Diagnoses. The family caregivers' primary goal may include relief of the problems related to this admission, but other goals may include concerns about the stress the illness is placing on the family, as well as a need for additional information about the disease. The child's age and ability for self-expression affect any goal-setting the child is able to do. The nurse's major goals are to relieve the child's immediate respiratory distress, improve nutritional status, protect the child from infection, and support and teach the child and family as needed.

Monitoring and Improving Respiratory Function. The mucus causes obstruction of the airways and diminishes gas exchange. The nurse must assess the child for signs of respiratory distress, monitoring dyspnea, tachypnea, labored respirations with or without activity, retractions, nasal flaring, and color of the nail beds. Aerosol treatments and CPT should be carried out every 2 to 4 hours as ordered. These treatments may be done by respiratory therapy technicians or physical therapists, but the nurse must observe the child after the treatment to assess effectiveness and determine if more frequent treatments may be needed. The child may be able to self-administer the nebulizer treatments but should be supervised by the nurse to ensure correct use. The child should be taught to cough effectively. The nurse examines the mucus produced, noting the color, consistency, and odor. Cultures are sent to the laboratory as appropriate. Increased fluid intake helps thin the mucus secretions. The nurse should encourage the child to drink extra fluids and ask the child (or the caregiver if the child is too young) what favorite drinks might be appealing. Intravenous fluids may be necessary. Humidified air is provided, either in the form of a cool mist humidifier or mist tent as prescribed. The child should be maintained in a semi-Fowler's or high-Fowler's position to promote maximum lung expansion. Pulse oximetry may be used. Oxygen saturation should be maintained higher than 90%. Oxygen should be administered if the oxygen saturation falls below this level for an extended period. The child benefits from mouth care administered every 2 to 4 hours, especially when oxygen is administered.

Preventing Infection. The child with CF has low resistance, especially to respiratory infections. For this reason, care must be taken to protect the child from any exposure to infectious organisms. Most important, good handwashing techniques should be practiced. The nurse should practice good handwashing and teach the child and family the importance of this first line of defense. Other good hygiene habits also should be observed. Medical asepsis must be carefully followed when the child and the equipment are taken care of. The child's vital signs should be monitored every 4 hours for any indication of an infectious process. People with an infection, including staff, family members, other patients, and visitors, should be restricted from contact with the child. The family should be advised to keep the child's immunizations up to date. Antibiotics should be administered in the hospital, and the child or caregiver is taught home administration as needed. The family also needs to be instructed on signs and symptoms to alert them to impending infection so that they can begin prophylactic measures at once. Adequate nutrition helps the child resist infections.

Maintaining Adequate Nutrition. The child needs to have greatly increased caloric intake to provide for impaired absorption of nutrients and adequate growth and development. In addition to increased caloric intake at meals, the child should have high-caloric, high-protein snacks, such as peanut butter and cheese. Newer low-fat products can be selected, if desired. The child always needs to take the pancreatic enzymes with meals and snacks. In addition, multiple vitamins and iron may be prescribed. Reinforcement for both the child and the family is important. The child also may require additional salt in the diet and can be encouraged to eat salty snacks. For instance, pretzels, salt bread sticks, and saltines. If the child has bouts of diarrhea or constipation, the dosage of enzymes may need to be adjusted. The change in bowels should be reported to the physician. The child should be weighed and measured and the growth plotted on a growth chart so that progress can easily be visualized.

Promoting Energy Conservation and Sensory Stimulation. The child's energy needs to be conserved. Plan nursing and therapeutic activities so that maximum rest time is provided for the child. Note dyspnea and respiratory distress in relation to any activities. Plan quiet diversional activities as the child's physical condition warrants (see the following paragraph). Help the child and family understand that activity is excellent for the child when not in an acute situation. Teach them that exercise helps loosen the thick mucus and also improves the child's self-image.

Reducing the Child's Anxiety. The child should have age-appropriate activities available to help alleviate anxiety and boredom, which also can come from enforced hospitalization. Activities such as reading, arts and crafts chosen according to age, and possibly school-work may help ease some of the anxiety. Some older children may enjoy a video game, if available; however, the child may need to be watched for overexcitement. Encouraging the parent or caregiver to stay with the child helps diminish some of the child's anxiety. Allowing the child to have familiar toys or mementos from home is also desirable. Staying with the child during acute episodes of coughing and dyspnea is essential in reducing anxiety. The child needs to be given information about CF that is at the child's level of understanding. Quizzing the child in a relaxed, friendly manner helps the nurse determine what the child knows and what teaching may be needed. Learning about CF can be turned into a game for some children, making it much more enjoyable.

Providing Teaching and Family Support. The family is faced with a long-term illness. Depending on the individual situation, the family may have already seen a deterioration in the child's health. An evaluation of the family's knowledge about CF is helpful in determining their needs. The family may need to have a complete reconfirmation of the information that they have already been given, or they may have just a few areas of need. The nurse should demonstrate an interest and willingness to talk to the family so that they do not feel as though they are intruding on time needed to do other things. Information should be provided for resources, such as the Cystic Fibrosis Foundation, the American Lung Association, and other local organizations. The family and the child need opportunities to voice their fears and anxieties. Responding with active-listening techniques helps authenticate the feelings expressed. The family may have questions about genetic counseling and may need referrals for counseling. Throughout the entire hospital stay, the child and the family need emotional support. The nurse is the person who can best provide overall support.

EVALUATION

- Airway is clear; child clears mucus from airway effectively
- Child exhibits no signs of infection as evidenced by vital signs within normal limits
- Child's intake promotes weight gain with no bouts of constipation or diarrhea
- Child rests quietly with no dyspnea
- Child engages in age-appropriate activities and appears relaxed with no signs of distress
- Family is able to cope as evidenced by demonstrating understanding of child's illness and therapy and becoming involved in available support groups

Accidents

Ingestion of Toxic Substances

Toddlers are natural explorers, examining their environment to learn all they can about it. One of the ways in which they find out about their environment is to taste the world around them. Toddlers and preschoolers are developing autonomy and initiative, which add to their tendency to examine their environment on their own. Substances that would repel an adult because of taste or smell are ingested by young children because their senses of taste and smell are not yet refined. This makes these age groups prime targets for ingestion of poisonous substances. The ordinary household has an abundance of poisonous substances in almost every room. The kitchen, bathroom, bedroom, and garage are the most common sites to harbor substances that are poisonous when ingested. Although most poisonings occur in the child's home, grandparents' homes offer many temptations to the young child. The grandparents tend to be less concerned about placing dangerous substances out of children's reach simply because the children are not part of the household, or the grandparents may place supplies where they are convenient, never giving the young grandchild's developmental stage and exploratory nature a thought.

When a child is found with a container whose contents the child has obviously sampled, action can be taken immediately. When a child manifests symptoms that are difficult to assess or that do not appear to relate specifically to any known cause, the possibility of poisoning should be suspected. Ingestion of a poisonous substance can produce symptoms that simulate an attack of an acute disease—vomiting, abdominal pain, diarrhea, shock, cyanosis, coma, and convulsions. If evidence of such a disease is lacking, acute poisoning should be suspected.

In instances of apparent poisoning, the family caregivers are asked to consider all medications in their home, if the substance is not known. Is it possible that any medication could have been available to the child, or did an older child or other person possibly give the child the container to play with? Is it possible that a parent inadvertently gave a wrong dose or wrong medication to a child? All such possibilities need to be considered. In the meantime, the most important priority is treatment for the child who shows symptoms of poisoning.

Emergency Treatment

The first step that the parent or caregiver should take when poison ingestion is suspected is to call the local poison control center. Most localities have a toll-free number available to those in remote areas. This number can be found in the local telephone directory and should be posted on every telephone in the house. Any obvious poison should be removed from the child's mouth before calling. The poison control center evaluates the situation and tells the caller whether the child can be treated at home or if the child needs to be transported to a hospital or treatment center.

Except when corrosive or highly irritant poisons have been swallowed, the first measure is to induce vomiting. If the child is convulsing or unconscious, however, vomiting should not be induced because of the danger of aspiration.

The approved method for producing vomiting is to have the child swallow 15 mL of syrup of ipecac. A second 15-mL dose can be given if vomiting does not occur within 15 to 30 minutes. Vomiting also may be induced by stimulating the child's posterior pharynx with the adult's finger. The child's head should be allowed to droop forward or turned to the side to avoid aspiration of the vomitus.

If the substance is unknown, all material vomited at home or on the way to the hospital or treatment center should be saved for analysis. If the substance that the child swallowed is known, the container should be taken along. If the container is left behind in the panic and confusion, someone will need to go to the home and retrieve it.

If the substance the child has swallowed is known, the ingredients can be found on the label. The poison control center can suggest an antidote if the name of the drug or other substance is known. If the substance is a prescription drug, the pharmacist who filled the prescription or who is familiar with the drug also can be contacted for information. In some instances, it may be necessary to analyze the residual stomach contents.

There are specific antidotes for certain poisons but not for all. Some antidotes react chemically with the poison to render it harmless; others prevent absorption of the poison. *Activated charcoal* given after vomiting absorbs many poisons. It is given in 6 to 8 ounces of water in a dose of 5 to 10 g per gram of ingested poison. This may be given through a nasogastric tube, if necessary.

Treatment Steps in Order of Importance. The treatment steps in order of importance are as follows:

1. Remove the obvious remnants of the poison.
2. Call the poison control center.
3. Prevent further absorption.
4. Administer appropriate antidote if known.
5. Administer general supportive and symptomatic care.

Further specific treatment is given according to the kind and amount of the toxic substance ingested. Examples of frequent types of poisoning and general treatment are described in Table 11-1. Complete listings of poisonous substances with the specific treatment for each are available from poison control centers, clinics, and pharmacies. All homes with young children should have this number posted by the telephone for quick reference.

Table 11-1. Commonly Ingested Toxic Substances

Agent	Symptoms	Treatment
Acetaminophen	Under 6 years—vomiting is the earliest sign Adolescents—vomiting, diaphoresis, general malaise. Liver damage can result in 48–96 h if not treated	Induce vomiting with syrup of ipecac. Gastric lavage may be necessary. Administer acetylcysteine (Mucomyst) diluted with cola, fruit juice, or water if plasma level elevated. Mucomyst may be administered by gavage, especially because its odor of rotten eggs makes it objectionable
Acetylsalicylic acid—aspirin	Hyperpnea (abnormal increase in depth and rate of breathing), followed by metabolic acidosis, hyperventilation, tinnitus, and vertigo are initial symptoms. Dehydration, coma, convulsions, and death follow untreated heavy dosage	Induce vomiting with syrup of ipecac. Gastric lavage may be necessary. Activated charcoal may be administered. Intravenous fluids, sodium bicarbonate to combat acidosis, and dialysis for renal failure may be necessary when large amounts are ingested
Ibuprofen (Motrin, Advil)	Similar to aspirin; metabolic acidosis, gastrointestinal bleeding, renal damage	Induce vomiting. Activated charcoal administered in emergency department. Observe for and treat gastrointestinal bleeding. Electrolyte determination to detect acidosis. Intravenous fluids
Ferrous Sulfate (iron)	Vomiting, lethargy, diarrhea, weak rapid pulse, hypotension are common symptoms. Massive dose may produce shock, erosion of small intestine, black, tarry stools, and bronchial pneumonia	Induce vomiting with syrup of ipecac. Deferoxamine, a chelating agent that combines with iron, may be used when child has ingested a toxic dose
Barbiturates	Respiratory, circulatory, and renal depression may occur. Child may become comatose	Establish airway, administer oxygen if needed, gastric lavage. Close observation of level of consciousness
Corrosives Alkali: lye, bleaches Acid: drain cleaners, toilet bowl cleaners, iodine, silver nitrate	Intense burning and pain with first mouthful; severe burns of mouth and esophageal tract; shock, possible death	*Never have child vomit.* Alkali corrosives such as ammonia, lye, and household bleach are treated initially with quantities of water, diluted acid fruit juices, or diluted vinegar. Acid corrosives, such as toilet bowl cleaners, iodine, and silver nitrate, are treated with alkaline drinks such as milk, olive oil, mineral oil, or egg white. *Lavage or emetics are never used.* Continuing treatment includes antidotes, gastrostomy or intravenous feedings, and specialized care. A tracheostomy may be needed
Hydrocarbons Kerosene, gasoline, furniture polish, lighter fluid, turpentine	Damage to the respiratory system is the primary concern. Vomiting frequently occurs spontaneously, which may cause additional damage to the respiratory system. Pneumonia, bronchopneumonia, or lipoid pneumonia often occur	Emergency treatment and assessment is necessary. Vital signs are monitored, oxygen administered as needed. Gastric lavage is performed only if the ingested substances contains other toxic chemicals that may threaten other body systems, such as the liver, kidneys, or cardiovascular system

Lead Poisoning (Plumbism)

Chronic lead poisoning has been a serious problem among children for many years. It is responsible for neurologic handicaps, including mental retardation, because of its effect on the central nervous system. Infants and toddlers are potential victims because of their tendency to mouth any object within their reach. In some children, this habit leads to **pica** (the ingestion of nonfood substances such as laundry starch, clay, paper, and paint). The unborn fetus of a pregnant mother who is exposed to lead (such as lead dust from renovation of an older home) also can be affected by lead contamination. Screening for lead poisoning is part of a complete well baby checkup between the ages of 6 months and 6 years.

Causes of Chronic Lead Poisoning. The most common causes of lead poisoning include the following:

- Lead-containing paint used on the outside or the inside of older houses
- Furniture and toys painted with lead-containing paint
- Drinking water contaminated by lead pipes or copper pipes with lead-soldered joints
- Dust containing lead salts from automotive exhaust, lead paint, or emission from lead smelters
- Storage of fruit juices or other food in improperly glazed earthenware
- Inhalation of motor fumes containing lead or burning of storage batteries
- Exposure to industrial areas with smelteries or chemical plants
- Exposure to hobbyists using lead, such as in stained glass

There are other causes, but the most common cause has been the lead in paint. Children tend to nibble on fallen plaster, painted wooden furniture (including cribs), or painted toys because they have a sweet taste. Fine dust that results from removing lead paint in remodeling also can cause harm to the young children in the household without parents becoming aware of it. When the danger of lead poisoning became apparent, attempts were made to control the sale of lead-based paint. In 1973, federal regulations banned the sale of paint containing more than 0.5% lead for interior residential use or use on toys. This has not eliminated the problem, however, because many homes built before to the 1960s were painted with lead-based paint, and they still exist, not only in the inner-city areas but also in small towns and suburbs. Older mansions in which upper-income families may live also have lead paint because of their age. Only contractors experienced in lead-based paint removal should do renovation.

Symptoms of Lead Poisoning. The onset of chronic lead poisoning is insidious. Some early indications may be irritability, hyperactivity, aggression, impulsiveness, or dis- interest in play. Short attention span, lethargy, learning difficulties, and distractibility also are signs of poisoning.

The condition may progress to **encephalopathy** (degenerative disease of the brain) because of intracranial pressure. Acute manifestations include convulsions, mental retardation, blindness, paralysis, coma, and death. Acute episodes sometimes develop sporadically and early in the condition.

Diagnosis. The nonspecific nature of the presenting symptoms make examination of the environmental history of the child important. Testing of erythrocyte protoporphyrin levels has been used as a screening method, but it is not accurate in identifying children with blood levels lower than 25 μg/dL; therefore, it is no longer an adequate method of screening. Finger sticks, or heel sticks for infants, can be used to collect a sample for lead level screening. In 1991, the Centers for Disease Control in Atlanta revised the blood lead level criteria to repeat testing on all children with blood levels greater than 10 μg/dL, with emphasis on primary prevention to reflect new information regarding safe levels.

Treatment. The most important aspect of treatment of a child with lead poisoning is to remove the lead from the child's system and environment. The use of a **chelating agent** (an agent that binds with metal) increases the urinary excretion of lead. Several chelating agents are available; individual circumstances and the physician's choice determine the particular drug used. Edetate disodium, known as EDTA, is usually given intravenously. Intramuscular administration is painful. Renal failure can occur with inappropriate dosage. Dimercaptopropanol (dimercaprol), also known as BAL, may be administered intramuscularly. BAL causes excretion of lead through bile and urine. Because of its peanut oil base, BAL should not be used in children allergic to peanuts. These two drugs may be used together in children with extremely high levels of lead.

The oral drug D-penicillamine can be used to treat children with blood lead levels lower than 45 μg/dL. The capsules can be opened and sprinkled on food or mixed in liquid for administration. This drug should not be administered to children with an allergy to penicillin. In 1991, the Food and Drug Administration approved succimer (Chemet), a new oral drug for treating children with blood lead levels higher than 45 μg/dL. Succimer comes in capsule form that can be opened and mixed with applesauce or other soft foods.

All of the chelating drugs may have toxic side effects, and children being treated must be carefully monitored with frequent urinalysis, blood cell counts, and renal function tests. Any child receiving chelation therapy should be under the care of an experienced health-care team.

Outcome. The prognosis after lead poisoning is uncertain. Early detection of the condition and removal of the

Parent Teaching

Tips to Prevent Lead Poisoning

1. If you live in an older home, make sure your child does not get any chips of paint or chew any surface painted with lead-based paint. Look for paint dust on window sills, and clean with a high phosphate sodium cleaner like Spic 'n Span.
2. Wet-mop hard-surfaced floors and woodwork with the cleaner at least once a week. Vacuuming hard surfaces scatters dust.
3. Wash child's hands and face before eating.
4. Wash toys and pacifiers frequently.
5. Prevent child from playing in dust near an old lead-painted house.
6. Prevent child from playing in dust near a busy highway. Lead from gasoline fumes will remain near an old lead-painted house.
7. If your water supply has high lead content, fully flush faucets before using for cooking, drinking, or formula.
8. Avoid contamination from hobbies or work.
9. Make sure your child eats regular meals. Food slows absorption of lead.
10. Encourage your child to eat foods high in iron and calcium.

From Centers for Disease Control. Preventing lead poisoning in young children: a statement by The Centers for Disease Control. Atlanta: Author, 1991.

child from the lead-containing surroundings offer the best hope. Follow-up should include routine examinations to prevent recurrence and to assess any residual brain damage not immediately apparent.

Although the incidence of lead poisoning has decreased, it is still prevalent. Measures to educate the public on the importance of preventing this disorder are essential if the problem is to be eliminated. Education of the family caregivers is an essential aspect of the treatment (see Parent Teaching: Tips to Prevent Lead Poisoning).

Ingestion of Foreign Objects

Young children are apt to put any small objects into their mouths, and these objects are too often swallowed. Normally, many of these objects will pass smoothly through the digestive tract and be expelled in the feces. Occasionally, however, something such as an open safety pin, a coin, a button, or a marble may lodge in the esophagus and need to be extracted. Foods such as hot dogs, pea-

nuts, carrot, popcorn kernel, apple piece, and round candy are frequent offenders.

Unless symptoms of choking, gagging, or pain are present, it is usually safe to wait and watch the feces carefully for 3 or 4 days. Any object, however, may pass safely through the esophagus and stomach only to become fixed in one of the curves of the intestine, causing an obstruction or fever due to infection. Also, sharp objects do present the danger of perforation somewhere within the digestive tract.

Diagnosis of a swallowed solid object may often, but not always, be made from the history. If a foreign object in the digestive tract is suspected, fluoroscopic and radiographic studies may be required.

Treatment

If a caregiver has seen an infant swallow an object and begin choking, the infant should be held along the rescuer's forearm with head lower than the chest and given several back blows. After the back blows are delivered, support the infant's back and head and turn the infant over onto the opposite thigh. Deliver up to five quick downward chest thrusts. Remove the foreign body if it is visualized. A child older than 1 year of age can be encouraged to continue to cough as long as the cough remains forceful. If the cough becomes ineffective (no sound with cough) or respirations become more difficult and stridor is present, the *Heimlich maneuver* can be attempted (Figure 11-5). If the child is not having respiratory problems and coughing has not resulted in removal of the object, the child needs to be transported to an emergency department to be assessed by a physician. Objects in the esophagus are removed by direct vision through an esophagoscope. Attempts to push the object down into the stomach or to extract it blindly can be dangerous. Some objects may need to be removed surgically. If the object is small and the physician believes that there is little danger to the child's gastrointestinal tract, the family caregiver may be advised to take the child home and watch the child's bowel movements over the next several days to confirm that the object has passed through the child's system.

Increasing respiratory difficulties indicate that the object has been aspirated rather than swallowed. Foreign objects aspirated into the larynx or bronchial tree may become lodged in the trachea or larynx. Deliver back blows and chest thrusts or the Heimlich maneuver as described. Open the child's airway, and try rescue breathing. If the child's chest does not rise, reposition the child and try again. If the airway is still obstructed, repeat these steps until successful in removing the object and establishing respirations. The child should be transported to the emergency department as quickly as possible. The caregiver should get emergency assistance while continuing to try to remove the offending object.

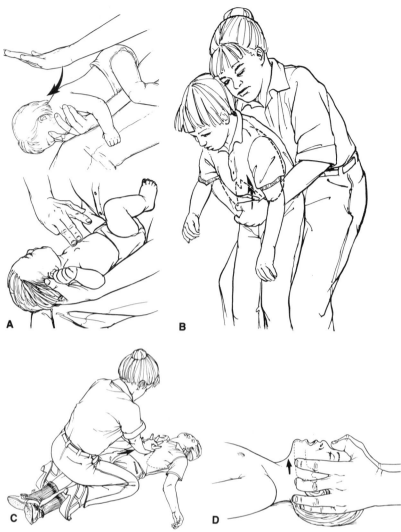

Figure 11-5. (**A**) Back blows (top) and chest thrusts (bottom) to relieve foreign-body airway obstruction in infant. Hold infant over arm as illustrated, supporting head by firmly holding jaw. Deliver up to 5 back blows. Turn infant over while supporting head, neck, jaw, and chest with one hand and back with other hand. Keep head lower than trunk. Give 5 quick chest thrusts with one finger below inter-mammary line. If foreign body not removed and airway remains obstructed, attempt rescue breathing. Repeat these 2 steps until successful. (**B**) Abdominal thrusts with child standing or sitting can be performed when child is conscious. Standing behind child, place thumb side of one fist against child's abdomen in midline slightly above navel and well below xiphoid process. Grab fist with other hand and deliver 5 quick upward thrusts. Continue until successful or child loses consciousness. (**C**) Abdominal thrusts with child lying can be performed on a conscious or unconscious child. Place heel of hand on child's abdomen slightly above the navel and below the xiphoid process and rib cage. Place other hand on top of first hand. Deliver 5 separate, distinct thrusts. Open airway and attempt rescue breathing if object not removed. Repeat until successful. (**D**) Combined jaw thrust-spine stabilization maneuver for a child trauma victim with possible head or neck injury. To protect from damage to cervical spine the neck is maintained in a neutral position and traction on or movement of neck is avoided. (From Pediatric Basic Life Support. JAMA 268[16]:2258, 1992.)

Adults must be aware of the power of example. A child who sees an adult hold pins or nails in his or her mouth may well follow this example, with disastrous and often fatal results.

Insertion of Foreign Bodies into the Ear or Nose

Children may insert small objects, such as peas or beans, crumpled paper, beads, and small toys, into their ears or noses. Irrigation of the ear may remove small objects, except paper, which becomes impacted as it absorbs moisture. The physician generally uses small forceps to remove objects not dislodged by irrigation.

A foreign body in the nose may have been placed just inside the nares by the child, but manipulation may push it in further. If the object remains in the nose for any length of time, infection may occur. Inspection with a speculum and removal of the object by a physician should be done promptly when discovered.

Drownings

Drowning is identified as the second leading cause of accidental death in children. Toddlers and older adolescents have the highest actual rate of death from drownings. The drownings in young children occur when the child has been left unattended in a body of water. Infants more frequently drown in a bathtub. Toddlers and preschoolers drown in pools or small bodies of water. A pail of water that becomes something for the toddler to investigate can become the lethal means of accidental death. A high number of deaths in this young age group occurs in home pools, including spas, hot tubs, and whirlpools.

All infants and young children must be continuously supervised by a responsible adult when near any source of water. Older children and adolescents should not play alone around any body of water. Swimming in undesignated swimming areas such as creeks, quarries, and rivers is hazardous for the older child and adolescent.

When a drowning victim of any age is discovered,

cardiopulmonary resuscitation (CPR) should be started immediately and continued until the victim can be transported to a medical facility for further care. Intensive care is carried out according to the needs of the patient. All adults who are involved with the care of children in any capacity must learn CPR to be ready to act immediately (Figure 11-6 and Table 11-2).

Burns

Among the many accidents that occur in the lives of children, burns are the most frightening. More than 70% of burn accidents happen to children younger than 5 years of age. Nearly all childhood burns are preventable, which causes considerable guilt for families and the child.

Carelessness of an adult, the child's exploring and curious nature, and failure to adequately supervise the child all contribute to the high incidence of burns in children. In addition, burns are a common form of child abuse.

Causes

Scalds from Hot Liquids. This is a frequent type of burn in small children, resulting from a dangling electric coffee maker cord, pans of hot liquid on the stove with handles turned out, cups of hot tea or coffee, bowls of soup or other hot liquids, or small children left alone in bathtubs. Dangerous and sometimes fatal burns can occur from these conditions.

Burns from Fire. The second most frequent kind of burn results from children playing with matches or being left alone in buildings that catch fire from any cause. Careless use of smoking materials are a frequent cause of house fires. Children are fascinated by fires and must be carefully supervised around fireplaces, campfires, room heaters, and outside barbecues.

Electricity. Although not common in children, infants and toddlers do suffer severe facial or mouth burns requiring extensive plastic surgery from biting on electrical cords that are still plugged into a socket. These burns may be more serious than they first appear because of the damage that may be done to underlying tissues.

Types of Burns

Burns are divided into types according to the depth of tissue involvement: superficial, partial thickness, or total thickness (Table 11-3 and Figure 11-7).

Superficial or First-Degree Burns. The epidermis is injured, but there is no destruction of tissue or nerve endings. Thus, there is erythema, edema, and pain but prompt regeneration.

Partial-Thickness or Second-Degree Burns. The epidermis and underlying dermis are both injured and devitalized or destroyed. There is generally blistering, with an escape of body plasma, but regeneration of the skin occurs from the remaining viable epithelial cells in the dermis.

Total-Thickness or Third-Degree Burns. The epidermis, dermis, and nerve endings are all destroyed. Pain is minimal, and there is no longer any barrier to infection or any remaining viable epithelial cells. Fourth-, fifth-, and sixth-degree burns have been described. They are extensions of full-thickness burns with involvement of fat, muscle, and bone, respectively.

Emergency Treatment

Cool water is an excellent emergency treatment for burns involving small areas. The immediate application of cool compresses or cool water to burn areas appears to inhibit capillary permeability and thus suppress edema, blister formation, and tissue destruction. Ice water or ice packs must not be used because of the danger of increased tissue damage. Immersion of a burned extremity in cool water alleviates pain and may prevent further thermal injury. This can be done after the airway, breathing, and circulation have been assessed but should not be done when large areas are involved because of the danger of hypothermia. In the case of a fire victim, special attention should be given to the airway to assess for smoke inhalation and respiratory passage burns. Clothing should be removed to inspect the whole body for burned areas and to remove clothing that may retain heat, causing further tissue damage. The child should be transported to a medical facility for assessment of the extent of the burns. If transported to a special burn unit, the child may be wrapped in a sterile sheet and the burn treated on arrival at the specialized facility.

Superficial Burns. Superficial burns can usually be treated on an outpatient basis because they heal readily unless infected. The area should be cleaned, an anesthetic ointment should be applied, and the burn should be covered with a sterile gauze bandage or dressing. An analgesic may be needed to relieve pain. Blisters should not be intentionally broken because of the risk of infection, but blisters that are already broken may be débrided (cut away). The child should be seen again in 2 days to inspect for infection. The caregiver must be instructed to keep the area clean and dry (no bathing the area) until the burn is healed, usually about a week to 10 days.

Partial- and Full-Thickness Burns. It is not always possible to distinguish between partial- and full-thickness burns. In the presence of infection, a partial-thickness burn may be converted into full thickness; also, with extensive burns, there is often a greater amount of full-thickness burn than had been estimated.

Full-thickness burns require the attention, skill, and conscientious care of a team of specialists. Children with mixed second- and third-degree burns, or with third-degree burns involving 15% or more of body surface,

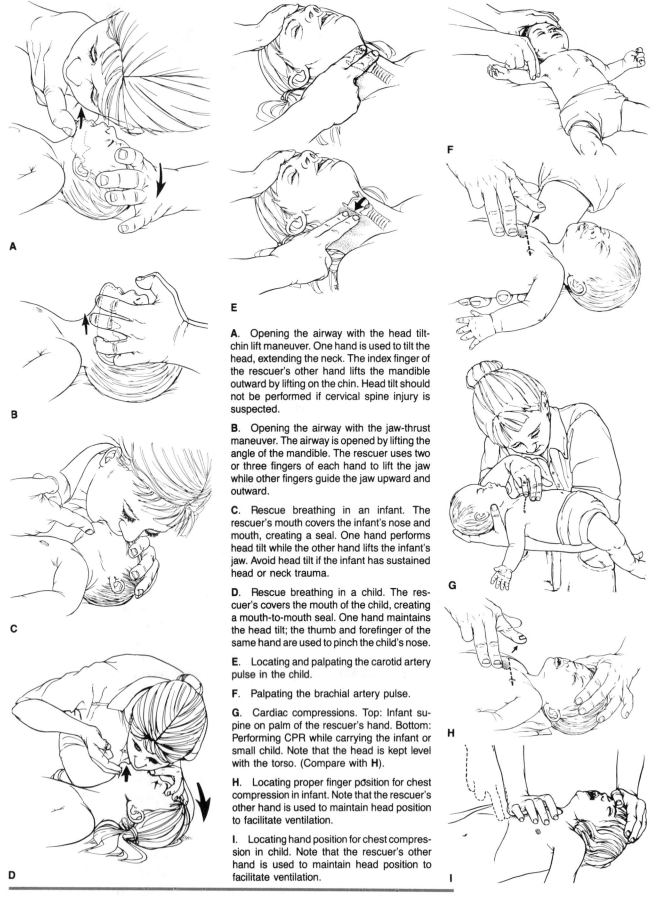

A. Opening the airway with the head tilt-chin lift maneuver. One hand is used to tilt the head, extending the neck. The index finger of the rescuer's other hand lifts the mandible outward by lifting on the chin. Head tilt should not be performed if cervical spine injury is suspected.

B. Opening the airway with the jaw-thrust maneuver. The airway is opened by lifting the angle of the mandible. The rescuer uses two or three fingers of each hand to lift the jaw while other fingers guide the jaw upward and outward.

C. Rescue breathing in an infant. The rescuer's mouth covers the infant's nose and mouth, creating a seal. One hand performs head tilt while the other hand lifts the infant's jaw. Avoid head tilt if the infant has sustained head or neck trauma.

D. Rescue breathing in a child. The rescuer's covers the mouth of the child, creating a mouth-to-mouth seal. One hand maintains the head tilt; the thumb and forefinger of the same hand are used to pinch the child's nose.

E. Locating and palpating the carotid artery pulse in the child.

F. Palpating the brachial artery pulse.

G. Cardiac compressions. Top: Infant supine on palm of the rescuer's hand. Bottom: Performing CPR while carrying the infant or small child. Note that the head is kept level with the torso. (Compare with **H**).

H. Locating proper finger position for chest compression in infant. Note that the rescuer's other hand is used to maintain head position to facilitate ventilation.

I. Locating hand position for chest compression in child. Note that the rescuer's other hand is used to maintain head position to facilitate ventilation.

Figure 11-6. Cardiopulmonary resuscitation. (From Pediatric Basic Life Support. JAMA 268[16]:2253, 2254, 2256, 2257, 2258, 1992.)

Table 11-2. Summary of Basic Life Support
Maneuvers in Infants and Children

Maneuver	*Infant (<1 y)*	*Child (1 to 8 y)*
Airway	Head tilt–chin lift (unless trauma present) Jaw thrust	Head tilt–chin lift (unless trauma present) Jaw thrust
Breathing Initial Subsequent	2 breaths at 1 to 1½ s/breath 20 breaths/min	2 breaths at 1 to 1½ s/breath 20 breaths/min
Circulation Pulse check Compression area Compression width Depth Rate Compression-ventilation ratio	Brachial/femoral Lower third of sternum 2 or 3 fingers Approximately ½ to 1 inch At least 100/min 5:1 (pause for ventilation)	Carotid Lower third of sternum Heel of 1 hand Approximately 1 to 1½ inch 100/min 5:1 (pause for ventilation)
Foreign-body airway obstruction	Back blows/chest thrusts	Heimlich maneuver

From Pediatric Basic Life Support. JAMA 268(16):2257, 1992.

require hospitalization. Burns are classified according to criteria of the American Burn Association (Table 11-4).

Treatment of Moderate to Severe Burns: First Phase—48 to 72 Hours

Hypovolemic shock is the major manifestation in the first 48 hours in massive burns. As extracellular fluid pours into the burned area, it collects in enormous quantities, dehydrating the body. Edema becomes noticeable, and symptoms of severe shock appear. Intense pain seldom is a major factor. Symptoms of shock are low blood pressure, rapid pulse, pallor, and often, considerable apprehension.

Intravenous Fluids. The primary concern is to replace body fluids that have been lost or immobilized at the burn areas. Because there is a distinct relationship between the extent of the surface area burned and the amount of fluid lost, the percentage of the skin area affected as well as the classification of the burns must be estimated to determine the medical treatment (Figure 11-8). The extent and depth of the burn and the expertise available within the hospital determine whether the child is treated at the general hospital or immediately transported to a burn unit.

An intravenous infusion site must be selected and fluids started, most often lactated Ringer's solution, isotonic saline, or plasma, using a large-bore catheter to administer replacement fluids and maintain total parenteral nutrition (TPN). Intravenous fluids for the maintenance and the replacement of lost body fluids are estimated for the first 24 hours, with half of this calculated requirement to be given during the first 8 hours. The

patient's needs may change rapidly, however, necessitating a change in the rate of flow or the amount or type of fluid. The urinary output, vital signs, and general appearance of the patient are all part of the information that the physician needs to determine the child's requirements. With TPN, fluids can be administered to provide the amino acids, glucose, fats, vitamins, and minerals that the child needs so that large amounts of foods do not need to be consumed orally. This nutrition is essential to adequately provide for the tissue repair and healing that must take place.

Airway. Adequacy of the patient's airway must be assessed in terms of a possible need for insertion of an endotracheal tube or (rarely) a tracheostomy. Inhalation injury is a leading cause of complications in burns. If burns are around the face and neck, or if the burns occurred in a small enclosed space, inhalation injury should be suspected. In fires, toxic substances and the heat produced can cause damage to the respiratory tract. All of these possibilities must be assessed.

Oral Fluids. The administration of oral fluids should either be omitted or kept to a minimum for 1 or 2 days. Delayed gastric emptying, causing acute gastric dilatation, is a common complication of burns and can become a serious problem, resulting in vomiting and anorexia. A nasogastric tube on low suction prevents vomiting. The child's thirst, which is usually severe, should be relieved by the intravenous fluids, and sips of water may be allowed. Oral feedings can be started when bowel sounds are heard. Nasogastric feedings may be needed to supple-

Table 11-3. Characteristics of Burns

Degree	Cause	Surface Appearance	Color	Pain Level	Histologic Depth	Healing Time
First (superficial)						
All are considered minor unless under 18 months, over 65, or with severe loss of fluids	Flash, flame, ultraviolet (sunburn)	Dry, no blisters, edema	Erythematous	Painful	Epidermal layers only	2 to 5 days with peeling, no scarring, may have discoloration
Second (partial thickness)						
Minor—less than 15% in adults, less than 10% in children Moderate—15%–30% in adults, or less than 15% with involvement of face, hands, feet, or perineum; minor chemical or electrical; in children, 10%–30% Severe—more than 30%	Contact with hot liquids or solids, flash flame to clothing, direct flame, chemical	Moist blebs, blisters	Mottled white to pink, cherry red	Very painful	Epidermis, papillary, and reticular layers of dermis; may include fat domes of subcutaneous layer	Superficial—5 to 21 days with no grafting Deep with no infection—21 to 35 days If infected, convert to full thickness
Third (full thickness)						
Minor—less than 2% Moderate—2%–10% any involvement of face, hands, feet, or perineum Severe—more than 10% and major chemical or electrical	Contact with hot liquids or solids, flame, chemical, electricity	Dry with leathery eschar until debridement, charred blood vessels visible under eschar	Mixed white (waxy-pearly), dark (khaki-mahogany), charred	Little or no pain, hair pulls out easily	Down to and includes subcutaneous tissue; may include fascia, muscle, and bone	Large areas require grafting that may take many months Small areas may heal from the edges after weeks

Adapted from Wagner MM. Emergency care of the burned patient. Am J Nurs 77:1788–1791, 1977.

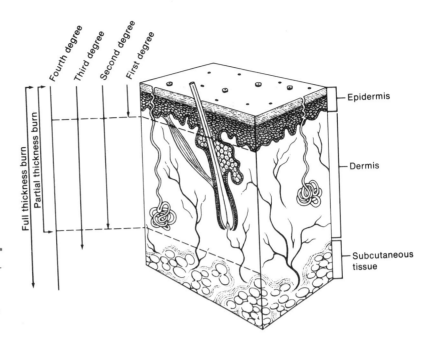

Figure 11-7. Cross section of the skin showing the relative depths of the types of burn injury. (From Scherer JC. Introductory Medical-Surgical Nursing. Philadelphia: JB Lippincott, 1991, p. 849.)

ment the child's intake. The caloric and nutritional requirements of the child are two or three times that needed for normal growth; thus, nutritional supplements will most likely be needed.

Diuresis. Urinary output must be monitored closely. The output may be decreased by the decrease in blood volume. Renal shutdown may be a threat. An output of 1 mL/kg of the child's weight per hour is desirable. An indwelling catheter facilitates the accurate measurement of urine and specific gravity. After the first hour, the volume of urine should be relatively constant. Any change in volume or specific gravity should be reported. Diuresis occurs in 48 to 72 hours.

After the initial fluid therapy has brought the burn shock under control, and after the extracellular fluid deficit has been made up, the patient faces another hazard with the onset of the diuretic phase. This occurs within 24 to 96 hours after the accident. The plasmalike fluid is picked up and reabsorbed from the "third space" in the burn areas, and the patient may rapidly become hypervolemic (exhibit an abnormal increase in the blood volume in the circulatory system), even to the point of pulmonary edema. This is the principal reason for the extremely close check on all vital signs, and for the close monitoring of intravenous fluids, which must now be slowed or stopped entirely.

The nurse needs to be alert for any signs of the onset of this phase to notify the physicians at once. Clues to the onset of the diuretic phase include the following:

1. Rapid rise in urinary output; may increase to 250 mL/h or higher
2. Tachypnea, followed by dyspnea
3. Increase in pulse pressure; mean blood pressure also may increase. Central venous pressure, if measured, is elevated.

Table 11-4. Classification of Burns

Classification	Description
Minor	First-degree burn or second degree <10% of body surface or third degree <2% of body surface; no area of the face, feet, hand, or genitalia is burned
Moderate	Second-degree burn between 10%–20% or on the face, hands, feet, or genitalia or third-degree burn <10% body surface or if smoke inhalation has occurred
Severe	Second-degree burn >20% body surface or third-degree burn >10% body surface

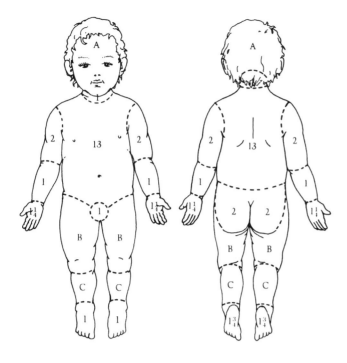

Relative Percentages of Areas Affected by Growth			
Area	Age 0	1	5
A = ½ of head	9½	8½	6½
B = ½ of one thigh	2¾	3¼	4
C = ½ of one leg	2½	2½	2¾

Figure 11-8. Determination of extent of burns in children.

drotherapy units, and patient care areas. In hospitals where there is no specific burn unit, a private room with a door that can be closed should be set up as a burn unit. "Reverse isolation," exercising the strictest aseptic technique, must be observed.

Wound Care. Two types of burn care are generally used: the open method and the closed method. The open method of burn care is most often used for superficial burns, burns of the face, and burns of the perineum. In open burn care, the wound is not covered, but antimicrobial ointment is applied topically. This type of care requires strict isolation precautions. In the closed burn method of burn care, nonadherent gauze is used to cover the burn. The child can be moved more easily, and there is less danger of added injury or pain. In the closed method, dressing changes are very painful, and infection may occur under the dressings. Occlusive dressings help minimize pain because of the reduced exposure to air.

In both methods, daily **débridement** (removal of necrotic tissue), usually preceded by **hydrotherapy** (use of water in treatment) is performed. Débridement is extremely painful, and the child must have an analgesic administered before the therapy. The child is placed in the tub of water to soak the dressings, which helps remove any sloughing tissue, **eschar** (hard crust or scab), exudate, and old medication (Figure 11-9). Often, the tissue is trapped in the mesh gauze of the dressing, easing its removal. Loose tissue is trimmed before the burn is redressed. Hosing instead of tub soaking is being used in some centers to reduce the risk of infection. Débridement is difficult emotionally for the child and the nurse. Diversionary activities may be used to help distract the child. Researchers also have found that children who are encouraged to participate actively in their burn care, even to help change dressings, experience healthy control over their situation and often suffer less anxiety than those who

Infection Control. The child has lost a portion of the integumentary system, which is a primary defense against infection. For this reason, measures must be taken to protect the child from infection. Antibiotics are not considered very effective in controlling infection of this type, most likely because of the injured capillaries that are unable to carry the antibiotic to the site. Antibiotics, if used, probably will be added to the intravenous fluids. Tetanus antitoxin or toxoid should be ordered according to the state of the child's previous immunization. If inoculations are up to date, a booster dose of tetanus toxoid is all that will be required.

To protect the child from infection introduced into the burn, sterile equipment must be used in the child's care. People caring for the child must wear a gown, a mask, and a head cover. Visitors are required to scrub, gown, and mask as well. Burn units are designed to be self-contained, with treatment and operating areas, hy-

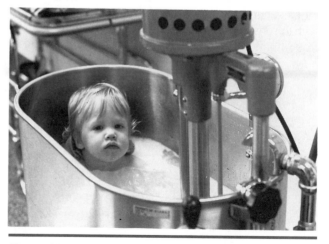

Figure 11-9. Child receiving hydrotherapy in Hubbard tank. (From Castiglia PT, Hardin RE. Child Health Care. Philadelphia: JB Lippincott, 1992, p. 986.)

are completely dependent on the nurse.[3] The child should never be scolded or reprimanded for uncooperative behavior. Praise for cooperation should be used generously.

Topical medications that may be used to reduce invading organisms are silver nitrate, mafenide acetate (Sulfamylon), silver sulfadiazine (Silvadene), gentamicin sulfate (Garamycin), and povidone-iodine (Betadine). Each of these agents have advantages and disadvantages. The choice of the agent used is made by the physician and is determined, at least partially, by the organisms that are found present in cultures of the burn area.

Grafting. Grafts may be either homografts, heterografts (xenografts), or autografts. The homografts and heterografts are temporary grafts. A **homograft** consists of skin taken from another person and is eventually rejected by the recipient tissue, sloughing off after 3 to 6 weeks. Skin from cadavers is often used, a procedure called an **allograft**; it can be stored and used up to several weeks, and permission for this use is seldom refused.

A **heterograft** is skin obtained from animals, usually pigs (called porcine). Both homografts and heterografts provide a temporary dressing after débridement and have proved to be lifesaving measures for children with extensive burns.

An **autograft**, consisting of skin taken from the child's own body, is the only kind of skin accepted permanently by recipient tissues, except for the skin from an identical twin. It is usually impossible to obtain enough healthy skin to cover a large area; therefore, homografts are of great value for immediate covering. If the donor site is kept free from infection and grafts of sufficient thinness are taken, the site should be ready for use again in 10 to 12 days.

After grafting, the donor as well as the graft sites are kept covered with sterile dressings.

Complications

Curling's ulcer (also called a "stress ulcer") is a gastric or duodenal ulcer that often occurs after serious skin burns. It can easily be overlooked when the attention of nurses and physicians is directed toward the treatment of the burn area and the prevention of infection.

Symptoms are those of any gastric ulcer but usually are vague, concerned with abdominal discomfort, with or without localization, or related to eating. Appearance of an ulcer, if it occurs, is during the first 6 weeks.

Blood may be present in the stools, an occurrence that, combined with abdominal discomfort, may be the basis for a diagnosis. If desired, roentgenograms can confirm the diagnosis. Treatment consists of a bland diet and the use of antacids and antispasmodics.

Contractures present another complication that must be carefully guarded against. If the burn extends over a movable body part, fibrous scarring that forms in the healing process can cause serious deformities and limit movement. Joints must be positioned, possibly in overextension, so that maximum flexibility is maintained. Splinting, exercise, and pressure also are used to prevent contractures. In severe burns, pressure garments, which help decrease hypertrophy of scar tissue, may need to be worn for 12 to 18 months (Figure 11-10). The child must wear these garments continuously, except when bathing.

Long-Term Care

The rehabilitative phase of care for the child is often long and difficult. Even after discharge from the hospital, the

Figure 11-10. Child continues to wear pressure garment for one year after burns occurred to avoid the contractures and scar formation. New suit required as child grows. **A**, Front view; **B**, side view; **C**, back view.

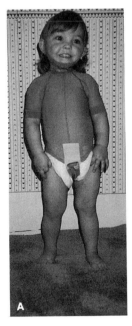
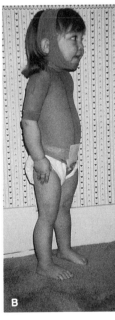
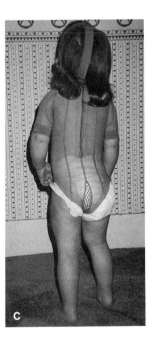

child may need to return for further treatment or plastic surgery to release the contractures and revise the scar tissue. The emotional scars of the family and the child must be evaluated, and therapy must be initiated or continued. The impact of scarring and disfigurement may need to be resolved by both the child and members of the family. If the child is of school age, school work and social interaction must be considered.

Nursing Process for the Child with a Burn

ASSESSMENT

Assessment of the child with a burn is complex and varies with the extent and depth of the burn, the stage of healing, and the age and general condition of the child. Initially, the primary concerns are the cardiac and respiratory state, the assessment of shock, and an evaluation of the burns.

After the first phase (the first 24 to 48 hours), the healing of the child's burns must be evaluated, the child's nutrition, signs of infection, and pain must be assessed. The emotional condition of the child and the family also must be evaluated.

NURSING DIAGNOSES

Many nursing diagnoses may be identified over the extended hospitalization of the child. Some of those that may be used are the following:

- High risk for infection related to the loss of a protective layer secondary to burn injury
- Altered nutrition: less than body requirements related to increased caloric needs secondary to burns and anorexia
- Pain related to tissue destruction and painful procedures
- High risk for impaired physical mobility related to pain and scarring
- Anxiety and fear related to body image disturbance secondary to thermal injury
- High risk for ineffective family coping related to the impact of the injury on the child's life
- Parental health-seeking behaviors regarding the long-term care required by the child

PLANNING AND IMPLEMENTATION

Initially, during the first phase of care, the major nursing goals will be directed toward cardiopulmonary stabilization, fluid and electrolyte balance, and infection control.

In the phase of care that follows the first 72 hours (sometimes called the management or subacute phase) more long-term goals must be developed. The child's goals will be limited by the child's age and ability to communicate. The goals may include relief of fear, pain and anxiety, and increased ability to move. The family may have additional goals of improved nutrition, optimum healing, decrease of complications with minimal permanent disability, and increased understanding of long term implications of care. The major nursing goals may be to relieve the anxiety, the fear, and the pain; to prevent infection; to promote optimum nutrition; improved mobility; avoidance of contractures; and helping the child and family prepare for long-term rehabilitation.

Preventing Infection. The fact that the child's immune system is immature, combined with the destruction of the layer of the skin and the ideal medium for bacterial growth that necrotic tissue provides, contributes to the significant danger of infection. Conscientious handwashing must be carried out by anyone who has contact with the child. Infection control precautions must be used, and sterile equipment and supplies are required. Vital signs, including temperature, must be monitored frequently, on a 1-, 2-, or 4-hour schedule. All people who have any contact with the child, including visitors, family, or staff caretakers, must be screened for any signs of upper respiratory or skin infection.

When caring for the burn, the nurse must wear a sterile gown, mask, and cap. Sterile gloves are worn or a sterile tongue blade is used to apply ointment to the burn. The room temperature should be maintained at around 80°F because evaporation of water through the denuded areas, and even through the leathery burn eschar, proceeds rapidly, with a consequent thermal evaporative loss. All drainage should be noted and documented. Any unusual odor should be reported immediately. Cultures should be done regularly, usually several times a week. Care should be taken to avoid injury to the eschar and the donor site. Hair on the tissue adjacent to the burn area should be shaved.

Assuring Adequate Nutrition. The child who has received extensive burns requires special attention regarding nutritional needs. The nutritional problem is much more complex than simply getting a seriously ill child to eat. The child is in negative caloric balance from a number of causes, including the following:

- Poor intake owing to anorexia, ileus, Curling's ulcer, or diarrhea
- External loss due to exudative losses of protein through the burn wound
- Thermal losses due to the burn itself; heat loss from the radiation of heat and water loss, responsible for large caloric losses
- Hypermetabolism due to fever, infection, and the state of "toxicity"

A diet high in protein (for healing and for replacement) and calories and bland is an essential component of therapy. Great efforts must be made to interest the child in foods essential for tissue building and repair. Large servings are not acceptable because of anorexia as well as the physical condition of the child. Foods are going to be of no value if the child refuses to eat them. Colorful trays, foods with eye appeal, and any special touches to spur a child's appetite should be tried. Allowing the child to have some control may be useful in gaining cooperation.

Foods that may appeal are flavored milk shakes, ice cream shakes, high-protein drinks containing eggs and extra dried protein milk, ice cream, milk and egg desserts, and pureed meats and vegetables.

Even with the best efforts of nurses, dietitians, and the child, the burn patient seldom can eat an amount of food sufficient to meet the increased needs. Hyperalimentation or tube feedings are frequently necessary as supplements to the daily intake. Commercial high-caloric formulas are available for tube feedings that meet the child's needs. Care must be taken to avoid making hyperalimentation or tube feedings a threat. The child must understand what is to be done and why. Demonstrating the tube feeding process with a doll may be helpful.

The child is weighed daily at the same time and with the same coverings. Intake and output should be monitored.

Recognizing and Relieving Pain and Providing Other Comfort Measures. The pain of a thermal injury can be severe. As a result of the pain, or the fear and anxiety that pain causes, the child may not sleep well, may suffer anorexia, and may be apprehensive and uncooperative during treatments and care. Analgesics must be administered to provide the most relief possible. Analgesics should be administered at least 20 to 30 minutes before dressing changes and débridement. The child's physiologic response to the pain and analgesics must be monitored. Pupil reaction, heart and respiratory rates, and behavior in response to pain and analgesics are documented. Administration of pain medications should be scheduled so that the child is not too sedated at mealtimes.

Support and comfort should be provided during painful procedures. Diversionary activities are important in helping the child focus on something other than the pain. A favorite activity can be promised after the dreaded procedure. Television may be helpful but should not be overused. The younger child may enjoy someone reading stories, learning new songs, and playing games that are age appropriate. The older child may enjoy video or computer games, tape recordings, books, and board or card games. At no time should the child be admonished for crying or behaving "like a baby." Acknowledging the child's pain, giving the child as much control as possible, and working with the child and the family to minimize the pain bring the greatest rewards for all involved.

Preventing Contractures. Care must be taken to avoid contractures and scarring that limit movement. No

two burned body surfaces, such as fingers, should touch. If the neck is involved, the child may have to be kept in a position with the neck hyperextended, arms may need to be placed in a brace to prevent underarm contractures, and joints of the knee or elbow must be extended to prevent scar formation from causing contractures that limit movement. Pressure dressings and pressure suits may be used for this purpose and may need to be worn for more than a year. Physical therapy may be needed, and splints may be used to position the body part to prevent contractures. All of these measures can add to the discomfort of the child.

Range of motion, early ambulation, and encouragement in self-help activities are additional means by which contractures can be prevented. With a little creativity the nurse can devise ways to involve the child in enjoyable activities that encourage movement of the affected part.

Reducing Anxiety About Changed Body Image. The age and level of understanding of the child influence the amount of anxiety and fear that the child has about scarring and disability related to the burn. If the child is in a burn unit with other children, seeing others may cause unrealistic fears. The child should be encouraged to explore his or her feelings about changes in body image. Therapeutic play with puppets or dolls may be helpful. The child needs continuous support from both the family and the nursing staff.

Promoting Family Coping. The family may feel guilty about the occurrence of the injury. One member may feel especially responsible. These feelings affect the coping abilities of the family. The family and the child should be given opportunities to discuss and express their feelings. Counseling may be necessary to assist family members to handle their feelings. Support groups also may be available and helpful to the family in working through problems. Family members should have care explained to them, and they can be involved in the care when possible. Caution is necessary to avoid saying anything that might add to the guilt or anxiety that the family members are feeling.

Providing Family Teaching. The family needs explanations about the whole process of burns, the care, the healing process, and the long-term implications. Information should be given to the family as they are ready for it and should not be thrust on them all at once. Preparation for home care involves teaching the family about the wound care; dressing changes; signs and symptoms to observe and report; and the importance of diet, rest, and activity. The family also needs guidance in finding resources for any necessary supplies and equipment. A referral to social services will assist them in home care planning. See Nursing Care Plan for toddler with a burn.

(text continued on page 278)

Nursing Care Plan
for the Toddler with a Burn

Nursing Diagnosis

High risk for infection related to loss of protective layer secondary to burn injury

Goal: Prevent infection

Nursing Interventions	*Rationale*	*Evaluation*
Carry out conscientious handwashing and follow other infection control precautions, including the use of sterile equipment and supplies. When providing direct burn care, wear a sterile gown, mask, and cap, and use sterile gloves.	Sterile technique lessens the introduction of microorganisms and reduces the risk of infection.	There are no signs and symptoms of infection as evidenced by vital signs within normal limits and no malodorous drainage.
Teach family and visitors sterile techniques, especially handwashing; stress importance of screening visitors for signs of upper respiratory or skin infection.	Infection control procedures must include all those who enter the child's room in order to be effective.	
Note and document all drainage and any unusual odor; take regular cultures.	Severe infection places an additional burden on an already overstressed system. Early detection and prompt treatment of infection is essential.	

Nursing Diagnosis

Altered nutrition: less than body requirements related to increased caloric needs secondary to burns and anorexia

Goal: Assure adequate nutrition

Nursing Interventions	*Rationale*	*Evaluation*
Administer a high-calorie, high-protein, bland diet in small servings.	Wound healing requires increased nutritional intake.	Child consumes at least 80% of diet high in calories and protein as evidenced by weight and intake and output records.
Make meals as appealing as possible. Provide small servings, and allow the child to have some control over choices.	Being allowed to make choices about the timing and types of foods will elicit the child's cooperation and will also help the child feel in control of at least one thing at a time when the child probably feels helpless; small servings are more likely to be appealing to the child than large servings and are easier for the child to eat.	The child's food likes, dislikes, and special habits regarding food and mealtime are clearly documented.
Weigh the child daily at the same time and with the same coverings. Monitor intake and output.	Provides vital data for continuous updating of nutritional therapy.	Weight and intake and output are documented and recorded at regular intervals.

(continued)

Nursing Care Plan
for the Toddler with a Burn (Continued)

Nursing Diagnosis
Pain related to tissue destruction and painful procedures

Goal: Relieve pain

Nursing Interventions	*Rationale*	*Evaluation*
Monitor the child's physiologic response to pain and analgesics.	Each individual responds differently to pain and analgesics. Knowledge of this child's unique responses will help the nurse plan the most effective pain reduction measures.	Pain is relieved promptly, as evidenced by the child's behavior and stable vital signs.
Administer analgesics promptly as ordered and 20 to 30 minutes before dressing changes and debridement.	This gives the analgesics time to reach optimum effectiveness during procedures when the child's pain is at its greatest.	
Support and comfort child during painful procedures; plan favorite diversional activities to follow procedures. Acknowledge the child's pain, and allow the child some control over timing or details of dressing change.	Distraction can help in getting through pain, but having control over some aspect of the hospitalization may prove even more beneficial to the child over the long treatment period.	

Nursing Diagnosis
High risk for impaired physical mobility related to pain and scarring

Goal: Prevent any permanent interference with mobility

Nursing Interventions	*Rationale*	*Evaluation*
Position child so that no two burned surfaces touch; this may require pressure dressings and suits or braces to hyperextended limbs.	Prevents scar formation that can lead to contractures and impair long-term physical mobility.	Child participates in range-of-motion activities; no evidence of contractures is present.
Encourage child to engage in safe activities, such as range-of-motion exercises and early ambulation, and to participate in self-care.	Provides opportunity for some physical mobility and helps prevent contractures.	

Nursing Diagnosis
Anxiety related to body image disturbance secondary to thermal injury

Goal: Reduce child's anxiety about changed body image

Nursing Interventions	*Rationale*	*Evaluation*
Encourage child to talk about fears regarding changed body image and disability related to the burn injury. Therapeutic play may be helpful.	Allows child to vent fears that may be exaggerated and to explore ways of dealing with those fears and the realistic changes that are expected.	Child expresses fears about body image and demonstrates a positive attitude of acceptance.

(continued)

Nursing Care Plan for the Toddler with a Burn (Continued)

Nursing Diagnosis
High risk for ineffective family coping related to the impact of burn injury on the child's life

Goal: Promote family coping

Nursing Interventions	Rationale	Evaluation
Provide opportunities for child and family to express fears and feelings about the injury and how it occurred.	Allows family members to explore fears and any feelings of guilt they have about the injury, which is a beginning step to improving positive coping skills.	Family members express guilt and anxieties, participate in care, and become involved in support groups when available.

Nursing Diagnosis
Parental health seeking behaviors related to long-term care for child

Goal: Provide family teaching

Nursing Interventions	Rationale	Evaluation
Explain the healing process, treatment, and long-term implications to family members, providing information in chunks as they are ready to hear about it rather than all at once.	A burn injury is an overwhelming experience in itself; people can only process so much information at a time during such a stressful event.	Family members demonstrate knowledge of how to care for the child and verbalize the principles of long-term management of the child's care.
Prepare family for home care by teaching individual family members about the importance of diet, rest, and activity and how to provide wound care and perform dressing changes. Instruct also on signs and symptoms to observe and report.	Family members need specific information and a chance to practice before the child is discharged.	Family members demonstrate care techniques successfully in nurse's presence.

EVALUATION

- No signs and symptoms of infection, as evidenced by vital signs within normal limits; no malodorous drainage
- Child consumes at least 80% of diet high in calories and protein as evidenced by weight and intake and output records
- Pain is relieved promptly, as evidenced by the child's behavior and stable vital signs
- Child participates in range of motion activities; no evidence of contractures is present.
- Child expresses fears about body image and demonstrates a positive attitude of acceptance
- Family members express guilt and anxieties, participate in the care, and become involved in support groups when available

- Family members demonstrate knowledge of how to care for the child and verbalize an understanding of the long-term management of the child's care

Summary

Toddlerhood is a time of exploring and learning, when mobility and communication influence what happens to the child. Autism may become evident if the child does not form relationships with parents and family. Respiratory infections may cause illness in the toddler, accounting for numerous sleepless nights. Upper respiratory infections can be the reason for hospital admission, if necessary. Hereditary diseases that affect nutrition are celiac syndrome and CF. CF also causes respiratory problems that contribute to the severity of the disease.

Because of the exploring nature of the toddler, an adult or another responsible person should supervise the toddler at all times. The toddler should not be left alone because the toddler's inquiring mind has not developed judgment about those things that are safe and those that are not. As a result of this curiosity and lack of judgment, the toddler may become involved in an accident. The accidents that occur to a toddler can be life threatening or cause permanent damage. Burns cause damage that may affect the child for the remainder of his or her life. The toddler likes to experience many things by "tasting" them. Therefore, the toddler may swallow either poisons or objects that can cause serious systemic damage.

Review Questions

1. Melanie is a toddler with infectious conjunctivitis. What principles of hygiene would you teach her caregiver, Ivor?
2. Which two conditions studied in this chapter cause fatty stools?
3. Carmella has idiopathic celiac disease. From the following list, select the foods that she may have in her meal plan. With the help of a nutrition text or by reading labels, identify the foods you will not recommend, and state the reason that each of those foods is not appropriate:

    ice cream
    corn flakes
    grits
    rice pudding
    whole wheat bread
    baked beans
    hamburger
    hot dog
    french fries
    fresh vegetables
    cream of tomato soup
    yogurt
    oatmeal
    Rice Krispies
    orange juice
    graham crackers
    corn chips
    peanut butter
    baked potato
    tuna salad
    pizza

4. Manuel, age 15 months, has episodes of croup (spasmodic laryngitis). What teaching can you give his grandmother, Rosita, who is his primary caregiver?
5. Draw a diagram to explain the heredity pattern of cystic fibrosis.
6. You discover your 18-month-old child with an empty bottle of children's acetaminophen. Tell what you would do in sequence.
7. What is meant by environmental follow-up of lead poisoning? Why is it important?
8. Make a list of all the water dangers you can find in an area around your home. Include those inside the home.
9. Thirteen-month-old Jessie unexpectedly reached from her high chair to a pan of hot vegetables. She grabbed it and spilled the hot liquid over her legs. Her mother immediately poured cool water over her legs, but Jessie still suffered moderate burns. How can you help her mother deal with the guilt?
10. Survey your house (or a house you select). List the hazards for ingestion of poisonous substances, drowning, and burns. Include all types of burns.
11. Two-year-old Omar has partial- and total-thickness burns from a wood stove accident. What can you tell the family about infection control and its importance?
12. Why are infants and young toddlers especially prone to ingestion of foreign objects?

References

1. American Psychiatric Association. Diagnostic and Statistical Manual of Mental Disorders, Third Edition, Revised. Washington, DC: Author, 1987.
2. Oski FA. Principles and Practices of Pediatrics. Philadelphia: JB Lippincott, 1990.
3. Kavanaugh C. A new approach to dressing change in the severely burned child and its effect on burn-related psychopathology. Heart Lung 12:612–619, 1983.

Bibliography

Adler R. Burns are different: The child psychiatrist on the pediatric burns ward. J Burn Care Rehabil 13(1):28–32, 1992.

Anson A, Weizman Z, Zeevi N. Celiac disease: Parental knowledge and attitudes of dietary compliance. Pediatrics 85(1): 98–103, 1990.

Attas AB, Orenstein SR, Orenstein DM. Pancreatitis in young children with cystic fibrosis. J Pediatr 120:756–759, 1992.

Bartholomew LK, Seilheimer DK, Parcel GS, et al. Planning patient education for cystic fibrosis: Application of a diagnostic framework. Patient Educ Counsel 13(1):57–68, 1989.

Bebko JM, Kostantareas MM, Springer J. Parent and professional evaluations of family stress associated with characteristics of autism. J Autism Dev Disord 17(4):565–576, 1987.

Berger OG, Gregg DJ, Succop PA. Using unstimulated urinary lead excretion to assess the need for chelation in the treatment of lead poisoning. J Pediatr 116:46–51, 1990.

Campbell LS, Thomas DO. Pediatric trauma: When kids get hurt. RN 54(9):32–38, 1991.

Castiglia PT, Harbin RE. Child Health Care: Process and Practice. Philadelphia: JB Lippincott, 1992.

DeRienzo-DeVivio S. Childhood lead poisoning: Shifting to primary prevention. Pediatr Nurs 18(6):565–567, 1992.

George MR. CF: Not just a pediatric problem anymore. RN 53(9):60–65, 1990.

Pillitteri A. Maternal and Child Health Nursing. Philadelphia: JB Lippincott, 1992.

Shukla R, Bornschein RL, Dietrich KN, et al. Fetal and infant lead exposure: Effects on growth in stature. Pediatrics 84(4):604–612, 1989.

Spock B, Rothenberg MB. Dr. Spock's Baby and Child Care. New York: Pocket Books, 1992.

Waite WW. Pharmacologic management of cystic fibrosis. J Pract Nurs 38(3):19–29, 1988.

Whaley LF, Wong DL. Nursing Care of Infants and Children, 4th ed. St. Louis: Mosby-Year Book, 1991.

Growth and Development of the Preschool Child: Ages 3 to 6 Years

Chapter 12

Student Objectives

Upon completion of this chapter, the student will be able to:

1. Briefly describe several social characteristics of the preschooler, and state the age group this includes.
2. Describe the growth rate of the preschooler.
3. State the age at which 20/20 vision usually is attained.
4. Relate preschool nutritional needs, including a.) Daily minimum needs; b.) Appetite variations; c.) Suggested snacks; d.) Television commercials and other influences.
5. State the recommended health maintenance schedule for the preschooler.
6. List guidelines for accident prevention in the preschool age population.
7. List nine health teachings for the preschooler concerning prevention of infection.
8. Identify the preschool social characteristic that increases the risk of infection.
9. List four factors that may delay language development.
10. Discuss the role of "magical thinking" and imagination in the preschooler.
11. Describe the characteristics of dreams, nightmares, and imaginary playmates.
12. Discuss the nurse's role in helping parents understand their preschooler's sexual curiosity.
13. Discuss masturbation in the preschool age.
14. List six types of play in which preschoolers engage, and define each.
15. Discuss aggression in the preschooler a.) Verbal aggression; b.) Physical aggression; c.) Parents' tasks; d.) Parents' example.
16. State the role of discipline for the preschooler a.) Caregiver behavior; b.) Effect on child; c.) Effect on caregiver.
17. Discuss the special needs of the disadvantaged school-age child.
18. Discuss the value of Head Start programs.

Marks MG: BROADRIBB'S INTRODUCTORY PEDIATRIC NURSING, 4th ed. © 1994 J.B. Lippincott Company.

Key Terms

associative play   onlooker play

cooperative play   parallel play

magical thinking   solitary independent
                          play
noncommunicative
    language   unoccupied behavior

*P*reschoolers are fascinating creatures. As their social circles enlarge to include peers and adults outside the family, their language, play patterns, and appearance change markedly. Their curiosity about the world around them grows as does their ability to explore the world in greater detail and see new meanings in what they find (Figure 12-1). Preschoolers can be said to soak up information "like a sponge." "Why?" and "how?" are favorite words. This curiosity also means that accidents are still a serious concern.

At 3 years of age, the child still has the chubby, baby-faced look of a toddler, but by age 5, a leaner, taller, better coordinated social being has emerged. The child works and plays tirelessly, "making things" and telling everyone about it. Although the child has some problem separating fantasy from reality, exploring and learning go on continuously. According to Erikson, the developmental task of the preschool age is initiative versus guilt. Preschoolers often try to find ways to do things to "help," but if they fail because of inexperience or lack of skill and get scolded, they may feel guilty.

Physical Development

Growth Rate

The preschool period is one of slow growth. The child gains about 3 to 5 lb each year (1.4 to 2.3 kg) and grows about 2½ inches (6.3 cm) taller. Because the increase in height is proportionately greater than the increase in weight, the 5-year-old child appears much thinner and

less babyish than the 3-year-old does. Boys tend to be leaner than girls during this time. Gross and fine motor skills continue to develop rapidly. Balance improves, and with that improvement the confidence to try new activities emerges. By age 5 the child generally is able to throw and catch a ball well, to climb effectively, and to ride a bicycle. Important milestones for growth and development are summarized in Table 12-1.

Dentition

By 6 years of age the child's skull is 90% of its adult size. The deciduous teeth have completely emerged by the beginning of the preschool period. Toward the end of the preschool stage, those teeth begin to be replaced by permanent teeth. This is an event that most children anticipate as an indication that they are "growing up." Pictures of smiling 5- and 6-year-olds typically show missing front teeth (Figure 12-2).

The age at which teeth erupt varies with individual children and with various ethnic and economic groups. Permanent teeth of African American children erupt at least 6 months earlier than those of American children of European ancestry. The central incisors are usually the first to go, just as they were the first to erupt in infancy. The child needs to be supervised in tooth brushing; the caregiver still should be responsible for flossing. Regular dental checkups are recommended every 6 months.

Visual Development

Although the preschooler's senses of taste and smell are acute, visual development is still immature at age 3. Eye-hand coordination is good, but judgment of distances generally is faulty, leading to many bumps and falls. During the preschool years, the child's vision should be checked to screen for amblyopia. Usually by age 6 the child has achieved 20/20 vision, but mature depth perception may not occur in some children until 8 to 10 years of age.

Skeletal Growth

Between the third and sixth birthdays, the greatest amount of skeletal growth occurs in the feet and legs. This contributes to the change from the wide-gaited, pot-bellied look

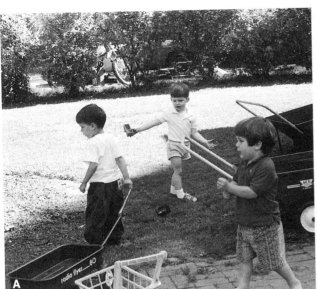
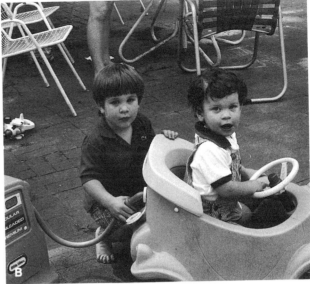
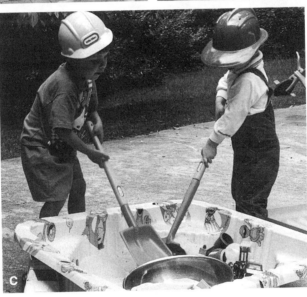

Figure 12-1. Children in the latter stages of preschool years engage in associative and dramatic play. **A**, They may act independently. **B**, They identify with adults. **C**, They enjoy dressing up to look like the people they are playing. (From Jackson DB, Saunders RB. Child Health Nursing. Philadelphia: JB Lippincott, 1993, p. 325.)

of the toddler into the slim, taller figure of the 6-year-old. In addition, the carpals and tarsals mature in the hands and feet, contributing to better hand and foot control.

Nutrition

The preschool period is not a time of rapid growth; therefore, children do not need large quantities of food. Nevertheless, protein needs continue to remain high to provide for muscle growth. The preschooler's appetite is erratic, however; at one sitting the preschooler may de-

vour everything on the plate and at the next be satisfied with just a few bites. Portions are smaller than adult-sized portions. The child may need to have meals supplemented with nutritious snacks. Some suggested snacks are listed in Box 12-1. Note that certain snacks are recommended only for the older child to avoid any danger of the younger child choking. Frequent, small meals with snacks in between generally are best accepted by the preschooler.

Among the preschooler's favorites are soft foods, grain and dairy products, raw vegetables, and sweets. Television commercials for sugar-coated cereals, snacks, and fast foods of questionable nutritional value exert a

Table 12-1. Growth and Development Chart: The Preschooler

Age (yr)	Personal-Social	Fine Motor	Gross Motor	Language	Cognition
3	Begins Erikson's stage of "initiative vs. guilt." It is at this time that conscience develops. Shy with strangers and inept with peers Sufficiently independent to be interested in group experiences with age mates (ie, nursery school)	Able to button clothes Copies ○ and + Uses pencils, crayons, paints Shows preference for right or left hand	Tends to watch motor activities before attempting them A jump of several feet is possible Uses hands in broad movements Rides tricycle Negotiates stairs well	Vocabulary up to 1000 words Articulates all vowels accurately Talks a lot Sings and recites Asks many questions	Continues in preoperational stage (2–7 years) characterized by: 1. *Centration* or the inability to attend to more than one aspect of a situation 2. *Egocentricity*, or the inability to consider the perception of others 3. The static and irreversible quality of thought that makes the child unable to perceive the processes of change
4	Boisterous and inflammatory Aggressive physically and verbally but developing behaviors to become socially acceptable Becomes socially acceptable Accepts punishment for wrongdoings because it relieves guilt	Can use scissors; copies a square Adds three parts to stick figures	Has some hesitations but tends to try feats beyond ability Greater powers of balance and accuracy Hops on one foot; can control movements of hands	Vocabulary of about 1500 words Constant questions Sentences of 4–5 words Uses profanity Reports fantasies as truth	Reality and fantasy are not always clear to the preschooler Believes that words make things real— "magical" thinking
5	Initiates contacts with strangers and relates interesting little tales Interested in telling and comparing stories about self Peer relations are important ("best friends" abound) Response to social values by assuming sex roles with rigidity	Ties shoelaces Copies a diamond and a triangle Prints a few letters or numbers May print first name Cuts food	Will not attempt feats beyond ability Throws and catches ball well Jumps rope Walks backward with heel to toe Skips and hops Adept on bicycle and climbing equipment	Vocabulary of 3000 words 90% of speech is intelligible Asks meanings of words Enjoys telling stores	Thinks feelings and thoughts can happen Intrusions into the body cause fear and anxiety (fear of mutilation and castration)

powerful influence on the preschooler and can make supermarket shopping an emotional struggle between the caregiver and child. Caregivers should read labels carefully before making a purchase.

Preschoolers need guidance in choosing foods and are strongly influenced by the example of family members and peers. Food should never be used as a reward or bribe; otherwise, the child will continue to use food as a means to manipulate the environment and the behavior of others.

To meet the minimum daily requirements, the preschooler should have two or three glasses of milk each day and several small portions from each food group. Preschoolers have definite food preferences. They generally do not like highly spiced foods, often will eat raw vegetables but not cooked ones, and prefer plain foods

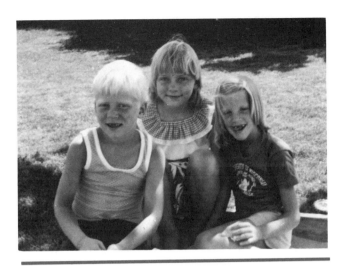

Figure 12-2. Five- and six-year-olds begin to lose their deciduous teeth. (Courtesy of E. Lundeen.)

rather than casseroles. New foods may be accepted but should be introduced one at a time to avoid overwhelming the child.

The preschooler shows growing independence and skill in eating. The 3-year-old child tries to mimic adult behavior at the table but often reverts to eating with his or her fingers, spilling liquids, and squirming. The 4-year-old is more skilled with the use of utensils, but an occa-

---

Box 12-1

Suggested Snacks for the Preschooler

Raw vegetables: such as carrots,* cucumbers, celery,* green beans, green pepper, mushrooms, turnips, broccoli, cauliflower, tomatoes

Fresh fruits: such as apples, oranges, pears, peaches, grapes,* cherries,* melons

Unsalted whole grain crackers

Whole grain bread: cut to finger-sized sticks; plain, toasted, or with peanut butter

Small sandwiches: cut into quarters

Natural cheese: cut in cubes

Cooked meat: cut in small chunks or sliced thinly

*Nuts**

*Sunflower seeds**

Cookies: made with lightly sweetened whole grains

*Plain popped corn**

Yogurt: plain or with fresh fruit added

*Children younger than 2 years of age may choke on nuts, seeds, popcorn, celery strings, or carrot sticks. Avoid offering until preschool years.

---

sional misjudgment of abilities results in a mess. The 5-year-old uses utensils well, even cutting his or her own food, and can be taught to practice sophisticated table manners. Rituals such as using the same plate, cereal bowl, cup, or placemat may become important to the child's mealtime happiness.

Psychosocial Development

Language Development

Between the ages of 3 and 5 years, language development is generally rapid. Most 3-year-old children can construct simple sentences, but they have many hesitations and repetitions as they search for the right word or try to make the right sound. Stuttering can develop during this period but usually disappears within 3 to 6 months. By the end of the fifth year, preschoolers use long, rather complex sentences; their vocabulary will have increased by more than 1500 words since age 2.

Preschoolers' use of language changes during this period. Three-year-old children often talk to themselves or to their toys or pets without any apparent purpose other than the pleasure of using words. Piaget called this egocentric, or **noncommunicative**, **language**. By 4 years of age, children increase their use of communicative language, using words to transmit information other than their own needs and feelings.

Four- and 5-year-old children delight in using "naughty" words or swearing. Bathroom words become favorites, and taunts such as "you're a big doo doo" bring heady excitement to them. Caregivers may become concerned by this turn of events, but the child simply may be trying words out to test their impact. A calm, matter-of-fact response that lets the child know that this is not language to use when in the company of others may help defuse some of its power. Development of preschoolers' verbal abilities is summarized in Table 12-2.

Delays or other difficulties in language development may be caused by one or more of the following:

- Hearing impairment or other physical problem
- Lack of stimulation
- Overprotection
- Lack of parental interest or rejection by parents

Good language skills are developed as the child is engaged regularly in conversation with caregivers and others. The conversation should be on a level that the child can understand. Reading to the child is an excellent method of contributing to language development. This can be enhanced by talking with the child about the pictures in the story books. Praise, approval, and encouragement are all part of supporting attempts at communication.

Family and cultural patterns also influence language

Table 12-2. Verbal Abilities of Preschoolers

Age (yr)	Characteristics of Language Usage	Expected Language Comprehension	Expected Correct Speech Articulation	Language Rhythm
3–4	Enjoys talking and talks a lot. Makes up words or may sing or recite own version of a song or rhyme. Enjoys new and special words. Asks many questions and demands answers. Sentences and concepts are not always logical. Comforts others with words. Vocabulary of 900–1000 words. Uses 4- to 5-word phrases. Aggression is displayed with words rather than physical force	3 years—up to 3600 words 4 years—up to 5600 words	3½ years—all vowels and p, m, and b sounds 4 years—speech is 100% intelligible, even though misarticulations may occur	3–5-year-olds may have many hesitations, repetitions, and revisions in an effort to produce adult speech. Stuttering may begin during this time. It disappears within 3–6 months but may continue as long as 2 years without permanent stuttering occurring
4–5	Understands words outside their usual context. Has difficulty finding the right word. Speech has high emotional content. Tells functions of things rather than names. Changes the subject rapidly. Boasts, brags, and quarrels. Fascinated with naughty words. Reports fantasies as truth. 90% of speech is intelligible. Uses complex phrase units. Vocabulary consists of 3000 words	5 years—up to 9600 words	5½ years—f, v, y, th, l, and wh sounds	

Adapted from Weiss CE, Lillywhite HS. Communicative Disorders: A Handbook for Prevention and Early Intervention. St. Louis: CV Mosby, 1976; and McElroy CW. Speech and Language Development of the Preschool Child. Springfield, Ill: Charles C Thomas, 1976, pp 179–185.

development. Some children come from bilingual families and are trying to learn the rules of both languages. Others may come from geographic or social communities that have dialects different from the general population.

Development of Imagination

Preschoolers have learned to think about something without actually seeing it—to visualize or imagine. This normal development, sometimes called **magical thinking**, makes it difficult for them to separate fantasy from reality. Preschoolers believe that words or thoughts can make things real, and this belief can have either positive or negative results. For example, in a moment of anger, a child wishes that a parent or a sibling would die; if that person later is hurt, the child feels responsible and suffers guilt. The child needs reassurance that this is not so.

Imagination makes preschoolers good audiences for storytelling, simple plays, and television, as long as the characters and events are not too frightening or sad. When preschoolers see a television character die, they believe it is real and often cry. The television viewing of the child should be supervised to avoid programs with negative impact or overstimulation.

During this stage, children often have imaginary playmates who are very real to them. This occurs particularly with only children, filling times of loneliness. The imaginary friend often has the characteristics that the child might wish for. Sometimes the imaginary friend is the one who gets the "blame" for breaking a toy or another act the child does not want to take credit for. Caregivers need assurance that this is normal behavior.

Dreams and nightmares are common during the preschool period. Caregivers need to explain that "it was only a dream" and offer love and understanding until the fear has subsided.

Fear of the dark is another common problem during these years. Children may be afraid to go to sleep in a dark bedroom. These are very real fears to the child. A small night light may be reassuring to the child. One mother solved this problem in an interesting fashion. The child was afraid of a "monster" in the closet or under the bed. The mother acknowledged the child's fears and purchased a spray can of room air freshener. At bedtime she ceremoniously sprayed around the room, in the closet, and under the bed. She assured the child that it was a special spray to kill "monsters" just like bug spray kills bugs. The child was reassured and slept without fear.

Sexual Development

The preschool period is the stage that Freud termed the *Oedipal* or *phallic* (genital) *period*. During these years, children become acutely aware of their sexuality, including sexual roles and organs. They generally develop a strong emotional attachment to the parent of the opposite sex. Curiosity about their own genitalia and those of peers and adults may make parents uncomfortable and evoke responses that indicate that sex is dirty and something to be ashamed and guilty about.

Despite today's abundance of sexually oriented literature, many families find it difficult to deal with the questions and actions of the young child. Nurses can help caregivers understand that the child's sexual curiosity is a normal, natural part of total curiosity about oneself and the surrounding world. The informed, understanding parent can help children develop positive attitudes toward sexuality and toward themselves as sexual human beings.

In addition to responsible teaching of sexual information, the caregiver also should teach the child about "good touch" and "bad touch." The child needs to understand that no one should touch the child's body in a way that is unpleasant.

Masturbation

Exploration of the genitalia is just as natural for the preschooler as thumbsucking is for the infant. This is one way the child learns to perceive the body as a possible source of pleasure and is the beginning of acceptance of sex as natural and pleasurable.

The caregivers can be reassured that this is not uncommon behavior, and a calm, matter-of-fact response to the child is the most effective approach. The child should be helped to understand that masturbation is not an activity that is appropriate in public. If the child seems to be masturbating excessively, counseling may be needed, especially if the child's life has been unsettled in other aspects.

Social Development

Preschoolers are outgoing, imaginative, social beings. They play vigorously and, in the process, learn about the world in which they live. Preschoolers have been charac-

terized as "sponges," soaking up all that goes on about them, influenced both positively and negatively. As they gain control over their environment, preschoolers try to manipulate it, which may lead to conflict with their caregivers. A preschool group of children are delightful to watch as they go about the business of growing and learning.

Play

Play activities are one way that children learn. Normally, by 3 years of age, children begin imitative play, pretending to be the mommy, the daddy, a policeman, a cowboy, an astronaut, or some well-known person or television character (Figure 12-3). Caregivers can gain good insight into the way their child interprets family behavior by watching the child play. Listening to a preschooler scold a doll or stuffed animal for "bothering me while I'm busy talking on the phone" lets the adults hear how they sound to the child.

Dramatic play allows a child to act out troubling situations and to control the final solution to the problem. This is important to remember when teaching children who are going to be hospitalized. Use of dolls and pup-

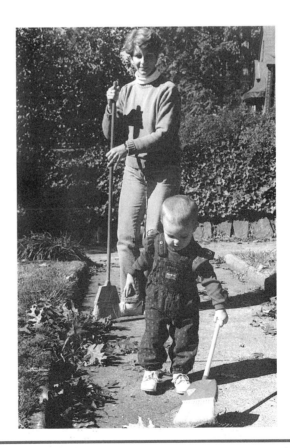

Figure 12-3. Toddlers learn by imitating adult activities. (From Jackson DB, Saunders RB. Child Health Care Nursing: A Comprehensive Approach to the Care of Children and Their Families. Philadelphia: JB Lippincott, 1993.)

pets to explain procedures makes the experience less threatening.

Drawing is another form of play through which children learn to express themselves. During the preschool years, as fine motor skills improve, children's drawings become much more complex and controlled and can be revealing about the child's self-concept and perception of his or her environment (Figure 12-4).

Preschoolers engage in various types of play: cooperative, associative, parallel, solitary independent, onlooker, and unoccupied behavior.[1]

In **cooperative play**, children play *with* each other, as in team sports. **Associative play** means being engaged in a common activity but without any sense of belonging. In **parallel play**, children play alongside each other but independently. Although common among toddlers, parallel play exists in all age groups, for example, in a scout troop where each member is working on an individual project or craft. **Solitary independent play** means playing apart from others without making an effort to be part of the group or their activity. Watching television is one form of **onlooker play**, in which there is an interest in observation without participation. In **unoccupied behavior**, the child may be daydreaming, fingering clothing or a toy, without apparent purpose.

Children need all types of play to aid in their total development. Too much of one kind may signal a problem; for example, a youngster who spends most of the time unoccupied may be troubled, depressed, or unstimulated. Cooperative play helps develop social interaction skills and often physical health as well.

Too much onlooker play, particularly television viewing, means that children are missing the benefits of other kinds of play and may be forming strong, highly inaccurate impressions of people and their behaviors. The amount of time that preschoolers spend watching television should be limited, and interactive play should be encouraged.

Aggression

Temper tantrums are an early form of aggression. The preschooler with newly developed language skills uses words aggressively in name-calling and threats. Four-year-old children use physical aggression as well, pushing, hitting, and kicking in an effort to manipulate the environment. The family caregivers' task during these years is to help the child understand that the anger and frustration that result in aggressive behavior are normal but need to be handled differently because aggressive behavior is not socially acceptable.

Children who come from unhappy home situations are likely to be more aggressive than those children from a comfortable family situation. Their caregivers have served as role models, and their aggressive behavior toward each other has said to the child, "this is acceptable."

Discipline

It is important for family caregivers to remember that preschoolers are developing initiative and a sense of guilt. They want to be good and follow instructions, and they feel bad when they do not, even though they are not physically punished. Discipline during this time should strive to teach the child a sense of responsibility and inner control. Spanking and other forms of physical punishment remove the responsibility from the child. Taking away a privilege from a child who has misbehaved until he or she can demonstrate that there has been an improvement in behavior is much more effective. Because the child's concept of time is not clear, the period should be comparatively brief (Table 12-3).

Nursery School or Day Care Experience

Group experiences with peers and adults outside the immediate family are important to a child's development. However, the transition to new experiences, new people, and new surroundings can be threatening to some preschoolers. Children vary in their willingness or ability to handle new situations, but being introduced gradually, according to individual readiness, produces the most

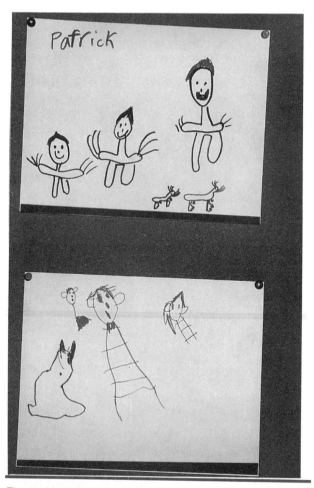

Figure 12-4. Drawings by preschoolers in Sibling Class representing family with new baby-to-be. (Drawings from Sibling Class, Lewistown Hospital.)

Table 12-3. Effects of Positive and Negative Caregiver Behavior

Behavior	Effect on Child	Effect on Adult
Attending only to desired behaviors Calm reasoning with expression of dislike of behavior Physical restraint with adult present Isolation of child for a period of time equal to 1 min per year of age Withholding of desired treats, outings, presents	Development of inner control	Feelings of adequacy as parents
Yelling, screaming, and implying guilt and punishment Telling child he or she is bad Physical punishment	Development of fears and compulsive behaviors	Feelings of guilt and inadequacy
Giving treats, presents, or food for lack of undesired behavior Physical punishment Threatening punishment from God or other authority figure	Development of control based on external forces	Feelings of being manipulated by child

satisfactory adjustment. Some children spend only a few hours each week in a nursery school or other day care program; others, because the adult family members work outside the home, must spend a great deal more time away from home and family. The family should understand that this probably means the child will demand more of their attention during the hours when they are together. As the child grows older and the attachment to peers becomes stronger, family caregivers sense a decrease in the need for adult attention and a greater sense of independence in the child.

The Disadvantaged Child
Discussions of normal growth and development assume that children come from a secure, well-adjusted home in which there is ample opportunity for social, cultural, and intellectual enrichment. This assumption ignores a sizable population that, for many reasons, is deprived of such a background. This population is the one most likely to have health problems and the need for health services.

Children who have not been able to achieve a sense of security and trust, for whatever reason, need special understanding, warm acceptance, and intelligent guidance to grow into self-accepting people. Society is gradually awakening to the needs of these children and trying to provide enriched nursery school and kindergarten experiences for those whose home life cannot do this for them, but much remains to be done. Further discussion of the problems of these children can be found in Unit IV: A Child in a Troubled Society.

Head Start Programs
Recognition that environmental enrichment is often not available in families of limited social, cultural, and economic resources led to the establishment of Head Start programs. Head Start programs are funded by federal and local money and are free of charge to the children enrolled. Children in such programs have an opportunity to broaden their horizons through varied experiences. Their understanding of the world in which they live is increased, and they are better prepared for a successful entry into the schoolroom. Family caregiver participation is a central component of the Head Start concept. Also, involvement of family caregivers often has a positive effect on other children in the household. In some programs, teachers go in to the home to help the caregiver teach the young child motor, cognitive, self-help, and language skills. Counseling and referral services are also provided through Head Start programs. Children who have had a background of Head Start enrichment are better prepared to enter kindergarten or first grade and compete successfully with their peers.

Health Maintenance

Preschoolers with up-to-date immunization schedules need boosters of diptheria-tetanus-pertussis, oral polio vaccine, and measles-mumps-rubella vaccine between 4 and 6 years of age, which are required as preschool boosters for entrance into kindergarten. An annual health examination is recommended to monitor the child's growth and development and to screen for potential health problems. The preschool child needs to be told in advance about the upcoming examination, with simple explanations and an opportunity to ask questions and voice anxieties. There are a number of books available through the public library that are excellent for this purpose. Children who attend nursery school or a day care program are required to have an annual examination, but children who stay at home may not have this advantage. Particular attention should be paid to the child's vision and hearing, so that any problems can be treated before he or she enters school at age 6 (Table 12-4).

Prevention of Accidents

Parents and caregivers of preschoolers need to be just as attentive as with toddlers because a child's curiosity at this stage still exceeds his or her judgment. Burns, poisoning, and falls are common accidents. Preschoolers are often victims of motor vehicle accidents, either because of darting into the street or driveway or as passengers without proper restraints. All states have vehicle restraint laws that define safety seat and restraint requirements for children. Adults must teach and reinforce these rules. One primary responsibility of adults is always to wear seat belts themselves and to make certain that the child always is in a safety seat or has a seat belt on. A child can be calmly taught that the vehicle "won't go" unless the child is properly restrained.

Parent Teaching

Preschooler Safety Teaching

1. Look both ways before crossing the street.
2. Cross street only with an adult.
3. Watch for cars coming out of driveways.
4. Never play behind a car or truck.
5. Watch for cars or trucks backing up.
6. Wear a safety helmet when bike riding.
7. Learn your name, address, and phone number.
8. Stay away from strange dogs.
9. Stay away from any dog while it's eating.
10. Only take medicine your caregiver gives you.
11. Don't play with matches or lighters.
12. Stay away from fires.
13. Don't run near a swimming pool.
14. Only swim when with an adult.
15. Don't go anywhere with someone you don't know.
16. Don't let anyone touch in a way you don't like.

By the age of 5 years, many preschoolers move from riding a tricycle to riding a bicycle. If the preschooler is not already wearing a bicycle helmet, it is important to

Table 12-4. Recommended Health Maintenance for Preschoolers by Age

	36 months (3 yr)	*48 Months (4 yr)*	*60 Months (5 yr)*
Examinations	Full physical examination First dental examination	Full physical examination Dental examination	Full physical examination Dental examination
Immunizations	Update if not current PPD	DTaP booster (between 4–6 yr) OPV booster (between 4–6 yr) MMR (second dose given at 4–6 or 10–12 yr) PPD	DTaP, OPV, and MMR boosters if not given previously PPD
Screening Procedures	Urinalysis Hematocrit Lead level Blood pressure Vision screening Hearing screening Denver Developmental Screening Test	Same as for 36 mo	Same as for 36 mo

PPD, purified protein derivative (of tuberculin); *DTaP*, diptheria-tetanus-pertussis; *OPV*, oral polio vaccine; *MMR*, measles-mumps-rubella.

educate caregivers that safety helmets are a necessary safety precaution. Lightweight, child-sized safety helmets that fit properly can be purchased, and the child should be taught that it must be worn when bike riding. Family caregivers or other adults who wear helmets provide the best incentive to children. Safety rules for bicycle riding should be reinforced. The preschool child should be limited to protected areas for riding and should have adult supervision.

The preschool age is an excellent time to begin teaching safety rules. The rules for crossing the street and playing in an area near traffic are of vital importance. The adults caring for or responsible for preschool children should be conscious of providing a good role model for the children. These safety rules should extend into all aspects of the child's life (see Parent Teaching: Preschooler Teaching for Safety).

Prevention of Infection

Preschoolers who enjoy sound nutrition, adequate rest, exercise, and shelter usually are not seriously affected by simple childhood infections. Children who live in less than adequate economic circumstances, however, can be severely threatened by even a simple illness, such as diarrhea and chickenpox. Immunizations are available for many childhood communicable diseases, yet some caregivers do not have their children immunized until it is required for entrance to school. As a result, some children suffer unnecessary illnesses.

Preschoolers are just learning to share, and that can mean sharing infections with the entire family—and playmates as well. Teaching them basic precautions can help

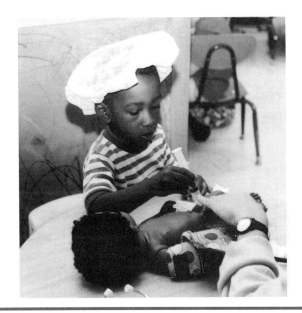

Figure 12-5. The child learns about interventions he will undergo by simulating the activity with a doll. This also may help him to be less afraid. (From Jackson DB, Saunders RB. Child Health Nursing: A Comprehensive Approach to the Care of Children and Their Families. Philadelphia: JB Lippincott, 1993.)

prevent spreading infections (see Parent Teaching: Teaching to Prevent Infections in the Preschooler).

Parent Teaching

Teaching to Prevent Infections

1. Cover your mouth when coughing or sneezing.
2. Throw away tissues used for nose blowing.
3. Wipe carefully after bowel movements (girls wipe front to back).
4. Wash hands after going to bathroom or blowing your nose.
5. Wash hands before eating.
6. Do not share food you've partly eaten.
7. If food or eating utensil falls on the floor, wash it right away.
8. Do not drink from another person's cup.
9. Do not share a toothbrush with someone else.

The Hospitalized Preschooler

The preschooler may look on hospitalization as an exciting new adventure or a frightening, dangerous experience, depending on the preparation by caregivers and health professionals. As mentioned earlier, play is an effective way to let children act out their anxiety and to learn what to expect from the hospital situation. Preschoolers are frightened about intrusive procedures; therefore, it is usually preferable to take the temperature with an oral or tympanic thermometer, if available, rather than a rectal type. Children are less anxious about procedures if they are allowed to handle equipment beforehand and perhaps "use" it on a doll or another toy (Figure 12-5).

The hospitalized preschooler may revert to bed-wetting and should not be scolded for it. The nurse should assure the family that this is normal. Explanations of where the bathrooms are and how to use the call light or bell to get help can help avoid problems with bed-wetting. If a child is afraid of the dark, a night light can be provided.

Hospital routines should follow home routines as closely as possible. The child should be allowed to partic-

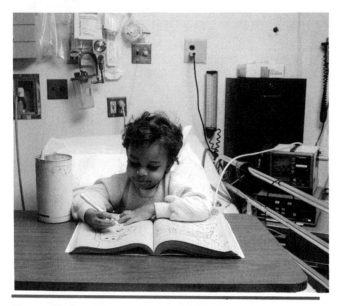

Figure 12-6. A preschooler plays while having hemo-dialysis. (From Jackson DB, Saunders, RB. Child Health Nursing: A Comprehensive Approach to the Care of Children and Their Families. Philadelphia: JB Lippincott, 1993.)

ipate in the care, even though this may take longer. All procedures should be carefully explained to the child in words that are at an appropriate level for the child's age, repeating if necessary.

If the child is ambulatory and not on infection control precautions, the playroom can offer diversionary activities. If not, play materials can be provided for use in bed (Figure 12-6).

Summary

Although physical growth slows during the preschool years, psychosocial growth is substantial. Endless questions, boundless energy, and an ongoing struggle to separate fantasy from reality make the preschooler stimulating to be with. Caregivers need to set limits within which the child can be free to explore and learn and to assert autonomy and initiative. Caregivers also need to serve as models for the kind of person they want the child to become, helping build confidence and self-esteem that will make easier the child's entrance into school and participation in a continually enlarging world.

Review Questions

1. The 4-year-old age group has sometimes been characterized as "the frustrating fours." After reviewing the preschool growth and development chart, identify the reasons you believe this may occur.
2. The parent of 3½-year-old Mario tells you that he is stuttering. With your knowledge of language development, what should you say to the parent?
3. Describe the progression of fine motor skills from 3 to 5 years of age.
4. Describe the progression of verbal ability in the preschooler.
5. What guidelines would you give the family to help children learn about food?
6. What accident prevention guidelines would you provide the caregiver of a preschooler?
7. Clara has noticed her 4-year-old son Theo masturbating. She is upset and comes to you for advice. Detail what you will tell her.
8. What are the various types of play? Give examples of each.
9. Why is regression normal for a hospitalized preschooler?

Reference

1. Schuster CS, Ashburn SS. The Process of Human Development, 3rd ed. Philadelphia: JB Lippincott, 1992.

Bibliography

Castiglia PT, Harbin RE. Child Health Care: Process and Practice. Philadelphia: JB Lippincott, 1992.

Christopherson ER. Discipline. Pediatr Clin North Am 39(3): 395–411, 1992.

Eschleman MM. Introductory Nutrition and Diet Therapy, 2nd ed. Philadelphia: JB Lippincott, 1991.

Howard BJ. Discipline in early childhood. Pediatr Clin North Am 38(6):1351–1369, 1991.

Pillitteri A. Maternal and Child Health Nursing. Philadelphia: JB Lippincott, 1992.

Schmitt BD. Does your child have a stuttering problem? Contemp Pediatr 8(3):83–84, 1991.

Spock B, Rothenberg MB. Dr. Spock's Baby and Child Care. New York: Pocket Books, 1992.

Whaley LF, Wong DL. Nursing Care of Infants and Children, 4th ed. St. Louis: Mosby-Year Book, 1991.

Health Problems of the Preschooler

Student Objectives

Upon completion of this chapter, the student will be able to:

1. Differentiate between the child who is hard of hearing and one who is deaf.
2. Differentiate between rubella and rubeola a.) Length of illness; b.) Signs and symptoms; c.) Complications.
3. State the contagious period for chickenpox.
4. List two nursing measures to increase comfort and decrease scarring in chickenpox.
5. Name the age group in which pertussis is most serious.
6. Describe cerebral palsy.
7. Discuss the causes of cerebral palsy a.) Prenatal; b.) Perinatal; c.) Postnatal.
8. Differentiate between spastic and athetoid cerebral palsy.
9. Identify the health care professionals involved in the care of the child with cerebral palsy.
10. List the causes of mental retardation a.) Prenatal; b.) Perinatal; c.) Postnatal.
11. Explain why Down syndrome is also called trisomy 21.
12. List ten signs and symptoms of Down syndrome.
13. Name the most common complication of a tonsillectomy, and list the signs to observe.
14. List four drugs commonly used in the treatment of acute lymphatic leukemia.
15. Name the most common type of hemophilia, and state how it is inherited.
16. Describe the symptoms of nephrotic syndrome.
17. Identify the cause of acute glomerulonephritis.
18. Name the most frequent presenting symptom of acute glomerulonephritis.
19. Compare nephrotic syndrome with acute glomerulonephritis.

Marks MG: BROADRIBB'S INTRODUCTORY PEDIATRIC NURSING, 4th ed. © 1994 J.B. Lippincott Company.

Key Terms

abdominal paracentesis	intercurrent infections
adenoids	intrathecal administration
adenopathy	leukemia
alopecia	leukopenia
ascites	lymphoblasts
astigmatism	lymphocytes
ataxia	monocytes
brachycephaly	myopia
clonus	oliguria
dysarthria	petechiae
granulocytes	purpura
hemarthrosis	refraction
hyperlipidemia	striae
hyperopia	tonsils

*T*oday's preschoolers have a better opportunity for good health than ever before. Immunizations have dramatically reduced the threat of communicable childhood diseases. Antibiotics can minimize the dangers of infection. Early detection and proper nutrition can prevent certain kinds of mental retardation. Simpler, more effective screening techniques help identify vision and hearing problems that need early treatment. Surgical advances make possible the early repair of life-threatening heart problems, yet serious health problems do occur during the preschool period. These problems must be recognized and treated as soon as possible so that the child can be in optimum physical and emotional health when it is time to enter school, a landmark in the child's total development.

Communicable Diseases

Half a century ago, growing up meant being able to survive measles, mumps, whooping cough, diphtheria, and often poliomyelitis. These diseases were expected almost as routinely as the loss of the deciduous teeth. Immunization has changed that outcome so drastically that some caregivers have become less conscientious about having their children immunized until the immunization is required for entrance to school. Nevertheless, the incidence of childhood diseases has decreased with an occasional outbreak in communities where a large number of children often are not immunized because of religious beliefs. One example of this is the measles epidemic in the eastern United States among Amish children in the late 1980s.

Understanding the various communicable diseases and their prevention, symptoms, and treatment (Table 13-1) requires knowledge of the definitions of the terms in Box 13-1. Some communicable diseases require isolation of the child to prevent spreading of the infection. Specific isolation procedures can be found in the procedure manuals of individual hospitals. (See Table 3-3 for types of isolation required).

The nurse should explain the reason for isolation procedures to protect the child from the threat of infection or to protect others from the infection the child has. Otherwise, the child may feel that the isolation is a form of punishment. Families are more likely to follow the correct procedures if they understand the need for them. Isolation increases the normal loneliness of being hospitalized, so the child needs extra attention and stimulation during this time.

Prevention

The recommended schedule of infant immunization is found in Chapter 8. Caregivers of children whose immunizations are incomplete must be urged to have the immunizations brought up to date. Various clinics where children can be immunized free of charge are available to families of limited means.

(text continued on page 298)

Table 13-1. Infectious Diseases of Childhood

Disease/Causative Organism	Incubation	Communicable Period; When/How	Immunization/Immunity	Symptoms	Treatment/Nursing Implications	Complications
Rubeola (measles) Measles virus	10–21 days	Fifth incubation day until first few days after rash erupts; direct or indirect contact with droplets	Attenuated live measles vaccine; (part of MMR vaccine); disease gives lasting natural immunity	Occurs in winter or spring; high fever; coryza (runny nose); cough; enlarged lymph nodes (head and neck); Koplik spots (small red spots with blue-white centers on oral mucosa, specific to rubeola); conjunctivitis; photophobia; maculopapular rash starts in hairline and spreads to entire body	Soothing measures for rash include tepid baths, soothing lotion, maintaining dry skin; dimly lighted room for comfort; encouraging fluids	Otitis media; pneumonia; encephalitis; airway obstruction
Rubella (German measles) Rubella virus	14–21 days	5–7 days before until about 5 days after rash appears Direct or indirect contact with droplets	Attenuated live vaccine; (part of MMR vaccine) disease gives lasting natural immunity	Low-grade fever; malaise; lymph glands of neck and head enlarged; pale small rash, disappears in 3 days	Symptomatic relief	Avoid contact with pregnant women; unborn fetus can suffer severe birth deformities if nonimmunized mother exposed, especially in first trimester
Parotitis (mumps) Paramyxovirus	14–21 days	Shortly before swelling appears until after it disappears Direct contact, droplet; indirect from contaminated articles	Attenuated live mumps vaccine; (part of MMR vaccine); disease gives natural immunity Passive: mumps immune globulin	Parotid glands swollen, unilaterally or bilaterally; may have fever, headache, malaise, and complain of earache before swelling appears; angle of jaw obliterated on affected side	Chewing is painful, so liquids and soft foods are given; sour foods cause discomfort; analgesics for pain; antipyretics for fever; local compresses of heat or cold may be soothing	In males past puberty, orchitis (inflammation of the testes); meningoencephalitis; may rarely cause severe hearing impairment
Varicella (chickenpox) Varicella-zoster virus	10–21 days	1 day before rash appears for about 6 days (until all vesicles crusted over) Direct or indirect contact with saliva or uncrusted vesicles	Lasting natural immunity; may reactivate in adult as herpes zoster; active artificial immunity available, but has undesirable side effects	Low-grade fever; malaise; successive crops of macules, papules, vesicles and crusts, all present at the same time; itching is intense; scarring may occur when scabs are "picked" off before ready to fall off	Antihistamines to reduce the itching; soothing baths and lotions may help; prevent scratching with short fingernails, mittens; acyclovir has been given to shorten the course of the disease *Aspirin must not be given*	Reye's syndrome can occur if child has had aspirin during illness; superinfection of lesions if scratched; encephalitis

(continued)

Table 13-1. Infectious Diseases of Childhood (Continued)

Disease/Causative Organism	Incubation	Communicable Period; When/How	Immunization/Immunity	Symptoms	Treatment/Nursing Implications	Complications
Pertussis (whooping cough) *Bordetella pertussis*	5–21 days	About 4–6 weeks Direct contact, droplet; indirect from contaminated articles	Pertussis vaccine is part of the DPT vaccine; disease gives natural immunity	Begins with mild upper respiratory symptoms; in second week progresses to severe paroxysmal cough with inspiratory whoop sometimes followed by vomiting; especially dangerous for young infants; may last 4–6 weeks	Bedrest; infants hospitalized; may need oxygen; observe for airway obstructions; provide high humidity; protect from secondary infections; encourage fluid intake; refeed child if vomiting occurs	Pneumonia (can cause death of infant); otitis media; hemorrhage; convulsions
Diphtheria *Corynebacterium diphtheriae*	2–5 days	As long as bacilli are present—2 to 4 weeks or less with antibiotic therapy Direct contact with infected person, carrier, or contaminated articles	Active immunity from diphtheria toxin in DPT vaccine; passive immunity diphtheria antitoxin	Mucous membranes of nose and throat covered by gray membrane; purulent nasal discharge; brassy cough; toxin from organism passes through blood stream to heart and nervous system	Strict isolation maintained; intravenous antitoxin and antibiotics administered; bedrest; liquid to soft diet; analgesics for throat pain; nonimmunized contacts should be immunized	Neuritis; carditis; congestive heart failure; respiratory failure
Poliomyelitis (infantile paralysis) Poliovirus types 1, 2, 3	5–14 days	Variable; 1 week after symptoms for respiratory contact, up to 6 weeks in feces	Trivalent live oral polio vaccine; disease causes active immunity against specific strain	Fever, headache, nausea, vomiting, abdominal pain; stiff neck, pain and tenderness in lower extremities that proceeds to paralysis	Strict isolation; bedrest; moist hot packs to extremities; range-of-motion exercises; supportive care; long-term ventilation if respiratory muscles involved	Permanent paralysis; respiratory arrest
Scarlet fever (scarlatina) Group a β-hemolytic streptococci	2–5 days	From onset of symptoms until 24 hours after antibiotic therapy and afebrile Direct contact, droplet	Disease gives lasting immunity; no immunization	Fine, pinpoint rash over trunk and extremities, face flushed with circumoral pallor, "strawberry tongue," fever, headache, abdominal pain, sore throat; hands and feet peel in sheets after the first week	Respiratory precautions during communicable period; penicillin administered (erythromycin in penicillin-sensitive children); all antibiotics must be taken; bedrest; encourage fluids; analgesics and antipyretics as needed	Glomerulonephritis; rheumatic fever
Tetanus (lockjaw) *Clostridium tetani*	3 days to 3 weeks	Not communicable person to person; direct contamination of closed wound	Tetanus toxoid administered as part of DPT; passive immunity from tetanus	Stiff neck and jaw; difficulty swallowing; muscular rigidity; clonic con-	Tetanus toxoid should be administered at time of injury if wound has	No long-term complications if treated promptly and adequately; can be fatal

Disease	Incubation	Communicability	Prophylaxis/Immunization	Clinical manifestations	Nursing care	Complications
(continued)		with contaminated soil or article	antitoxin or tetanus immune globulin	vulsions; irritability; respiratory obstruction; asphyxia	been contaminated with soil or feces; no booster necessary if wound is clean and booster given within 10 years; tetanus immune globulin or tetanus antitoxin should be administered if immunizations are incomplete. Wound should be thoroughly cleaned and debrided; seizure precautions; decrease external stimulation; maintain airway; respiratory ventilation may be necessary. Prevention by complete immunizations is essential	None
Erythema infectiosum (fifth disease) Parvovirus B19	6–14 days	Period of communicability uncertain, possibly few days before onset until few days after Respiratory droplet	None	Rash on face gives "slapped face" appearance with circumoral pallor, much like scarlet fever; rash moves to arms, trunk, buttocks; rash may last for 1 week or more; rash may reappear in sunlight, heat or cold for several more weeks; may have complaints of arthralgia (pain in joints);	Supportive nursing care; reassurance of benign nature; immunosuppressed child placed in protective isolation	
Erythema subitum (roseola) Herpesvirus 6	Unknown	Unknown	None	Fever 40°C (104°F) to 40.6°C (105°F) initially; child appears well; fever drops and rubella-like rash appears first on trunk; may be mistaken for heat rash; no other symptoms; rash disappears in 1–2 days	Antipyretics for fever; anticonvulsive precautions in child with history of febrile convulsions; supportive care; reassurance of benign nature	Febrile seizures

MMR, measles-mumps-rubella; *DPT*, diphtheria-pertussis-tetanus.

Box 13-1

Common Terms in Communicable Disease Nursing

Antibody: a protective substance in the body produced in response to the introduction of an antigen.

Antigen: a foreign protein that stimulates the formation of antibodies.

Antitoxin: an antibody that unites with and neutralizes a specific toxin.

Carrier: a person in apparently good health whose body harbors the specific organisms of a disease.

Enanthem: an eruption on a mucous surface.

Endemic: Habitual presence of a disease within a given area.

Epidemic: an outbreak in a community of a group of illnesses of similar nature in excess of the normal expectancy.

Erythema: redness of the skin produced by congestion of the capillaries.

Exanthem: an eruption appearing on the skin during an eruptive disease.

Host: a human, animal, or plant that harbors or nourishes another organism.

Immunity: passive—immunity acquired by administration of an antibody. Active—immunity acquired by an individual as the result of his or her own reactions to pathogens. Natural—resistance of the normal animal to infection.

Incubation period: the time interval between the infection and the appearance of the first symptoms of the disease.

Macule: a discolored skin spot not elevated above the surface.

Pandemic: a world-wide epidemic.

Papule: a small, circumscribed, solid elevation of the skin.

Pustule: a small elevation of epidermis filled with pus.

Toxin: a poisonous substance produced by certain organisms such as bacteria.

Toxoid: a toxin that has been treated to destroy its toxicity but that retains its antigenic properties.

Vaccine: a suspension of attenuated or killed microorganisms administered for the prevention of a specific infection.

Sensory Disorders

Hearing Impairment

Hearing loss is one of the most common disabilities in the United States, affecting an estimated 1 million children. Depending on the degree of hearing loss and the age at which it is detected, a child's development can be moderately to severely impaired. Development of speech, human relationships, and understanding of the environment all depend on the ability to hear. Infants at high risk for hearing loss should be screened when they are between 3 and 6 months of age.

Hearing loss ranges from mild (hard of hearing) to profound (deaf) (Table 13-2). A child who is hard of hearing has a loss of hearing acuity but has been able to learn speech and language by imitation of sounds. A deaf child has no hearing ability. Children who are profoundly deaf are more likely to be diagnosed before 1 year of age than are children with mild to moderate hearing losses.

Deafness, mental retardation, and autism are sometimes incorrectly diagnosed because the symptoms can be similar. Deaf children may fail to respond to sound or to develop speech because they cannot hear. Mentally retarded or autistic children may show the same lack of response and development even though they do not have a hearing loss.

Types of Hearing Impairment

There are four types of hearing loss: conductive, sensorineural, mixed, and central.

Conductive Hearing Loss. In this type of impairment, middle ear structures fail to carry sound waves to the inner ear. Most often, conductive hearing loss is the result of chronic serous otitis media or other infection, and it can make hearing levels fluctuate. Chronic middle ear infec-

Table 13-2. Levels of Hearing Impairment

Decibel Level	Hearing Level Present
Slight (<30dB)	Unable to hear whispered words or faint speech No speech impairment present May not be aware of hearing difficulty Achieves well in school and home by compensating by leaning forward, speaking loudly; turns TV volume up
Mild (30–50 dB)	Beginning speech impairment may be present Difficulty hearing if not facing speaker; some difficulty with normal conversation
Moderate (55–70 dB)	Speech impairment present; may require speech therapy Difficulty with normal conversation
Severe (70–90 dB)	Difficulty with any but nearby loud voice Hears vowels easier than consonants Requires speech therapy for clear speech
Profound (>90 dB)	Hears almost no sound

Adapted from Pilliteri A. Maternal and Child Health Nursing. Philadelphia: JB Lippincott, 1992.

tion can destroy part of the ear drum or the ossicles, thus leading to conductive deafness. This type of deafness is seldom complete and responds well to treatment.

Sensorineural (Perceptive) Hearing Loss. This type of hearing loss may be caused by damage to the nerve endings in the cochlea or to the nerve pathways leading to the brain. It is generally severe and unresponsive to medical treatment. Diseases such as meningitis and encephalitis, hereditary or congenital factors, and toxic reactions to certain drugs (such as streptomycin) may cause sensorineural hearing loss. Maternal rubella is believed to be the most common cause of sensorineural deafness in children.

Mixed Hearing Loss. Some children have both conductive and sensorineural hearing impairment. In these instances, the conduction level determines how well the child is able to hear.

Central Auditory Dysfunction. Although this child may have normal hearing, damage to or faulty development of the proper brain centers makes the child unable to use the auditory information he or she receives.

Detection and Evaluation of Hearing Loss

Mild to moderate hearing loss often remains undetected until the child moves outside the family circle into nursery school or kindergarten. The hearing loss may have been gradual, but the child may have become such a skilled lip reader that neither the child nor the family is aware of the partial deafness. Caregivers and teachers should be aware of the possibility of hearing loss in children who appear to be inattentive, noisy, and creators of disturbances in the classroom.

Certain reactions and mannerisms characterize a child with hearing loss. The child should be observed for an apparent inability to locate a sound and turning of the head to one side when listening. The child who fails to comprehend when spoken to, who gives inappropriate answers to questions, who consistently turns up the volume on the television or radio, or who cannot whisper or talk softly may have hearing loss.

Audiologic Assessment. The child who is suspected of having a hearing loss should be referred for a complete audiologic assessment, including pure-tone audiometric, speech reception, and speech discrimination tests. Children with sensorineural impairment generally have a greater loss of hearing acuity in the high-pitched tones. The loss may vary from slight to complete. Those children with a conductive loss are more likely to have equal losses over a wide range of frequencies.

A child's hearing should be tested at all frequencies by a pure-tone audiometer in a soundproof room. Speech reception and speech discrimination tests measure the amount of hearing impairment for both speech and communication. Accurate measurements usually can be made in children who are as young as 3 years of age if the test is introduced as a game (Figure 13-1).

Infants and very young children must be tested in a different way. An infant with normal hearing should be able to locate a sound at 28 weeks, imitate sounds at 36 weeks, and associate sounds with people or objects at 1 year of age. A commonly used screening test for very young children employs noisemakers of varying intensity and pitch. The examiner stands beside or behind the child, who has been given a toy. As the examiner produces sounds with a rattle, buzzer, bell, or other noise-

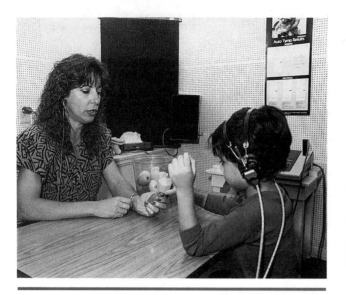

Figure 13-1. Hearing testing. Using a game-like model, the child is taught to respond to hearing a sound by taking a toy from the test assistant. (Courtesy John Tracy Clinic, Los Angeles, CA.)

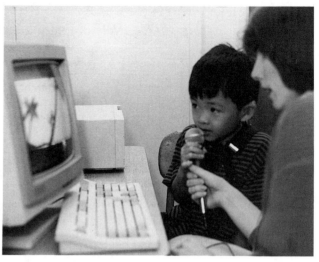

Figure 13-2. A young deaf boy (wearing hearing aids and a FM amplifier to increase the loudness of his teacher's voice) makes speech sounds into the microphone. As he changes the volume or pitch of the sound, the images on the Speech Viewer screen change. This gives him immediate feedback about his own voice and is very useful in speech development. (Courtesy John Tracy Clinic, Los Angeles, CA.)

maker, a hearing child is distracted and turns to the source of the new sound, whereas a deaf child does not react in a particular way.

Treatment and Education

When the type and degree of hearing loss have been established, the child, even an infant, may be fitted with a hearing aid. Hearing aids are helpful only in conductive deafness, not in sensorineural or central auditory dysfunction. These devices only amplify sound; they do not localize or clarify it. Many types of models are available, including those in the ear, behind the ear, incorporated in glasses, or on the body with a wire connection to the ear. FM receiver units are also available that can broadcast the speaker's voice from a greater distance, cutting out the background noise. When the FM transmitter is turned off, this type of unit functions as an ordinary hearing aid.

It is believed that deaf children can best be taught to communicate by a combination of lip reading, sign language, and oral speech (Figure 13-2). The family members are the child's first teachers, and they must be aware of all phases of development—physical, emotional, social, intellectual, and language—and then seek to aid this development.

A deaf child depends on sight to interpret the environment and to communicate. Thus, it is important to be sure that the child's vision is normal, and if not, to correct that problem. The probability is twice as great that the child with a hearing loss also will have some vision impairment. Training in the use of all the other senses—sight, smell, taste, and touch—make the deaf child better able

to use any available hearing. It is believed that most deaf children do have some hearing ability.

Preschool classes for deaf children exist in many large communities. These seek to create an environment in which a deaf child can have the same experiences and activities that normal preschoolers have. Children are generally enrolled at age 2½ years.

The John Tracy Clinic in Los Angeles is dedicated to young children (birth through age 5) who have been born with a severe hearing loss or who have lost hearing through illness before acquiring speech and language.* The Clinic's purpose is "to find, encourage, guide, and train the parents of deaf and hard of hearing children first in order to reach and help the children, and second to help the parents themselves." With early diagnosis and intervention, hearing-impaired children can develop language and communication skills in the critical preschool period that enable many of them to speech-read and to speak.

All services to parents and children are given without charge. The Clinic has existed since 1943 to help all deaf children. Full audiologic testing, parent–infant education, demonstration nursery school, parent education classses, and parent groups are offered. Many medical residents, nurses, and allied health care professionals come to observe the model programs at the Clinic to see for themselves the benefits of early diagnosis.

*John Tracy Clinic, 806 West Adams Boulevard, Los Angeles, CA 90007.

The Clinic also provides a correspondence course to parents who live anywhere in the world that can be reached by mail. There are three courses available in both English and Spanish: deaf infants, deaf preschoolers, and deaf–blind children. These courses, which include materials and videotape, guide parents in encouraging their child to develop auditory awareness, speech-reading skills, and expressive language. Information about the services of the Clinic can be obtained by calling toll free 1-800-522-4582.

Free and appropriate education for all disabled children is required by federal law. Children with a hearing loss who cannot successfully function in regular classrooms are provided with supplementary services (speech therapy, speech interpreter, signer) in special classrooms or a residential school.

Nursing Care for the Deaf Child in the Hospital

When deaf children must be hospitalized, it is ideal for their primary caregiver to room-in with them, not as a convenience to the nursing staff but for the child's benefit in being able to communicate his or her needs and feelings.

The deaf child's anxiety about unfamiliar situations and procedures can be greater than that of the child with normal hearing. Always be certain that deaf children can see you before you touch them. Each procedure must be demonstrated before it is performed, showing the child equipment or pictures of equipment to be used. Keeping a night light in the child's room is helpful because sight is such a critical sense to the deaf child. By imagining being in a dark room with no sound, the nurse may achieve some understanding of the helpless feeling the child has. Signing classes are also available in many communities for those working with hearing-impaired children and adults.

When speaking to the deaf child, the nurse should be face to face on the child's level. Explanations should be followed by demonstrations to be sure the child understands.

Nurses need to be familiar with the care and maintenance of hearing aids because the aids are expensive. Care should be taken to put the aids in a safe place when not worn. Linens should be checked before being put into the laundry to eliminate the possibility of discarding the hearing aids with the dirty linens. Family members can be used as important resources about the child's habits and communication patterns.

Vision Impairment

Like hearing, good vision is essential to a child's normal development. How well a child sees affects the child's learning process, social development, coordination, and safety. One in 1000 children of school age has a serious vision impairment. The sooner these impairments are corrected, if possible, the better a child's chances for normal or near-normal development.

Children with vision impairments are classified as sighted with eye problems, partially sighted, and legally blind.

Types of Vision Impairment

Eye Problems in Sighted Children. Among sighted children with eye problems, errors of **refraction** (the way light rays bend as they pass through the lens to the retina) are the most common. Approximately 10% of the children of school age have myopia. **Myopia** means that the child can see objects clearly at close range but not at a distance. When proper lenses are fitted, vision is corrected to normal. If uncorrected, this defect may cause a child to be labeled inattentive or retarded. Myopia tends to be familial and often progresses into adolescence, then levels off.

Hyperopia is a refractive condition in which the person can see objects better at a distance than close up. It is a common condition of young children and often persists into the first grade or even later. Whether corrective lenses are needed must be decided on an individual basis by the ocular specialist examining the child. Usually, correction is not needed in the preschool-age group. Teachers and parents should be aware of the considerable eye fatigue that may result from efforts at accommodation for close work.

Astigmatism may occur with or without myopia or hyperopia and is caused by unequal curvatures in the cornea of the eye that bend the light rays in different directions, producing a blurred image. Slight astigmatism often does not require correction; moderate degrees usually require glasses for reading, television, and movies, and severe astigmatism requires that glasses be worn at all times.

Blindness. Blindness is legally defined as a corrected vision of 20/200 or less or peripheral vision of less than 20 degrees in the better eye. Many of the causes of blindness have been reduced or eliminated, such as retrolental fibroplasia due to excessive oxygen concentrations in newborns and trachoma, a viral infection. Maternal infections are still a common cause of blindness, although the incidence of maternal rubella has decreased because of immunization.

Between the ages of 5 and 7 years, children begin to form and retain visual images; they have memory with pictures. Children who become blind before 5 years of age are missing this crucial element in their development. Blindness can seriously hamper the child's ability to form human attachments; learn coordination, balance, and locomotion; distinguish fantasy from reality; and interpret the surrounding world. How well the blind child learns to cope depends on the family's ability to communicate, teach, and foster a sense of independence in the child.

Partial Sight. Children with partial sight have a visual acuity between 20/20 and 20/200 in the better eye after all necessary medical or surgical correction. These children also have a high incidence of refractive errors, particularly myopia. Eye injuries also cause loss of vision, as do conditions such as cataracts that can be improved by treatment but result in diminished sight.

Detection and Evaluation of Vision Impairment

Squinting and frowning while trying to read a blackboard or other material at a distance, tearing, red-rimmed eyes, holding work too close to the eyes while reading or writing, and rubbing the eyes are all signs of possible vision impairment. Although blindness is likely to be detected in early infancy, partial sightedness or correctable vision problems may go unrecognized until a child enters school, unless vision screening is part of routine health maintenance.

A simple test kit for preschoolers is available for home use by parents or visiting nurses (Figure 13-3). This kit is an adaptation of the Snellen E chart used for testing children who have not learned to read. The child covers one eye and then points his or her fingers in the same direction as the "fingers" on each E, beginning with the largest. These are also referred to as "legs on a table" by some examiners.

The Snellen Chart. This is the familiar test in which the letters on each line are smaller than those on the line above. If the child can read the 20 ft-line standing 20 ft away from the chart, visual acuity is stated as 20/20. If the child can read only the line marked 100, acuity is stated as 20/100. The chart should be placed at eye level with good lighting and in a room free from distractions. One eye is tested at a time with the other eye covered. Normal preschool acuity is 20/30.

Picture charts for identification also are used but are not considered to be as accurate. An intelligent child can memorize the pictures and guess from the general shape without seeing distinctly.

Treatment and Education

Significant medical and surgical advances have occurred in the treatment of cataracts, strabismus, and amblyopia. The earlier the treatment, the better the child's chances of adequate vision for normal development and function. Errors of refraction largely are correctable. Corrective lenses for minor vision impairments should be prescribed early and checked regularly to be sure that they are still providing adequate correction.

Children who are partially sighted or totally blind benefit from association with normally sighted children. In most communities, education for these special children is provided within the regular school or in special classes that offer the child more specialized equipment and instruction (Figure 13-4).

Special equipment includes printed material with large print, pencils with large leads for darker lines, tape recordings, magnifying glasses, and typewriters. For children with a serious impairment whose participation in regular activities is sharply curtailed, talking books, raised maps, and Braille equipment are needed as well (Figure 13-5). These devices prevent isolation of the visually impaired child and minimize any differences from the other children.

Nursing Care for the Visually Impaired Child in the Hospital

Children with visual impairment or other disabilities have the same needs as other children, and these should not be overlooked in dealing with the specific disability. The child who is blind needs emotional comfort and sensory stimulation, much of which must be communicated by touch, sound, and smell. It is important for the nurse to explain sounds and other sensations that are new to the hospitalized child and to let him or her touch equipment that will be used in any procedures. A tactile tour of the room helps orient the child to the location of furniture and other facilities. Awareness of safety hazards is particularly important when caring for the blind or partially sighted child.

It is essential for the nurse and other personnel to identify themselves when they enter the child's room and to tell the child when they leave. Explanations of what is going to happen reduce the child's fear and anxiety and the possibility of being startled by an unexpected touch.

The child with a visual impairment should be involved with as many peers and their activities as possible. The child also should be encouraged to be as independent as possible. One step is to provide the child with finger foods and encourage self-feeding after orienting the child to the plate. A small bowl, instead of a plate, is useful so that food can be scooped against the side to get it on the spoon. Eating is a time-consuming and messy affair, but it is essential to the growth of independence in all children.

Central Nervous System Disorders

Reye Syndrome

Reye syndrome (rhymes with "eye") is characterized by acute encephalopathy and fatty degeneration of the liver and other abdominal organs. It occurs in children of all ages but is seen more in young school-age children than any other age group. Reye syndrome usually occurs after a viral illness, particularly appearing after the child has had varicella (chickenpox) or an upper respiratory infection. Administration of aspirin during the viral illness has

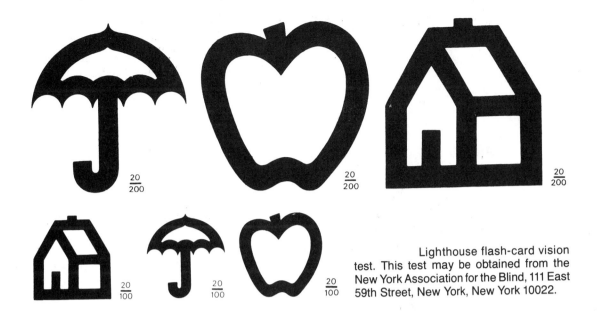

Lighthouse flash-card vision test. This test may be obtained from the New York Association for the Blind, 111 East 59th Street, New York, New York 10022.

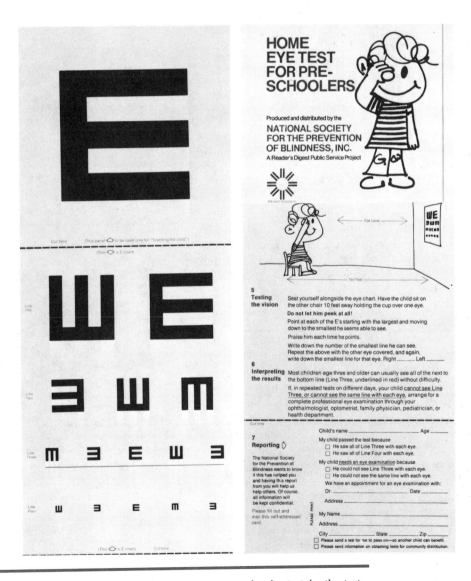

Figure 13-3. Home testing kit. This allows the very young preschooler to take the test in more familiar surroundings. The test may be obtained from the National Society to Prevent Blindness, 79 Madison Avenue, New York, NY 10016.

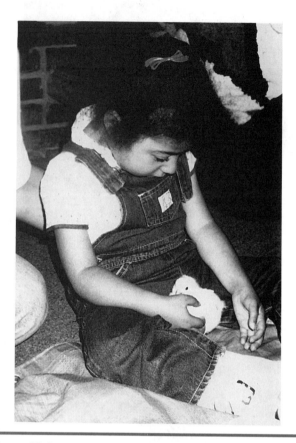

Figure 13-4. A trip to a farm provides this visually impaired child a chance to experience it—through touch, sound, and smell. (Courtesy Perkins School for the Blind, Watertown, MA.)

been implicated as a contributing factor. As a result, the American Academy of Pediatrics (AAP) recommends that aspirin or aspirin compounds not be given to children with viral infections.

Clinical Manifestations

The symptoms appear 1 to 3 weeks after the initial illness. The child is recuperating unremarkably when symptoms of severe vomiting, irritability, lethargy, and confusion occur. Immediate intervention is needed to prevent serious insult to the brain, including respiratory arrest (Table 13-3).

Diagnosis

The history of a viral illness is an immediate clue. Liver function tests, including serum glutamic oxaloacetic transaminase, serum glutamic pyruvic transaminase, lactic dehydrogenase, and serum ammonia levels are elevated because of poor liver function. The patient is hypoglycemic.

Nursing Care

The child with Reye syndrome is cared for in the intensive care unit with specialized nursing care. The treatment is determined by the staging of the symptoms. Neurologic

evaluation is essential in assessing the progression of the illness. Respiratory function, reduction of cerebral edema, and control of hypoglycemia are major concerns. Low blood glucose levels can lead to seizures quickly in young children. Osmotic diuretics (eg, mannitol) are administered to reduce cerebral edema.

This hospitalization period is a traumatic time for the family. The nurse must give the family opportunities to deal with their feelings. In addition, the family needs to be kept well informed about the progress of the child's care. Having a child in intensive care is a frightening experience, and every effort must be made to reassure the family with sincerity and honesty.

Since the AAP made the recommendation to avoid the administration of aspirin to children, especially during viral illnesses, there has been a steady decrease in the number of cases of Reye syndrome. The prognosis of children with Reye syndrome is greatly improved with early diagnosis and vigorous treatment.

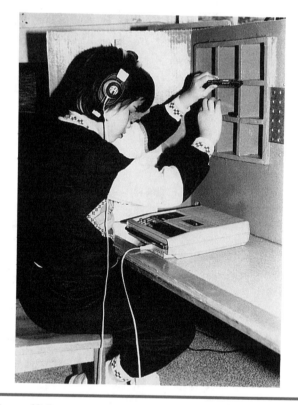

Figure 13-5. Interaction with a stimulating environment is necessary for every child's development. For visually impaired, developmentally delayed, or multi-impaired children, it is often necessary to create special environments to meet unique learning needs. Through the use of a realistic skills table, with a mailbox, door handle with lock and key, and rewired telephone, and various nooks and crannies filled with cherished objects, this child is developing the concept of spatial organization and receiving positive reinforcement about her ability to have an impact on what happens around her. (Courtesy Perkins School for the Blind, Watertown, MA.)

Table 13-3. Staging of Reye Syndrome

Stage	Signs and Symptoms
I	Lethargy; follows verbal commands; normal posture; purposeful response to pain; brisk pupillary light reflex; and normal oculocephalic reflex
II	Combative or stuporous; inappropriate verbalizing; normal posture; purposeful or nonpurposeful response to pain; sluggish pupillary reflexes; and conjugate deviation on doll's eye maneuver
III	Comatose; decorticate posture; decorticate response to pain; sluggish pupillary reaction; conjugate deviation on doll's eye maneuver
IV	Comatose; decerebrate posture and decerebrate response to pain; sluggish pupillary reflexes and inconsistent or absent oculocephalic reflex
V	Comatose; flaccid; no response to pain; no pupillary response; no oculocephalic reflex

Terhune PE. Reye's syndrome. In Oski FA, DeAngelis CD, Feigin RD, Warshaw JB (eds.). Principles and Practice of Pediatrics. Philadelphia: JB Lippincott, 1990, p. 1883.

Cerebral Palsy

Cerebral palsy is a term used to denote a group of disorders arising from a malfunction of motor centers and neural pathways in the brain. It is one of the most complex of the common permanent disabling conditions and often can be accompanied by seizures, mental retardation, various sensory defects, and behavior disorders. Research in this area is directed at adapting biomedical technology to help people with cerebral palsy cope with the activities of daily living and gain maximum function and independence.

Causes

Cerebral palsy is caused by damage to the parts of the brain that control movement and generally occurs during the fetal or perinatal period, particularly in premature infants.

Prenatal Causes. The following prenatal causes are commonly identified:

1. Any process that interferes with the oxygen supply to the brain, such as separation of the placenta, compression of the cord, and bleeding
2. Maternal infection (eg, cytomegalovirus, toxoplasmosis, and rubella)
3. Nutritional deficiencies that may affect brain growth
4. Kernicterus (brain damage caused by jaundice) resulting from Rh incompatibility
5. Teratogenic factors such as drugs and radiation

Perinatal Causes. The following perinatal causes are commonly identified:

1. Anoxia immediately before, during, and after birth

2. Intracranial bleeding
3. Asphyxia or interference with respiratory function
4. Maternal analgesia (eg, morphine) that depresses the sensitive neonate's respiratory center
6. Birth trauma
7. Prematurity because immature blood vessels predispose the neonate to cerebral hemorrhage

Postnatal Causes. The following postnatal causes are commonly identified:

1. Head trauma (eg, due to a fall)
2. Infection (eg, encephalitis and meningitis)
3. Neoplasms
4. Cerebral vascular accident

Prevention

Because brain damage in cerebral palsy is irreversible, prevention is the most important aspect of care. Prevention of cerebral palsy is directed to the following:

Prenatal care to improve nutrition, prevent infection, and decrease the incidence of prematurity

Perinatal monitoring with appropriate interventions to decrease birth trauma

Postnatal prevention of infection through breast feeding, improved nutrition, and immunizations

Clinical Manifestations and Types

Difficulty in controlling voluntary muscle movements is one manifestation of the central nervous system damage. Seizures, mental retardation, hearing and vision impairments, and behavior disorders frequently accompany the major problem. Delays in gross motor development; abnormal motor performance, such as poor sucking and feeding behaviors; abnormal postures; and persistence of primitive reflexes are other signs of cerebral palsy. Diagnosis of cerebral palsy seldom occurs before 2 months of age and may be delayed until the second or third year, until walking is attempted and an obvious lag in motor development is evident. Diagnosis is based on observations of delayed growth and development through a process that rules out other diagnoses.

There are several major types of cerebral palsy, each with distinctive clinical manifestations.

Spastic Type. This is the most frequent type, characterized by a hyperactive stretch reflex in associated muscle groups; an increased activity of the deep tendon reflexes; **clonus** (rapid involuntary muscle contraction and relaxation); contractures affecting the extensor muscles, especially the heel cord; and scissoring caused by severe hip adduction. When scissoring is present, the child's legs are crossed and the toes are pointed when the child is standing.

Athetoid Type. Athetoid cerebral palsy is marked by involuntary, incoordinate motion with varying degrees of muscle tension (Figure 13-6). Children with this disorder are constantly in motion, and the whole body is in a state of slow, writhing, muscular contractions whenever voluntary movement is attempted. Facial grimacing, poor swallowing, and tongue movements causing drooling and **dysarthria** (poor speech articulation) are also present. These children are most likely to possess average or above average intelligence, despite their abnormal appearance. Hearing loss is most common in this group.

Ataxia Type. **Ataxia** is essentially a lack of coordination caused by disturbances in the kinesthetic and balance senses. The least common type of cerebral palsy, ataxia may not be diagnosed until children start to walk. Their gait is awkward and wide based.

Rigidity Type. This type is uncommon. It is characterized by rigid postures and lack of active movement.

Mixed Type. Children with signs of more than one type of cerebral palsy are usually severely disabled. The disorder may have been caused by postnatal injury.

Diagnosis

Children with cerebral palsy may not be diagnosed with certainty until they have difficulties when attempting to walk. They may show signs of mental retardation, attention deficit disorder, or recurrent convulsions.

Treatment and Special Aids

Treatment of cerebral palsy focuses on helping the child make the most complete use of residual abilities and achieve maximum satisfaction and enrichment in his or her life. A team of health care professionals—physician, surgeon, physical therapist, occupational therapist, speech

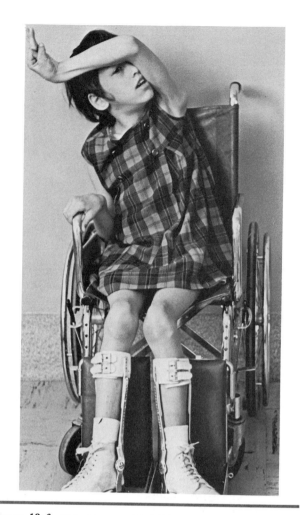

Figure 13-6. This 11-year-old child with athetosis wears short leg braces and special shoes to keep her feet fairly flat. She shows the random movements characteristic of this type of cerebral palsy.

therapist, and perhaps a social worker—works with the family to set realistic goals. Dental care is important in the care of these children because enamel hypoplasia is common, and those children whose seizure disorders are controlled with phenytoin (Dilantin) are likely to develop gingival hypertrophy. Medications such as baclofen, diazepam, and dantrolene may be used to help decrease spasticity.

Physical Therapy. Control of the body needed for purposeful physical activity is learned automatically by a normal child but must be consciously learned by a child who has problems with physical mobility. Physical therapists attempt to teach a child activities of daily living that the child has been unable to accomplish. Methods must be suited to the needs of the individual child as well as to the general needs arising from his or her condition. These methods are based on principles of conditioning, relaxation, use of residual patterns, stimulation of contraction and relaxation of antagonistic muscles, and other pertinent principles. A variety of techniques is used. Because there are many variations in the disabilities in cerebral palsy, each child must be evaluated individually and treated appropriately.

Orthopedic Management. Braces are used as supportive and control measures to facilitate muscle training, to reinforce weak or paralyzed muscles, or to counteract the pull of antagonistic muscles. Various types are available, each designed for a specific purpose. Orthopedic surgery sometimes is used to improve function and correct deformities, such as the release of contractures and the lengthening of tight heel cords.

Technologic Aids for Daily Living. Biomedical engineering, particularly in the field of electronics, has perfected a number of devices to help make the disabled person more functional and less dependent on others. The devices range from simple items, such as wheelchairs and specially constructed toilet seats, to completely electronic cottages furnished with a computer, a tape recorder, a typewriter, a calculator, and other equipment that facilitate independence and useful study or work. Many of these devices can be controlled by a mouth stick, an extremely useful feature for people with poor hand coordination.

A child who has difficulty maintaining balance while sitting may need a high-backed chair with side pieces and a foot platform. Feeding may be a challenge. Feeding aids include spoons with enlarged handles for easy grasping or with bent handles that allow the spoon to be brought easily to the mouth (Figure 13-7). Plates with high rims and suction devices to prevent slipping enable a child to eat with little assistance. Covered cups set in holders, with a hole in the lid to admit a straw, help a child who does not have hand control. A nasogastric or a gastrostomy tube may be necessary for the severely disabled child.

Manual skill can be aided by games, such as pegboards and cards, that must be manipulated. Typing is an ego-boosting alternative for a child whose disability is too severe to permit him or her to write legibly. Computer programs have been designed to enable these children to communicate and improve their learning skills. Special keyboards, joysticks, and electronic devices help the child have fun and gain a sense of achievement while learning. Computers also have expanded the opportunities for future employment for these children.

Nursing Care

The child with cerebral palsy may be seen in the health care setting at any age level. The nurse must assess the child and the family to determine the child's needs, the level of development, and the stage of family acceptance and to set realistic long-range goals. The newly diagnosed child and family may have more potential nursing diagnoses than the child and family who have been successfully dealing with cerebral palsy for a long time.

The nurse needs to assess the family to learn as much as possible about the child's activities at home to ease the

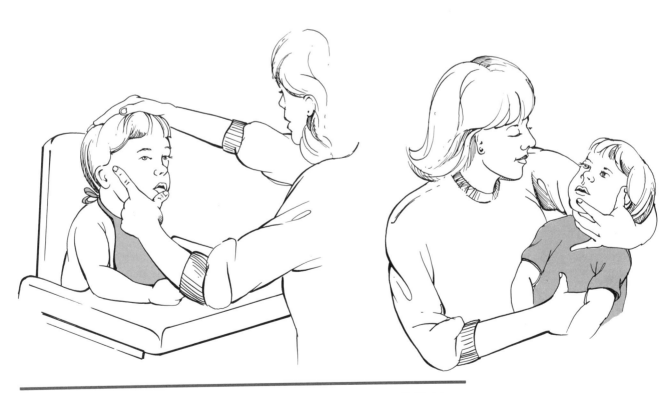

Figure 13-7. Feeding techniques to promote jaw control. (From Castiglia PT, Harbin R. Child Health Care. Philadelphia: JB Lippincott, 1992.)

change of environment. The child should be encouraged to maintain current self-care activities and set goals for attaining new ones. Positioning to prevent contractures, providing modified feeding utensils, and suggesting educationally sound play activities are all important aspects of the child's care. If the child has been admitted for surgery, the child and family will need appropriate preoperative and postoperative teaching, emotional support, and assistance in setting realistic expectations. The family may need assistance in exploring educational opportunities for the child.

Like any chronic condition, cerebral palsy can become a devastating drain on the family's emotional and financial resources. The child's future depends on many variables: family attitudes, economic and therapeutic resources, the intelligence of the child, and the availability of competent, understanding health care professionals. Some children, given the emotional and physical support they need, are able to achieve a satisfactory degree of independence. Some have been able to attend college and find fulfilling work. Vocational training is also available to an increasing number of these young people. Some people with cerebral palsy will always need a significant amount of nursing care, with the possibility of institutionalized care when their family can no longer care for them. The outlook for these children and their families is improving, but a great deal of work must be done. Working as a community member, the health care professional can play a vital role in promoting educational opportunities, rehabilitation, and acceptance for disabled children.

Mental Retardation

Mental retardation is defined in the American Psychiatric Association's *Diagnostic and Statistical Manual, Third Edition, Revised* using two criteria: significant subaverage general intellectual functioning—an intelligence quotient (IQ) of 70 or lower—and concurrent deficits in adaptive functioning. *Adaptive functioning* refers to how well people are able to meet the standards of independence (activities of daily living) and social responsibility expected of them for their age and the cultural group to which they belong. Mental retardation frequently occurs in combination with other physical disorders.

Causes

Many factors can cause mental retardation. The most common causes are outlined.

Prenatal Causes. Prenatal causes include:

- *Inborn errors of metabolism*, such as phenylketonuria, galactosemia, or congenital hypothyroidism damage often can be prevented by early detection and treatment.

- *Prenatal infection*, such as toxoplasmosis, and cytomegalovirus infections—microcephaly, hydrocephalus, cerebral palsy, and other brain damage–can result from intrauterine infections.
- *Teratogenic agents*, such as drugs, radiation, and alcohol, can have devastating effects on the central nervous system of a developing fetus.
- *Genetic factors*—inborn variations of chromosomal patterns result in a variety of deviations, the most common of which is Down syndrome.

Perinatal Causes. Birth trauma, anoxia from various causes, prematurity, and difficult birth can all cause mental retardation. In some instances, prenatal factors may have influenced the perinatal complications.

Postnatal Causes. Postnatal causes include:

- *Poisoning*, such as lead poisoning. Children who develop encephalopathy from chronic lead poisoning usually have significant brain damage.
- *Infections and trauma* such as meningitis, convulsive disorders, and hydrocephalus often lead to mental retardation.
- *Impoverished early environment*, such as lack of sensory stimulation and adequate nutrition, can result in mental retardation. Emotional rejection in early life may do irreparable damage to a child's ability to respond to the environment.

The Mentally Retarded Child

About 3% of all children born in the United States have some level of cognitive impairment. Approximately one fifth of these are so severely retarded that diagnosis is made at birth or during the first year. Most of the other children are diagnosed as retarded when they begin school.

The most common classification of mental retardation is based on IQ. Although controversy exists about the validity of tests that measure intelligence, this system is still the most useful for grouping these children.

The child with an IQ of 70 to 50 is considered mildly mentally retarded. This child is a slow learner but is capable of acquiring basic skills. The child can learn to read, write, and do arithmetic to a 4th or 5th grade level but is slower than average in learning to walk, talk, and feed himself or herself. Retardation may not be obvious to casual acquaintances. With support and guidance, this child usually can develop social and vocational skills that are adequate for self-maintenance. Approximately 80% of retarded children are classified in this category.

The moderately retarded child whose IQ is 55 to 35 has little, if any, ability to attain independence and academic skills and is referred to as *trainable*. Motor development and speech are noticeably delayed, but training in self-help activities is possible. This child may be able to learn repetitive skills in sheltered workshops. Some children may learn to travel alone, but few become capable of assuming complete self-maintenance. This category accounts for about 10% of retarded children.

The child considered severely retarded tests in the IQ range of 40 to 20. This child's development is markedly delayed during the first year of life. The child is not capable of learning academic skills but may be able to learn some self-care activities if sensorimotor stimulation is begun early. Eventually, this child will probably learn to walk and develop some speech; however, a sheltered environment and careful supervision always will be required.

The profoundly retarded child has an IQ lower than 20. This child has minimal capacity for functioning and needs continuing care. Eventually, the child may learn to walk and develop a primitive speech but will never be able to perform self-care activities. Only about 1% of retarded children are in this category.

Nursing Process for the Child with Cognitive Impairment

ASSESSMENT

The child who has a cognitive impairment is seen in the health care setting for diagnosis, treatment, and follow-up, as well as for the usual health maintenance visits that any child has. During these visits, health care personnel may be challenged to communicate with the child. A thorough assessment accomplished through an interview with the child's caregiver can be most helpful. The nurse must listen carefully to the caregiver, paying particular attention to any comments or concerns that are voiced.

The assessment may be lengthy and detailed, depending partially on the circumstances of the child's admission to the health care facility. Aside from the assessment that is dictated by the reason for the current admission, the nurse also needs information about the child's habits, routines, and personal terminology (such as nicknames and toileting terms). The nurse must be careful to communicate at the child's level of understanding and not "talk down" to the child during the assessment interview. It is important to treat the child with respect. This approach helps gain cooperation from both the family and the child. The nurse should arrange the assessment interview so that it can be conducted with an unhurried atmosphere to avoid placing undue stress on the child or the family.

NURSING DIAGNOSES

The appropriate nursing diagnoses vary with the primary reason for the child's admission to the hospital. Often, the child with mental retardation also has physical disabilities that must be considered when a plan of care is being developed. The nurse should work with the child's caregiver to set goals that are realistic for the child. Some

nursing diagnoses that are useful with the retarded child are the following:

- Self-care deficit in basic hygiene, grooming, nutrition, and toileting related to cognitive or neuromuscular impairment or both
- Impaired communication related to impaired receptive or expressive skills
- High risk for social isolation (family or child) related to fear of and embarrassment about the child's behavior or appearance
- Altered growth and development related to physical and mental disability
- High risk for injury related to physical or neurologic impairment, or both

PLANNING AND IMPLEMENTATION

Promoting Self-Care. Teaching the mentally retarded child can be time consuming, frustrating, challenging, and rewarding. When the child is admitted to the hospital, a teaching program can be set up that reflects the developmental level of the child. All personnel who care for the child, as well as any family members who are involved in caring for the child, should be aware of the program. Each element of care that is to be taught must be broken into small segments and repeated over and over. Patience is one of the most important aspects of teaching the mentally retarded. Generous use of praise and small material rewards are useful tools that aid in teaching. The child should be challenged, but the immediate small goals should be such that they are realistic and attainable. Brushing teeth, brushing or combing the hair, bathing, washing the hands and face, feeding oneself, dressing independently, and basic safety are all self-care areas in which the child needs instruction and positive reinforcements.

Teaching the mentally retarded child requires the same principles as teaching any child at a level appropriate to the stage of the child's maturation, not the chronologic age. If the child has physical disabilities in addition to retardation, the rate of development is also affected. One factor that makes the child with cognitive impairment different from the average child is the lack of ability to reason abstractly. This prevents transfer of learning or application of abstract principles to varied situations. Learning takes place by habit formation, emphasizing the "three R's": routine, repetition, and relaxation. Most cognitively impaired children increase in mental age, although slowly, and to a limited level. Therefore, each child needs to be watched for evidence of readiness for a new skill.

Environmental stimulation is essential for everyone's development. The cognitively impaired child needs much more environmental enrichment than the average child. Suggested activities for providing this enrichment are summarized in Table 13-4.

Table 13-4. Examples of Developmental Stimulation and Sensorimotor Teaching for Retarded Infants and Young Children

Developmental Sequence	Possible Activities to Encourage Development
Sitting	
1. Sit with support in caretaker's lap	Hold child in sitting position on lap, supporting him or her under armpits. Do several times a day gradually lessening the support
2. Sit independently when propped	Place child in sitting position against firm surface with pillow behind his or her back and on either side. Leave the child alone several times a day
3. Sitting with increasingly less support	Allow child to sit on equipment that provides increasingly less support such as baby swing, feeder, walker, high chair
4. Sit in chair without assistance	Place child in a chair with arms. Provide balance support at first, then gradually withdraw. Leave for 10 minutes at a time
5. Sit without support	Place child on floor. Gradually withdraw assistance
Self-Feeding	
1. Sucking	Encourage child to suck by putting food on pacifier, putting a drop on tongue, and so forth
2. Drink from a cup	Put small amount of fluid in a baby cup. Raise cup to his or her mouth by placing hands under child's
3. Grasp piece of food and place in mouth	Place bit of favorite food in child's hand. Guide hand and food to mouth. Gradually reduce support
4. Transfer food from spoon to mouth	Move spoon to child's mouth with hand supporting baby's. Gradually withdraw support
5. Scoop up food and transfer to mouth	Have child hold spoon by handle, scoop up food, and transfer to mouth. Do not allow child to use fingers. Progress from bowl to flat plate
Stimulation of Touch	
1. Body sensation	Hold, cuddle, rock child
2. Explore environment through touch	Brush skin with objects of various textures (feathers, silk, sandpaper). Place objects of different textures near child. Move hand to object
3. Explore environment through mouth	Give child objects that can be chewed. Guide hand to mouth at first
4. Explore tactile sensations	Expose child to hard, soft, warm, and cold objects
5. Explore with water	Place hands and/or feet in water

Adapted from Johnson V, Werner R. A Step-by-Step Learning Guide for Retarded Infants and Children. Syracuse, Syracuse University Press, 1975; and Eddington C, Lee T. Sensory-motor stimulation for slow to develop children. Am J Nurs 75(1):59–62, 1975.

Whether at home or in the hospital, the child with cognitive impairment needs to know which behavior is acceptable and which is unacceptable. Discipline is as important to this child as to any other.

The limited ability of these children to adapt to varying circumstances makes it essential that discipline be consistent, with instructions given in simple, direct, concise language. A positive approach that relies heavily on example and demonstration produces better results than a constant "don't touch" or "stop that." Obedience is an important part of discipline, especially for the child with faulty reasoning ability, but the objectives of discipline should be much broader. The child needs to know what to expect and finds security and support in routines and consistency. Kindness, love, understanding, and physical comforting are also part of discipline.

If discipline is needed, it must follow the misdeed immediately, so that the cause-and-effect relationship is made clear. Taking the child away from the group for a short time can help restore self-control. Retaliation can confuse and anger the child. If the child is using misbehavior to get attention, praise and approval for good behavior may eliminate the need for wrongdoing.

Fostering Communication Skills. The child with cognitive impairment often has major problems with language skills. The child may have problems forming various speech sounds because of an enlarged tongue or other physical deviations, including hearing impairment. These problems can frustrate attempts at communication. In addition, the child may not be able to mentally process the words that have been spoken, which compounds communication problems.

A speech therapist can evaluate the child and develop a program to help caregivers work with the child to improve both the child's understanding of what is said and the child's ability to use language.

Promoting Family Coping. Before effective treatment can begin, the family must accept the reality of the child's problem and want to cope with the difficult task of helping the child develop his or her full potential. Diagnosis made at birth or during the first year affords the greatest hope of early acceptance and beginning education and training.

The family's first reaction to learning that the child may have cognitive impairment is grief—this is not the perfect child of their dreams. A parent may feel shame at the assumed inability to produce a perfect child. Some rejection of the child is almost inevitable, at least in the initial stages, but this needs to be worked through for the family to cope. Some parents compensate for their early hostile feelings by overprotection or overconcern, making the child unnecessarily helpless and perhaps taking out their anger and frustration on the normal siblings. Only when the family accepts the child as another member of the family, to be helped, loved, and disciplined as the others, can they begin to function effectively.

The family needs to know that their feelings are normal. Talking with other families of impaired children can offer some of the best support and guidance as they seek information to help them deal with the problem. One group that includes both families and health care professionals is the National Association of Retarded Citizens, a volunteer organization with local chapters in many communities. The National Down Syndrome Society is an excellent resource for the family of a child with Down syndrome.

Promoting Growth and Development. The child with cognitive impairment often has physical disabilities that affect growth and development. All but the most profoundly impaired children go through the sequence of normal development, with delays at each stage and leveling off of ability as they reach the limits of their capabilities. A cognitively impaired child, however, proceeds according to mental age rather than chronologic age. Thus, an impaired 6-year-old child may be functioning on a mental level of 2 years, and the expected behavior must be essentially that of a 2-year-old child. Adequate knowledge of the important landmarks of normal growth and development is essential to understanding the progressive nature of maturation.

Preventing Injury. The child with cognitive impairment has faulty reasoning ability and a short attention span. As a result, the adult caregivers must be responsible for protecting the child. The hospital environment as well as the home environment must be made safe. Elementary safety rules can be taught but must be reinforced regularly.

EVALUATION

- The child will practice basic hygiene habits with support and supervision.
- The child's communication with staff and family shows improvement.
- The family voices their feelings about the child; the family establishes relationships with families of other children with cognitive impairment.
- Family caregivers demonstrate knowledge of normal growth and development.
- The child is protected from injury by caregivers; the child learns basic safety rules.

Down Syndrome

Down syndrome is the most common of the chromosomal anomalies, occurring in about 1 in 700 to 1000 births. The condition was first described by Langdon Down in 1866, but its cause was a mystery for many years. In 1932, it was suggested that a chromosomal anomaly might be the cause, but the anomaly was not demonstrated until 1959.

Down syndrome has been observed in nearly all countries and races. The old term mongolism is not appropriate and is no longer used. Most people with Down syndrome have trisomy 21 (see Figure 4-6); a few have partial dislocation of chromosomes 15 and 21. Women older than 35 years of age are at a greater risk of bearing a child with Down syndrome, but children with Down syndrome are born to women of all ages. Older women are more likely to choose to have an amniocentesis to determine if they are carrying a child with Down syndrome and may decide to have an abortion. The growing trend toward routine screening of all pregnant women for an elevated maternal serum alphafetoprotein level may have an impact on the number of children with Down syndrome who are born because the parents have the option to elect to abort the pregnancy. All forms of the condition show a variety of abnormal characteristics. Mental status is usually within the moderate to severe range of retardation, with most being moderately retarded.

The most common anomalies include the following:

- **Brachycephaly** (shortness of head)
- Retarded body growth
- Upward and outward slanted eyes (almond shaped) with an epicanthic fold at inner angle
- Short, flattened bridge of the nose
- Thick, fissured tongue
- Dry, cracked, fissured skin that may be mottled
- Hair may be dry and coarse
- Hands are short, with an incurved fifth finger
- A single palmar crease
- Wide space between the first and second toes
- Lax muscle tone (often referred to as "double jointed" by others)
- Frequent heart and eye anomalies
- Susceptibility to leukemia greater than in the general population

Not all of these physical signs are present in all people with Down syndrome. Some may have only one or two characteristics; others may show nearly all the characteristics (Figure 13-8).

Treatment and Education

Knowledge about mental retardation has increased dramatically during the last half of the 20th century, and new teaching methods have begun to yield encouraging results. Mildly and moderately retarded people are being taught in increasing numbers to perform tasks that enable them to achieve some degree of independence and usefulness. More and better services are being provided for all retarded children and adults.

The child with cognitive impairment may not be identified until well into the preschool stage. Slow development often can be excused in one way or another. The family may be the best judge of the child's development, and health care personnel must listen carefully to any concerns or questions they express. When family members are faced with the facts of mental retardation, they will need to go through a grieving process, as do family members of any other child with a serious disorder. They need to mourn the loss of the normal child that was expected and resolve to give this child the best opportunities to develop to his or her potential.

Early diagnosis and intervention are important tools to use in the care of the mentally retarded. Early infant tests are difficult to administer, and results are not accurate, but the family may get some idea about the possible potential of the child. The family must be aware that these are only predictions based on unreliable test data. The child is usually kept at home in the family environment. At one time families were advised to place their retarded children in an institution. In many instances, these people were kept there until their death. Little learning took place in these situations. The current philosophy of care for the retarded child is to approach teaching in an aggressive manner, encouraging learning in a supportive home environment where the child can relate closely to a few people whose role is to stimulate and encourage maximum development. The individual attention, security, and sense of belonging to a family are important factors in every child's growth and development.

Each family must decide individually whether it is able to manage the child at home. Depending on their physical, emotional, and financial resources, it may be better for the family to place the child outside the home. The profoundly retarded child can take so much time and strength from one or more family members that the other children are neglected. A retarded child who is undisciplined or improperly supervised may threaten the safety of others in the home and the neighborhood. Caring for a retarded child may demand so much sacrifice from other family members that the family eventually disintegrates. Health care professionals must be realistic in providing information on which the family can base their decision.

Respiratory System Disorders

Tonsillitis

Tonsillitis is a common illness in childhood, resulting from pharyngitis. Frequently, the cause of tonsillitis is viral, although β-hemolytic streptococcal infection also may be the cause. Throat cultures are performed to determine the causative organism.

Pathophysiology

A brief description of the placement and functions of the tonsils and adenoids serves as an introduction to the discussion of their infection and medical and surgical treatment.

A ring of lymphoid tissue encircles the pharynx, forming a protective barrier against upper respiratory infection. This ring consists of groups of lymphoid tonsils.

The faucial tonsils, the commonly known **tonsils**, are two oval masses attached to the side walls of the back of the mouth between the anterior and posterior pillars.

The pharyngeal tonsil, known as **adenoids**, is a mass of lymphoid tissue in the nasal pharynx, extending from the roof of the nasal pharynx to the free edge of the soft palate.

The lingual tonsils are two masses of lymphoid tissue at the base of the tongue.

There is a normal progression of enlargement of lymphoid tissue in childhood between the ages of 2 and

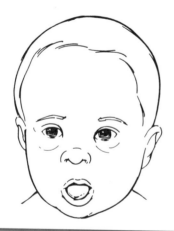

Figure 13-8. Typical facial features of a child with Down syndrome. (From Oski F et al. Principles and Practice of Pediatrics. Philadelphia: JB Lippincott, 1990.)

10 years and reduction during the preadolescence. If the tissue itself becomes a site of acute or chronic infection, it may become hypertrophied and can interfere with breathing, causing partial deafness, or it may become a source of infection in itself.

Treatment
Medical treatment of tonsillitis consists of analgesics for pain, antipyretics for fever, and in the case of streptococcal infection, an antibiotic. A standard 10-day course of antibiotics is recommended. The importance of completing the full prescription of antibiotic should be stressed to the caregiver to ensure that the streptococcal infection is completely eliminated. The child will find that a soft or liquid diet is easier to swallow and should be encouraged to maintain good fluid intake. A cool-mist vaporizer may be used to ease respirations.

Tonsillectomies and adenoidectomies are controversial. A tonsillectomy or an adenoidectomy can be performed independent of the other, but they are often done together. No conclusive evidence has been found that a tonsillectomy, in itself, improves a child's health by reducing the number of respiratory infections, increasing the appetite, or improving general well-being. Currently, tonsillectomies generally are not being performed unless other measures are ineffective or the tonsils are so hypertrophied that breathing and eating are difficult. Tonsillectomies are not performed while the tonsils are infected.

The adenoids are more susceptible to chronic infection. An indication for adenoidectomy is hypertrophy of the tissue to the extent of impairing hearing or interfering with breathing. An increasingly common practice is to perform only an adenoidectomy if tonsil tissue appears to be healthy.

A tonsillectomy is postponed until after the age of 4 or 5 years, except in the rare instance when it appears urgently needed. Often, when a child has reached the acceptable age, the apparent need for the tonsillectomy has disappeared.

Nursing Process for the Child Having a Tonsillectomy

ASSESSMENT
Much of the presurgical preparation, including complete blood count, bleeding and clotting time, and urinalysis often are done on a preadmission outpatient basis. In many hospitals, the child is admitted to the hospital on the day of surgery. Psychological preparation is often accomplished through preadmission orientation. Acting out the forthcoming experience, particularly in a group, with the use of puppets, dolls, and play-doctor or play-nurse material helps the child develop security. The amount and the timing of preparation before admission depends on the child's age. The child may become frightened

about losing a body part. Telling the child that the troublesome tonsils are going to be "fixed" is a much better choice than to say that they are going to be "taken out."

The child and the caregiver are included in the admission assessment. The history should include information on any bleeding tendencies because postoperative bleeding is a concern. The nurse must be careful to explain all procedures to the child and be sensitive to the child's apprehension. Taking and recording vital signs will establish a baseline for postoperative monitoring. The temperature is important as part of the assessment to determine that the child has no upper respiratory infection. Assessing the child for loose teeth that could cause a problem during administration of anesthesia is also necessary.

NURSING DIAGNOSES
Using the information gathered in the assessment, the appropriate nursing diagnoses can be determined. Preoperative nursing diagnoses are generally those for any child undergoing a surgical procedure. Postoperative nursing diagnoses may include the following:

- High risk for aspiration postoperatively related to unswallowed saliva and bleeding at the operative site
- High risk for fluid volume deficit related to blood loss from surgery and inadequate oral intake
- Pain related to surgical procedure
- High risk for altered health maintenance related to caregivers' knowledge deficit of postdischarge care

PLANNING AND IMPLEMENTATION
Preventing Aspiration Postoperatively. Immediately following a tonsillectomy, the child is placed in a partially prone position, head turned to one side, until completely awake. This position can be accomplished by turning the child partially over and by flexing the knee on which the child is not resting to help maintain the position. Pillows placed under the chest and abdomen may embarrass respiration and so are usually avoided. The child should be encouraged to expectorate all secretions and should be provided with an ample supply of tissues with a handy waste container close by. The child should be discouraged from coughing.

Monitoring Vital Signs and Fluid Intake. Vital signs are checked every 10 to 15 minutes until the child is fully reacted, then every 30 minutes or 1 hour. The nurse should be aware of the child's preoperative baseline vital signs to interpret the vital signs correctly. Hemorrhage is the most common complication of tonsillectomies. Any unusual restlessness or anxiety, frequent swallowing, or rapid pulse may indicate bleeding and should be reported. Vomiting of dark, old blood may be expected, but bright, red-flecked emesis or oozing indicates fresh bleeding. The nurse should observe the pharynx with a flashlight each time vital signs are checked. When the child is fully awake from surgery, small amounts of clear fluids or ice chips are given. Synthetic juices, carbonated beverages that are "flat," and juice popsicles are good choices. Liquids that are red are avoided to eliminate any possible confusion with bloody discharge. Irritating liquids such as orange juice and lemonade also are avoided. Milk and ice cream products tend to cling to the surgical site and make swallowing more difficult, thus they are poor choices, despite the old tradition of offering ice cream after tonsillectomies. Intravenous fluid administration and recording of intake and output are continued until adequate oral intake is established.

Providing Comfort and Relieving Pain. An ice collar may be used postoperatively; however, if the child is uncomfortable with it, the collar should be removed. Pain medication is administered as ordered. Frequently, liquid acetaminophen with codeine is prescribed. Rectal or intravenous analgesics may be used. The child's caregiver is encouraged to remain at the bedside to provide soothing reassurance. Crying irritates the raw throat and increases the child's discomfort; thus, it should be avoided, if possible. The nurse can tell the caregiver what may be expected in drainage and signs that should be reported immediately to the nursing staff.

Providing Family Teaching. The child is discharged on the day after surgery if no complications are present. The child should be kept relatively quiet for a few days after discharge. The family should be told that there is a danger of hemorrhage between the fifth and tenth postoperative days, so the child must be observed for any bleeding during this time. If bleeding should occur, the pediatrician or emergency department should be notified at once. Soft foods and nonirritating liquids should be given during the first few days. The caregivers are advised that a transient earache may be expected about the third day. If the child has recurring, severe earache, cough, or fever the child should be evaluated by the physician. See Nursing Care Plan for the child having a tonsillectomy.

EVALUATION

- The child expectorates saliva and drainage with no breathing difficulties.
- No evidence of bleeding is noted. The child's fluid intake increases as the child recovers.
- The child rests with minimal discomfort.
- Caregivers demonstrate an understanding of postoperative care through responses and appropriate questions.

Blood Disorders

There are several blood dyscrasias, or abnormalities of the blood, that may manifest themselves in the child of preschool age. Although leukemia, purpura, and hemo-

philia may be diagnosed at either an earlier or a later age, they are commonly associated with the preschool years. Children with these disorders are often chronically ill and require long-term care.

Acute Leukemia

Leukemia is the most common type of cancer in children, accounting for approximately 30% of all childhood cancers. *Acute lymphatic leukemia* (ALL) is responsible for about 85% of the childhood leukemias; fortunately, ALL is also considered to be the most curable of all the major forms of leukemia. The incidence of ALL is greatest between the ages of 3 and 5 years, is higher among boys than girls, and is seen more frequently in white children than in African American children.

Pathophysiology

Leukemia is the uncontrolled reproduction of deformed white blood cells. Despite intensive research, its cause is not known. Mature leukocytes (white blood cells) are made up of three types of cells

Monocytes—(5% to 10% of white blood cells) defend the body against infection

Granulocytes—divided into eosinophils, basophils, and neutrophils; neutrophils (60% of the white blood cells) can pass through capillary walls to surround and destroy bacteria

Lymphocytes—(30% of white blood cells) divided into T cells, which attack and destroy virus-infected cells, foreign tissue, and cancer cells, and B cells, which produce antibodies (proteins that help destroy foreign matter)

An immature lymphocyte is called a lymphoblast. Leukemia occurs when lymphocytes reproduce so fast that they are mostly in the "blast," or immature, stage. This rapid increase in lymphocytes causes crowding that, in turn, decreases the production of red blood cells and platelets. The decrease in red blood cells, platelets, and normal white blood cells causes the child to be easily fatigued and susceptible to infection and increased bleeding.

Clinical Manifestations

Clinical manifestations of leukemia appear with surprising abruptness in many affected children, with few, if any, warning signs. Each of the symptoms are a result of a response to the proliferation of lymphoblast cells. Presenting manifestations are frequently lassitude, pallor, and low-grade fever caused by anemia. Other early or presenting symptoms are bone and joint pain caused by lymphocytes invading the periosteum, widespread **petechiae** (pinpoint hemorrhages beneath the skin), and

Nursing Care Plan
for the Child Having a Tonsillectomy

Nursing Diagnosis

High risk for aspiration postoperatively related to unswallowed saliva and bleeding at the operative site

Goal: Prevent postoperative aspiration

Nursing Interventions	Rationale	Evaluation
Place child in partially prone position, head turned to one side immediately following surgery.	Prevents unswallowed saliva and blood from draining into pharynx, where it could be aspirated.	Child expectorates saliva and drainage with no breathing difficulties.
Encourage child to spit out all secretions, and provide an ample supply of tissues with a waste container nearby.	The child needs instruction in and constant encouragement to expectorate.	

Nursing Diagnosis

High risk for fluid volume deficit related to blood loss from surgery and inadequate oral intake

Goal: Maintain adequate hydration

Nursing Interventions	Rationale	Evaluation
Monitor vital signs every 10 to 15 minutes until the child is fully reacted, then every 30 minutes to 1 hour. Observe for and promptly report any signs of bleeding or hemorrhage—restlessness, anxiety, frequent swallowing, or rapid pulse.	Hemorrhage is the most frequent complication of tonsillectomies.	No evidence of bleeding is noted; child's fluid intake increases as child recovers.
Offer the child small amounts of clear fluids or ice chips once fully awake, then synthetic juices or flat carbonated beverages; avoid milk and other dairy products (including ice cream), red liquids, and irritating liquids like orange juice and lemonade.	Clear fluids won't irritate surgical site; milk products tend to cling and thus could irritate the throat; red liquids might be confused with bloody discharge.	

Nursing Diagnosis

Pain related to surgical procedure

Goal: Provide comfort and relieve pain

Nursing Interventions	Rationale	Evaluation
Apply an ice collar unless the child finds it uncomfortable.	Ice reduces swelling in the throat.	Child rests with minimal discomfort.
Encourage caregiver to remain at child's bedside if possible.	The soothing presence of someone the child knows and loves can be reassuring and also may prevent the child from crying, which irritates the raw throat.	

(continued)

Nursing Care Plan
for the Child Having a Tonsillectomy (Continued)

Nursing Diagnosis

High risk for altered health maintenance related to caregivers' lack of knowledge of post-discharge care

Goal: *Provide family teaching*

Nursing Interventions	Rationale	Evaluation
Provide caregivers with care instructions in terms they can understand; inform caregivers that the danger for hemorrhage occurs between the 5th and 10th postoperative day, and discuss whom they should contact if bleeding does occur.	Caregivers may feel uneasy about being able to provide safe care at home. Understanding the healing process and normal signs of healing as well as potential complications and information about whom to contact for questions or problems will give them confidence about being able to take care of their child.	Caregivers demonstrate understanding of postoperative care through responses and appropriate questions.

purpura (hemorrhages into the skin or the mucous membranes) as a result of a low thrombocyte count.

Anorexia, nausea and vomiting, headache, diarrhea, and abdominal pain, although seldom presenting signs, often occur during the course of the disease as a result of enlargement of the liver and spleen. Easy bruising is a constant problem. Ulceration of the gums and throat develops as a result of bacterial invasion and contributes to anorexia. Intracranial hemorrhages are not uncommon. Anemia becomes increasingly severe.

Diagnosis

In addition to the history, symptoms, and laboratory blood studies, a bone marrow aspiration must be done to confirm the diagnosis of leukemia. The preferred site for bone marrow aspiration in children is the iliac crest. Radiographs of the long bones demonstrate changes caused by the invasion of the lymphoblasts.

Treatment

The advances in the treatment of ALL have dramatically improved long-term survival. In children whose initial prognosis is good, approximately 90% have long-term survival. For those children who have a relapse, survival rates are greatly reduced. Each succeeding relapse reduces the probability of survival.

Intensive chemotherapy is initially divided into the following three phases:

Induction—geared to achieving a complete remission with no leukemia cells

Sanctuary—preventing invasion of the central nervous system by leukemia cells (no sanctuary is given to the leukemia cells)

Maintenance—maintaining the remission

A combination of drugs is used during the induction phase to bring about remission. Among the drugs used are vincristine, prednisone, and L-asparaginase. During the sanctuary phase, **intrathecal administration** (injected into the cerebrospinal fluid by lumbar puncture) of methotrexate is used to eradicate leukemia cells in the central nervous system. The maintenance phase may last 2 or 3 years and includes treatment with methotrexate, vincristine, prednisone, and 6-mercaptopurine. The drugs frequently are administered through a double-lumen catheter (Broviac) placed in the subclavian vein. Two additional phases are instituted for those children who suffer a relapse, as follows:

Reinduction—drugs previously used, plus additional drugs are administered; each relapse decreases the child's chance of survival

Bone marrow transplant—usually recommended after the second remission in children with ALL

Nursing Process for the Child with Leukemia

ASSESSMENT

The nursing assessment of the child with leukemia varies according to the stage of the child's illness. The assessment interview should be conducted with the family caregiver and the child. The nurse must avoid having the caregiver monopolize the interview. The child needs an opportunity to express feelings and fears and answer the nurse's questions. Physical assessment of the child should include examination for **adenopathy** (enlarged lymph glands); vital signs; especially observing for a low-grade fever; careful assessment for signs of bruising; petechiae; bleeding from or ulcerations of mucous membranes; abdominal pain or tenderness; and bone or joint pain. The child should be observed for lethargic behavior, and the caregiver should be questioned about this. Signs of local infection, including edema, redness, and swelling, or any indication of systemic infection should be noted.

The emotional state of the child and the family must be assessed. The diagnosis of leukemia is devastating. The child and family's emotional states must be evaluated so that a plan can be made to assist them in working through and resolving their feelings and fears.

NURSING DIAGNOSES

Depending on the results of the nursing assessment and the interview with both the child and the caregiver, the nursing diagnoses are developed. Some of the diagnoses that may be appropriate are the following:

- High risk for infection related to immunosuppression
- High risk for injury related to bleeding tendencies
- Pain related to the effects of chemotherapy and the disease process
- Activity intolerance related to fatigue
- High risk for altered growth and development related to impaired ability to achieve developmental tasks secondary to limitations of disease and treatment
- Body image disturbance related to alopecia and weight loss
- Anticipatory grieving of family related to the prognosis

PLANNING AND IMPLEMENTATION

Nursing goals for the child with leukemia vary, depending on individual circumstances. The goals should be determined with the participation of the child and caregiver. Prevention of infection and bleeding and relief of pain are primary concerns.

Preventing Infection. The immune system is weakened by the uncontrolled growth of lymphoblasts that overpower the normal production of granulocytes (particularly neutrophils) and monocytes. In addition, the chemotherapy that is necessary to inhibit this proliferation of lymphoblast cells causes immunosuppression. Thus, these children are susceptible to infection, especially during chemotherapy. Infections such as meningitis, septicemia, and pneumonia are the most frequent causes of

death. The organism most often responsible is *Pseudomonas*. Other organisms that can be dangerous for the child are *Escherichia coli, Staphylococcus aureus, Klebsiella, Pneumocystis carinii, Candida albicans*, and *Histoplasmosis*. These infectious organisms can threaten the child's life.

To protect the child from infectious organisms, reverse isolation precautions must be maintained. Staff, family, and visitors must be carefully screened to eliminate any known infection. Handwashing, gowning, and masking are necessary. The social isolation that this imposes on the child can be difficult for the child to understand and tolerate. The nurse should make an effort to spend time with the child in addition to the time that is necessary for direct care. Playing games, coloring, reading stories, and doing puzzles are all good activities that the child will enjoy. This also can give the caregiver, who may be staying with the child, a much needed "time out" break.

Preventing Bleeding. The mucous membranes bleed easily, therefore care must be taken to be gentle when oral hygiene is done, using a soft, sponge-type brush or gauze strips wrapped around the nurse's finger. Mouthwash composed of 1 part hydrogen peroxide to 4 parts saline solution or a normal saline solution may be used. Epistaxis (nosebleed) is a common problem. Usually, this can be handled by applying external pressure to the nose. Pressure should be applied to sites of injections or venipunctures to prevent excessive bleeding. Observations must be made at least every 4 hours to assess the child for other signs of bleeding, such as petechiae, ecchymosis, hematemesis (bloody emesis), tarry stools, and swelling and tenderness of the joints. The child must be protected from injury by external forces to prevent the possibility of hemorrhage from the injury. Extra caution must be taken when the child's platelet count is especially low.

Reducing Pain. Pain from the invasion of lymphoblasts into the periosteum and bleeding into the joints can be excruciating. Gentle handling, sheepskin pads under bony prominences, and positioning can help relieve discomfort and skin breakdown. Painful procedures are also a concern. The nurse should explain to the child that these procedures are necessary to help and are not a form of punishment of the child. The child needs help to communicate how great the pain is. A pain scale can help the child rate the pain and communicate its intensity. The Oucher Scale[1] and the Faces Scale[2] are useful with children 3 years of age and older (see Figure 3-19). The child needs analgesics administered to achieve maximum comfort.

Promoting Energy Conservation and Relieving Anxiety. As a result of anemia, the child will experience fatigue. Procedures should be paced so that the child has as much uninterrupted rest as possible. Stress adds to the child's feelings of exhaustion; therefore, efforts to help the child deal with feelings of stress caused by the illness and treatments may help decrease fatigue. Encouraging the child to talk about feelings and acknowledging the child's feelings as valid are ways in which the nurse can help.

Promoting Normal Growth and Development. During treatment, the child may be prevented from normal activity much of the time. The social isolation that accompanies reverse isolation often interferes with normal development. Physical activities often are limited simply because of the child's lack of energy. Knowledge of normal growth and development expectations is important to consider when planning developmental activities. Conscious effort must be made to stimulate growth and development within the child's physical capabilities. Positive developmental tasks can be stressed, for example, practicing or improving reading skills and learning or increasing computer skills. The family should be encouraged to help the child return to normal activities as much as possible during the maintenance phase of the treatment when the child has been discharged from the hospital.

Promoting a Positive Body Image. The drugs that are administered in chemotherapy cause **alopecia** (loss of hair). The child and the family need to be psychologically prepared for this change in appearance. The child may want to have a wig that can be worn, especially when the child is ready to return to school. The wig should be chosen before chemotherapy is started so that it matches the child's hair and the child has time to get used to it. A cap or scarf often has an appeal to a child, particularly if it carries special meaning for that child. The child and the family can be reassured that the hair will grow back in about 3 to 6 months. The scalp must be washed regularly to avoid cradle cap. Prednisone therapy may cause the child to have a moon-faced appearance, which may be upsetting to either the child or the family. Reassure them that this is temporary and will disappear when the drug is no longer needed.

The child may be hesitant for peers to see these changes. Visits from peers should be encouraged before discharge, if possible, so the child can be prepared to handle reactions and questions. A school teacher can be invaluable in preparing classmates to welcome the child back with minimal reaction to the child's physical changes. Families can be encouraged to enlist the assistance of the child's teacher, school nurse, and pediatrician to ease the transition. Meeting other children who are undergoing chemotherapy and are in various stages of recovery is often helpful to the child. This helps relieve the feeling that no one else has ever looked like this. Both the child and the family need opportunities to express their feelings and apprehensions.

Promoting Family Coping. Family members often are devastated when they first learn that their child has leukemia. They need support from the moment of the first diagnosis, through the hospitalization, and continuing through the maintenance phase. Families live one day at a time, hoping that the remission will not end and that their child will be one who does not have a relapse and is finally considered cured. The family needs opportunities to freely express its feelings about the illness and treatment. The family will find comfort in having a consistent nurse caring for the child. This consistency helps give them a feeling of stability.

Caregivers need to be involved in the care of the child during hospitalization and should be given complete information about what to expect when caring for the child at home during the maintenance phase. The family needs a contact person who can be called to answer questions during this phase. The family needs to work though feelings of overprotectiveness toward the child so that the child can lead as normal a life as possible. The family also needs to consider how siblings can fit into the return of the child to the home. Siblings may have many questions about the seriousness of the child's illness and about the possible death of the child. Families need support in dealing with these concerns and benefit from counseling. Most hospitals that provide care for pediatric oncology patients have caregiver support groups that meet regularly and provide support. Candlelighters is a national organization for parents of young cancer patients that also provides support.

EVALUATION

- The child remains free of superimposed infection.
- The child evidences no signs of bleeding.
- The child rests quietly and indicates that the pain is tolerable.
- The child has extended periods of rest.
- The child is involved in age-appropriate activities within limitations of energy.
- The child and the family express feelings about changes in physical appearance and evidence acceptance by demonstrating pride and adjustments in grooming.
- The family expresses feelings and fears about the child's prognosis and accepts counseling as needed.

Idiopathic Thrombocytopenic Purpura

Purpura is a blood disorder associated with a deficit of platelets in the circulatory system. The most common type of purpura is idiopathic thrombocytopenic purpura. Purpura is preceded by a viral infection in about half of the diagnosed cases.

The onset of idiopathic thrombocytopenia purpura is frequently acute. Bruising and a generalized rash occur. In severe cases, hemorrhage may occur in the mucous membranes; epistaxis, which is difficult to control, or hematuria may be present. Rarely, a serious complication of intracranial hemorrhage occurs. In most cases, spontaneous disappearance of symptoms occurs in a few weeks without serious hemorrhage. A few cases may continue in a chronic form of the disease.

In idiopathic thrombocytopenia purpura, the platelet count may be as low as 20,000/mm³ or lower. The bleeding time is prolonged, and the clot retraction time is abnormal. The white blood cell count remains normal, and anemia is not present unless excessive bleeding has occurred.

Treatment and Nursing Care
Corticosteroids are useful in reducing the severity and shortening the duration of the disease in some, but not all, cases of idiopathic thrombocytopenia purpura. Intravenous gamma globulin has been used to increase the production of platelets until recovery occurs spontaneously. If the platelet count is higher than 20,000/mm³, treatment may be delayed to see if a spontaneous remission occurs. Nursing care consists of protecting the affected child from falls and trauma, observing for signs of external or internal bleeding, regular diet, and general supportive care.

Hemophilia

Hemophilia is one of the oldest known hereditary diseases. Recent research has demonstrated that hemophilia is a syndrome of several distinct inborn errors of metabolism, all resulting in the delayed coagulation of blood. Defects in the synthesis of protein lead to deficiencies in any of the factors in the blood plasma needed for thromboplastic activity. The principal factors involved are factors VIII, IX, and XI.

Mechanism of Clot Formation
The mechanism of clot formation is complex. In a simplified form, it can best be described as occurring in three stages:

1. Prothrombin is formed through plasma–platelet interaction.
2. Prothrombin is converted to thrombin.
3. Fibrinogen is converted into fibrin by thrombin.

Fibrin forms a mesh that traps red and white blood cells and platelets into a clot, closing the defect in an injured vessel. A deficiency in one of the thromboplastin precursors may lead to hemophilia. This progression of events is diagrammed in Figure 13-9.

Reference to one of the specialized texts on the circulatory system is necessary for a detailed discussion and for better understanding of the clot-forming mechanism.

Clinical Manifestations
Hemophilia is characterized by prolonged bleeding, with frequent hemorrhages externally and into the skin, the joint spaces, and the intramuscular tissues. Bleeding from tooth extractions, brain hemorrhages, and crippling disabilities are serious complications. Death during infancy or in early childhood is not unusual in severe hemophilia and results from a great loss of blood, intracranial bleeding, or respiratory obstruction caused by bleeding into the neck tissues.

A young infant beginning to creep or walk bruises easily and often may cause serious hemorrhages from minor lacerations. Bleeding often occurs from lip biting or from sharp objects put in the mouth. Tooth eruption seldom causes bleeding, but extractions require specialized handling and should be avoided by preventive care, if at all possible. Family caregivers have to be careful not to overprotect the child, however. The preschooler is active and plays hard, and injuries are practically unavoidable.

Clinical manifestations in any type of hemophilia are similar and are treated by administration of the deficient factor and by measures to prevent or treat complications. In severe bleeding, the quantities of fresh blood or frozen plasma needed may easily overload the circulatory system. Factor VIII concentrate eliminates this problem.

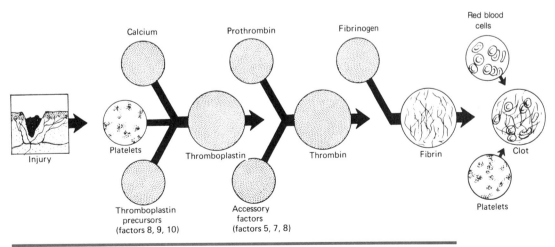

Figure 13-9. The mechanism of the formation of a blood clot is complex.

Diagnosis

A careful examination of family history and of the type of bleeding the patient presents is conducted. Abnormal bleeding beginning in infancy, in combination with a family history, suggests hemophilia. A markedly prolonged clotting time is characteristic of severe factor VIII or IX deficiency, but mild conditions may have only a slightly prolonged clotting time. The partial prothrombin time (PTT) is the test that most clearly demonstrates that factor VIII is low.

Recognized Types of Hemophilia

Factor VIII Deficiency (Hemophilia A; Antihemophilic Globulin Deficiency; Classic Hemophilia). Classic hemophilia is inherited as a sex-linked recessive Mendelian trait with transmission to affected males by carrier females. Hemophilia A (classic hemophilia) is the most commonly found type, occurring in about 1 in 10,000 people, and is also the most severe. It is caused by a deficiency of antihemophilic globulin—the factor VIII necessary for blood clotting.

Factor IX Deficiency (Hemophilia B; Plasma Thromboplastin Component Deficiency; Christmas Disease). Christmas disease was named after a 5-year-old boy who was one of the first patients diagnosed as having a deficiency in factor IX. This deficiency constitutes about 15% of the hemophilias. It is a sex-linked recessive trait appearing in male offspring of carrier females, caused by a deficiency of one of the necessary thromboplastin precursors, factor IX, the plasma thromboplastin component. In either hemophilia A or B, as many as 25% or more of the affected people can trace no family history of the disease. It is assumed that spontaneous mutations have occurred in some of these cases. Hemophilia B (Christmas disease) is indistinguishable from classic hemophilia in its clinical manifestations, particularly in its severe form. It also may exist in a mild form, probably more frequently than in hemophilia A.

Factor XI Deficiency (Hemophilia C; Plasma Thromboplastin Antecedent Deficiency). This exists as an autosomal dominant trait, appearing in both males and females. Sporadic cases also may be observed, as in the other hemophilias. The deficient factor is plasma thromboplastin antecedent (factor XI). Bleeding is generally milder than in the antihemophilic globulin and the plasma thromboplastin component deficiencies, hemorrhage usually being by trauma and rarely spontaneous.

Von Willebrand Disease (Vascular Hemophilia; Pseudohemophilia). Von Willebrand disease is classified with the hemophilias. It is a Mendelian dominant trait present in both sexes and is characterized by prolonged bleeding times.

Treatment

For many years the only treatment for bleeding in hemophilia was the use of fresh blood or plasma. When fresh frozen plasma came into use, it became the mainstay in hemophilia management. It has been particularly helpful in emergency situations.

Frozen plasma does, however, have several shortcomings. One major problem has been the large volumes needed to control bleeding. Another is the danger that injections of large amounts of plasma may lead to congestive heart failure. In addition, plasma must be given within 30-minutes because factor VIII loses its potency at room temperature.

Several factor VIII concentrates for the treatment of hemophilia are now available. One of these, called cryoprecipitate, resulted from the discovery that the precipitate remaining undissolved when frozen plasma thawed slowly could be used to stop bleeding.

Commercial preparations are now available that supply higher potency factor VIII than previous preparations. These concentrates are supplied in dried form together with diluent for reconstitution. Directions for mixing and administration are included with the package. The preparations can be stored for a long time but have the disadvantage of exposing the recipient to a large number of donors.

One of the serious problems with blood products of any kind has been the risk of exposure to hepatitis B and human immunodeficiency virus (HIV), the causative organism of acquired immunodeficiency syndrome (AIDS). Currently, blood is screened thoroughly for viral contamination, greatly diminishing the danger of transmission of HIV. However, large numbers of hemophiliacs treated before the late 1980s were exposed to HIV and now test positive for HIV antibodies.

Researchers continue to explore new ways to replace the missing factor while protecting the recipient from the threat of contracting an unknown illness.

Nursing Process for the Child with Hemophilia

ASSESSMENT

The nursing assessment begins with a review of the child's history with the caregiver. This should include previous episodes of bleeding, the usual treatment, medications the child takes, and the current episode of bleeding. The child should be included in the interview if he or she is old enough to answer questions. The child should be carefully observed for any signs of bleeding. The nurse inspects the mucous membranes, examines the joints for tenderness and swelling, and checks the skin for evidence of bruising. The child or caregiver should be questioned about hematuria, hematemesis, headache, or black tarry stools.

NURSING DIAGNOSES

After a careful nursing assessment, a selection of appropriate nursing diagnoses is made. Some nursing diagnoses that may be useful are the following:

- Pain related to joint swelling and limitations secondary to hemarthrosis
- High risk for physical immobility related to pain and tenderness of joints
- High risk for injury related to hemorrhage secondary to trauma
- High risk for altered health maintenance related to insufficient knowledge of condition, treatments, and hazards
- High risk for ineffective family coping related to treatment and care of the child

PLANNING AND IMPLEMENTATION

Using the information gathered from the nursing assessment, goals are set with the cooperation and input of the caregiver and the child. Mutual goals are set for the child's and the family's care.

Relieving Pain. Bleeding into the joint cavities often occurs following some slight injury and seems nearly unavoidable if the child is to be allowed to lead a normal life. Pain, caused by the pressure of the confined fluid in the narrow joint spaces, is extreme, requiring the use of sedatives or narcotics. Prompt immobilization of the involved extremity is essential to prevent contractures of soft tissues and the destruction of the bone and joint tissues (Figure 13-10). Immobilization helps relieve pain and decrease bleeding. A bivalve plaster cast may be applied in the hospital for immobilization of the affected part. Drugs containing aspirin and nonsteroidal anti-inflammatory drugs, such as ibuprofen and indometha-

cin, should not be given to the child because of the danger of prolonging bleeding. Cold packs may be used to stop bleeding. The affected limb may be elevated above the level of the heart to slow blood flow. Using age-appropriate diversionary activities may help the child deal with the pain. Careful handling of the affected joints prevents additional pain.

Preventing Joint Contracture. Passive range of motion exercises help prevent the development of joint contractures. Many patients who have had repeated **hemarthrosis** (bleeding into the joints), however, have developed functional impairment of their joints despite careful treatment. Splints and devices should be used to position the limb in a functional position. Physical therapy is helpful after the bleeding episode is under control. Joint contractures are a serious risk, and every effort should be made to avoid them.

Preventing Injury. The child with hemophilia is continuously at risk for additional injury. The nurse must protect the child from trauma caused by procedures necessary in caring for the child. Invasive procedures should be limited as much as possible. Blood sample collection should be done by means of a finger stick, if possible. Intramuscular injections should be avoided. When an invasive procedure must be done, the site should be compressed for 5 minutes or longer after the procedure, and cold compresses should be applied.

The child's hospital environment should be made safe by eliminating any sharp objects. If the child is young, the cribsides should be padded to protect from bumping and bruising. Toys must be examined for sharp edges and hard surfaces. Soft toys are best for the young child. For mouth care, a soft toothbrush or sponge-type brush decreases the danger of causing bleeding of the gums. During daily hygiene, the nails should be trimmed to prevent scratching, and adequate skin care should be given to prevent irritation.

Providing Family Teaching. The family may need a thorough explanation of hemophilia or reinforcement of information that they already have. The nurse should review the family's knowledge about the disease and give additional information when needed. A child with hemophilia is healthy between bleeding episodes, but the fact that bleeding may occur as the result of slight trauma, or often without any known injury, causes considerable anxiety. For an unknown reason, bleeding episodes are more common in the spring and fall. There also appears to be some evidence that emotional stress can initiate bleeding episodes.

Topical fluoride applications to the teeth are of particular importance in these children. Particular attention should be paid to proper oral hygiene, a well-balanced diet, and proper dental treatment. The family needs to carefully select a dentist who understands the problems presented and who will set up an appropriate program of preventive dentistry.

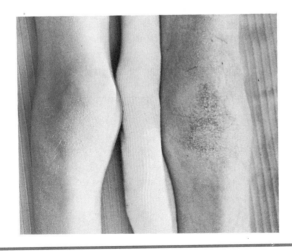

Figure 13-10. The hemophiliac can suffer from bleeding into the joints and painful swollen knees.

Safety measures for the home and the child's lifestyle must be discussed. A young child may need a protective helmet and elbow and knee pads for everyday wear, especially when first becoming mobile. Carpeting in the home, when possible, helps soften the fall of a toddler just learning to walk. An older child may need to wear the protective devices when playing outdoors. Playground areas can be treacherous for these children, but within reason, normalcy should be maintained. The family also needs instruction in giving medications, range of motion exercises, emergency measures to stop or limit bleeding, and all aspects of the child's care. Emergency splints are available and should be kept in the home of every person with hemophilia. Ice packs also should be available for instant use. If possible, the bleeding area can be raised above the level of the heart. Before leaving for the hospital, a splint and cold packs should be applied, and factor replacement may be indicated, according to the protocol established with the child's physician.

The family experiences continuous anxiety over how much activity to allow their child, how to keep from overprotecting, how to help the child achieve a healthy mental attitude, and yet prevent mishaps that may cause serious bleeding episodes. They must help the child toward autonomy and independence within the framework of necessary limitations. There certainly will be times when the emotional effect of social deprivation and restrained activity must be weighed against possible physical harm.

The financial strain on the family is considerable, as it is with most families with a child who has a chronic condition. Children who have had several episodes of hemarthrosis may be disabled to the extent of needing crutches and braces or wheelchairs. Measures toward rehabilitation require hospitalization, with possible surgery, casts, and other orthopedic appliances.

A hemophiliac child usually loses much school time. The child who must frequently interrupt his or her schooling, for whatever reason, experiences a considerable handicap. Each child should be considered individually and provided with as normal an environment as possible.

Promoting Family Coping. Both the child and family must accept the limitations and yet realize the importance of normal social experiences. School, health, and community agencies must be prepared to assist the family with counseling and encouragement and enable them to raise their affected child in a healthy manner, both emotionally and physically. The family should be informed that the National Hemophilia Foundation is a resource for a number of services and publications.

The nurse needs to review all of these concerns with the family, and through discussion, questions, and demonstrations the nurse will confirm that the family understands the information provided. Counseling may be required for the family to learn to cope with the child's needs. The nurse should encourage the family to express their feelings about the impact this has on their lifestyle. The family may have fears about the child dying from hemorrhaging. Guilt may play an important part in the family's reactions to the child. Recognizing and validating the feelings are important aspects of active listening that the nurse must use. During hospitalization, the family can be involved in the care of the child to learn how to help the child without causing additional pain.

EVALUATION

- The child rests quietly with minimal signs of discomfort.

- There is no evidence of new joint contractures; range of motion is maintained.

- No injuries or bleeding episodes occur as a result of procedures or treatments.

- The family demonstrates knowledge of the disease and discusses the child's home care, asking and answering appropriate questions.

- Family members express their feelings and demonstrate good coping mechanisms by seeking help from appropriate support systems.

Genitourinary System Disorders

Nephrotic Syndrome

A number of different types of nephrosis in the nephrotic syndrome have been identified. The most common type in children is called *lipoid nephrosis, idiopathic nephrotic syndrome*, or *minimal change nephrotic syndrome* (MCNS). All forms of nephrosis have early characteristics of edema and proteinuria; therefore, definite clinical differentiation cannot be made early in the disease.

The chief clinical manifestation of nephrotic syndrome is generalized edema that becomes so great that the child may double his or her normal weight (Figure 13-11). It has a course of remissions and exacerbations, usually lasting for months. The recovery rate is generally good with the use of intensive steroid therapy and protection against infection.

The cause of MCNS, the nephrotic syndrome most often seen in children, is not known. In rare cases, it may be associated with other specific diseases. The nephrotic syndrome is present in as many as 7 children per 100,000 population younger than 9 years of age. The age of onset, on the average, is $2\frac{1}{2}$ years, with most occurring between the ages of 2 and 6 years.

Clinical Manifestations

Edema is usually the presenting symptom, appearing first around the eyes and ankles. As the swelling advances, the edema becomes generalized, with a pendulous abdomen

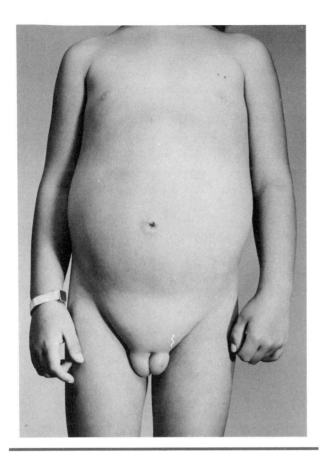

Figure 13-11. A child with nephrotic syndrome. Notice the distended abdomen caused by iscites and the edematous labia. (From Pillitteri A. Maternal and Child Health Nursing. Philadelphia: JB Lippincott, 1992.) (Courtesy of the Department of Medical Photography, Children's Hospital, Buffalo, NY.)

Treatment

The management of nephrotic syndrome is a long process, with remissions and recurrence of symptoms. The use of corticosteroids has induced remissions in most cases and reduced recurrences. Corticosteroid therapy usually produces diuresis in about 7 to 14 days, but the drug is continued until a remission occurs. Prednisone is the drug most commonly used. After the diuresis occurs, intermittent therapy is continued every other day, or for 3 days a week. Daily urine testing for protein is continued whether the child is at home or in the hospital.

Diuretics may not be necessary when diuresis can be induced with steroids. Diuretics have not been effective in reducing the edema of nephrotic syndrome, although a loop diuretic (furosemide) may be administered if edema causes respiratory embarrassment.

Immunosuppressant therapy may be used to reduce symptoms and prevent further relapses in children who do not respond adequately to corticosteroid administration. Cyclophosphamide (Cytoxan) is the drug most commonly used. Because cyclophosphamide has serious side effects, the family caregivers need to be fully informed before therapy is started. **Leukopenia** (leukocyte count less than 5000 mm^3) can be expected as well as other common side effects of immunosuppressant therapy, such as gastrointestinal symptoms, hematuria, and alopecia. The length of therapy is usually a brief period of 2 or 3 months.

A general diet, appealing to the child's poor appetite with frequent, small feedings if necessary, is recommended. The addition of salt is discouraged. Family caregivers need encouragement and support for the long months ahead. Relapses usually become less frequent as the child gets older.

full of fluid. Respiratory embarrassment may be severe, and edema of the scrotum on the male is characteristic. The edema shifts with change of position of the child when lying quietly or walking about. Anorexia, irritability, and loss of appetite develop. Malnutrition may become severe. The generalized edema masks the loss of body tissue, causing the child to present a chubby appearance, but after diuresis, the malnutrition becomes apparent. These children are usually susceptible to infection, and repeated acute respiratory conditions are the usual pattern. This is intensified by the immunosuppression caused by the administration of prednisone.

Diagnosis

Laboratory findings include marked proteinuria, especially albumin, with large numbers of hyaline and granular casts in the urine. Hematuria is not usually present, although a few red blood cells may appear in the urine. The blood serum protein level is reduced, and there is an increase in the level of cholesterol in the blood (**hyperlipidemia**).

Nursing Process for the Child with Nephrotic Syndrome

ASSESSMENT

The nursing assessment of the child with nephrotic syndrome must include evaluation of the child for edema. The child should be weighed, and the abdominal measurement should be taken and recorded to serve as a baseline. Vital signs, including blood pressure, need to be assessed. Swelling about the eyes and swelling of the ankles and other dependent parts should be noted and the degree of pitting recorded. The skin must be carefully inspected for pallor, irritation, or breakdown. The scrotal area of the young boy should be examined carefully for swelling, redness, and irritation. The caregiver should be questioned about the onset of symptoms, the child's appetite, urine output, and signs of fatigue or irritability.

NURSING DIAGNOSES

The nursing diagnoses vary with the outcome of the nursing assessment. The caregiver should be consulted when the nurse is determining suitable diagnoses so that the child's and the family's needs are met. Among the nursing diagnoses that may be included are the following:

- Fluid volume excess related to fluid accumulation in tissues and third spaces
- High risk for altered nutrition: less than body requirements related to anorexia
- High risk for impaired skin integrity related to edema
- Activity intolerance related to fatigue
- High risk for infection related to immunosuppression
- Parental health-seeking behaviors related to home care of a child with chronic illness

PLANNING AND IMPLEMENTATION

The primary nursing goal for the child with nephrotic syndrome is the monitoring and management of the child's fluid balance. Other nursing goals can be determined after the assessment, and the goals of the family must be integrated into the plan.

Monitoring Fluid Intake and Output. Accurate assessment and documentation of the child's intake and output are a must. The child should be weighed at the same time every day, on the same scale, wearing the same clothing. The output must be accurately measured. If the child is not toilet trained, the diapers may be weighed before being applied and after wetting to determine the amount of urine excreted (1 g = 1 mL). The child's abdomen should be measured daily, and measurement is usually done at the level of the umbilicus. Making certain that all staff personnel are measuring at the same level is essential. The desired location for measuring must be noted on the nursing care plan so that everyone follows the same practice. The urine should be tested regularly for albumin and specific gravity. Albumin can be tested with reagent strips for this purpose that can be dipped into the urine and read by comparison with a color chart on the container.

The abdomen may be greatly enlarged with **ascites** (edema in the peritoneal cavity). The abdomen can even become marked with **striae** (stretch marks). Before the common use of corticosteroids, an **abdominal paracentesis** (surgical puncture into the abdomen to drain fluid) was frequently necessary to drain the fluid. This used to be a traumatic experience for the child but is rarely needed with current therapy.

Improving Nutritional Intake. Although the child may look plump, underneath the edema is a thin, possibly malnourished child. The child's appetite is poor for several reasons: (1) the ascites diminish the appetite because of the full feeling in the abdomen; (2) the child may

be lethargic and apathetic and simply not interested in eating; (3) a no-added-salt diet may be unappealing to the child; and (4) corticosteroid therapy may decrease the appetite. A visually appealing and nutritious diet must be offered. The child and the family should be consulted to learn those foods that are appealing to the child. Catering to the child's wishes as much as possible may perk up a lagging appetite. A dietitian can help plan appealing meals for the child. Serving six small meals may help increase the child's total intake better than the customary three daily meals.

Promoting Skin Integrity. The child's skin is stretched with edema and becomes thin and fragile. All skin surfaces should be inspected regularly for breakdown. Because the child may be lethargic, he or she needs to be turned and positioned every 2 hours. Care should be taken to protect skin surfaces from pressure by means of pillows and padding. Overlapping skin surfaces should be protected from rubbing by careful placement of cotton gauze. The child should be bathed regularly, and skin surfaces that touch each other must be washed thoroughly with soap and water and completely dried. A sheer dusting of cornstarch may be soothing. Because the scrotum of a male child may be edematous, a soft cotton support may be used to provide comfort, if necessary.

Promoting Energy Conservation and Sensory Stimulation. Bed rest is common during the edema stage of the condition. The child rarely protests because of his or her fatigue. The sheer bulk of the edema makes movement difficult. When the diuresis occurs, in several days after the beginning of the administration of prednisone, the child may be allowed more activity. Care should be taken to balance the activity with rest periods. The nurse can plan quiet, age-appropriate activities that interest the child. Most children love being read to, and coloring is a quiet activity, as are dominoes, puzzles, and some kinds of computer and board games. The family should be involved in providing some of these activities. Avoid using the television excessively as a diversion; the child should be encouraged to rest when fatigue occurs.

Preventing Infection. The child with nephrotic syndrome is especially at risk for respiratory infections. The edema and the corticosteroid therapy lower the body's defenses. The child should be protected from anyone with an infection—staff, family, visitors, and other children. Handwashing and strict medical asepsis are essential. The child's vital signs should be monitored every 4 hours and evaluated for any early signs of infection.

Providing Parent Teaching. Children with nephrotic syndrome are usually hospitalized for diagnosis, thorough evaluation of their general health and specific condition, and institution of therapy. If the child has an infection, a course of antibiotic therapy may be given, and unless unforeseen complications develop, the child is discharged with complete instructions for management.

A written plan is most useful to help family caregivers

follow the program successfully. They must keep a careful record of home treatment and bring it to the clinic or the physician's office at regular intervals.

Family caregivers must be aware of reactions that may occur with the use of steroids and the adverse effects of abrupt discontinuance of these drugs. If these aspects are well understood, the incidence of forgetting to give the medication or of neglecting to refill the prescription should be reduced or eliminated entirely. Family caregivers also need to be encouraged to report promptly any symptoms that they consider caused by the medication.

Special care to keep the child in optimum health is important, and **intercurrent infections** (occurring during the course of an already existing disease) must be reported promptly. Exacerbations are common, and family caregivers need to understand that these will probably occur and that they should report rapidly increasing weight, increased proteinuria, or signs of infections for a possible alteration in the therapeutic regimen and the specific antibiotic agents as indicated.

Caring for the child at home follows the same pattern as that for any chronically ill child. Bed rest is not indicated, except in the event of an intercurrent illness. Activity is restricted only by edema, which may slow the child down considerably, but otherwise normal activity is beneficial. Sufficient food intake may be a problem, as it is in other types of chronic illness. Fortunately, there are usually no food restrictions, and the appetite can be tempted by attractive, appealing foods.

Just as the name implies, MCNS results in few changes in the kidneys, and the children have a good prognosis. Complications from kidney damage necessarily alter the course of treatment. Failure to achieve satisfactory diuresis, or the need to discontinue the use of steroids because of adverse reactions, requires a reevaluation of treatment. The presence of gross hematuria suggests renal damage. In a small percentage of children, persistence of abnormal urinary findings following diuresis presents a less hopeful outlook. A child who has frequent relapses lasting into adolescence or adulthood may develop renal failure and eventually be a candidate for kidney transplant.

EVALUATION

- Edema is decreased as evidenced by the child's weight loss and abdominal measurement.
- The child eats 80% or more of his or her meals.
- The skin remains free of breakdown as evidenced by absence of redness and irritation.
- The child rests as needed and engages in quiet activities.
- There are no signs or symptoms of infection as evidenced by normal vital signs, no respiratory symptoms, and no gastrointestinal symptoms.

- The family demonstrates an understanding of the disease and home care, asking and answering appropriate questions.

Acute Glomerulonephritis

Acute glomerulonephritis is a condition that appears to be an allergic reaction to a specific infection, most often group A β-hemolytic streptococcal infection, as in rheumatic fever.

Acute glomerulonephritis has a peak incidence in children 6 and 7 years of age and occurs twice as often in boys as in girls. The disease is discussed in this chapter to provide an easy means to compare it with nephrotic syndrome.

The antigen–antibody reaction in acute glomerulonephritis causes a response that blocks the glomeruli, permitting red blood cells and protein to escape into the urine. The prognosis of this condition is usually excellent. In a small number of children, chronic nephritis may develop.

Clinical Manifestations

Presenting symptoms appear 1 to 3 weeks after the onset of a streptococcal infection, such as "strep" throat, otitis media, tonsillitis, or impetigo. Most frequently, the presenting symptom is grossly bloody urine. The caregiver may describe the urine as smoky colored or bloody. Periorbital edema may accompany or precede hematuria. Fever may be as high as 39.4 or 40°C (103 or 104°F) at the onset but decreases in a few days to about 37.8°C (100°F). Slight headache and malaise are usual, and there may be vomiting. Hypertension appears in 60% to 70% of patients during the first 4 or 5 days. Both hematuria and hypertension disappear within 3 weeks.

Oliguria (production of a subnormal volume of urine) is usually present, and the urine has a high specific gravity and contains albumin, red and white blood cells, and casts. The blood urea nitrogen and serum creatinine levels and sedimentation rates are all elevated.

Cerebral symptoms occur in connection with hypertension in a small percentage of cases, consisting mainly of headache, drowsiness, convulsions, and vomiting. When the blood pressure is reduced, these symptoms disappear. Cardiovascular disturbance may be revealed in electrocardiogram tracings, but few have clinical signs. In most children, this condition is short term, but in some, it progresses to congestive heart failure. Table 13-5 compares the features of acute glomerulonephritis with those of nephrotic syndrome.

Treatment

Although the child usually feels well in a few days, activities should be limited until the clinical manifestations subside. This generally occurs 2 to 4 weeks after the onset. Penicillin may be given during the acute stage to

Table 13-5. Comparison of Features of Acute Glomerulonephritis and Nephrotic Syndrome

Assessment Factor	Acute Glomerulonephritis	Nephrotic Syndrome
Cause	Immune Reaction to group A β-hemolytic streptococcal infection	Idiopathic; possibly a hypersensitivity reaction
Onset	Abrupt	Insidious
Hematuria	Grossly bloody	Rare
Proteinurea	3+ or 4+, but not massive	Massive
Edema	Mild	Extreme
Hypertension	Marked	Mild
Hyperlipidemia	Rare or mild	Marked
Peak age frequency	5–10 y	2–3 y
Interventions	Limited activity; antihypertensives as needed; symptomatic therapy if congestive heart failure occurs	Bed rest during edema stage Corticosteroid administration Possible cyclophosphamide administration
Diet	Normal for age; no added salt if child is hypertensive	Nutritious for age; no added salt; small, frequent meals may be desirable
Prevention	Prevention through treatment of group A β-hemolytic streptococcal infections	None known
Course	Acute—up to 2–3 weeks	Chronic—may have relapses

Adapted from Pilliteri A. Maternal and Child Health Nursing. Philadelphia: JB Lippincott, 1992.

eradicate any existing infection; however, it does not affect the recovery from the disease because the condition is an immunologic response. The diet is generally not restricted, but additional salt may be limited if edema is excessive. Treatment of complications is symptomatic.

Nursing Care

Bed rest frequently is maintained until acute symptoms and gross hematuria have disappeared. The child should be protected from chilling and from contact with people with infections. When the child is allowed out of bed, it is important that he or she not become fatigued.

Urinary output must be carefully checked and recorded every 8 hours. The child is weighed daily at the same time, on the same scale, wearing the same clothes. The amount of fluid the child is allowed may be based on output as well as on evidence of continued hypertension and oliguria. Careful recording of the child's fluid intake is essential, as is careful attention to keep the intake within prescribed limits.

Blood pressure must be monitored regularly using the same arm and properly fitting cuff. If hypertension develops, a diuretic may help reduce the blood pressure to normal levels. An antihypertensive drug may be added if needed. A diastolic pressure of 90 mm Hg or higher is an indication for the administration of antihypertensive drugs. The urine must be tested regularly for protein. This can be done with a dipstick test. The presence of hematuria also can be tested by means of a dipstick test. Tests, such as the Addis count and urine concentration, require preparation.

Traces of protein in the urine may persist for months after the acute symptoms disappear, and an elevated Addis count, indicating urinary red blood cells, persists as well. Family caregivers are taught to test for urinary protein routinely. If the urinary signs persist for more than 1 year, the disease has probably assumed a chronic form.

In spite of such grave implications, a recovery rate of 95% or higher is reported.

Summary

Most preschool children have few health problems. Immunizations have helped eliminate many diseases that caused illness in the past. However, preschoolers do get sick, and illnesses that are serious enough to warrant hospitalization can be frightening to the child and the family. The preschooler may view any illness as punishment for wrongdoing and must be reassured that an illness is not punishment. The preschool child can begin to understand simple explanations. Fear of bodily harm is common, so the child needs to be reassured about procedures that must be performed. Allowing the child to handle the equipment and act out procedures with dolls when possible can be helpful. Words that the nurse uses must be carefully thought out so that the child does not misunderstand and perceive them as threatening. Magical thinking can cause anxieties and fears that are real to the child. The nurse needs to be alert for these perceptions so the child can be helped to acknowledge and deal with them. During hospitalization, the child may regress to bedwetting, thumbsucking, and fussiness. Encouraging and involving the child in bathing, dressing, feeding, and other activities of daily living can help preserve the child's developing independence.

The preschool child is active physically. Illness that requires the child to be restricted to bed rest is difficult. The nurse and the family must summon all their expertise to keep the child as content as possible. The nurse needs to have plans for age-appropriate diversional activities to interest the child. In the case of the mentally retarded child, the nurse must be aware of the child's cognitive level and adjust the plans accordingly.

Disorders that have been discussed in this chapter are not limited to the preschool-age group, but many are first seen during this age. Health disorders that affect children's senses have a major impact on their ability to learn. Illnesses that require isolation precautions either to protect the child, as in leukemia and nephrotic syndrome, or to prevent infection of other children, as in the infectious diseases, cause feelings of rejection and separation. Thoughtful nursing care can decrease the trauma that children suffer when they are isolated for any reason.

Many of the disorders described in this chapter have a much improved prognosis through new technology. Research on new methods of treatment is ongoing, and children will benefit from these findings.

Review Questions

1. You are caring for 3½-year-old Missy, who is mildly hearing impaired. How will you adapt your nursing care to improve your communication with her?
2. Name five childhood diseases that are caused by viruses. Which of these diseases can be prevented by routine immunization?
3. Four-year-old Todd is blind. You are helping with his hospital admission. Tell how you will prepare him for his hospital stay.
4. What is the association between Reye syndrome and aspirin?
5. Your friend asks you if cerebral palsy is inherited. Give a complete answer to this friend about the causes of cerebral palsy.
6. What can you tell your friend who says that all children with cerebral palsy are mentally retarded.
7. Make a list of aids that can be used to assist a child with cerebral palsy.
8. What are the "three R's" you must follow when teaching new self-care practices to a child with cognitive impairment?
9. Jeremy is a 6-year-old boy with Down syndrome. His mental age is that of a 3-year-old child. How will you prepare him for a tonsillectomy?
10. The Marino family has just been told that their 4-year-old daughter, Angi, has ALL. What can you tell them about ALL, its treatment, and her long-term outlook?
11. What can you tell the family of Seth, a 3-year-old boy with hemophilia, to relieve their concerns that Seth might get AIDS from his treatments?
12. Make a list of safety measures to protect Seth from injury in the hospital and at home.
13. What are the three names given to the most common type of nephrotic syndrome in children?
14. Why is it important to protect the child with MCNS from infection?
15. What nursing care would you plan for a child with generalized edema?
16. How does the onset of acute glomerulonephritis differ from the onset of MCNS? Give a full explanation.

References

1. Beyer JE. The Oucher: A User's Manual and Technical Report. Denver: University of Colorado, 1988.
2. Wong D, Baker C. Pain in children: Comparison of assessment scales. Pediatr Nurs 14(1):9–17, 1988.

Bibliography

Baker MH. Jennifer's life is a success story. RN 53(2):30–34, 1990.

Binder H, Eng GD. Rehabilitation management of children with spastic diplegic cerebral palsy. Arch Phys Med Rehabil 70(6): 482–489, 1989.

Bossert E, Martinson IM. Kinetic drawings—revised: A method of determining the impact of cancer on the family as perceived by the child with cancer. J Pediatr Nurs 5(3):204–213, 1990.

Carpenito LJ: Handbook of Nursing Diagnosis. Philadelphia: JB Lippincott, 1991.

Castiglia PT, Harbin RE. Child Health Care: Process and Practice. Philadelphia: JB Lippincott, 1992.

Clements DA, Wilfert CM, MacCormack JN, et al: Pertussis immunization in eight-month-old children in North Carolina. Am J Public Health 80(6):734–736, 1990.

Consolvo CA. Jeff's last wish . . . A dying child wanted to go home to his rocking chair. Nursing 20(9):152, 1990.

Damrosch S, Perry L. Self-reported adjustments, chronic sorrow, and coping of parents of children with Down syndrome. Nurs Res 38(1):25–29, 1989.

Eagan J. Measles: An infection control nightmare. RN 54(6): 26–29, 1991.

Edwards SJ, Yuen HK. An intervention program for a fraternal twin with Down syndrome. Am J Occup Ther 44(5):454–458, 1990.

Fletcher M. Haemophilia research. Nursing (Lond) 4(6):38, 1990.

Frenkel LD. Routine immunizations for American children in the 1990s. Pediatr Clin North Am 37(3):531–548, 1990.

Frick SB, Del Po EG, Keith JA, et al. Chemotherapy-associated nausea and vomiting in pediatric oncology patients. Cancer Nurs 11(2):118–124, 1988.

Garvin JM. Reye's syndrome. Emerg Med Serv 19(3):33, 53, 1990.

Griffin MR, Ray WA, Mortimer EA, et al. Risk of seizures and encephalopathy after immunization with the diphtheria-tetanus-pertussis vaccine. JAMA 263(12):1641–1645, 1990.

Hinojosa J. How mothers of preschool children with cerebral palsy perceive occupation therapists and their influence on family life. Occup Ther J Res 10(3):144–162, 1990.

Hockenberry MJ, Coody DK, Bennett BS. Childhood cancers: Incidence, diagnosis, and treatment. Pediatr Nurs 16(3): 234–246, 256–257, 1990.

Holman RC, Gomperts ED, Jason JM, et al. Age and human immunodeficiency virus infection in persons with hemophilia in California. Am J Public Health 80(8):967–969, 1990.

Hymovich DP. A theory for pediatric oncology nursing practice and research. J Pediatr Oncol Nurs 7(4):131–138, 1990.

Irwin B. Eight precious words. Nursing 20(9):81, 1990.

Johnson DL. Nephrotic syndrome: A nursing care plan based on current pathophysiologic concepts. Heart Lung 18(1):85–93, 1989.

Jones SH, Jenista JA. Fifth disease: Role for nurses in pediatric practice. Pediatr Nurs 16(2):148–150, 1990.

Jurgrau A. Why aren't we protecting our children? . . .Childhood immunization. RN 53(11):30–35, 1990.

Lee CV, McDermott SW, Elliott C. The delayed immunization of children of migrant farm workers in South Carolina. Public Health Rep 105(3):317–320, 1990.

Levine BE, Lavi S. Perils of childhood immunization against measles, mumps, and rubella. Pediatr Nurs 17(2):159–161, 1991.

Long SS, Deforest A, Smith DG, et al. Longitudinal study of adverse reactions following diphtheria-tetanus-pertussis vaccine in infancy. Pediatrics 85(3):294–302, 1990.

Markova I, Wilkie PA. Self- and other-awareness of the risk of HIV/AIDS in people with haemophilia and implications for behavioural change. Soc Sci Med 31(1):73–79, 1990.

Mayers M. Clinical care plans: Pediatric nursing. Philadelphia: Markham McKenzie, 1991.

McAnear S. Parental reaction to a chronically ill child. Home Health Nurse 8(3):35–40, 1990.

Mossberg KA, Friske K. Ankle-foot orthoses: Effect on energy expenditure of gait in spastic diplegic children. Arch Phys Med Rehabil 71(7):490–494, 1990.

Munet Vilaro F, Vessey JA. Children's explanation of leukemia: A Hispanic perspective. J Pediatr Nurs 5(4):274–282, 1990.

Phillips WE, Audet M. Use of serial casting in the management of knee joint contractures in an adolescent with cerebral palsy. Phys Ther 70(8):521–523, 1990.

Pillitteri A. Maternal and Child Health Nursing. Philadelphia: JB Lippincott, 1992.

Ragab A. Growth factors in leukemia: How it all begins. J Pediatr Oncol Nurs 7(2):56, 1990.

Rothman JG. Understanding of conservation of substance in youngsters with cerebral palsy. Phys Occup Ther Pediatr 9(3): 119–125, 1989.

Schmitt BD. Masturbation in preschoolers: Should you worry? Contemp Pediatr 9(3):71–72, 1992.

Shanwick M. Development and chronic illness. Nursing (Lond) 4(16):24–27, 1990.

Shiminski-Maher T. Selective posterior rhizotomy in the pediatric cerebral palsy population: Implications for nursing practice. J Neurosci Nurs 21(5):308–312, 1989.

Suderman JR. Pain relief during routine procedures for children with leukemia. MCN 15(3):163–166, 1990.

Tate M. Deafness in babies. Midwives Chron 10212:382–383, 1989.

Tate M. Deafness in children. Midwife Health Visit Commun Nurse 25(10):438, 440–441, 1989.

Tate M. Radio hearing aids for school children. Midwife Health Visit Commun Nurse 26(7/8):268, 270, 1990.

Weinstein BD, De Neffe LS. Hemophilia, AIDS, and occupational therapy. Am J Occup Ther 44(3):228–232, 1990.

Whaley LF, Wong DL. Nursing Care of Infants and Children, 4th ed. St. Louis: Mosby-Year Book, 1991.

Wood S, McCormick B. Use of hearing aids in infancy. Arch Dis Child 65(9):919–920, 1990.

Wood SL, White GL Jr. Advances in pediatric immunizations. Physician Assist 12(5):22, 27–29, 32, 1988.

Yasukasa A. Upper extremity casting: Adjunct treatment for a child with cerebral palsy. Am J Occup Ther 44(9):480–486, 1990.

Growth and Development of the School-Age Child: Ages 6 to 10 Years

Chapter 14

Student Objectives

Upon completion of this chapter, the student will be able to:

1. State the major developmental task of the school-age group according to Erikson.
2. Discuss the physical growth patterns during school-age a.) Girls; b.) Boys.
3. Describe dentition in this age group.
4. Describe practices that contribute to good dental hygiene for this age group.
5. Identify nutritional influences on the school-age child, including a.) Family attitudes; b.) Mealtime atmosphere; c.) Snacks; d.) School's role.
6. List three factors that contribute to obesity in the school-age child.
7. State two appropriate ways to help an obese child control weight.
8. State the usual amount of sleep the school-age child needs.
9. Describe safety education appropriate for the school-age group.
10. Discuss the need for sex education in the school-age group a.) Family's role; b.) School's role; c.) Others.
11. State factors that may deter successful completion of the developmental task of industry versus inferiority.
12. Describe the psychosocial characteristics of the 6- to 7-year-old child.
13. Discuss the importance of groups of "gangs" in the 7- to 8-year-old child.
14. Briefly describe the progression in the 6- to 10-year-old child's concept of biology a.) Birth; b.) Death; c.) Human body; d.) Health; e.) Illness.
15. State several factors that may influence the school-age child's hospital experience.

Marks MG: BROADRIBB'S INTRODUCTORY PEDIATRIC NURSING, 4th ed. © 1994 J.B. Lippincott Company.

Key Terms

classification	hierarchical arrangement
conservation	reversibility
decentration	scoliosis
epiphyses	

*T*he first day of school marks a major milestone in a child's development, opening a new world of learning and growing. Between the ages of 6 and 10 years, dramatic changes occur in the child's thinking process, social skills, activities, attitudes, and use of language. The squirmy, boisterous 6-year-old child with a limited attention span bears little resemblance to the more reserved 10-year-old child who can become absorbed in a solitary craft activity for several hours.

Moving from the small circle of family into school and community, children begin to see differences in their own lives and the lives of others. They constantly compare their families with other children's families and observe the way other children are disciplined, the foods they eat, the way they dress, and the houses they live in. Every aspect of lifestyle is subject to comparison with that of other children.

Most children reach school age with the necessary skills, abilities, and independence to function successfully in this new environment. They are able to feed and dress themselves, use the primary language of their culture to communicate their needs and feelings, and separate from their caregivers for extended periods. They show increasing interest in group activities and in making things. Erikson called this the period of industry versus inferiority. Children of this age "work" at many activities, involving motor, cognitive, and social skills. Success in these activities provides the child with self-confidence and a feeling of competence. Those children who are unsuccessful during this stage, whether from physical, social, or cognitive disadvantages, develop a feeling of inferiority.

The health of the school-age child is no longer the exclusive concern of the family but of the community. Prior to entrance, most schools require that children have a physical examination and that immunizations meet state requirements. Generally, this is a healthy period in the child's life, although minor respiratory disorders and other communicable diseases can spread quickly within a classroom. Few major diseases have their onset during this period. Accidents still pose a serious hazard; therefore, safety measures are an important part of learning.

Physical Development

Growth

Between the ages of 6 and 10 years, growth is slow and steady. Average annual weight gain is about 7 lb (about 3 kg). By age 7, the child weighs approximately seven times as much as at birth. Annual height increase is about 2½ inches (6 cm) per year. This period ends in the preadolescent growth spurt in girls at about age 10 and in boys at about age 12.

Dentition

At about age 6, the child starts to lose the deciduous ("baby") teeth, usually beginning with the incisors. At about the same time, the first permanent teeth, the 6-year molars, appear directly behind the deciduous molars (Figure 14-1).

These 6-year molars are of the utmost importance; they are the key or pivot teeth that help to shape the jaw and affect the alignment of the permanent teeth. If they are allowed to decay so severely that they must be removed, the child will encounter dental problems later.

Education for the care of the teeth, with particular attention to the 6-year molars, is important. Proper dental hygiene includes a routine inspection with cleaning and application of fluoride at least twice a year and conscientious brushing after meals. A well-balanced diet with plenty of calcium and phosphorus and minimal sugar is important to healthy teeth. Foods containing sugar should be eaten only at mealtimes and should be followed immediately by proper brushing (Figure 14-2).

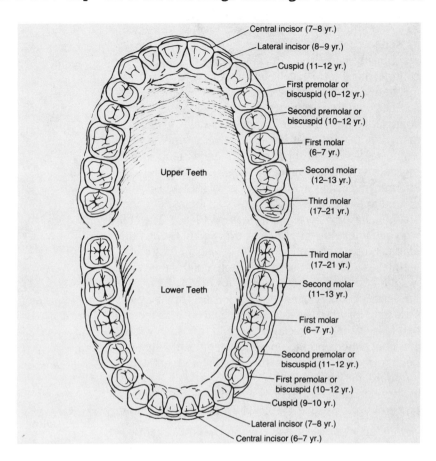

Central incisor (7–8 yr.)
Lateral incisor (8–9 yr.)
Cuspid (11–12 yr.)
First premolar or biscuspid (10–12 yr.)
Second premolar or biscuspid (10–12 yr.)
First molar (6–7 yr.)
Second molar (12–13 yr.)
Third molar (17–21 yr.)

Upper Teeth

Third molar (17–21 yr.)
Second molar (11–13 yr.)
First molar (6–7 yr.)
Second premolar or biscuspid (11–12 yr.)
First premolar or biscuspid (10–12 yr.)
Cuspid (9–10 yr.)

Lower Teeth

Lateral incisor (7–8 yr.)
Central incisor (6–7 yr.)

Figure 14-1. Chart showing the sequence of eruption of permanent teeth.

Skeletal Growth

The 6-year-old silhouette is characterized by a protruding abdomen and lordosis ("swayback"). By the time the child has reached the age of 10 years, the spine is straighter, the abdomen flatter, and the body generally more slender and long-legged (Figure 14-3).

Bone growth occurs mostly in the long bones and is gradual during the school years. Cartilage is being replaced by bone at the **epiphyses** (growth centers at the end of long bones and at the wrists). Skeletal maturation is more rapid in girls than in boys and in African Americans than in whites. Growth and development of the school-age child is summarized in Table 14-1.

Nutrition

As coordination improves, the child becomes increasingly active and requires more food to supply the necessary energy. Increased appetite and a tendency to go on food "jags" are typical of the 6-year-old child. This stage soon passes and is unimportant if the child generally gets the necessary nutrients. Allowing the child to express food dislikes and permitting refusal of the disliked food item are usually the best ways to handle this phase. As the child's tastes develop, once-disliked foods may become favorites unless earlier "battles" have been waged over eating a particular food. Children are more likely to learn to eat most foods if everyone else accepts them in a matter-of-fact way.

Children learn by the examples caregivers and others set for them. They will accept more readily the importance of manners, calm voices, appropriate table conversation, and courtesy if they see them carried out consistently at home. Mealtime should never be used for nagging, finding fault, correcting manners, or discussing a poor report card. Hygiene should be taught in a cheerful but firm manner, even if the child must leave the table more than once to wash his or her hands adequately.

Most children prefer simple, plain foods and are good judges of their own needs if they are not coaxed, nagged, bribed, rewarded, or influenced by television commercials. Disease or strong emotions may cause loss of appetite, but force helps little and can have harmful effects.

Caregivers need to carefully supervise children's snacking habits to be sure that snacks are nutritious and not too frequent, avoiding junk food and continual nibbling that can cause lack of interest at mealtime. Children should be encouraged to eat a good breakfast to provide the energy and nutrients needed to perform well in school. Children need a clearly planned schedule that allows time for a good breakfast and brushing of teeth before leaving for school.

Obesity can be a concern during this age. Some children may have a genetic tendency to obesity; environment and a sedentary lifestyle also play a part. In many families, children are urged to "clean your plate" or encouraged to belong to the "clean plate club." In addition, many families now eat fast foods several times a week, which reinforces the problem. Fast foods tend to have high fat and calorie content, contributing to obesity. Other children, especially in the later elementary grades, can be unkind to overweight children, teasing them, not choosing them in games or avoiding them as friends. The child who becomes sensitive to being overweight is often miserable. Encouraging physical activity and limiting dietary fat intake to 35% of total calories help control the child's weight. Popular fad diets must be avoided because they do not supply adequate nutrients for the growing child. Care must be taken to avoid nagging and creating feelings of inferiority or guilt because the child may simply rebel. The child who is pressured too much to lose weight may become a food "sneak," setting up patterns that will be harmful later in life.

Health teaching at school should reinforce the importance of a proper diet (Table 14-2). Family and cultural

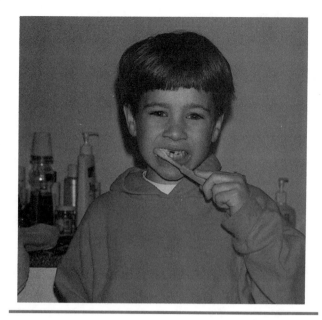

Figure 14-3. The school-age child needs encouragement to brush after meals and at bedtime as part of a good dental hygiene program.

food patterns are strong, however, and tend to persist despite nutritional education. Some families are making a positive effort to reduce fat and cholesterol when preparing meals. Most schools have lunch programs, subsidized for those children who are eligible, and some have breakfast programs. These provide well-balanced meals, but often children eat only part of what they are offered.

Health Maintenance

Disease Prevention

The school-age child should have a physical examination by a physician or health care provider every year. Additional visits are commonly made throughout the year for minor illness.

Most states have immunization requirements that must be met when the child enters school. A booster of tetanus-diphtheria vaccine is recommended every 10 years for the remainder of life. In addition, physical and dental examinations may be required at specific intervals during the elementary school years. During a physical examination at about the age of 10 to 11 years, the child is examined for signs of **scoliosis** (lateral curvature of the spine). Vision and hearing screening should be performed before entrance to school and on a periodic basis (annual or biannual) thereafter. These examinations often are conducted by the school nurse.

Elementary school-age children generally are healthy, with only minor illnesses, usually respiratory or gastroin-

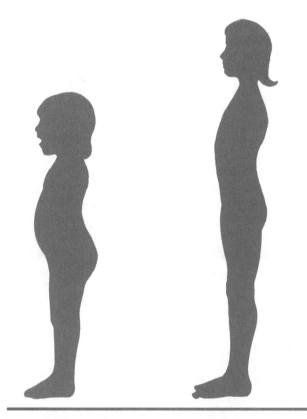

Figure 14-2. **Left**, Profile of a 6-year-old showing protuberant abdomen. **Right**, Profile of a 10-year-old showing flat abdomen and four curves of adultlike spine. (Courtesy of S. Robbins.)

Table 14-1. Developmental Milestones for the School-Age Child

Age (yr)	Physical	Motor	Social	Language	Perceptual	Cognitive
6	Average height 116 cm (45 in) Average weight 21 kg (46 lb) Loses first tooth (upper incisors) Six-year molars erupt Food "jags" Appetite increased	Ties shoes Can use scissors Runs, jumps, climbs, skips Can ride bicycle Can't sit for long periods Cuts, pastes, prints, draws with some detail	Increased need to socialize with same sex Egocentric— believes everyone thinks as they do Still in preoperational stage until age 7	Uses every form of sentence structure Vocabulary of 2500 words Sentence length about 5 words	Knows right from left May reverse letters Can discriminate vertical, horizontal, and oblique Perceives pictures in parts or in whole but not in both	Recognizes simple words Conservation of number Defines objects by use Can group according to an attribute to form subclasses
7	Weight is seven times birth weight Gains 2–3 kg/yr (4.4–6.6 lb) Grows 5–6 cm/yr (2–2½ in)	More cautious Swims Printing smaller than 6-year-old's Activity level lower than 6-year-olds	More cooperative Same-sex play group and friend Less egocentric	Can name day, month, season Produces all language sounds	b, p, d, q confusion resolved Can copy a diamond	Begins to use simple logic Can group in ascending order Grasps basic idea of addition and subtraction Conservation of substance Can tell time
8	Average height 127 cm (49½ in) Average weight 25 kg (55 lb)	Movements more graceful Writes in cursive Can throw and hit a baseball Has symmetric balance and can hop	Adheres to simple rules Hero worship begins Same-sex peer group	Gives precise definitions Articulation is near adult level	Can catch a ball Visual acuity is 20/20 Perceives pictures in parts and whole	Increasing memory span Interest in causal relationships Conservation of length Seriation
9–10	Average height 132–137 cm (51½–53½ in) Average weight 27–35 kg (59½–77 lb)	Good coordination Can achieve the strength and speed needed for most sports	Enjoys team competition Moves from group to best friend Hero worship intensifies	Can use language to convey thoughts and look at other's point of view	Eye-hand coordination almost perfected	Classifies objects Understands explanations Conservation of area and weight Describes characteristics of objects Can group in descending order

Adapted from Castiglia PT, Harbin RE. Child Health Care: Practice and Process. Philadelphia: JB Lippincott, 1992, p. 321.

testinal in nature. Chickenpox will continue as a common communicable disease until a vaccine is readily available to the general public. The leading cause of death in this age group continues to be accidents. Health teaching, both in the home and at school, is essential. Caregivers have a responsibility to teach the child basic hygiene, safety, substance abuse, and sexual functioning. Schools have an obligation to include these topics in the school curriculum, also, because many families are not well informed enough themselves to cover the topics ade-

quately. Some schools offer health classes at each grade level taught by a health educator. In other schools, health and sex education are integrated into the curriculum and taught by each classroom teacher. Nurses should become active in their community to ensure that these kinds of programs are available to the children.

School-age children need between 10 and 12 hours of sleep per night. The 6-year-old child needs 12 hours of sleep and should be provided with a "quiet" time after school to recharge after a busy day in the classroom.

Table 14-2. Foods to Meet the Nutritional Needs
of the Six- to Ten-Year-Old

Food	Serving Size
Milk, Vitamin-D fortified	2–3 cups
Eggs	3–4 per wk
Meat, poultry, fish	2–3 oz (small serving)
Dried beans, peas, or peanut butter	2 servings each week. If used as an alternative for meat, allow ½ cup cooked beans or peas or 2 tbsp peanut butter for 1 oz meat
Potatoes, white or sweet (occasionally spaghetti, macaroni, rice or noodles, etc.)	1 small or ⅓ cup
Other cooked vegetable (green leafy or deep yellow 3–4 times per wk)	¼ cup
Raw vegetable (salad greens, cabbage, celery, carrots, etc.)	¼ cup
Vitamin C food (citrus fruit, tomato, cantaloupe, etc.)	1 medium orange or equivalent
Other fruit	1 portion or more as: 1 apple, 1 banana, 1 peach, 1 pear, ½ cup cooked fruit
Bread, enriched or whole grain	3 slices or more
Cereal, enriched or whole grain	½ cup
Additional foods	Butter or margarine, desserts, etc., to satisfy energy needs

Adapted from Robinson CH, Lawler MR, Chenoweth WL, et al. Normal and Therapeutic Nutrition, 17th ed. New York: Macmillan, 1986.

Safety

As stated earlier, accidents continue to be a leading cause of childhood death during this period. Even though school-age children do not require constant supervision, they must be taught certain safety rules and practice them until they are routine. They should understand the function of traffic lights and should have watched family members obeying them as a matter of course. Example is the best teacher for any child. Children should know their full name, their caregivers' names, and their own home address and telephone number. Children should be taught how to get help, using the universal 911 number in communities where this is available. In communities that do not have a 911 system, children should be taught the appropriate way to call for emergency help in that community. Many communities have safe-home programs that designate homes to which children can go if they have a problem on the way home from school. These homes are clearly marked in a way that the children are taught to recognize. In some communities, the local police or fire fighters are interested in coming into the classroom to help teach safety. Children gain from meeting police officers and understanding that they have a duty to help children, not to punish them. Safety rules should be stressed at home and at school (Figure 14-4). The Parent Teaching display summarizes important safety considerations for school-age children.

Sex Education

Children learn about femininity and masculinity from the time they are born. Behaviors, attitudes, and actions of the men and women in the child's life toward the child and toward each other form impressions in the child that last a lifetime. There has been much controversy about the proper time and place for formal sex education. Part of the problem seems to stem from the fact that many people automatically think that sex education means adult sexuality and reproduction. However, sex education includes helping children develop positive attitudes toward their own bodies, their own sex, and their own sexual role to achieve optimum satisfaction in being a boy or a girl.

In some schools sex education is limited to a class,

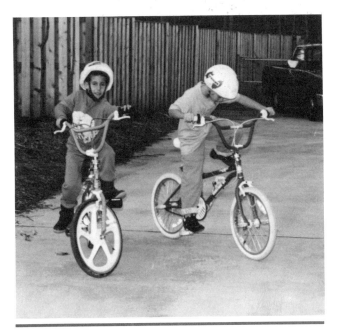

Figure 14-4. Outdoor activities that encourage physical activity are recommended for school-age children. Helmets are an important part of bike safety. (From Jackson DB, Saunders RB. Child Health Nursing. Philadelphia: JB Lippincott, 1993, p. 353.)

Parent Teaching

Safety Topics for Elementary School-Age Children

1. Traffic signals and safe pedestrian practices
2. Safety belt use for car passengers
3. Bicycle safety
   a. Wearing a helmet
   b. Use of hand signals
   c. Riding with traffic
   d. Being sure others see you
4. Skateboard and roller blade safety
   a. Wearing helmet
   b. Wearing elbow and knee pads
   c. Safe skating areas
5. Swimming safety
   a. Learn to swim
   b. Never swim alone
   c. Always know the water depth
   d. Don't dive head first
   e. No running or "horseplay" at a pool
6. Danger of projectile toys
7. Danger of all-terrain vehicles
8. Use of life jacket when boating
9. Stranger safety
   a. Who is a stranger
   b. Never accept a ride from someone you don't know
   c. Never accept food or gifts from someone you don't know
   d. Check the license number and try to remember it
10. Good touch–bad touch

usually in the fifth grade, in which children are shown films about menstruation and their developing bodies. Often these are taught in separate classes for boys and girls. Some health educators strongly recommend that sex education should be started in kindergarten and developed gradually over the proceeding grades. Learning about reproduction of plants and animals, about birth and nurturing in other animals, and about the roles of the male and the female in family units can lead to the natural introduction of human reproduction, male and female roles, families, and nurturing. If all children grew up in secure, loving, ideal families, much of this could be learned at home. However, many children do not have this type of home, so they need healthy, positive information to help them develop healthy attitudes about their own sexuality. Feelings of self-worth also are woven into these lessons, helping children to feel good about themselves and who they are.

Caregivers who feel uncomfortable discussing sex with their children may find it helpful to use books or pamphlets available for various age groups. Generally, a female caregiver finds it easier to discuss sex with a girl, and a male caregiver feels more comfortable with a boy. This can pose special problems for the single caregiver with a child of the opposite sex. Again, printed materials may be helpful. Nurses often may be called on to help a caregiver provide information for his or her child. Nurses need to be comfortable with their own sexuality to handle these discussions well.

At a young age, children are exposed to a great amount of sexually provocative information through the media. Children who do not get accurate information at home or in the school will learn what they want to know from their peers, but this information is often inaccurate, making adequate sexual education even more urgent. In addition, the Centers for Disease Control currently recommends that elementary school-age children should be taught about acquired immunodeficiency syndrome and how it is spread. Many school districts are working hard to integrate this information into the health curriculum at all grade levels in a sensitive and age-appropriate manner.

In addition to nutrition, health practices, safety, and sex education, school-age children also need substance abuse education. Programs that teach children to "just say no" are one way in which children can learn that they are in control. Teaching children the unhealthy aspects of tobacco and alcohol use and drug abuse should be started in elementary school as a good foundation for more advanced information in adolescence.

Psychosocial Development

The sense of duty and accomplishment occupies the years from 6 to 12 years. This is the period Erikson calls *industry versus inferiority*, during which the child is interested in engaging in real projects and seeing them through to completion. The child applies the energies earlier put into play toward accomplishing tasks, often spending numerous sessions on one project. With these attempts comes the refinement of motor, cognitive, and social skills and development of a positive sense of self. Some school-age children, however, may not be ready for this stage because of environmental deprivation, a dysfunctional family, insecure attachment to parents, or immaturity, among other possible reasons. Entering school at a disadvantage, these children may not be not ready to be productive. Excessive or unrealistic goals set by a teacher or caregiver who is not sensitive to the child's needs will defeat such a child, leading to the possible development of a feeling of inferiority rather than self-confidence. Effective completion of several personality developmental tasks should take place during these years, providing that environmental support is adequate (Table 14-3).

During the school-age years, the child's cognitive skills develop, and at about the age of 7 years, the child enters the concrete operational stage identified by Piaget. Significant in this stage are the skills of conservation. **Conservation** (the ability to recognize that change in shape does not necessarily mean change in amount or mass) begins with the conservation of numbers, when the child understands that a number of cookies does not change, even though they may be rearranged, to conservation of mass when the child can see that an amount of cookie dough is the same whether it is in a ball or flattened out for baking, and is followed by conservation of weight in which the child recognizes that a pound is a pound, regardless of whether plastic or bricks are being weighed. Conservation of volume (1/2 cup of water is the same amount regardless of the shape of the container) does not come until late in the concrete operational stage, at about 11 or 12 years of age.

Each child is a product of personal heredity, environment, cognitive ability, and physical health. Every child needs love and acceptance, with understanding, support, and concern when mistakes are made. Children thrive on praise and will work to earn more praise and recognition.

The Child from Ages 6 to 7 Years

Children in the age group of 6 to 7 years are still characterized by magical thinking—the tooth fairy, Santa Claus, the Easter Bunny, and others. Keen imaginations contribute to fears, especially at night, about remote, fanciful, or imaginary events. Trouble distinguishing fantasy from reality can contribute to lying to escape punishment or boost self-confidence.

Children who have attended nursery school, kinder-

Table 14-3. Personality Developmental Tasks of the School-Age Child

Task	Environmental Support
Development of coping mechanisms	Stable home environment Examples of positive coping by caretakers and peers

Development of a sense of right and wrong by
  Gaining a sense of the future
  Recognition of authority
  Feeling guilty about acts not sanctioned by authority
  Validation of feelings and actions with others in environment
	Consistent limits with gradual lessening of restrictions
	Future-oriented home environment
	Exposure to authority outside the home
	Delineation of "rules of the game" by authority figures
	Opportunity to question the rules
	Opportunity to validate own feelings and actions with others

Strengthening of a feeling of self-esteem by
  Gaining a sense of fit with the outside world
  Learning when to accommodate these forces
  Gaining a feeling of satisfaction through the completion of projects
	Exposure to different ways of living
	Opportunity to discuss these ways with peers and family
	Positive reinforcement for opinions and actions
	Opportunity to adjust ways of living to fit with others despite differences
	Exposure to new experiences and activities
	Development of competence in some of these activities
	Opportunity to complete projects of own choosing

Assuming body independence through
  Unconscious control of bladder
  Ability to care for own body
  Independence in eating and satisfaction with food itself
	Demonstration of faith in ability to care for self
	Opportunity for self-care
	Pleasant eating experiences
	Role modeling

Wieczorek RR, Natapoff J. A Conceptual Approach to the Nursing of Children: Health Care from Birth Through Adolescence. Philadelphia: JB Lippincott, 1981.

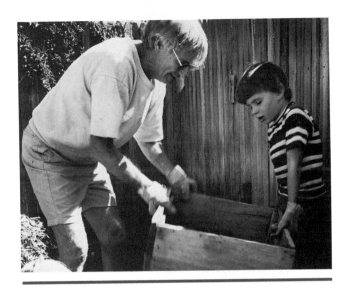

Figure 14-5. An 8-year-old helps his grandfather sift compost. (Photo by Elizabeth McKinney Chmiel.)

garten, or a Head Start program usually make the transition into first grade with pleasure, excitement, and little anxiety. Those who have not may find it helpful to visit the school and to experience separation from home and parents and getting along with other children on a trial basis. Most 6-year-old children are able to sit still for short periods and understand about taking turns. Those who have not matured sufficiently for this experience will find school unpleasant and may not do well.

Group activities are important to most 6-year-old children, even if the groups comprise only two or three children. They delight in learning and show an intense interest in every experience. Judgment about acceptable and unacceptable behavior is not well developed, so this may result in name calling and the use of vulgar words.

Between the ages of 6 and 8 years, children begin to enjoy participating in real-life activities, helping with gardening, housework, and other chores (Figure 14-5). They love making things, such as drawings, paintings, and craft projects.

The Child from Ages 7 to 10 Years

Between the seventh and eighth birthdays, children begin to shake off their acceptance of parental standards as the ultimate authority and become more impressed by the behavior of their peers. Interest in group play increases, and acceptance by the group or gang is tremendously important. These groups quickly become all-boy or all-girl groups and are often project oriented, such as scout troops and athletic teams. Private "clubs" with home-made clubhouses, secret codes, and languages are popular. Individual friendships also are formed, and "best friends" are intensely loyal, if only for short periods. Table games, arts and crafts requiring skill and dexterity, school

science projects, and science fairs are popular, as are more active pursuits (Figure 14-6). This period includes the beginning of many neighborhood team sports, including Little League, softball, football, and soccer. Both boys and girls are actively involved in many of these sports (Figure 14-7).

Even though parents are no longer considered the ultimate authority, their standards have become part of the child's personality and conscience. Although the child may cheat, lie, or steal on occasion, he or she suffers considerable guilt if he or she learns that these are unacceptable behaviors.

Important changes occur in a child's thinking processes at about age 7 years, when there is movement from preoperational, egocentric thinking to concrete, operational, decentered thought. For the first time, children are able to see the world from someone else's point of view. **Decentration** means being able to see several aspects of a problem at the same time and understand the relationship of various parts to the whole situation. Cause and effect relationships become clear; consequently, magical thinking begins to disappear.

During the seventh or eighth year, children have an increased understanding of the conservation of continuous quantity. Understanding conservation depends on **reversibility**, the ability to think in either direction. Children aged 7 years can add and subtract, count forward and backward, and see how it is possible to put something back the way it was. A child aged 7 or 8 years can understand that illness is probably only temporary, whereas a 6-year-old child may think it is permanent.

Another important change in thinking during this period is **classification**, the ability to group objects into a **hierarchical arrangement** (grouping by some common system). Children in this age group love to collect baseball cards, insects, rocks, stamps, and coins. These collections may be only a short-term interest, but some can develop into lifetime hobbies.

The Hospitalized School-Age Child

Increased understanding of their bodies, continuing curiosity about how things work, and development of concrete thinking all contribute to helping school-age children tolerate hospitalization better than younger children. They can communicate better with health care providers, understand cause and effect, and tolerate longer separations from their family.

Nurses who care for school-age children should understand how concepts about birth, death, the body, health, and illness change between the ages of 6 and 10 years (Table 14-4). All procedures must be explained to children and their families, showing the equipment and materials to be used (or pictures of these) and outlining

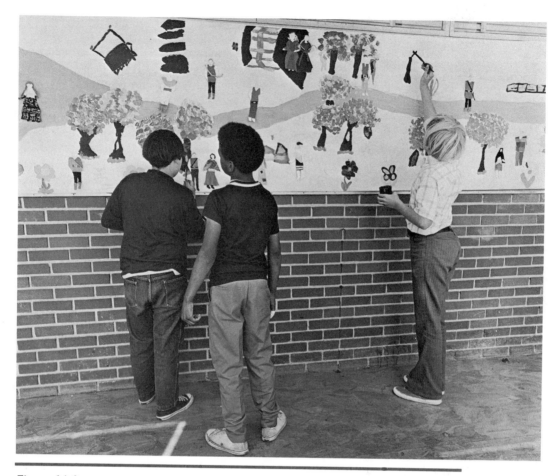

Figure 14-6. Cooperation and creativity are achieved. (Photo by Carol Baldwin.)

realistic expectations of procedures and treatments. Children's questions should be answered truthfully, including those about pain. Children of this age have anxieties about looking different from other children. An opportunity to verbalize these anxieties will help a child deal with them. School-age children need privacy more than younger children and may not want to have physical contact with adults, a wish that should be respected. Boys may be uncomfortable having a female nurse bathe them, and girls may feel uncomfortable with a male nurse. These attitudes should be recognized and handled in a way that will ensure as much privacy as possible. Family caregivers may feel guilty about the child's need for hospitalization and, as a result, may overindulge the child. The

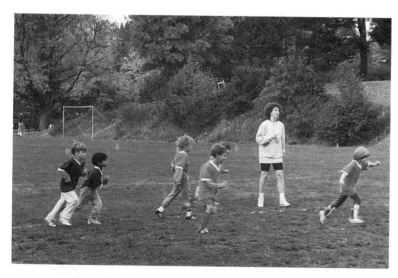

Figure 14-7. Boys playing hard during soccer game. (Courtesy of Ann West.)

Table 14-4. Children's Concept of Biology

Concept	6 to 8 Years	8 to 10 Years	Implications for Nursing
Birth	Gradually see babies as the result of three factors—social and sexual intercourse and bio-genetic fusion Tend to see baby as emerging from female only; many still see baby as manufactured by outside force—created whole Boys are less knowledgeable about baby formation than girls	Begin to put three components together; recognize that sperm and egg come together but may not be sure why Fewer discrepancies in knowledge based on sex differences	Cultural and educational factors play a part in development of where babies come from Nurse should assess children's ideas about birth and whether they can understand where babies come from and how before teaching Explanations about role of both parents can begin, but the idea of sperm and egg union may not be understood until 8 or 9 years of age
Death	May be viewed as reversible Animism (attribution of life) may be seen in some children—death viewed as result of outside force Experiences with death facilitate concept development	Considered irreversible Ideas about what happens after death unclear—related to concreteness of thinking and socio-religious upbringing	Change from vague view of death as reversible and caused by external forces to awareness of irreversibility and bodily causes Fears about death more common at 8—adults should be alert to this Explanations about death, the fact that their thoughts will not cause a death, and they will not die (if illness is not fatal) are needed
The human body	Know body holds everything inside Use outside world to explain inside Aware of major organs Interested in visible functions of body	Can understand physiology; utilize general principles to explain body functions; interested in invisible functions of body	Cultural factors may play a part in ability and willingness to discuss bodily function Educational programs can be very effective because of natural interest Assess knowledge of body by using diagrams before teaching
Health	See health as doing desired activities List concrete practices as components of health Many do not see sickness as related to health; may not consider cause and effect	See health as doing desired activities Understand cause and effect Believe it is possible to be part healthy and part not at the same time; can reverse from health to sickness and back to health	Need assistance in seeing cause and effect Capitalize on positiveness of concept—health lets you do what you really want to do Young children who are sick may feel they will never get well again
Illness	Sick children may see illness as punishment; evidence suggests that healthy children do not see illness as punishment Highly anxious children more likely to view illness as disruptive Sickness is a diffuse state; rely on others to tell them when they are ill	Same as 6–8 years of age; can identify illness states; report bodily discomfort; recognize illness is caused by specific factors	Social factors play a part in illness concept Recognize that some see illness as punishment Encourage self-care and self-help behavior, especially in older children

Wieczorek RR, Natapoff J. A Conceptual Approach to the Nursing of Children: Health Care from Birth Through Adolescence. Philadelphia: JB Lippincott, 1981.

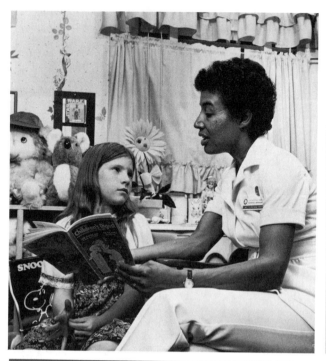
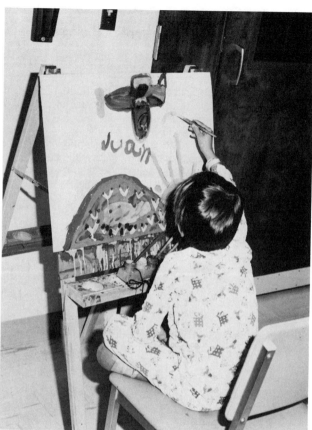

Figure 14-8. **A,** Eight-year-olds still like to listen to stories. **B,** Young artist in the hospital playroom. (Courtesy of J Nurs Care, Westport, CT.)

child may regress in response to this, but this regression should not be encouraged. Sometimes, families need as much reassurance as the children.

Discipline and rules do have a place on a pediatric unit. Families and children must be informed about the rules as part of the admission routine. Opportunity for interaction with peers, learning experiences, crafts, and projects can help make hospitalization more tolerable (Figure 14-8).

Summary

The ages between 6 and 10 years are an exciting time for children and families. Growth and development is steady at all levels—emotional, social, intellectual, and physical. Normally, this is a less turbulent time than either the preschool period or the adolescent period that is soon to follow. The school-age child gains a real sense of self, with individualized moral standards and conscience. Although much time is spent with peers in activities outside the home, the family is still the major sustaining force. Whether a child succeeds or fails in efforts during this period can have life-long impact on attitudes and performance.

Review Questions

1. When does a child usually begin to lose baby teeth? Give another name for "baby" teeth. Which teeth are usually lost first? Which molars come in first?
2. Delsey is upset that 6-year-old Jasmine is a "picky" eater and often does not want to eat what Delsey has prepared. What advice or reassurance can you give her?
3. Sue tells you she is really worried that 9-year-old Rachel needs to lose weight. How can you respond to Sue to help her solve her problem?
4. Using materials available to you, make a safety poster or teaching aid to use in an elementary school classroom. Perhaps you can make this a class project and donate the posters to your pediatric unit or nearby school.
5. Make a classroom presentation talking about the safety practice(s) illustrated in the poster or teaching aid you completed in question 4.

6. Steve is the primary family caregiver of 8-year-old Carolyn. He feels a responsibility for her sex education and asks your advice. What will you tell him?

7. Substance-abuse education, including alcohol and tobacco, should be included in the school health program. What are effective methods that you believe should be used to present these programs to children?

8. Explain the characteristics of school-age children that illustrate Piaget's stage of concrete operation.

9. What are several characteristics of school-age children that affect how you will care for them in the hospital?

Bibliography

Brooks RB. Self-esteem during the school years: Its normal development and hazardous decline. Pediatr Clin North Am 39(3):537–550, 1992.

Brown J. Be headstrong! Start a bicycle helmet campaign! Contemp Pediatr 9(7):54–73, 1992.

Castiglia PT, Harbin RE. Child Health Care: Process and Practice. Philadelphia: JB Lippincott, 1992.

Eschleman MM. Introductory Nutrition and Diet Therapy, 2nd ed. Philadelphia: JB Lippincott, 1991.

Jackson DB, Saunders RB. Child Health Nursing. Philadelphia: JB Lippincott, 1993.

Maloney MJ, McGuire J, Daniels SR, et al. Dieting behavior and eating attitudes in children. Pediatrics 84:482–489, 1989.

Pillitteri A: Maternal and Child Health Nursing. Philadelphia: JB Lippincott, 1992.

Schuster CS, Ashburn SS. The Process of Human Development, 3rd ed. Philadelphia: JB Lippincott, 1992.

Spock B, Rothenberg MB. Dr. Spock's Baby and Child Care. New York: Pocket Books, 1992.

Whaley LF, Wong DL. Nursing Care of Infants and Children, 4th ed. St. Louis: Mosby-Year Book, 1991.

Winkelstein ML. Fostering positive self-concept in the school-age child. Pediatr Nurs 15(3):229–233, 1989.

Health Problems of the School-Age Child

Chapter 15

Student Objectives

Upon completion of this chapter, the student will be able to:

1. Identify 10 characteristics that may be seen in a child with attention deficit hyperactivity disorder.
2. Describe a grand mal (tonic-clonic) seizure; an absence (petit mal) seizure.
3. List factors that can trigger an asthmatic attack, and describe the physiologic response that occurs in the respiratory tract.
4. List the symptoms of appendicitis; differentiate symptoms of the older and the younger child.
5. Identify three intestinal parasites common to children, and state the route of entry for each.
6. Develop a teaching plan for an 8-year-old child with diabetes mellitus; include skin care, insulin administration, and exercise.
7. Describe scoliosis, and identify four methods of correction.
8. Identify the most common form of muscular dystrophy; describe its characteristics.
9. Name the drug of choice in the treatment of juvenile rheumatoid arthritis, and state its primary purpose.
10. List and define the five P's necessary to observe, record, and report when caring for a child in a cast.
11. Describe the treatment for pediculosis of the scalp, and state the protection the nurse must use when treating a child in the hospital with this condition.

Marks MG: BROADRIBB'S INTRODUCTORY PEDIATRIC NURSING, 4th ed. © 1994 J.B. Lippincott Company.

Key Terms

allergen	lordosis
ankylosis	metered dose inhaler
anthelmintic	nebulizer
arthralgia	polyarthritis
aura	polydipsia
carditis	polyphagia
chorea	polyuria
desensitization	school phobia
diabetic acidosis	seizure
encopresis	skeletal traction
enuresis	skin traction
halo traction	soft neurologic signs
hirsutism	synovitis
insulin reaction	tinea
kussmaul breathing	traction
kyphoscoliosis	wheezing

*E*ntering school is a stressful time for every child, but especially so for the child with a chronic health problem. Imitation of one's peers is important during this time, but sometimes this is impossible for the child with a learning disorder, severe allergies, or a problem that limits physical mobility or makes the child feel "different" from peers. These children must cope with all the normal developmental stresses and the additional stress the health problem causes.

School-age children can learn to manage their health problems. Given enough information and guidance, children can understand and cope with problems such as diabetes and asthma. Nurses and caregivers who care for these children should foster maximum independence and a life as normal as possible.

Behavioral Problems

A number of behavioral problems are common in the school-age group. These problems can interfere with socialization, education, and development of the child. Some of these have definite organic causes; in others, causes are not clearly defined. School phobia is discussed in the following section. Attention deficit disorder is discussed in the subsequent section.

School Phobia

School absenteeism is a national problem. Children are absent from school for a variety of reasons. One cause of the absenteeism is **school phobia**. Children who develop school phobia may be good students and are more frequently girls than boys. School teachers and nurses can help detect the occurrence of school phobia by close attention to absence patterns. School-phobic children may have a strong attachment to one parent, usually the mother, and they fear separation from that parent, perhaps because of anxiety about losing the parent while away from home. Another factor may be that the child has a problem at school that seems overwhelming and unconsciously handles it in this way. The parent can unwittingly reinforce the school phobia by permitting the child to stay home. These children have genuine symptoms caused by anxiety that may approach panic. The symptoms include vomiting, diarrhea, abdominal or other pain, and even a low-grade fever. The symptoms disappear with relief of the immediate anxiety after the child has been given permission to stay home.

Treatment includes complete medical examination to rule out any organic cause for the symptoms and school–family conferences to facilitate the return of the child to school. The school nurse, the teacher, and other professionals, such as a social worker, a psychologist, and a psychiatrist, all may contribute to the resolution of this problem. If a specific factor in the school setting is feared, such as an overly critical teacher, the child may need to be moved to another class or school.

343

Central Nervous System Disorders

Although the health problems discussed in this section may not be classified simply as central nervous system disorders, the central nervous system most certainly plays an important part in each of them. All three of the conditions have a great impact on the success of the child in school and in society in general. As research continues, more knowledge will help identify causes and improve treatment. The future holds great promise for children with these conditions.

Attention Deficit Hyperactivity Disorder

Attention deficit hyperactivity disorder (ADHD), also called attention deficit disorder (ADD), is the terminology currently used to describe the syndrome characterized by certain behavioral and perceptual problems. Boys are more frequently affected than girls. The disorder affects every part of the child's life. The child with ADHD may be described in the following ways:

- Is impulsive
- Is easily distracted
- Often fidgets or squirms
- Has difficulty sitting still
- Has problems following through on instructions despite being able to understand them
- Is inattentive when spoken to
- Often loses things
- Goes from one uncompleted activity to another
- Has difficulty taking turns
- Often talks excessively
- Often engages in dangerous activities without considering the consequences

Diagnosis can be made after the child is 3 years old but often is not made until the child reaches school and has trouble settling into the routine.

Although these children have poor success in the classroom because of their inability to attend, they are not intellectually impaired. The child's poor impulse control also contributes to disciplinary problems in the classroom. Some children with ADHD may have learning disorders, such as dyslexia and perceptual deficits. The self-confidence of the child can suffer from the child's feeling inferior to the other children in the class. Special arrangements can be made to provide an educational atmosphere that is supportive to the child without the child leaving the classroom.

Diagnosis
Diagnosis of ADHD can be difficult and also may be controversial. Many of the symptoms are subjective and rely on the assessment of caregivers and teachers. Some authorities have expressed concern that children are incorrectly labeled as hyperactive by teachers. The symptoms may be a result of environmental factors, which can include broken homes, stress, and nonsupportive caregivers. A careful, detailed history, including school and social functioning, and a neurologic examination are necessary to help determine the diagnosis. These children often demonstrate **soft neurologic signs** (signs of clumsiness or poor coordination that may be appropriate for a younger child).

Treatment
Treatment also is controversial. Learning situations should be structured so that the child has minimal distractions and a supportive teacher. Home support is necessary, requiring structured, consistent guidance from the caregivers. Medication is used for some children, and this, too, has been controversial. Stimulant medications, such as methylphenidate (Ritalin) and dextroamphetamine (Dexedrine), have been frequently used. When given in large amounts, these medications may cause appetite suppression and affect the child's growing. Promelet (Cylert) has been used but generally with less success than methylphenidate and dextroamphetamine. Using stimulants for a hyperactive child seems strange, but these drugs apparently stimulate the area of the child's brain that helps them achieve more concentration, thus enabling the child to have better control.

In the health care setting, the nurse should maintain a calm, patient attitude toward the child with ADHD. The child should be given only one simple instruction at a time. Distractions should be eliminated from the child's environment. Regular routine with limitations, consistency, and praise for accomplishments are invaluable methods of working with these children. The families of children with ADHD need a great deal of support. Primary family caregivers, in particular, can become frustrated and upset by the constant challenge of dealing with a child with ADHD. The development of the child's self-esteem, confidence, and academic success must be the primary goal of all who work with these children.

Convulsive Disorders

Convulsive disorders are not uncommon in children and may result from a variety of causes. A common form of seizure is the febrile convulsion that occurs with fevers and acute infections.

Types of Epilepsy (Recurrent Convulsive Disorders)
Epilepsy can be classified as primary (idiopathic), with no known cause, or secondary, resulting from infection, head trauma, hemorrhage, tumor, or other organic or degenerative factor. Primary epilepsy is the most common; its onset generally is between ages 4 and 8 years.

Seizures are the characteristic clinical manifestation of both types of epilepsy and may be either generalized or partial (focal).

Generalized Seizures. Types of generalized seizures include grand mal (major motor), absence (petit mal), akinetic, myoclonic, and infantile spasms.

Grand mal (major motor) seizures consist of a sudden loss of consciousness, with generalized tonic and clonic movements. The seizure may be preceded by an **aura** (a sensation that signals impending attack), although young children may have difficulty describing it. The initial rigidity of the tonic phase (contraction of extensor and flexor muscles) changes rapidly to generalized jerking movements of the muscles (clonic phase). The child may bite the tongue or lose control of bladder and bowel functions. The contraction of respiratory muscles during the tonic phase may cause the child to become cyanotic, appearing briefly to have respiratory arrest. The jerking movements gradually diminish, then disappear, and the child relaxes. The seizure can be brief, lasting less than 1 minute, or it can last 30 minutes or longer. Following the episode, some children return rapidly to an alert state, many have a period of confusion, and others experience a prolonged period of stupor. The period following the tonic-clonic phase is called the postictal period.

Absence (petit mal) seizures last a few seconds, rarely longer than 20 seconds. The child loses awareness and stares straight ahead but does not fall. Immediately following the seizure, the child is alert and continues conversation but does not know what was said or done during the episode. Absences can recur frequently, sometimes as often as 50 to 100 in a single day. They often decrease significantly or stop entirely at adolescence.

Akinetic seizures cause a momentary loss of consciousness, muscle tone, and postural control and can result in serious facial, head, or shoulder injuries. They may recur frequently, particularly in the morning.

Myoclonic seizures are characterized by a sudden jerking of a muscle or group of muscles without loss of consciousness. Myoclonus occurs during the early stages of falling asleep in people who are nonepileptic.

Infantile spasms occur between 3 and 12 months of age and almost always indicate a cerebral defect and poor prognosis despite treatment. These seizures occur twice as often in boys as in girls and are preceded or followed by a cry. Muscle contractions are sudden, brief, and symmetric, accompanied by rolling eyes. Loss of consciousness does not always occur.

Diagnosis

Differentiation between types of seizures may be made through the use of electroencephalograms, skull radiography, computed tomography scan, brain scan, and physical and neurologic assessment.

Treatment

The main goal of treatment is complete control of seizures, which can be achieved for most people through the use of anticonvulsant drug therapy. A number of anticonvulsant drugs are available and are used according to their effectiveness in controlling seizures and to their degree of toxicity (Table 15-1). The oldest and most popular of these is phenytoin (Dilantin), which can cause hypertrophy of the gums after prolonged use. A small number of children may be candidates for surgical intervention when the focal point of the seizures can be determined to be in an area of the brain that is accessible surgically and is not an area critical to functioning. Ketogenic diets (high in fat and low in carbohydrates and protein) have been prescribed, but they are difficult to follow and unappealing to the child, so long-term maintenance is difficult.

Education and counseling of the child and the family caregivers are important parts of treatment. They need complete, accurate information about the disorder and the results that can be realistically expected from treatment. Epilepsy does not lead inevitably to mental retardation, but continued and uncontrolled seizures increase the possibility of mental retardation. This emphasizes the importance of early diagnosis and control of seizures.

Although the outlook for a normal, well-adjusted life is favorable, the child and family need to be aware of the restrictions that may be encountered. Children with epilepsy should be encouraged to participate in physical activities but should not participate in sports in which a fall could cause serious injury, such as rope climbing, and they may have to be careful in contact sports. Unsupervised swimming or underwater swimming should not be permitted. In many states a person with uncontrolled epilepsy is legally forbidden to drive a motor vehicle. This could limit choice of vocation and lifestyle. Despite attempts at educating the general public about epilepsy, many people remain prejudiced about this disorder, which can limit the epileptic person's social and vocational acceptance.

Allergic Reactions

Millions of Americans suffer from allergic diseases, most of which begin in childhood. An allergic condition is caused by sensitivity to a specific substance, such as pollen, mold, certain foods, and drugs. That substance is called an **allergen** (antigen that causes an allergy). Allergens may enter the body through a variety of routes, the most common being the nose, throat, eyes, bronchial tissues in the lungs, the skin, and the digestive tract. The first time the child comes in contact with an allergen, no response may be evident, but an immune response is stimulated through the lymphocytes (white blood cells):

Table 15-1. Antiepileptic-Anticonvulsive Therapeutic Agents

Drug	Indication	Side Effects	Nursing Implications
Carbamazepine (Tegretal)	Generalized grand mal, complex partial, focal motor seizures, mixed seizures	Drowsiness, dry mouth, vomiting, double vision, leukopenia, GI upset, thrombocytopenia	There may be dizziness and drowsiness with initial doses. This should subside within 3–14 days.
Ethosuximide (Zarontin)	Absence seizures, myoclonic (petit mal)	Dry mouth, anorexia, dizziness, headache, nausea, vomiting, GI upset, lethargy, bone marrow depression	Use with caution in hepatic or renal disease.
Clonazepam (Klonopin)	Absence seizures, myoclonic (petit mal)	Double vision, drowsiness, increased salivation, changes in behavior, bone marrow depression	Obtain periodic liver function tests and complete blood count. Monitor for over-sedation.
Phenobarbital (Luminol)	Tonic-clonic, generalized	Drowsiness, alteration in sleep patterns, irritability, respiratory and cardiac depression, restlessness, headache	Alcohol can enhance the effects of phenobarbital. Blood studies and liver tests are necessary with prolonged use.
Primidone (Mysoline)	Tonic/clonic generalized, complex and simple partial seizures	Behavior changes, drowsiness, hyperactivity, ataxia, Bone marrow depression	Adverse effects are the same as for phenobarbital. Sedation and dizziness may be severe during initial therapy—dosage may need to be adjusted by the physician.
Valproic acid (Depakene)	Tonic/clonic, myoclonic absence seizures, mixed seizures	Nausea, vomiting or increased appetite, tremors, elevated liver enzymes, constipation, headaches, depression, lymphocytosis, leukopenia, increased prothrombin time	Physical dependency may result when used for prolonged period. Tablets and capsules should be taken whole. Elixir should be taken alone, not mixed with carbonated beverages. Increased toxicity may occur with administration of salicylates (aspirin).
Phenytoin (Dilantin)	Tonic-clonic generalized, complex and simple partial	Double vision, blurred vision, slurred speech, nystagmus, ataxia, gingival hyperplasia, hirsutism, cardiac arrhythmias, bone marrow depression	Alcohol, antacids, and folic acid decrease the effect of Dilantin. Instruct the child or the family caregivers to notify the dentist that he or she is taking Dilantin in order to monitor hyperplasia of the gums. Inform the child or family caregivers that the drug may color the urine pink to red-brown.

General Nursing Considerations with Anticonvulsant Therapy

General nursing considerations with anticonvulsant therapy that apply to all or most of drugs given to children include:

1. Warn the patient and family that patients should avoid activities that require alertness and complex psychomotor coordination (eg, climbing).
2. Medication can be given with meals to minimize gastric irritation.
3. The anticonvulsant medications should not be discontinued abruptly as this can precipitate status epilepticus.
4. Anticonvulsant medications generally have a cumulative effect, both therapeutically and adversely.
5. Alcohol ingestion increases the effects of anticonvulsant drugs, exaggerating the CNS depression.
6. Many of the drugs can cause bone marrow depression (leukopenia, thrombocytopenia, neutropenia, megaloblastic anemia.) Regular CBC are necessary to evaluate bone marrow production.
7. The child receives periodic blood tests to determine drug levels in order to monitor therapeutic levels as opposed to toxic blood levels.

Adapted from Castiglia PT, Harbin RE. Child Health Care: Practice and Process. Philadelphia: JB Lippincott, 1992.

T-helper lymphocytes stimulate B lymphocytes to make immunoglobulin E (IgE) antibody. The IgE antibody attaches to mast cells and macrophages. When contacted again, the allergen attaches to the IgE receptor sites, and a response occurs in which certain substances, such as histamine, are released; these substances produce the symptoms known as allergy.

Millions of children with allergies are hampered by poor appetite, poor sleep, restricted physical activity in play and at school, often resulting in altered physical and personality development.

Children whose parents or grandparents have allergies are more likely to become allergic than other children. There are thousands of allergens; some of the most common are pollen, mold, dust, animal dander, insect bites, tobacco smoke, nuts, chocolate, milk, fish, and shellfish. Drugs can be allergens also, particularly aspirin and penicillin. Some plants and chemicals cause allergic reactions on the skin that are discussed later in this chapter in the section on skin allergies.

Diagnosis of an allergy requires a careful history and physical examination and possibly skin tests and blood tests, including complete blood count, serum protein electrophoresis, and immunoelectrophoresis. Skin testing is generally done when removal of obvious inhalants is not possible or has not brought relief. If a food allergy is suspected, an "elimination" diet may help identify the allergen. When specific allergens have been identified, patients can either avoid them or, if this is not possible, undergo immunization therapy by injection, called **desensitization** or immunotherapy.

Desensitization is performed for those allergens that produced a positive reaction on skin testing. The allergist sets up a schedule for injections in gradually increasing doses until a maintenance dose is reached. The patient should remain in the physician's office for 20 to 30 minutes following injection in case any reaction occurs. Reactions are treated with epinephrine. Severe reactions in children are uncommon, and desensitization is considered a safe procedure with considerable benefit for some children.

Symptomatic relief in allergic reactions can be gained through antihistamine or steroid therapy; however, the best treatment is prevention.

Allergic Rhinitis (Hay Fever)

Allergic rhinitis in children is most often due to sensitization to animal dander, house dust, pollens, and molds. Pollen allergy seldom appears before 4 or 5 years of age.

Symptoms
A watery nasal discharge, postnasal drip, sneezing, and allergic conjunctivitis are the usual symptoms of allergic rhinitis. Continued sniffing, itching of the nose and palate, and the "allergic salute" (Figure 15-1) are common

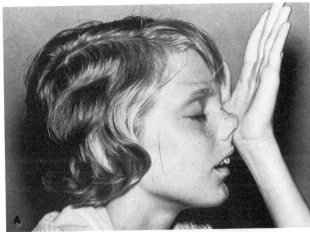

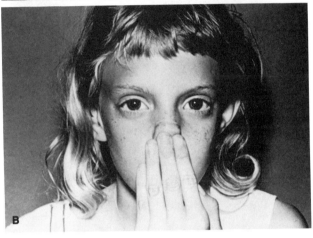

Figure 15-1. Allergic salute. **A,** The allergic child often pushes his or her nose upward and backward to relieve itching and to free edematous turbinates from contact with the septum. This allows for free passage of air. **B,** The allergic salute induces transverse nasal crease. (Courtesy of the Upjohn Company, Kalamazoo, MI, and M. B. Marks, MD, Miami, FL.)

complaints. Dark circles under the eyes are typical (Figure 15-2).

Treatment
When possible, offending allergens are avoided or removed from the environment. Antihistamine-decongestant preparations, such as Dimetapp and Actifed, can be helpful for some patients. Desensitization can be implemented, particularly if antihistamines are not helpful or are needed chronically.

Asthma

Asthma is a spasm of the bronchial tubes due to hypersensitivity of the airways in the bronchial system and inflammation that leads to mucosal edema and mucus hypersecretion. This reversible obstructive airway dis-

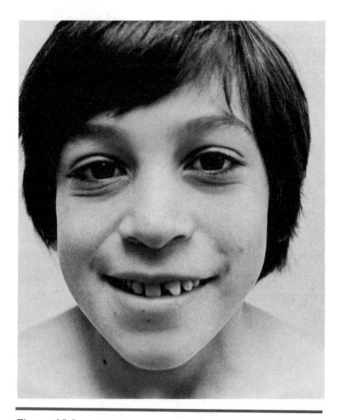

Figure 15-2. Typical facies of allergic rhinitis. (Photo by Marcia Lieberman.)

ease affects at least 10 million people in the United States, with 5% to 10% of all children in the United States being affected.

Asthma attacks are often triggered by a hypersensitive response to allergens; in young children, asthma may be the response to certain foods. Asthma can frequently be triggered by exercise, exposure to cold weather, or such irritants as wood burning stoves, cigarette smoke, dust, pet dander, and foods such as chocolate, milk, eggs, nuts and grains. Infections, such as bronchitis and a urinary tract infection, frequently can provoke asthma attacks. In children who have asthmatic tendencies, emotional stress or anxiety can trigger an attack. Some children with asthma may have no evidence of an immunologic cause for the symptoms. Asthma can be either intermittent, with extended periods when the child has no symptoms and does not need medication, or chronic, with the need for frequent or continuous therapy. Chronic asthma affects the child's school performance and general activities and may contribute to poor self-confidence and dependency. Asthma is the most common single cause of school absence.[1]

Pathophysiology

Spasms of the smooth muscles cause the lumina of the bronchi and bronchioles to narrow. Edema of the mucous membrane lining these bronchial branches, and increased production of thick mucus within them, combine with the spasm to cause respiratory obstruction (Figure 15-3).

Clinical Manifestations

The onset of an attack may be very abrupt, or it may progress over several days, evidenced by a dry, hacking cough, wheezing, and difficult breathing. Asthmatic attacks frequently occur at night, waking the child from sleep. The child has to sit up and is totally preoccupied with efforts to breathe. Attacks may last for only a short time or may continue for several days. Thick, tenacious mucus may be coughed up or vomited after a coughing episode. In some asthmatic patients, coughing is the major symptom, and wheezing occurs rarely, if at all. Many children no longer have symptoms after puberty, but this is not predictable. Other allergies may develop in adulthood.

Diagnosis

The child's history and physical examination are of primary importance in establishing a diagnosis of asthma. When listening to the child's breathing (auscultation), the examiner hears dyspnea and **wheezing** (sound on expiration of air being pushed through obstructed bronchioles), usually generalized over all lung fields. Mucus production may be profuse. Pulmonary function tests are valuable diagnostic tools. These tests indicate the amount of obstruction in the bronchial airways, especially in the smallest airways of the lungs. A definitive diagnosis of asthma is made when the obstruction in the airways is reversed with bronchodilators.

Treatment

Prevention is the most important aspect in the treatment of asthma. Children and their families must be taught to recognize the symptoms that lead to an acute attack so that they can be treated as early as possible. These symptoms include increasing cough at night, in the early morning, or on activity; respiratory retractions; and wheezing.[2] Use of a peak flow meter is an objective way to measure airway obstruction, and children as young as 4 or 5 years of age can be taught to use one (Parent Teaching: How to Use a Peak Flow Meter). A peak flow diary should be maintained, which also can include symptoms, exacerbations, actions taken, and outcomes. Families also must make every effort to eliminate any possible allergens from the home.

Drug Treatment. Bronchodilators are the drugs of choice for treatment of asthma. These drugs are classified into two major groups: (1) theophylline preparations and (2) adrenergic, or sympathomimetic, drugs. Corticosteroid drugs and cromolyn sodium, a mast cell stabilizer, also are used in addition to the bronchodilators. Epinephrine may be administered subcutaneously in an acute attack.

Theophylline preparations are available in short-acting and long-acting forms. The short-acting forms, such

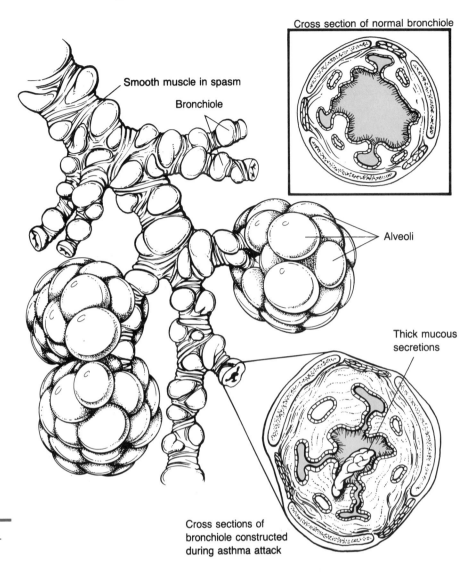

Cross section of normal bronchiole

Smooth muscle in spasm

Bronchiole

Alveoli

Thick mucous secretions

Cross sections of bronchiole constructed during asthma attack

Figure 15-3. Bronchiole airflow obstruction in asthma.

as Theon and Elixicon liquids and aminophylline rectal suppositories, are given approximately every 6 hours. These are most effective when used by the patient, as needed, for intermittent episodes of asthma because they enter the blood stream quickly. Side effects are nervousness, insomnia, muscular spasms, irritability, palpitations, upset stomach, anorexia, perspiration, and frequent urination.

Long-acting preparations of theophylline, such as Theo-Dur tablets and Theophyl SR capsules, are given every 8 to 12 hours. They are helpful in patients who continually need medication because these drugs sustain more consistent theophylline levels in the blood than do the short-acting forms. Patients hospitalized for status asthmaticus receive theophylline intravenously.

The beta-adrenergic, or sympathomimetic, drugs are being used with cromolyn sodium (Intal) replacing the use of theophylline more recently. Frequently used beta-adrenergic drugs are metaproterenol sulfate (Alupent or

Metaprel) and terbutaline sulfate (Brethine). They are short-acting and available in liquid, inhalant, or pill form. These drugs are administered every 6 to 8 hours if breathing difficulty continues despite theophylline administration. In severe attacks, epinephrine by subcutaneous injection often affords quick relief of symptoms. Metaproterenol or isoetharine hydrochloride (Bronkosol) are administered in inhalant form only. Terbutaline can cause tremors in skeletal muscles and increased awareness of one's heartbeat. These are normal side effects and not a cause for alarm. Often these effects diminish with continued use of the medication or a decrease in dosage.

Cromolyn sodium prevents mast cells from releasing chemical mediators that cause bronchospasm and mucous membrane inflammation. It is used to decrease daily wheeze and exercise-induced asthma attacks. A beta-adrenergic drug that functions to open the airways is administered with cromolyn sodium. The beta-adrenergic drug is administered first so that cromolyn sodium is

How to Use a Peak Flow Meter

Introduction

Early changes in the airway cannot be felt by your child. By the time the child feels tightness in the chest or starts to wheeze, he or she are already far into an asthma episode. The most reliable early sign of an asthma episode is a drop in the child's peak expiratory flow rate, or the ability to breathe out quickly, which can be measured by a peak flow meter. Almost every asthmatic child over the age of 4 years can and should learn to use a peak flow meter (Figs. A and B.)

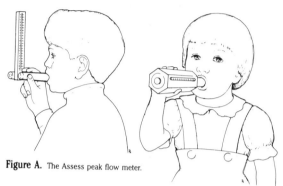

Figure A. The Assess peak flow meter.

Figure B. The Mini-Wright peak flow meter.

Steps to Accurate Measurements

1. Remove gum or food from the mouth.
2. Move the pointer on the meter to zero.
3. Stand up and hold the meter horizontally, with fingers away from the vent holes and marker.
4. With mouth wide open, slowly breathe in as much air as possible.
5. Put the mouthpiece on the tongue and place lips around it.
6. Blow out as hard and fast as you can. Give a short, sharp blast, not a slow blow. The meter measures the fastest puff, not the longest.
7. Repeat steps 1–6 three times. Wait at least 10 seconds between puffs. Move the pointer to zero after each puff.
8. Record the best reading.

Guidelines for Treatment

Each child has a unique pattern of asthma episodes. Most episodes begin gradually, and a drop in peak flow can alert you to start medications before the actual symptoms appear. This early treatment can prevent a flare from getting out of hand. One way to look at peak flow scores is to match the scores with three colors:

Green	Yellow	Red
80%–100% personal best No symptoms	50%–80% personal best Mild-to-moderate symptoms	Below 50% personal best Serious distress
Full breathing reserve	Diminished reserve	Pulmonary function is significantly impaired
Mild trigger may not cause symptoms	A minor trigger produces noticeable symptoms	Any trigger may lead to severe distress
Continue current management	Augment present treatment regimen	Contact physician

Remember, treatment should be adjusted to fit the individual's needs. Your physician will develop a home management plan with you. When in doubt, consult your physician.

most effective. The child may dislike the taste, which can be minimized with sips of water before and after administration. Cromolyn sodium is not useful in severe asthmatic attacks and can actually worsen an attack, but it is effective as a preventive drug. Side effects are minimal.

Steroids are used in severe or very chronic cases of asthma, but they must be used with great care. They are often prescribed only after other medications have failed to produce the desired effects. Steroids may be given in inhaled form, such as beclomethasone dipropionate (Beclovent), to decrease systemic effects that accompany oral steroid administration.

Many of these drugs can be given either by a **nebulizer** (tube attached to a wall unit or cylinder that delivers moist air via a face mask) or a **metered dose inhaler** (hand-held plastic device that delivers a premeasured dose) (Figure 15-4).

Chest Physiotherapy. Because asthma has multiple causes, treatment and continuing management of the disease require more than medication. Chest physiotherapy includes breathing exercises, physical training, and inhalation therapy. Studies have shown that breathing exercises to improve respiratory function and help control asthma attacks can be an important adjunct to treatment. These exercises teach children how to help control their own symptoms and thereby build self-confidence, sometimes lacking in asthmatic children. If the exercises can be taught as part of play activities, children are more likely to find them fun and to practice them more often.

Nursing Process for the Child with Asthma

ASSESSMENT

An interview with the caregiver of the child should include questions about the child's asthmatic history, the medications the child takes, and the medications taken within the last 24 hours. The nurse should ask if the child has vomited because vomiting would prevent absorption of oral medications. Other information that should be obtained is a history of respiratory infections; possible allergens in the household, such as pets; type of furniture and toys; whether there is a damp basement (mold spores); and a history of breathing problems after exercise. Physical examination should include vital signs, observation for diaphoresis and cyanosis, position, type of breathing, alertness, chest movement, intercostal retractions, and breath sounds. Any wheezing must be noted.

If the child is old enough and alert enough to cooperate, the nurse should involve the child in gathering the

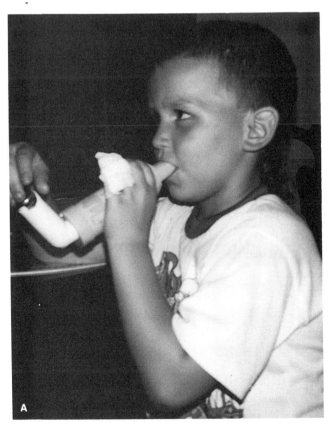

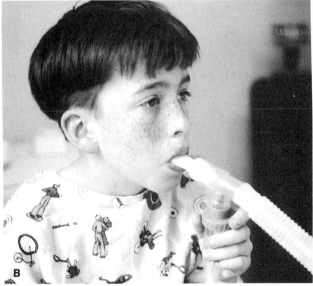

Figure 15-4. **A,** Five-year-old child using metered dose inhaler with spacer. **B,** Nine-year-old child using nebulizer. (From Jackson DB, Saunders RB. Child Health Nursing. Philadelphia: JB Lippincott, 1993, p. 940.)

history and encourage the child to add any information desired. Asking questions that can be answered "yes" or "no" may be less tiring to a child in distress.

NURSING DIAGNOSES

Nursing diagnoses can be formulated working with the child and the child's caregiver. Apprehensions of both the child and the family must be considered. Nursing diagnoses may include the following:

- Ineffective airway clearance related to bronchospasm and increased pulmonary secretions
- High risk for fluid volume deficit related to insensible water loss from tachypnea, diaphoresis, and reduced oral intake
- Fatigue related to dyspnea
- Fear related to sudden attacks of breathlessness
- Parental health-seeking behaviors related to management of home care, disease process, treatment, and control

PLANNING AND IMPLEMENTATION

The nursing goals are aimed initially at relieving the child's breathing distress. Quiet, relaxed reassurance of the child and the family is important. Constant teaching of the child and the family is essential throughout the child's hospitalization.

Monitoring Respiratory Function. During the time that the child is in acute distress in an asthma attack, the child should be continuously monitored with pulse oximetry and a cardiopulmonary monitor. If this equipment is not available, the child's respirations should be taken every 15 minutes during an acute attack and every 1 or 2 hours after the crisis is over. Observations include nasal flaring, chest retractions, and skin for color and diaphoresis. The child's head should be elevated, and an older child may be more comfortable resting forward on a pillow placed on an overbed table. The child should be monitored for response to medications and their side effects, such as restlessness, gastrointestinal upset, and seizures. Humidified oxygen and suction may be needed during periods of acute distress.

Monitoring and Improving Fluid Intake. During an acute attack the child may lose a lot of fluids through the respiratory tract and may have a poor oral intake because of coughing and vomiting. Theophylline administration also has a diuretic effect, which compounds the problem. Monitoring the child's intake and output is necessary. Oral fluids that the child likes should be encouraged. Intravenous fluids may be administered and must be monitored. The child's skin turgor and mucous membranes must be assessed at least every 8 hours. A daily weight can help determine fluid loss.

Promoting Energy Conservation. The child may become extremely tired from the exertion of trying to breathe. Activities should be spaced so that maximum periods of uninterrupted rest are provided. Quiet activities should be provided when the child needs diversion. Visitors should be kept to a minimum and a quiet environment maintained.

Reducing Child and Parent Anxiety. The sudden onset of an asthmatic attack can be frightening. Family caregivers may tend to overprotect the child because of the fear that an attack may occur when the child is with a babysitter, at school, or anywhere that the caregiver is not present. The child's fear of attacks can be increased by the behavior of the caregiver. The child's and the caregiver's fears can be lessened by teaching them the signs and symptoms of an impending attack and the immediate response needed to decrease the threat of an attack.

Providing Family Teaching. Child and family caregiver teaching is of primary importance in the care of asthmatic children. Asthmatic attacks can be prevented or decreased by prompt and adequate intervention. Aspects that must be taught to the caregiver and child (within the scope of the child's ability to understand) are the disease process, recognition of symptoms of impending attack, environmental control, avoidance of infection, exercise, drug therapy, and chest physiotherapy.

The caregiver and the child must be taught how to use the metered dose inhaler medications and be able to demonstrate the correct usage (see Parent Teaching: How to Use a Metered Dose Inhaler). Instructions should be given on home use of a peak flowmeter and maintenance of a diary recording the peak flow as well as asthma symptoms, onset of attacks, action taken, and results.

Parent Teaching

How to Use a Metered Dose Inhaler

1. When ready to use, shake the inhaler well with the cap still on. The child should stand, if possible.
2. Remove the cap.
3. Hold the inhaler with the mouthpiece down, facing the child.
4. Be sure the child's mouth is empty.
5. Hold the mouthpiece 1–2 inches from the lips.
6. Breathe out normally. Open mouth wide and begin to breathe in.
7. Press top of medication canister firmly while inhaling deeply. Hold breath as long as possible (at least 10 seconds—teach child to count slowly to 10).
8. Breathe out *slowly* through nose or pursed lips.
9. Relax 2–5 minutes, and repeat as directed by physician.

Instructions should be given about premedication before the child is exposed to situations in which an attack may occur.

Family caregivers must be informed of possible allergens that may be in the child's environment and encouraged to eliminate or control them as needed. The importance of quick response when the child has a respiratory infection must be stressed to the caregiver. Instructions should be given for exercise and chest physiotherapy.

Family caregivers should be made aware of the importance of informing the child's school teacher, physical education teacher, school nurse, babysitter, and others who are responsible for the child for periods of time. With a physician's order, including directions for use, the child should be permitted to bring medications to school and keep them so they can be used when needed.

The nurse should provide information on support groups available in the area. The American Lung Association has many materials available to families and can provide information about support groups, camps, and workshops. *Superstuff*, an excellent booklet geared to the elementary- and middle school-age child, is available from the American Lung Association. The Asthma and Allergy Foundation of America and the National Asthma Education Program are also excellent resources.

EVALUATION

- Breath sounds clear, no retractions or nasal flaring, skin color good, pulse rate within normal limits
- Intake and output measurements indicate adequate fluid intake for size; mucous membranes moist, skin turgor good, weight returns to pre-illness level
- Achieves extended periods of rest, dyspnea kept to minimum
- Child or caregiver states signs and symptoms of impending attack and appropriate response
- Child or caregiver demonstrates understanding and knowledge of disease process, treatment and control through interaction with health care personnel, asking and answering relevant questions and demonstrating techniques as appropriate; caregiver obtains information to make contact with support groups

Gastrointestinal System Disorders

The school-age child may have periodic complaints about stomachache or abdominal pain. Usually these are minor complaints that are benign and self-limiting. However, the child's complaints should not be dismissed without being assessed, especially if they seem to be acute, have a regular pattern, or are accompanied by other symptoms.

Appendicitis

Most cases of appendicitis in childhood occur in the school-age child. In young children, the symptoms may be difficult to evaluate.

The appendix is a blind pouch located in the cecum near the ileocecal junction. Obstruction of the lumen of the appendix is the primary cause of appendicitis (inflammation of the appendix). The obstruction is usually caused by hardened fecal matter or a foreign body. This obstruction causes circulation to be slowed or interrupted, resulting in pain and necrosis of the appendix. The necrotic area can rupture, causing escape of fecal matter and bacteria into the peritoneal cavity and resulting in the complication of peritonitis.

Clinical Manifestations

Symptoms in the older child may be the same as in an adult: pain and tenderness in the right lower quadrant of the abdomen, nausea and vomiting, fever, and constipation. These symptoms are infrequent in young children, however, because many children already have a ruptured appendix when first seen by the physician. The young child has difficulty localizing pain, may act restless and irritable, and have a slight fever, flushed face, and rapid pulse. Usually the white blood cell count is slightly elevated. It may take several hours to rule out other conditions and make a positive diagnosis. When appendicitis is suspected, laxatives and enemas are contraindicated because they increase peristalsis and thereby increase the possibility of rupturing an inflamed appendix.

Treatment

Surgical removal of the appendix is the necessary procedure and should be performed as soon as possible after diagnosis. If the appendix has not ruptured prior to surgery, the operative risk is nearly negligible. Even after perforation has occurred, the mortality rate is less than 1%.

Food and fluids by mouth are withheld prior to surgery. If the child is dehydrated, intravenous fluids are ordered. If fever is present, temperature should be reduced to below 38.9°C (102°F).

Recovery is rapid and usually uneventful. The child is ambulated early and is able to leave the hospital a few days after surgery. In the instance when peritonitis or a localized abscess is a complication, gastric suction, parenteral fluids, and antibiotics may be ordered.

◣ Nursing Process of the Child with Appendicitis

ASSESSMENT

When a child is admitted with a diagnosis of possible appendicitis, an emergency situation exists. The family caregiver who brings the child to the hospital is often upset and anxious. The admission assessment must be performed quickly and skillfully. Gathering information about the child's condition for the last several days is important to obtain a picture of how the condition has developed. Particular emphasis should be placed on gastrointestinal complaints, appetite, bowel movements for the last few days, and general activity level. Physical assessment includes vital signs, especially noting any elevation of temperature, presence of bowel sounds, abdominal guarding, and nausea or vomiting. Diminished or absent bowel sounds should be reported immediately. The child and caregiver need careful explanations about all procedures that are to be performed. The level of anxiety requires special empathy and understanding on the part of the nurse.

NURSING DIAGNOSES

As soon as the medical diagnosis of appendicitis has been confirmed, the child is prepared for surgery. Some nursing diagnoses might include the following:

- Anxiety of child and family caregiver related to emergency surgery
- Pain related to necrosis of appendix and surgical procedure
- High risk for fluid volume deficit related to decreased intake
- Caregiver health-seeking behaviors related to lack of knowledge about postoperative care

PLANNING AND IMPLEMENTATION

Because of the urgent nature of the child's admission and preparation for surgery, great efforts must be taken to provide calm, reassuring care, both to the child and the caregiver. Nursing goals must be determined with this in mind.

Reducing Child and Parent Anxiety. Although procedures must be performed quickly, care must be taken to consider both the child's and the family's anxieties. The child may be extremely frightened by the sudden change of events. The child also may be in considerable pain. The family caregiver may be apprehensive about impending surgery. Introducing various health care team members by name and title as they come into the child's room to perform procedures can help to reassure the child and the family. Explaining to the child and the family what is happening, and why, may help to alleviate some of their anxiety. Explaining the post anesthesia care unit (recovery room) to the child and the family is important. The family and child should be encouraged to verbalize fears, and the nurse should try to allay these fears as much as possible. Family members should be given information about where to wait while the

child is having surgery, how long to the surgery will last, where dining facilities are located, and where the surgeon will expect to find them after surgery. If possible, the nurse should demonstrate deep breathing, coughing, and abdominal splinting to the child and practice it. Throughout the preoperative care, the nurse must be sensitive to anxieties, whether verbalized or not, and provide understanding care.

Reducing Pain. Preoperatively, analgesics should not be given to the child because of concern for concealing signs of tenderness that are important for diagnosis. Providing comfort through positioning and gentle care while performing preoperative procedures are important. Heat to the abdomen is contraindicated because of the danger of rupture of the appendix. Postoperatively, the child should be assessed hourly for pain and analgesics administered. Providing quiet diversional activities can be helpful. The child may fear ambulation postoperatively because of pain. Many children (and adults, too) are worried that the "stitches will pull out." The child must be reassured that the nurse understands this worry but that the sutures (or clamps) are secure and are intended to withstand the strain of walking and moving about. Activity is essential to the child's recovery but should be as pain free as possible. The nurse can help the child understand that as activity increases, the pain will decrease. The child whose appendix had ruptured before surgery may also have pain related to the nasogastric tube, abdominal distention, or constipation.

Monitoring Fluid Intake. Dehydration can be a concern, especially if the child has had bouts of nausea and vomiting preoperatively. On admission to the hospital, the child is maintained on NPO until after surgery. The child's intake and output is measured and recorded. Intravenous fluids are administered with appropriate nursing measures. Postoperatively, dressings should be checked to detect evidence of excessive drainage or bleeding, indicating loss of fluids. Clear oral fluids are usually ordered early postoperatively, and after the child takes and retains fluids successfully, a progressive diet is ordered. Bowel sounds should be assessed and reported at least every 4 hours because the physician may use this as a gauge to determine when the child can have solid food.

Providing Family Teaching. The child who has had an uncomplicated appendectomy that has not ruptured convalesces quickly and returns to school within 1 or 2 weeks. The incision is kept clean and dry. Activities should be limited according to the recommendations of the physician. The child who has had a ruptured appendix is hospitalized for a week or more and is more limited in activities postoperatively. The family should be instructed to observe for signs and symptoms of complications postoperatively, including fever, abdominal distention, and pain. Instructions on follow-up appointments must be emphasized before discharge.

EVALUATION

- Child and family verbalize fears and ask questions preoperatively; child cooperates with health care personnel
- Child's pain is at a tolerable level as evidenced by child's verbalization of pain level
- Child's skin turgor is good, vital signs are within normal limits, weight remains stable
- Caregiver will discuss expected recovery and ask appropriate questions, demonstrate wound care as needed, and review signs and symptoms that should be reported

Intestinal Parasites

A few intestinal parasites are commonly found in the United States. They are especially frequent in the young and school-age population. Frequent hand-to-mouth practices contribute to infestations. Several of the more common are discussed in the following section.

Enterobiasis (Pinworm Infection)

The pinworm, *Enterobius vermicularis*, is a white, thread-like worm that invades the cecum and may enter the appendix. Pinworms are spread from person to person by articles contaminated with pinworm eggs. The infestation is common among children. Infestation occurs when the pinworm eggs are swallowed. The eggs hatch in the intestinal tract and grow to maturity in the cecum. The female worm, when ready to lay her eggs, crawls out of the anus and lays the eggs on the child's perineum.

Itching around the anus causes the child to scratch and trap new eggs under his or her fingernails, which causes frequent reinfection when the child's fingers go into his or her mouth. Clothing, bedding, food, toilet seats, and other articles become infected, and the infestation spreads to other members of the family. Pinworm eggs can also float in the air and be inhaled.

The life cycle of these worms is from 6 to 8 weeks, after which reinfestation commonly occurs unless treated. The condition appears most frequently in school-age children and next highest in preschool-age children. All members of the family are susceptible.

Diagnosis. Capturing the eggs from around the anus by the use of cellophane tape and examining them under a microscope is the usual method of identification. As they emerge from the anus, adult worms also may be seen when the child is lying quietly or sleeping.

The cellophane tape test for identifying worms is performed in the early morning just before, or as soon as, the child wakens and is carried out as follows:

1. Wind clear cellophane tape around the end of a tongue blade, sticky side outward.

2. Spread the child's buttocks, and press the tape against the anus, rolling from side to side.

3. Transfer the tape to a microscope slide and cover with a clean slide to send to the laboratory. The tongue blade can be placed in a plastic bag, if the caregiver does not have slides or a commercially prepared kit.

4. The tape is examined microscopically in the laboratory for eggs.

Prevention and Treatment. The child should be taught to wash his or her hands after bowel movements and before eating and to observe other hygienic measures, such as regular bathing and daily change of underclothing. Fingernails should be kept short and clean. Bedding also should be changed frequently to avoid reinfestation. All bedding and clothing, especially underclothing, should be washed in hot water.

Treatment consists in the use of an **anthelmintic** (medication that expels intestinal worms—vermifuge). Mebendazole (Vermox) is the most commonly used product. Medication should be repeated in 2 or 3 weeks to eliminate any parasites that hatch after the initial treatment. All family members should be treated.

Roundworms

Ascaris lumbricoides is a large intestinal worm found only in humans. Infestation is from the feces of infested people. It is usually found in areas where sanitary facilities are lacking and human excreta is deposited on the ground.

The adult worm is pink and from 9 to 12 inches in length. The eggs hatch in the intestinal tract, and the larvae migrate to the liver and lungs. The larvae reaching the lungs ascend up through the bronchi, are swallowed, and reach the intestine, where they grow to maturity and mate. Eggs are then discharged into the feces. Full development requires about 2 months. In tropical countries where infestation may be heavy, bowel obstructions may present serious problems. Generally, however, no symptoms are present in ordinary infestations. Identification is made by means of microscopic examination of feces for eggs. Pyrantel pamoate (Antiminth) is the medication commonly used. Improved hygienic conditions with sanitary disposal of feces, including diapers, are necessary to prevent infestation.

Hookworms

The hookworm lives in the human intestinal tract, where it attaches itself to the wall of the small intestine. Eggs are discharged in the feces of the host.

These parasites are prevalent in areas where infected human excreta is deposited on the ground and when the soil, moisture, and temperature are favorable for the development of infective larvae of the worm. In the southeastern United States and tropical West Africa, the prevailing species is *Necator americanus*.

After feces containing eggs are deposited on the ground, larvae hatch, where they can survive as long as 6 weeks. Usually, they penetrate the skin of barefoot people. They produce an itching dermatitis on the feet (ground itch). The larvae pass through the blood stream to the lungs and into the pharynx, where they are swallowed and reach the small intestine. In the small intestine, they attach themselves to the intestinal wall, where they feed on blood. Heavy infestation may cause anemia through loss of blood to the worms. Chronic infestation produces listlessness, fatigue, and malnutrition. Identification is made by examination of the stool under the microscope.

Treatment. Pyrantel pamoate or mebendazole may be used in the treatment of hookworms. Caregivers should keep children from running barefoot where there is any possibility of ground contamination with feces.

The infected child needs a well-balanced diet with additional protein and iron. Transfusions are rarely necessary.

Giardiasis

Giardiasis is not caused by a worm but by a protozoan parasite, *Giardia lamblia*. It is a common cause of diarrhea in world travelers and is also prevalent in children who attend day care centers and other types of residential situations; it may be found in contaminated mountain streams or pools frequented by diapered infants. The child ingests the cyst containing the protozoa. The cyst is activated by stomach acid and passes into the duodenum, where it matures, causing diarrhea, weight loss, and abdominal cramps. Identification and diagnosis are made through examination of stool under the microscope.

Treatment. Metronidazole (Flagyl) or quinacrine (Atabrine) are effective in treating the infestation. Quinacrine causes a yellow discoloration of the skin, about which the nurse should alert the caregiver.

Disorders of Elimination

Although difficulties with diarrhea or constipation may occur commonly in the school-age child, the most common cause for stress in the child and the caregiver is a problem with continence. Enuresis or encopresis can cause many days of frustration and discouragement for both the child and the caregiver.

Enuresis

Enuresis is the term used for involuntary urination beyond the age when control of urination commonly is acquired. Many children do not acquire complete night-time control before 5 to 7 years of age, and an occasional bed wetting may be seen in children as late as 9 or 10 years of age. Boys have more difficulty than girls, and in some instances, enuresis may persist into the adult years.

Enuresis may have a physiologic or psychologic cause and can indicate a need for further exploration and treatment of this problem. Physiologic causes may include a small bladder capacity, urinary tract infection, and lack of awareness of the signal to empty the bladder because of sleeping too soundly.

Persistent bed-wetting in a 5- or 6-year-old child may be a result of rigorous toilet training before the child was physically or psychologically ready. Enuresis in the older child may express resentment toward family caregivers or a desire to regress to an earlier level to receive more care and attention. Emotional stress also can be a precipitating factor. The health care team also needs to consider the possibility that enuresis can be a symptom of sexual abuse.

If a physiologic cause has been ruled out, efforts should be made to discover possible causes, including emotional stress. If the child is interested in achieving control, for instance in order to go to camp or visit friends overnight, waking the child during the night to go to the toilet or limiting fluids before retiring may be helpful. However, these measures should not be used as a replacement for searching for the cause. Help from a pediatric mental health professional may be needed.

The family caregiver may become extremely frustrated about having to deal with smelly, wet bedding every morning. Health care personnel must take a supportive, understanding attitude toward the problems of the caregiver and the child, allowing each of them to ventilate feelings and providing a place where emotions can be freely expressed.

Encopresis

Encopresis is the chronic involuntary fecal soiling beyond the age when control is expected (about 3 years of age). Speech and learning disabilities may accompany this problem. If there are no organic causes, (eg, worms or megacolon), encopresis indicates a serious emotional problem and the need for counseling the child and the family caregivers. It is believed that overcontrol or undercontrol by a caregiver can cause encopresis. Recommendations for treatment differ; the most important aspect, however, is recognition of the problem and referral for treatment and counseling.

Cardiovascular System Disorders

The child's cardiovascular system experiences a period of slow growth with few problems through the school-age years. The primary threat to the cardiovascular system during this age is rheumatic heart disease as a complication of rheumatic fever.

Rheumatic Fever

Rheumatic fever is a chronic disease of childhood, affecting the connective tissue of the heart, joints, lungs, and brain. An autoimmune reaction to group A beta-hemolytic streptococcal infections, rheumatic fever occurs throughout the world, particularly in the temperate zones. Rheumatic fever has become less common in developed countries, but there have been recent indications of increased occurrences in some areas of United States.

Rheumatic fever is precipitated by a streptococcal infection such as a "strep throat," tonsillitis, scarlet fever, or pharyngitis, which may be undiagnosed or untreated. The resultant rheumatic fever manifestation may be the first indication of trouble. An elevation of antistreptococcal antibodies, indicative of recent streptococcal infection, however, can be demonstrated in about 95% of the rheumatic fever patients tested within the first 2 months of onset. An antistreptolysin-O titer measures these antibodies.

Clinical Manifestations

Following the initial infection, a latent period of 1 to 5 weeks follows. The onset is frequently slow and subtle. The child may be listless, anorectic, and pale and may lose weight, complaining of vague muscle, joint, or abdominal pains. Frequently, a low-grade late afternoon fever occurs. None of these is diagnostic by itself, but if such signs persist, the child should have a medical examination.

Major manifestations of rheumatic fever are **polyarthritis**, **chorea**, and **carditis**. The onset may be acute rather than insidious, with severe carditis or arthritis as the presenting symptom. Chorea generally has an insidious onset.

Polyarthritis. Polyarthritis is a migratory arthritis that moves from one major joint to another: the ankles, knees, hips, wrists, elbows, and shoulders. The joint becomes hot, swollen, and painful to either touch or movement. Body temperature is moderately elevated; the erythrocyte sedimentation rate (ESR) is increased. Although extremely painful, this type of arthritis does not lead to the disabling deformities that occur in rheumatoid arthritis.

Chorea (Sydenham's Chorea). This manifestation involves the central nervous system. Chorea is characterized by emotional instability, purposeless movements, and muscular weakness. The onset is gradual, with increasing incoordination, facial grimaces, and repetitive involuntary movements. Movements may be mild and remain so, or they may become increasingly violent. Active arthritis is rarely present when chorea is the major manifestation. Carditis occurs, although less frequently

than when polyarthritis is the major condition. Attacks tend to be recurrent and prolonged but rare after puberty. It is seldom possible to demonstrate an increase in antistreptococcal antibody level because of the generally prolonged latency period.

Corticosteroids and salicylates are of little value in the treatment of uncomplicated chorea. Sedation with phenobarbital for relaxation or the use of medications, such as chlorpromazine (Thorazine), phenobarbital, haloperidol (Haldol), or diazepam (Valium), help relax the child. Bed rest is necessary, with protection such as padding the bed sides if the movements are severe.

Carditis. Carditis is the major cause of permanent heart damage and disability among children with rheumatic fever. Carditis may occur singly, or it may occur as a complication of either arthritis or chorea. Presenting symptoms may be vague enough to be missed. A child may have a poor appetite or pallor, perhaps a low-grade fever, listlessness, and a moderate degree of anemia. Careful observation may reveal slight dyspnea on exertion. Physical examination shows a soft systolic murmur over the apex of the heart. Unfortunately, such a child may have been in poor physical health for some time before the murmur is discovered.

Acute carditis may be the presenting symptom, particularly in young children. An abrupt onset of high fever, perhaps as high as 40°C (104°F), tachycardia, pallor, poor pulse quality, and a rapid decrease in hemoglobin are characteristic. Weakness, prostration, cyanosis, and intense precordial pain are frequently present. Cardiac dilatation usually occurs. The pericardium, the myocardium, or the endocardium may be affected.

Diagnosis

Rheumatic fever is difficult to diagnose and sometimes impossible to differentiate from other diseases. The possible serious effect of the disease demands early and conscientious medical treatment. However, caution should be taken to avoid causing apprehension and disrupt the child's life because the condition could prove to be something less serious. The nurse should not attempt a diagnosis but should understand the criteria on which a presumptive diagnosis is based.

The criteria of the modified Jones criteria is generally accepted as a useful rule for guidance when making a decision as to whether to treat the patient for rheumatic fever. The criteria are divided into major and minor categories (Figure 15-5). The presence of two major, or one major and two minor, criteria is accepted as an indication of a high probability of rheumatic fever if supported by evidence of a preceding streptococcal infection. It is not infallible because no one criterion is specific for the disease, and other additional manifestations are helpful aids toward a confirmed diagnosis.

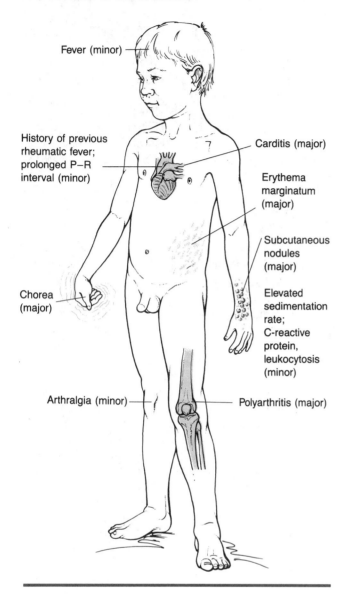

Fever (minor)

History of previous rheumatic fever; prolonged P–R interval (minor)

Carditis (major)

Erythema marginatum (major)

Subcutaneous nodules (major)

Chorea (major)

Elevated sedimentation rate; C-reactive protein, leukocytosis (minor)

Arthralgia (minor)

Polyarthritis (major)

Figure 15-5. Major and minor manifestations of rheumatic fever.

Treatment

The chief concern in caring for a child with rheumatic fever is prevention of residual heart disease. As long as the rheumatic process is active, progressive heart damage is possible. Bed rest, therefore, is essential to reduce the workload of the heart. How long the period of bed rest should last cannot be arbitrarily stated. Guidelines for bed rest are outlined in Table 15-2.

Residual heart disease is treated in accordance with its severity and its type with digitalis, restricted activities, diuretics, and a low-sodium diet as indicated.

Laboratory appraisal tests, although nonspecific, are useful for an evaluation of the activity of the disease to guide in the treatment. Two commonly used indicators are the ESR and the presence of C-reactive protein. The

ESR is elevated in the presence of an inflammatory process and is nearly always increased in the polyarthritis or in the carditis manifestations of rheumatic fever. It remains elevated until clinical manifestations have ceased and any subclinical activity has subsided. It seldom increases in uncomplicated chorea. Therefore, ESR elevation in a choreic patient may indicate cardiac involvement.

C-reactive protein is not normally present in the blood of healthy people, but it does appear in the serum of acutely ill people, including those ill with rheumatic fever. As the patient improves, C-reactive protein disappears.

Leukocytosis is also an indication of an inflammatory process. Until the leukocyte count returns to a normal level, the disease probably is still active.

Drug Therapy. Medications used in the treatment of rheumatic fever include penicillin, salicylates, and corticosteroids. Penicillin is administered to eliminate the hemolytic streptococci. If the child is allergic to penicillin, erythromycin is used. Penicillin administration continues for long-term follow-up after the acute phase of the illness to prevent the recurrence of rheumatic fever.

Salicylates are given in the form of acetylsalicylic acid (aspirin) to children, with the daily dosage calculated according to the child's weight. Aspirin provides relief of pain and reduction of inflammation of polyarteritis. It is also used for its antipyretic effect. The continued administration of a relatively large dosage may cause toxic effects because individual tolerance differs greatly.

In the presence of mild or severe carditis, corticosteroids appear to be the drug of choice because of their prompt, dramatic action. Administration of salicylates or corticosteroids is not expected to alter the course of the disease, but the control of the toxic manifestations enhances the child's comfort and sense of well being and helps reduce the burden on the heart. This is of particular importance in acute carditis with congestive heart failure. Diuretics may be administered when needed in severe carditis.

Prevention

Because rheumatic fever is a condition that has its peak of onset in school-age children, health services for this age group assume an added importance. The overall approach is to promote continuous health supervision for all children, including the school-age child. Establishment and use of well-child conferences or clinics needs to increase among school-age children to provide continuity of care. The nurse who has contact in any way with school-age children must be aware of the importance of teaching the public about the necessity to have upper respiratory infections evaluated for group A beta-hemolytic streptococcus and the need for treatment with penicillin. The nurse also should stress the necessity of taking the complete prescription of penicillin (usually 10 days' supply) even though the symptoms disappear and the child feels well.

Table 15-2. Bedrest Guidelines in Children
with Acute Rheumatic Fever

Cardiac Status	Management
No carditis	Bed rest for 2 weeks and gradual ambulation for 2 weeks even if on salicylates
Carditis, no heart enlargement	Bed rest for 4 weeks and gradual ambulation for 4 weeks
Carditis, with enlargement	Bed rest for 6 weeks and gradual ambulation for 6 weeks
Carditis, with heart failure	Strict bedrest for as long as heart failure is present and gradual ambulation for 3 months

Behrman RE, Vaughan VC (eds). Nelson's Textbook of Pediatrics, 13th ed. Philadelphia: WB Saunders, 1987.

Nursing Process for the Child with Rheumatic Fever

ASSESSMENT

The nurse must conduct a thorough evaluation of the child's physical condition, beginning with a careful review of all systems. The nurse notes any indication of signs or symptoms that may be classified as major or minor manifestations. Physical assessment includes observation for elevated temperature and pulse and careful examination of the child's body to observe for erythema marginatum, subcutaneous nodules, swollen or painful joints, or signs of chorea. A throat culture determines if there is an active infection. Obtaining a complete, up-to-date history from the child and the caregiver is also important. Careful questioning about a recent sore throat or upper respiratory infection must be included. The nurse should find out when the symptoms began, the extent of the illness, and what, if any, treatment was obtained. The school-age child is able to help contribute to the history and should be included in the nursing interview.

NURSING DIAGNOSES

The nursing diagnoses vary depending on the manifestations of rheumatic fever that the child displays. The nursing assessment helps the nurse determine the diagnoses that are appropriate. Some of the diagnoses that may be included are the following:

- Altered comfort related to **arthralgia** (painful joints)
- Diversional activity deficit related to prescribed bed rest
- High risk for injury related to choreic (chorealike) movements
- High risk for noncompliance with prophylactic drug

therapy related to financial or emotional burden of lifelong therapy
- Activity intolerance related to carditis or arthralgia
- High risk for altered health maintenance related to knowledge deficit about the condition, need for long-term therapy, and risk factors

PLANNING AND IMPLEMENTATION

The goals for the nursing care are determined in cooperation with the child and the caregiver. Throughout planning, the child's developmental stage should be considered, and implementation must be modified with this in mind.

Providing Comfort Measures and Reducing Pain. Positioning of the child to relieve joint pain is important. Large joints usually are involved, including the knees, ankles, wrists, and elbows. Careful handling of the joints when moving the child helps minimize the pain. Even the weight of blankets may cause the child pain, therefore the nurse must be alert to this possibility and improvise covering as needed. Warm baths and gentle range-of-motion exercises may help to alleviate some of the joint discomfort. A pain scale indicator can be given to the child to express the level of pain being experienced (see Figure 3-19). Salicylates are administered in the form of aspirin to reduce fever and relieve joint inflammation and pain. Because of the long-term administration of salicylates, the nurse must note any signs of toxicity and report them promptly. Tinnitus, nausea, vomiting, and headache are all important signs of toxicity. Aspirin administered after meals or with a glass of milk causes less gastrointestinal irritation. Enteric-coated aspirin is also available for patients who are sensitive to its effects. Large doses may alter the prothrombin time and thus interfere with the clotting mechanism. Salicylate therapy is usually continued until all laboratory findings are normal. The child whose pain is not well-controlled with salicylates may be administered corticosteroids. Side effects such as **hirsutism** (abnormal hair growth) and "moon face" may be upsetting to the child and family. Toxic reactions such as euphoria, insomnia, gastric irritation, and growth suppression must be watched for and reported. Because premature withdrawal of a steroid drug is likely to cause a relapse, it is gradually discontinued by decreasing dosages.

Providing Diversional Activities. Children vary greatly in how ill they feel during the acute phase of rheumatic fever. For those children who do not feel very ill, bed rest can cause distress or resentment. The nurse must be creative in finding ways in which diversional activities can be provided that adhere to the bed rest but prevent restlessness and boredom. Quiet games can provide some entertainment. Use of a computer can be beneficial to the child because both entertaining and educational games are available, and most children enjoy working with a computer. Simple needlework or model building are also diversional activities that may be useful. During the school year, efforts should be made to provide the child with a tutor and work from school that helps with boredom and also maintains a contact with peers. Care must be taken not to use the television as an all-day "babysitter." All activities should be planned with the child's developmental age in mind.

Preventing Injury. The child who has chorea may be frustrated with his or her lack of control of movements. The nurse must provide an opportunity for the child to express feelings. The child must be protected from injury by maintaining siderails up, padding siderails, not leaving a child with chorea unattended in a wheelchair, and employing all appropriate safety measures.

Promoting Compliance with Drug Therapy. A child does not become immune from future attacks of rheumatic fever after the first illness. Rheumatic fever can recur at any time a child has a group A beta-hemolytic streptococcal infection if the child is not properly treated. For this reason, the child who has had rheumatic fever must be maintained on prophylactic doses of penicillin for 5 years or longer. Anytime the child is to have oral surgery, including dental work, extra prophylactic precautions should be taken, even into adulthood. Because of this long-term therapy, noncompliance can become a problem for both financial and emotional reasons. Oral penicillin is usually prescribed, but in cases when compliance is poor, monthly injections can be substituted. Encouraging the family to contact the local chapter of the American Heart Association for help in finding economical sources of penicillin may be helpful. Other resources may be available in the individual community, and the nurse should become informed about these resources. Stressing to the child and the family the need to prevent recurrence of the disease with the danger of heart dam-

age is essential. Follow-up care must be ongoing, even into adulthood.

Providing Sensory Stimulation and Promoting Energy Conservation. The pain of arthralgia may be so great that the child will not want to be involved in any kind of activity. Administration of analgesics helps decrease the inflammation of the joints and decrease the pain. Providing rest periods for the child between activities helps pace the child's energies and provide for maximum comfort. During times of increased cardiac involvement or exacerbations of joint pain, the child may want to rest and perhaps have someone read a story. This may be a good time to choose a book that involves the child's imagination and that has enough excitement to create ongoing interest. Peers may be encouraged to visit, but these visits must be monitored so that the child is not overly tired. A school classroom could be encouraged to write to the child to provide contact with everyday school activities and keep the child in touch. If the child has chorea, visitors need to be informed that the child is not able to control these movements and that the unexpected movements are as upsetting to the child as to others.

Providing Family Teaching. The family and child should be informed about the importance of having all upper respiratory infections checked by a health care provider to prevent another bout of a streptococcal infection. The nurse must be certain that they understand that the child can have recurrences and that a future recurrence could have much more serious effects. If the child has had carditis and heart damage has occurred, the child must be regularly followed to evaluate the damage. The child may need to be maintained on cardiac medications, about which the family will need full information. Mitral valve dysfunction is a common aftereffect of severe carditis. A girl who has had mitral valve damage from cardiac involvement may have problems in adulthood during pregnancy. She should be informed that heart failure is a possibility during pregnancy and be given the option to have a mitral valve replacement if needed.

The nurse has an excellent opportunity to stress the importance of prevention of rheumatic fever during teaching. There may be other children in the family who will benefit from the caregivers having this information.

EVALUATION

- Child voices that his or her pain level is bearable, using a pain scale to express degree of pain
- Child is involved in age-appropriate activities
- Child remains free of injury
- Child and family voice understanding of the importance of prophylactic medication and identify means for obtaining the medication
- Child rests quietly during rest periods and is actively involved in diversional therapy

■ Child and family voice understanding of need for follow-up care and indicate how they will obtain it

Endocrine System Disorders

Diabetes mellitus is the most significant endocrine disorder that affects children of school age. Other conditions that may affect school children are disorders of the pituitary gland that alter the growth of children and diabetes insipidus. The incidence of these latter conditions is low.

Juvenile Diabetes Mellitus (Insulin-Dependent Diabetes Mellitus)

At least 10 to 12 million Americans have been diagnosed with diabetes; a significant number of these are children. Although specific statistics are not available, it is estimated that diabetes mellitus affects 1 in 600 children between the ages of 5 and 15 years. Incidence of this condition continues to increase.

Diabetes is often considered an adult disease, but at least 5% of cases begin in childhood, with the greatest incidence at approximately 6 years of age and around the time of puberty. Management of diabetes in children is different from adults and requires conscientious care that is geared specifically to the developmental stage of the child.

Classification of diabetes includes two major types: type 1 insulin-dependent diabetes mellitus (IDDM) and type 2 non–insulin dependent diabetes mellitus (NIDDM). As noted in Table 15-3, diabetes in children is type 1 (IDDM).

Pathogenesis

The exact pathophysiology of diabetes is not completely understood; however, it is known to result from dysfunction of the beta (insulin-secreting) cells of the islets of Langerhans in the pancreas. It is believed that the presence of an acute infection during childhood may trigger a mechanism in genetically susceptible children, activating beta-cell dysfunction, thus disrupting insulin secretion. Other conditions that may contribute to IDDM are pancreatic tumors, pancreatitis, and long-term corticosteroid use.

Table 15-3. Comparison of Type 1 and Type 2 Diabetes

Assessment	Type 1 (Insulin Dependent)	Type 2 (Noninsulin Dependent)
Age of onset	5–7 y or at puberty	40–65 y
Type of onset	Abrupt	Gradual
Weight changes	Marked weight loss is often initial sign	Associated with obesity
Other symptoms	Polydipsia	Polydipsia
	Polyuria (often begins as bed-wetting)	Polyuria
	Fatigue (marks fall in school)	Fatigue
	Blurred vision (marks fall in school)	Blurred vision
	Glycosuria	Glycosuria
	Polyphagia	
	Pruritus	Pruritus
	Mood changes (may cause behavior problems in school)	Mood changes
Therapy	Hypoglycemia agents never effective; insulin must be administered	Managed by insulin injection or diet alone; oral hypoglycemic agents a possibility
	Diet only moderately restricted; no dietary foods used	Diet tends to be strict
	Common-sense foot care for growing children	Good skin and foot care necessary
Period of remission	Period of remission for 1–12 mo generally follows initial diagnosis	Not demonstrable

Adapted from Pillitteri A. Maternal and Child Health Nursing. Philadelphia: JB Lippincott, 1992, p. 1529.

Normally, the sugar derived from digestion and assimilation of foods is burned to provide energy for the body's activities. Excess sugar is converted into fat or glycogen and stored in the body tissues. Insulin, a hormone secreted by the pancreas, is responsible for the burning and storing of sugar. In diabetes, the secretion of insulin is inadequate or nonexistent, allowing sugar to accumulate in the blood stream and spill over into the urine. In children, diabetes causes an abrupt, pronounced decrease in insulin production, resulting in decreased ability to derive energy from the food eaten. Large amounts of protein and fat are used to supply the energy needs of the child, causing loss of weight and slowed growth. This combination of failure to gain weight and lack of energy may be the initial reason the child is brought to the attention of the health care provider. However, the child may not be seen by a health care provider until symptoms of acidosis are evident.

Clinical Manifestations

Classic symptoms of diabetes mellitus are **polyuria** (dramatic increase in urinary output, probably with enuresis), **polydipsia** (abnormal thirst), and **polyphagia** (increased food consumption). These symptoms are usually accompanied by weight loss or failure to gain weight and lack of energy. Symptoms of diabetes in children often have an abrupt onset.

If the child's symptoms are not noted and referred for diagnosis, the disorder is likely to progress to diabetic acidosis and eventually to diabetic coma.

Because of inadequate insulin production, carbohydrates are not converted into fuel for energy production. Fats are then mobilized for energy, but, in the absence of glucose, are incompletely oxidized. Ketone bodies (acetone, diacetic acid, and oxybutyric acid) accumulate. They are readily excreted in the urine, but in this excretion the acid–base balance of body fluids is upset, resulting in acidosis.

Diabetic acidosis is characterized by drowsiness, dry skin, flushed cheeks and cherry red lips, acetone breath with a fruity smell, and **Kussmaul breathing** (abnormal increase in the depth and rate of the respiratory movements). Nausea and vomiting may occur. If untreated, the child lapses into coma and exhibits dehydration, electrolyte imbalance, rapid pulse, and subnormal temperature and blood pressure.

Treatment for acidosis includes keeping the patient warm. The child needs skilled nursing care and may be admitted to a pediatric intensive care unit, if available. Blood and urine are tested to evaluate the degree of acidosis. If the child is unable to urinate, a catheter is inserted. Gastric lavage may be performed to relieve abdominal distention and eliminate the danger of aspiration. Regular insulin is given intravenously along with intravenous electrolyte fluids.

Diagnosis

Early detection and control are of critical importance in postponing or minimizing later complications of diabetes. The nurse should observe carefully for any signs or symptoms in all members of a family that has a history of diabetes. The family also should be taught to observe the children for frequent thirst, urination, and weight loss. All relatives of diabetics are considered a high-risk group and should have periodic testing.

Children who have a family history of diabetes should be monitored by fingerstick glucose monitoring or dipstick testing for glycosuria at each visit to a health care provider. If the blood glucose level is elevated or glycosuria is present, a fasting blood sugar (FBS) is performed. An FBS of 200 mg/gL or higher almost certainly is diagnostic for diabetes when other signs such as polyuria and weight loss despite polyphagia are present. Although glucose tolerance tests are performed in adults to confirm diabetes, they are not commonly used in children. The traditional oral glucose tolerance test is often unsuccessful with children because they may vomit the concentrated glucose that must be swallowed.

Treatment

Management of diabetes in children includes insulin therapy, a meal plan, and an exercise plan. Treatment of the diabetic child involves the family and child and a number of health team members, such as the nurse, the pediatrician, the nutritionist, and the diabetic nurse educator. After diabetes is diagnosed, the child is usually hospitalized for a period to stabilize the condition under supervision. The nurse must remember that this is a trying time for all and plan care with an understanding of the emotional impact of the diagnosis. Plans need to be made to inform the child's school teacher, school nurse, and others who are involved in supervising the child during daily activities.

Insulin. Insulin therapy is an essential part of the treatment of diabetes in children. The dosage of insulin is based on monitoring of blood glucose levels so that the child's levels are maintained near normal. Two kinds of insulin are often combined for the best results. Insulin can be grouped into rapid acting, intermediate acting, and long acting (Table 15-4). An intermediate-acting and a rapid-acting insulin often are given together. Some preparations come in a premixed proportion of 70% intermediate-acting and 30% rapid-acting insulins that eliminates the need for mixing insulins.

Insulin reaction (insulin shock, hypoglycemia) is caused by insulin overload, resulting in too rapid metabolism of the body's glucose. This may be due to a change in the body's requirement; carelessness in diet, such as failure to eat proper amounts of food; an error in insulin measurement; or excessive exercise. Because diabetes in children is very labile (unstable, fluctuating), the child is

Table 15-4. Types of Insulin: Onset, Peak, Duration

Action	Preparation	Onset	Peak	Duration
Rapid Acting	Regular iletin Pork, beef	½–1 h	2–4 h	6–8 h
	Humulin R Human (Lilley)	½–1 h	2–4 h	6–8 h
	Novolin Human (Squibb)	½ h	2½–5 h	8 h
	Semilente	½–1 h	5–10 h	12–16 h
Intermediate Acting	NPH Pork, beef	1½–2 h	6–12 h	24 h
	Humulin N Human (Lilley)	1–2 h	6–12 h	18–24 h
	Novolin N Human (Squibb)	1½ h	4–12 h	24 h
	Lente Beef, pork	2–4 h	6–12 h	18–26 h
	Humulin 70/30 70% N, 30% R	½ h	4–8 h	24 h
	Novolin 70/30 70% N, 30% R	½ h	4–8 h	24 h
Long Acting	Protamine zinc Beef, pork	4–8 h	14–24 h	28–36 h
	Ultralente Beef, pork	4–8 h	14–24 h	28–36 h

subject to insulin reactions. Some of the symptoms of impending insulin shock in children are any type of odd, unusual, or antisocial behavior, headache and malaise, blurred vision and faintness, and undue fatigue or hunger. Frequently, children have hypoglycemic reactions during the early morning hours. The nurse must observe the child at least every 2 hours during the night, note the tossed bedding that would indicate restlessness, note any excessive perspiration, and if necessary, try to arouse the child. As the child becomes regulated and observes a careful diet at home, parents need not watch so closely but should have a thorough understanding of all aspects of this condition. Often, blood glucose monitoring is scheduled for this early morning time, especially while the child is hospitalized.

Treatment of insulin reaction should be immediate, allowing the child to take sugar, candy, orange juice, or one of the commercial products designed for this emergency. Repeated or impending reactions require consultation with the physician.

If the child is unable to take a sugar source orally, glucagon should be administered subcutaneously to bring about a prompt increase in blood glucose level. Every adult responsible for a diabetic child should clearly understand the procedure for administering this drug and should have easy access to it. Glucagon is a hormone produced by alpha cells of the pancreatic islets. An elevation in the blood glucose level results in an insulin release (in a normal person), but a decrease in the blood glucose level stimulates glucagon release. The released glucagon in the blood stream acts on the liver to promote glycogen breakdown and glucose release.

Glucagon is available as a pharmaceutical product, packaged as a powder in individual dose units. A person preparing the dose need only add the diluent, which comes with the powdered drug, by using a sterile syringe and needle. The solution is then drawn up into the syringe and administered in the same manner as insulin.

Glucagon acts within minutes to restore a child to consciousness, after which the child can take candy or sugar. This treatment prevents the long delay in waiting for a physician to come and administer glucose intravenously or for an ambulance to reach the hospital emergency department. It is, however, one form of emergency treatment and not a substitute for proper medical supervision.

Insulin Regimen. Most newly diagnosed diabetic children show a decreased need for insulin during the first weeks or months after control is established. This is often referred to as the "honeymoon period," and it should be explained to the family in advance to avoid the false hope that the child is "getting better." As the child grows, the need for insulin increases and continues to do so until the child reaches full growth. Again, this needs to be explained; the child's condition is not getting worse.

Methods of Giving Insulin. The child may not be able to take over the management of the insulin dose as early as blood glucose monitoring but can watch the preparation of the syringe and learn the technique for drawing up the dosage. Encouraging the child to watch until it becomes routine may be helpful. By 8 or 9 years of age, the child should be thinking out the dose and getting the feel of the syringe. The child also may draw up the dose and prepare for self-administration. Just when that is possible cannot be stated arbitrarily. There are automatic injection devices that can help the child self-administer insulin at a younger age. No two children mature at the same rate; some may be able to do this much earlier than others. The child should be encouraged, however, to take over the management of the therapy when ready. The child can learn the importance of the routine and accept the restrictions the disease imposes if encouraged to help make the decisions.

Insulin Pumps. An insulin pump is a method of continuous insulin administration that is useful for some diabetics. The pump is about the size of a transistor radio and can be worn strapped to the waist or on a shoulder strap. It delivers a steady low dose of insulin through a syringe housed in the pump and connected by polyethylene tubing to a small-gauge subcutaneous needle implanted in the abdomen. Extra insulin is released at mealtimes and other times when needed by pressing a button. The pump does not sense the blood glucose level, therefore careful blood glucose monitoring is necessary to adjust the dosage as needed. The pump must be removed to bathe, go swimming, or shower. Because the pump is always present, the child may want to wear loose clothing that will hide it. The needle site must be regularly observed for redness and irritation.

Unique Needs of the Adolescent. Adolescence is an extremely trying period for many diabetics, as it is for other young people. Just as a normal adolescent has to work through from dependence to independence, so does the diabetic. Even when an adolescent has accepted responsibility for self-care, it is not unusual to see the adolescent rebel against the control that this condition demands, become impatient, and appear to ignore future health. The adolescent may skip meals, drop diet controls, or neglect glucose monitoring. Going barefoot and neglecting proper foot care also can cause problems for the diabetic adolescent. It can be a difficult time for both the family and the adolescent. The caregivers naturally become concerned and are apt to give the adolescent more controls to rebel against. Special care should be taken by the family, teachers, nurses, and physicians to see that these young people find enough maturing satisfaction in other areas and do not need to rebel in this vital area.

The adolescent who completely understands all aspects of the condition (especially if allowed to assume control of treatment previously) should be allowed to continue. Should the adolescent run into difficulty, this is a time when an adolescent clinic can be of great value. In this area the adolescent can discuss problems with understanding people who respond with care, providing dignity and attentive listening.

Nursing Process for the Child with Diabetes Mellitus

ASSESSMENT

Nursing assessment of the child with diabetes includes an interview with the child's family caregiver to discover the signs and symptoms that the child had leading up to the present illness. The caregiver should be asked about the child's appetite, weight loss or gain, evidence of polyuria or enuresis in a previously toilet-trained child, polydipsia, dehydration that may include constipation, irritability, and fatigue. The child should be included in the interview and encouraged to contribute information. An assessment of the child's developmental stage is necessary to determine appropriate nursing diagnoses and plan effective care (Table 15-5). If the child is first seen in diabetic coma, the nursing assessment needs to be adjusted initially.

Physical assessment of the child includes measurement of height and weight and examination of skin for evidence of dryness or slowly healing sores; signs of hyperglycemia must be noted, vital signs should be recorded, and a urine specimen collected. A blood glucose level using a bedside glucose monitor provides useful information.

NURSING DIAGNOSES

Nursing diagnoses should be based on the nursing assessment with adjustments for the child's developmental stage and may include the following:

- High risk for injury related to excess carbohydrate intake
- Health-seeking behaviors related to home management of hypoglycemia and hyperglycemia
- Anxiety of child and caregiver related to insulin administration
- Altered nutrition, less than body requirements related to decrease in insulin production
- High risk for infection related to circulatory or sensory impairment
- Anxiety of child and caregiver related to diagnosis of diabetes and complications

Table 15-5. Developmental Guidelines for Diabetic Child Responsibilities*

Issues	Under 4	4–5	6–7	8–10	11–13	14+
				Age (yr)		
Food	Teaching focuses on parents	Knows likes and dislikes	Can begin to tell sugar content of food and know foods they should *not* have	Has more ability to select foods according to criteria—like exchange lists	Knows if foods fit own diet plan	Helps plan meals and snacks
Insulin	Parents take responsibility for care	Can tell where injection should be. Can pinch the skin	Can begin to help with aspects of injections	Gives own injections with supervision	Can learn to measure insulin	Can mix two insulins
Testing		Can choose finger for fingerstick. Can wash finger with soap and water. Collects urine; should watch caregiver do testing; helps with recording	Can do own fingerstick using automatic puncture device. Can help with some aspects of the blood test. Can do own urine test and record results	Can do blood tests with supervision	Can see test results forming a pattern	Can begin to use test results to adjust insulin
Psychological		Identifies with being "bad" or "good"—these words should be avoided. A child this age may think he or she is bad if the test is said to be "bad"	Needs many reminders and supervision	Needs reminders and supervision. Understands only immediate consequences, not long-term consequences, of diabetes control. "Scientific" mind developing—intrigued by tests	May be somewhat rebellious Concerned with being "different"	Understands long-term consequences of actions including diabetes control Independence and self-image are important Rebellion continues and some supervision and continued support is still needed

*These are only guidelines. Each child is an individual. Talk to your health care provider about any concerns you may have.

Adapted from Hess V. Diabetes: Stuff and More Stuff. Lincoln, NE: HERC Publishing, 1989.

- Altered self-concept related to chronic illness, insulin dependency

PLANNING AND IMPLEMENTATION

Preventing Injury. The child who is admitted to the hospital with diabetes may be newly diagnosed or may be experiencing an unstable episode as a result of illness or changing needs. The child's blood glucose level must be monitored to be maintained within normal limits. The blood glucose level should be assessed at least in the morning before breakfast and before the evening meal by means of bedside glucose monitoring. On initial diagnosis of diabetes, until some stability is achieved, the child's blood glucose level may be assessed as often as every 4 hours. Because this procedure involves a fingerstick, the child may object and resist this testing. The nurse needs to offer encouragement and support, helping the child to express fears and acknowledging that the fingerstick does hurt and it is acceptable to express dislike for it. The nurse needs to consider the child's developmental stage when performing the testing. School-age children can be involved in much of the process. The child can choose the finger to be used and clean it off with soap and water. Automatic-release instruments make it easier for the child to do the fingerstick. The child can be taught to read results and learn the desired ranges of blood glucose level. School-age children are in the stage of industry versus inferiority and usually are interested in learning new information. The nurse can appeal to this developmental characteristic to gain the child's cooperation.

The child must be monitored at least every 4 hours for signs of hyperglycemia or hypoglycemia (see Parent Teaching: Signs of Hyperglycemia and Hypoglycemia). If the blood glucose level is higher than 240 mg/dL, the urine may be tested for ketones. The nurse should be aware of the most probable times for an increase or decrease in blood glucose level in relation to the insulin the child is receiving. Regular monitoring of the blood glucose level is necessary to detect either hyperglycemia or hypoglycemia.

Providing Family Teaching on Monitoring of Blood Glucose Levels. Regular monitoring of the blood glucose level is necessary to detect either hyperglycemia or hypoglycemia. The child and the caregiver must be taught the signs of both hyperglycemia and hypoglycemia and be prepared to take the appropriate action, if necessary. They must be alert to signs of hypoglycemia, especially at times when insulin is at peak action (see Table 15-4). Blood glucose levels lower than 60 mg/dL should be treated with juice, sugar, or nondiet soda. If the blood glucose level cannot be checked promptly, the child should still consume a simple carbohydrate. If the child is unable to swallow, glucagon or dextrose should be administered following orders of the physician. Glucagon is commercially available and can be administered intramuscularly. The child's caregiver should be taught how to mix and administer glucagon. The child and the family caregiver should be taught the signs that indicate hypoglycemia. The child should be taught to get help immediately when signs of hypoglycemia occur and to carry and take sugar cubes, Lifesavers, gumdrops, or a small tube of cake frosting. The reaction should be followed with a snack of a complex carbohydrate, such as crackers, and a protein, such as cheese, peanut butter, or half of a meat sandwich. The snack is needed to maintain the increase in blood glucose level created by the simple carbohydrates and prevent another hypoglycemic reaction.

The caregiver and the child can be reassured that hypoglycemia is much more apt to occur than hyperglycemia. If there is any doubt as to whether the child is having a hypoglycemic or a hyperglycemic reaction, the safer plan is to treat as though it is hypoglycemia. A record should be kept of the hypoglycemic reactions to determine if there is a pattern and if an adjustment needs to be made to the child's insulin schedule or food plan. Periods of exercise have a decreasing effect on the child's blood glucose level because the carbohydrates are being burned for energy. Adjustments should be made to the child's therapeutic program to allow for this increase in energy requirements to avoid hypoglycemia. Adjustments also may need to be made in the child's school schedule. For instance, physical education should never be scheduled right before lunch for a diabetic child. Also, the diabetic child should not be scheduled for a late lunch period at school.

Many children are subject to minor infections and illnesses throughout the school years with little long-term effect. However, the diabetic child is more susceptible to long-term complications. When the diabetic child has an infection and fever, the temperature and metabolic rate increases, the body needs more sugar and therefore more insulin to make the sugar available to the body. Although a child may not be eating because of vomiting or anorexia, the body's insulin needs continue. Insulin should never be skipped during illness. Blood glucose levels should be checked every 2 to 4 hours during this time. Fluids need to be increased. The physician should be

---

Parent Teaching

Signs of Hyperglycemia and Hypoglycemia

Signs of Hyperglycemia
- Polyphagia (excessive hunger)
- Polyuria (excessive urination)
- Dry mucous membranes
- Poor skin turgor
- Lethargy
- Change in level of consciousness

Signs of Hypoglycemia
- Shaking
- Irritability
- Hunger
- Diaphoresis
- Dizziness
- Drowsiness
- Pallor
- Changed level of consciousness
- Feeling "strange"

contacted when the child becomes ill, especially if the child is vomiting, cannot eat, or has diarrhea, so that close supervision can be maintained. Guidelines for care of an ill child should be given to the caregiver with the initial diabetic instructions.

It is extremely important that the child wear a Medic Alert identification medal or a bracelet, with information about diabetic status. Identification cards, such as those carried by many adult diabetics, are seldom practical for a child.

Providing Family Teaching on Insulin Administration. The family caregiver and the child are taught the correct way to give insulin and are supervised until it is certain that they are measuring and injecting the insulin correctly. Disposable syringes make caring for equipment relatively easy. A doll may be used to practice the actual administration until the caregiver (and child, if age appropriate) is comfortable and confident. Direct supervision must be given until proficiency is demonstrated. The nurse should recognize that this part of the treatment is probably the most threatening aspect of the illness. Perhaps the nurse may do well to remember personal feelings at the time of the first injection administered while in nursing school. A great deal of empathy and warm support are needed by the child and family.

Rotating injection sites is also a matter of considerable importance. If insulin is given frequently in the same location, the area is apt to become indurated and is eventually fibrosed, hindering proper insulin absorption. The atrophic hollows in the skin, or the lumps of hypertrophied tissue, are unsightly as well. Some people, however, appear to have a greater skin sensitivity than others.

Clear instructions should be given concerning the importance of rotating sites (Figure 15-6). Areas on both the upper arms, upper thighs, abdomen, and buttocks can be used, allowing several weeks between the use of the same site, if a plan is carefully mapped out. Starting from the inner, upper corner of the area, each injection is given 1/2 inch below the preceding one, going down in a vertical line, with the next series starting 1/2 inch outward at the upper level. If there is any sign of induration, the local site should be carefully avoided for weeks after all signs of irritation have disappeared. A chart recording the sites used and the rotation schedule is helpful and recommended.

Assuring Adequate and Appropriate Nutrition. The child with diabetes needs to have a sound nutritional program that provides adequate nutrition for normal growth while it maintains the blood glucose at near normal levels. The food plan should be well balanced with food choices that take into consideration the food preferences, cultural customs, and lifestyle of the child (see Parent Teaching: Child's Diabetic Food Plan). The child and caregiver need to understand the importance of eating regularly scheduled meals. Special occasions can be planned so that the child does not feel left out of celebrations. If a particular

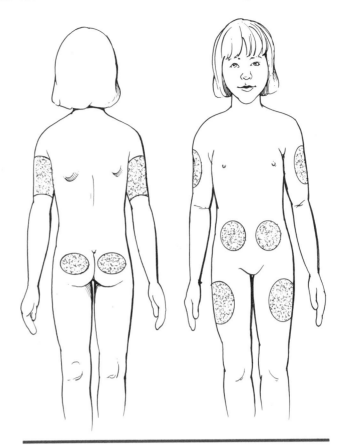

Figure 15-6. Subcutaneous injection sites. (From Castiglia PT, Harbin RE. Child Health Care. Philadelphia: JB Lippincott, 1992, p. 904.)

meal is going to be late, the child should have a complex carbohydrate and protein snack. Children need to be included in meal planning when possible so that they learn what is permissible and what is not. In this way they will be able to handle eating when they are on their own in school and in social situations.

Preventing Infection and Skin Breakdown. Skin breakdowns, such as blisters and minor cuts, can become major problems for the diabetic child. The caregiver and child should be taught to inspect the child's skin daily and promptly treat even small breaks in the skin. Daily bathing should be encouraged. The skin should be dried well after bathing, with careful attention given to any area where skin touches skin, such as the groin, axilla, or other skin folds. Good foot care should be emphasized. This includes wearing well-fitting shoes, inspecting between toes for cracks, trimming nails straight across, wearing clean socks, and not going barefoot. Establishing these habits early will help the child prepare for lifelong care of diabetes.

Diabetic children may be more susceptible to urinary tract and upper respiratory infections. The child and caregiver should be taught to be alert for signs of urinary tract

Parent Teaching

Child's Diabetic Food Plan

1. Plan well-balanced meals that are appealing to your child.

2. Be positive with child when talking about foods that child can eat; downplay the negatives.

3. Space three meals and three snacks throughout the day. Daily caloric intake is divided to provide 20% at breakfast, 20% at lunch, 30% at dinner, and 10% at each of the snacks.

4. Calories should be made up of 50%–60% carbohydrates, 15%–20% protein, and no more than 30% fat.

5. Avoid concentrated sweets such as jelly, syrup, pie, candy bars, and soda pop.

6. Artificial sweeteners may be used.

7. Child must not skip meals. Make every effort to plan meals with foods that child likes.

8. Include foods that contain dietary fiber, such as whole grains, cereals, fruits and vegetables, nuts, seeds and legumes. Fiber helps prevent hyperglycemia.

9. Dietetic food is expensive and not necessary.

10. Teach your child day by day about the food plan to encourage independence in food selections when at school or away from home.

infection, such as itching and burning on urination. Signs of urinary tract or upper respiratory infections should be reported to the physician promptly.

Reducing Child and Family Anxiety. When the diagnosis of diabetes is confirmed, the family caregiver may feel devastated. A young child will not understand the implications, but the school-age or adolescent child will experience a great amount of fear and anxiety. The caregiver may have feelings of guilt, resentment, or denial. Other family members also may experience strong feelings about the illness. All of these feelings and concerns must be recognized and resolved to work successfully with the diabetic child. The nurse needs to encourage the family to express feelings and fears. Involving the caregiver in caring for the child during hospitalization may be helpful. Questions are carefully listened to and answered completely and honestly. Many materials are available to give to the caregiver to read; the nurse must be sure that the caregiver is able to read and understand these materials. Videos are also available that are helpful in education of the diabetic and the family. The nurse can recommend community support groups that

are available. Home care must be covered in detail. The family caregiver also needs a support person to contact when questions arise after discharge. Because so much information must be absorbed in a brief time, they may seem forgetful or confused. Careful, patient repetition of all aspects of diabetes and the child's care is necessary. When anxiety levels are high, information is often heard but not digested. Giving them as much written material in a form that they can easily understand is necessary. Having them repeat information is helpful, and asking them questions to confirm that they understand is also useful.

Promoting Self-Care and Positive Self-Concept. The school-age or older child may experience some strong feelings of inadequacy or being "sick." These feelings must be expressed and dealt with. Teaching the child as much as is age appropriate helps allay some of the fears. Telling the child about athletes and other famous people who are diabetic can be encouraging. When possible, another child who is diabetic may visit so that the child does not feel so alone. The child must be encouraged to become active in helping with self-care. Questions need to be answered concerning how diabetes affects the activities in which the child is involved. Summer camps for children with diabetes are available in many areas and can serve to develop the child's self-assurance.

The diabetic child can participate in normal activities. However, at least one friend should be told about the diabetic condition, and the child should not go swimming or hiking without a responsible person nearby who knows what to look for and what to do if the child should have a reaction.

Some older children are sensitive about their condition and fear that they seem "different" from their friends. Even with the best instruction and preparation, they may feel this way and wish to keep their condition secret. They must understand that a teacher or some other adult in their environment must be acquainted with their condition. Classroom teachers need to know which of their students have such a condition and should understand the signs of an impending reaction.

Diabetic children under good control need not be kept from such activities as campouts, overnight trips with the school band, or other similar activities away from home. Of course, these children must be capable of measuring their insulin and giving their own injections. Some young people may find that a desire to participate in such an activity can be the factor that helps them overcome reluctance to measure and administer their own insulin. See nursing care plan for the child with diabetes mellitus.

EVALUATION

- Child's blood glucose level within normal limits, urine negative for acetone, no signs or symptoms of hyperglycemia

Nursing Care Plan
for the Child with Diabetes Mellitus

Nursing Diagnosis
Altered nutrition, less than body requirements related to decrease in insulin production

Goal: Assure adequate and appropriate nutrition

Nursing Interventions	*Rationale*	*Evaluation*
Emphasize the importance of following the prescribed nutritional program, explaining why it is necessary and stressing the need for well-balanced meals eaten at regular intervals; teach how to improvise with a complex carbohydrate and protein snack if meals are delayed.	If the parents and child understand the disease and the relationship of food to blood glucose, they will be in a better position to make well informed decisions about the child's diet in different situations.	Child eats food at meals and snack times; child and/or caregiver demonstrate understanding of the food plan by making appropriate menu selections.
Help child and family plan diet for home, school, and restaurant settings.	Planning diet options for settings other than home will encourage the family to help their child to lead a normal active life. Including the child in meal planning will prepare the child for independent decision-making about food choices when away from the family.	

Nursing Diagnosis
High risk for infection related to circulatory/sensory impairment with diabetes mellitus

Goal: Prevent infection

Nursing Interventions	*Rationale*	*Evaluation*
Teach caregiver and child to inspect skin daily and promptly treat even small breaks in the skin.	Infections occur more frequently in the diabetic child. In addition, decreased circulation may lead to more frequent skin breakdown, especially in the feet.	No signs and symptoms of infection, skin clear and intact; child and/or caregiver demonstrate skin inspection and care, discuss importance of promptly reporting infections.
Teach careful skin hygiene, with an emphasis on foot care.	Teaching good habits early in the child's life will help to prepare the child for lifelong care of diabetes. Diabetics are at a high risk for foot problems, therefore daily foot care is essential.	
Teach child and caregiver to be alert for signs of urinary infection and to report these or signs of respiratory infection to physician promptly.	Bacterial and fungal infections are more frequent in diabetics than in nondiabetics, and they can become more severe if not promptly treated.	

(continued)

Nursing Care Plan
for the Child with Diabetes Mellitus (Continued)

Nursing Diagnosis
Caregiver anxiety related to diagnosis of diabetes in child

Goal: *Reduce caregiver anxiety*

Nursing Interventions	Rationale	Evaluation
Encourage the family to express feelings and fears about diabetes and what it may be like to have a child with a chronic illness.	Helps the caregivers begin to cope with the diagnosis.	Child and/or caregivers talk about fears and anxieties related to diabetes.

Nursing Diagnosis
Altered self-concept related to chronic illness

Goal: *Promote positive self-concept in child*

Nursing Interventions	Rationale	Evaluation
Encourage the child to become active in selfcare.	Gives the child some control over the illness.	As appropriate for age, child discusses adjustments to daily schedule and activities; names several people to inform about diabetic condition.
Teach the child and parent that the child can engage in normal activities, including overnight trips away, as long as they or a responsible adult, is able to measure and give the injections.	Assures the child that activities don't need to stop because of their illness. May motivate the child to take responsibility for self-care.	

Nursing Diagnosis
Health-seeking behaviors related to home management of hypoglycemia and hyperglycemia

Goal: *Provide family teaching*

Nursing Interventions	Rationale	Evaluation
Provide information in small doses, with written back-up, in a form caregivers can easily understand. Ask caregivers to repeat information or ask them questions about what you have taught.	Information may be heard, but not digested, when anxiety levels are high.	Child and/or caregiver(s) discuss diabetes, its physiology and treatment; list signs and symptoms of hyperglycemia and hypoglycemia and how to handle each; ask questions to clarify information; and clearly discuss home care.
Teach child and caregiver the signs of hyperglycemia and hypoglycemia and appropriate actions for each. Discuss the effects of exercise and routine childhood illnesses on the child's blood sugar and adjustments	Both caregivers and child need the same information. Information needs to address the normal activities the child is likely to engage in during school so that the	

(continued)

Nursing Care Plan
for the Child with Diabetes Mellitus (Continued)

Nursing Interventions	Rationale	Evaluation
that may need to be made in therapeutic plan.	family can feel prepared and confident about their ability to handle changes in their child's metabolism.	
Teach the correct way to give insulin and supervise until you are certain that the procedure is being done correctly. Teach about the rotation of injection sites.	Giving injections may be the most threatening part of the illness to the child or family. Patience and practice will go far in helping the family gain confidence in this aspect of their child's care.	Caregiver or child or both demonstrates insulin injection technique, identifies injection sites, and demonstrates knowledge about choosing sites and rotation schedule.
Stress importance of child's wearing of Medic Alert identification medal or bracelet.	Children are often reluctant to wear a bracelet advertising their illness. However, both child and family will feel more confident that appropriate care will be given in an emergency if the child is wearing something that identifies her or him as having diabetes.	

- Child's blood glucose level higher than 60 mg/dL, no signs or symptoms of hypoglycemia; prompt response to any hypoglycemic reaction
- Child or caregiver, or both, discuss diabetes, its physiology and treatment; lists signs and symptoms of hyperglycemia and hypoglycemia and how to handle each; asks questions to clarify information; and clearly discusses home care
- Child eats food at meals and snack times; child or caregiver, or both, demonstrate understanding of the food plan by making appropriate menu selections
- No signs and symptoms of infection, skin clear and intact; child or caregiver, or both, demonstrate skin inspection and care, discuss importance of promptly reporting infections
- Child or caregiver, or both, express fears and anxieties and participate in hospital care and planning for home care
- As appropriate for age, child discusses adjustments to daily schedule and activities; names several people to inform about diabetic condition

Musculoskeletal System

The long bones of the extremities grow rapidly during the school-age period. "Growing pains" are a frequent complaint of this stage but rarely indicate serious disease. School age is a time of increasing physical activity, including team sports. Peer approval and group or team participation at school and in after-school activities are important to the school-age child. Minor skeletal injuries, such as sprains and minor fractures, may make the child a temporary celebrity. However, a serious skeletal defect or injury may influence the child's ability to cope with peer relationships and create social adjustment problems.

Scoliosis

Scoliosis is a lateral curvature of the spine that appears more frequently in young girls during the rapid growth period before puberty. It occurs in two forms, structural and nonstructural (functional), the latter being the more common. Structural scoliosis is caused by rotated and malformed vertebrae. Nonstructural scoliosis can have several causes: poor posture, muscle spasm due to trauma, or unequal length of legs. When the primary problem is corrected, elimination of the functional scoliosis has begun.

Most cases of structural scoliosis are idiopathic (no known cause); a few are caused by congenital deformities or infection. Although mild curves occur as frequently in boys as in girls, idiopathic scoliosis requiring treatment occurs eight times more frequently in girls than in boys.[3]

During examination, the undressed child is observed from a posterior view, and any lateral curvature is noted. The examiner then should have the child bend at the hips (ask the child to touch toes) and observe the child for prominence of the scapula on one side (Figure 15-7). Many states require regular examination of students for scoliosis beginning in the fifth or sixth grade. A school nurse may do the initial screening. Idiopathic scoliosis is seen in late school age at 10 years and older. Curvatures of less than 25 degrees are observed closely but not treated. Curvatures between 25 and 40 degrees are corrected with electrical stimulation or a Milwaukee brace, and those more than 40 degrees are usually corrected surgically.

Treatment is by application of electrical stimulation, braces, traction, casts, and spinal fusion, which may include internal fixation with rods. Treatment is long term and lasts usually through the remainder of the child's growth cycle. The brace most commonly used is the Milwaukee brace, which exerts pressure on certain areas to maintain correct posture or immobilization.

Electrical Stimulation

Electrical stimulation may be used as an alternate to bracing for the child with a mild to moderate curvature. These electrodes may be applied to the skin or surgically implanted. Treatment takes place at night during the child's sleeping hours. The leads are placed to stimulate muscles on the convex side of the curvature to contract as impulses are transmitted. This causes the spine to straighten. If external electrodes are used, the skin under the leads must be checked regularly for irritation. This treatment is the least disruptive to the child's life.

Braces

The Milwaukee brace (Figure 15-8) is considered the most effective spinal brace for treatment of scoliosis. It exerts lateral pressure and longitudinal traction, thus achieving vertical alignment. The brace does not correct the existing curvature but serves to prevent further progression of the curve.

The brace should be worn constantly, except during bathing or swimming. It should be worn over a T-shirt or undershirt to protect the child's skin and the leather of the brace. The throat mold of the brace can be covered with soft cloth if sweating or irritation occurs.

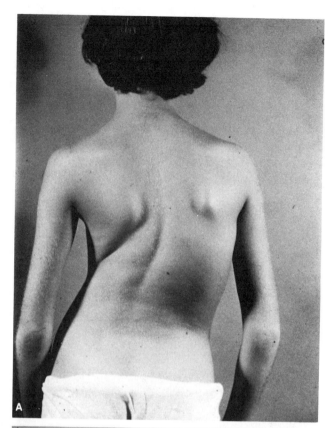

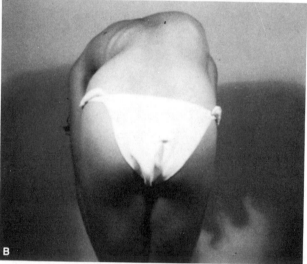

Figure 15-7. **A**, Posterior view of child's back with lateral curvature. **B**, View of child bending over with prominence of scapular area and asymmetry of flank demonstrated. (From O'Connor BJ. Scoliosis: Classification and diagnosis in pediatric orthopedics. ONAJ 3:84, 1976.)

Wearing the Milwaukee brace creates a distinct change in body image, usually in adolescence, a time when body consciousness is at an all-time high. Acceptance of the brace and its limitations may cause anger; the change in cation hook-up with the school. Casts need to be changed periodically to continue the correction as the child grows.

Halo traction may be added to the body cast using stainless steel pins inserted into the skull and into the femurs (Figure 15-9). Weights are increased gradually to promote correction. When the curvature has been corrected, spinal fusion is performed.

The strange appearance of the halo traction apparatus magnifies the problems of body image, in addition to which the head may need to be shaved. The child needs a thorough explanation of what will occur during the procedure and, if possible, have the opportunity to talk with a child who has had this kind of traction. The nurse can help the child ventilate any feelings of fear, anger, depression, and embarrassment. Family members also need support in managing their own feelings about the child in halo traction.

Frequent shampooing, cleansing of the pin sites, and observation for signs of complications are critical in the

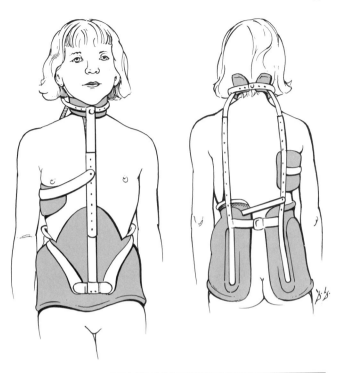

Figure 15-8. Milwaukee brace. (From Castiglia PT, Harbin RE. Child Health Care. Philadelphia: JB Lippincott, 1992, p. 945.)

body image can cause a grief reaction. Working through these feelings successfully requires understanding support from the nurse, family, and peers. Sometimes it is helpful for the patient in a Milwaukee brace to talk with other scoliosis patients and learn how they have coped. Understanding the disorder itself and the important benefits of treatment also can ease the adjustment.

Casts and Traction

Some orthopedic surgeons continue to use casts with varying success. Casts are sometimes combined with halo traction in cases of severe curvature to provide correction.

Before the cast is applied, the child should be given an explanation of the procedure and what the treatment is intended to accomplish. The adolescent girl needs reassurance that the cast will not interfere with breast development.

Care of the child in this type of cast is similar to the care of a child in any kind of cast: regular observation and recording of color, temperature, presence or absence of edema, sensation and motion; proper positioning; meticulous skin care; and patient teaching. When ready for discharge, the child will need an understanding of cast care, a firm mattress (and probably a bed board), and family support. If return to school is not possible, arrangements need to be made for a tutor at home or a communi-

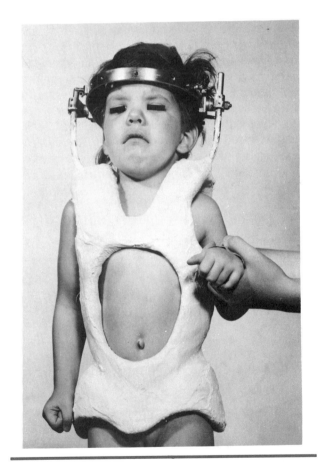

Figure 15-9. Halo traction applied to a body cast. Although this appears top heavy, the child can ambulate with traction in place. (From Pillitteri A. Maternal and Child Health Nursing. Philadelphia: JB Lippincott, 1992; Courtesy of J. H. Moe, MD.)

care of children in halo traction. Any sign of infection, cyanosis, respiratory distress, diplopia (double vision), pupil irregularity, numbness, paralysis, or inability to void should be documented and reported at once. Particular care should be taken to prevent bumping the halo because it magnifies sounds. Turning the child at least every 2 hours and performing skin care with alcohol every 4 hours help prevent tissue breakdown. Breathing exercises and range-of-motion activities reduce the possibility of other complications.

Rod Implantation

Rigid stainless steel rods may be implanted along the spinal column to maintain reduction of the curvature, combined with spinal fusion. This procedure, which is done only in severe curvatures, is frightening to the child and to the family. This is major surgery, and the child and family will need to be well prepared for it. The child can expect to experience postoperative pain, days when it is necessary to remain flat in bed, being turned only in a log-rolling fashion. Because this is an elective procedure, thorough preoperative teaching can be carried out for the child and the family. The child may be given a patient-controlled analgesia pump to control pain. A Foley catheter is most often inserted in surgery because of the need to remain flat. The rods remain in place permanently. About 6 months after surgery, the child will be able to take part in most activities except contact sports, such as tackle football, gymnastics, and wrestling. Because bones are fused and rods are implanted, this procedure arrests the child's growth in height, which contributes to the emotional adjustment that the child and family must make.

Nursing Process for the Child with Scoliosis

ASSESSMENT

Nurses serve an important role in the screening for scoliosis. School nurses, and others who contact children in a health care setting at age 10 and beyond, should conduct or assist in the conduct of screening programs in the fifth or sixth grade through at least eighth grade (see Figure 15-5).

- The child should remove all clothes above the waist, except girls may wear a bra.
- The child is viewed from the back; the examiner looks for
  - One shoulder higher than the other
  - A more prominent shoulder blade
  - Unequal distance between the child's arms and waist
  - One hip higher or more prominent than the other
  - Curvature of the spinal column

- The child is asked to bend over, touching his or her toes; the examiner then looks for
  - A rib hump
  - Curvature of the spinal column

This is a sensitive age for children, when privacy and the importance of "being like everyone else" are top priorities. The nurse must keep this in mind when assessing the child. Privacy must be provided and modesty protected.

The child who is admitted to the hospital for application of a Milwaukee brace or other instrumentation may be carrying a lot of unseen "emotional baggage." The nurse must be sensitive to this emotional state. The family caregivers also may be upset but may be trying to hide it for the child's sake. In addition to routine assessment, the nurse should look for clues to the emotional state of both the child and family caregivers.

NURSING DIAGNOSES

Assessing the emotional states of the child and caregiver is necessary to determine effective nursing diagnoses. The particular type of treatment that the child is to have also contributes to the determination of nursing diagnoses. Some diagnoses for application of a Milwaukee brace that may be desirable are the following:

- Impaired physical mobility related to restricted movement
- High risk for impaired skin integrity related to mechanical irritation of brace
- High risk for noncompliance related to long-term treatment
- High risk for body image disturbance related to wearing a brace continuously

PLANNING AND IMPLEMENTATION

The child and caregiver should be consulted when establishing nursing goals. The nurse must be especially sensitive to the child's needs. Goals of the child may include minimum disruption of activities and maintenance of self-image. Nursing goals include maintenance of skin integrity and compliance with treatment.

Promoting Mobility. The child needs assistance to practice moving about with safety. Exercises are prescribed that the child must practice and perform as directed. Encouragement and support are needed while these exercises are performed. The child may need to be in traction for 1 or 2 weeks before the brace is applied. This can be emotionally traumatic.

After the brace has been applied the child's environment should be evaluated and precautions taken to prevent injury. The child needs to practice moving about: going up and down stairs safely; avoiding hazardous surfaces; getting in and out of vehicles, chairs, or desks;

and getting out of bed. The nurse should listen carefully to the child and the family caregiver to determine any other hazards that may be in the child's home or school environment. Comfortable, supportive seating at school and the adjustments in the physical education program must be arranged for by the family caregiver with school personnel.

Preventing Skin Irritation. When the brace is first applied, the child needs to be checked regularly to confirm the proper fit. Any areas of rubbing, discomfort, or skin irritation must be assessed, and the brace must be adjusted as necessary. The child must be taught to inspect all areas under the brace daily. Reddened areas should be reported to the physician so that adjustments can be made. Skin under the pads should be massaged daily. Daily bathing is essential, and clean cotton underwear or a T-shirt should be worn under the brace to provide protection.

Promoting Compliance with Therapy. The child must wear the brace for years, until the spinal growth is completed, and needs to be weaned from it gradually for another 1 or 2 years, wearing it only at night. During this period, the family caregivers and the child need emotional support from the nursing staff. The child and the family caregivers must have a complete understanding of the importance of continual wearing of the brace. Teaching them about the complications that may occur if correction is not successful may help improve compliance. The family caregiver must be informed about the necessity to monitor the child for compliance. The nurse may need to help the family caregiver be empathic to the child's need to be like others during this period of development and offer ways in which the caregiver can help the child deal with adjustment to the therapy.

Promoting Positive Body Image. The child should be involved in all aspects of planning of care. Self-image and the need to be like others is so important at this age. Learning to be confident enough to handle the comments of peers can be difficult for the child. The child should be given frequent opportunities to ventilate feelings about being different. Help the child to select clothing that blends with current styles but is loose enough to hide the brace. The child needs to be encouraged to find extracurricular activities with which the brace will not interfere. Active sports are not permitted, but many other activities are available. Helping the child focus and enhance a positive attribute, such as hair and complexion, may be useful. Encourage the child and family caregiver to discuss accommodations with school personnel together.

EVALUATION

- Child ambulates without injury
- Skin remains irritation free
- Compliance is maintained, as reported by caregiver and evidenced by child's condition

- Child is self-confident; appearance is attractive and well groomed

Legg-Calvé-Perthes Disease (Coxa Plana)

Legg-Calvé-Perthes disease is an aseptic necrosis of the head of the femur, occurring four to five times more often in boys than in girls and ten times more often in whites than in African Americans. It can be caused by trauma to the hip but generally the cause is unknown. Symptoms first noticed are pain in the hip or groin and a limp, accompanied by muscle spasms and limitation of motion. These symptoms mimic **synovitis** (inflammation of a joint, most commonly the hip in children), which makes immediate diagnosis difficult. Radiographic examination may need to be repeated several weeks after the initial visit to demonstrate vascular necrosis for a definitive diagnosis.

There are three stages of the disease. In the first stage, radiographic studies show opacity of the epiphysis. In the second stage, the epiphysis becomes mottled and fragmented, and during the third stage, reossification occurs. Each stage lasts from 9 months to 1 year.

In the past, immobilization of the hip was considered essential for recovery without deformity. The use of braces and crutches, bedrest with traction, or casting were used to achieve this. However, restricting activity for a child for a period of 2 years or more was extremely difficult. Current treatment focuses on containment of the femoral head within the acetabulum during the revascularization process so that the new femoral head will form to make a smooth functioning joint. The method of containment varies with the portion of the head affected. Use of a brace which holds the necrotic portions of the head in place during healing is considered an effective method of containment. Reconstructive surgery is now possible that enables the child to return to normal activities within 3 to 4 months. Complete recovery without difficulty later in life depends on the age of the child at the time of onset, the amount of involvement, and the cooperation of the child and the family caregivers.

Osteomyelitis

Osteomyelitis is an infection of the bone usually caused by *Staphylococcus aureus*. Acute osteomyelitis is twice as common in boys and results from a primary infection such as a staphylococcal skin infection (impetigo), burns, a furuncle (boil), a penetrating wound, or a fracture. The bacteria enter the blood stream and are carried to the metaphysis of a bone, where an abscess forms, ruptures, and spreads the infection along the bone under the periosteum.

Clinical Manifestations and Diagnosis

Symptoms usually begin abruptly with fever, malaise, and pain and localized tenderness over the metaphysis of the affected bone. There is limitation of joint motion. Diagnosis is based on laboratory findings of leukocytosis of 15,000 to 25,000 cells or more, increased ESR, and positive blood cultures. Radiographic examination does not reveal the process until 5 to 10 days after the onset. The child may have fever, general malaise, irritability, and pain, especially on movement.

Treatment

Treatment for acute osteomyelitis must be immediate. Intravenous antibiotic therapy is started at once and is continued for at least 6 weeks. Depending on the physician, and the compliance of the child and family, a short treatment of intravenous antibiotics may be followed by administration of oral antibiotics for the complete treatment. Surgical drainage of the involved metaphysis may be performed. If the abscess has ruptured into the subperiosteal space, chronic osteomyelitis follows.

If prompt specific antibiotic treatment is vigorously employed, acute osteomyelitis may be brought under rapid control, and extensive bone destruction of chronic osteomyelitis is prevented. Relief of pain and immobilization of the affected joint are other aspects of treatment. If extensive destruction of bone has occurred before treatment, surgical removal of necrotic bone becomes necessary.

Muscular Dystrophy

Muscular dystrophy is a hereditary, progressive, degenerative disease of the muscles. The most common form of muscular dystrophy is Duchenne (pseudohypertrophic) muscular dystrophy. Duchenne muscular dystrophy, an X-linked recessive hereditary disease, occurs almost exclusively in males and is carried by females. When muscular dystrophy has been diagnosed in a child, the mother and the siblings should be tested to see if they have the disease or are carriers.

First signs are noted in infancy or childhood when the child finds it difficult to stand or walk, usually at about 3 years of age; later, trunk muscle weakness develops. Mild mental retardation often accompanies this disease. The child is unable to rise easily to an upright position from a sitting position on the floor. The child rises by "climbing up" his or her lower extremities with his or her hands (Figure 15-10). Weakness of leg, arm, and shoulder muscles progresses gradually. Increasing abnormalities in gait and posture appear by school age with **lordosis** (forward curvature of lumbar spine—swayback), pelvic waddling, and frequent falling (Figure 15-11). The child becomes progressively weaker, usually becoming wheelchair bound by 10 to 12 years of age (middle school or junior high school age). The disease continues into ado-

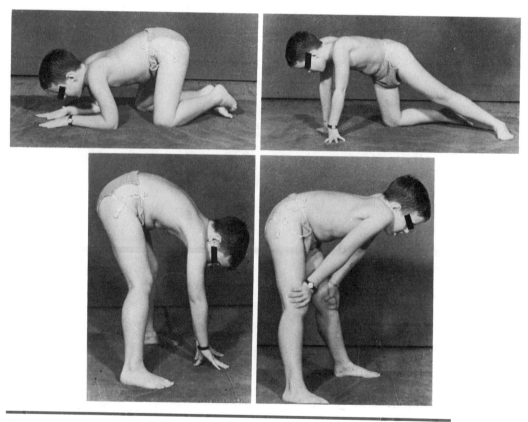

Figure 15-10. Progressional photos of child "climbing up" lower extremities (Gower sign). (From Morrisey RT [ed]. Lovell and Winter's Pediatric Orthopedics, 3rd ed, vol 1. Philadelphia: JB Lippincott, 1990.)

The family is advised to make the child's life as normal as possible, which may be difficult. This disease can drain the emotional and financial reserves of the entire family. Some assistance can be found through the Muscular Dystrophy Association of America (810 7th Avenue, New York, NY 10019), through local chapters of this organization, and through talking with other parents who face the same problem. No effective treatment for the disease has been found, but research is rapidly closing in on genetic identification, which promises exciting changes in treatment in the future.

Juvenile Rheumatoid Arthritis

Juvenile rheumatoid arthritis (JRA) is the most common connective tissue (tissues that provide supportive framework and protective covering for the body, such as the musculoskeletal system and skin and mucous membranes) of childhood. Joint inflammation occurs first, and if untreated, leads to irreversible changes in joint cartilage, ligaments, and menisci (crescent-shaped fibrocartilage in the knee joints), eventually causing complete immobility. The occurrence of JRA appears to peak at two age levels: 1 to 3 years and 8 to 12 years. JRA can be subdivided into three different types: systemic, polyarticular (involving five or more joints), and pauciarticular (involving four or fewer joints, most often the knees and the ankles) (Table 15-6).

Treatment

The goal of treatment of JRA is to maintain mobility and preserve joint function. Treatment can include drugs, physical therapy, and surgery. Early diagnosis and drug therapy to control inflammation and the other systemic changes that occur in JRA can reduce the need for other types of treatment.

Enteric-coated aspirin is the drug of choice for JRA; an effective anti-inflammatory drug, it is inexpensive, easily administered, and has few side effects when carefully regulated. Administering aspirin with food or milk is important to decrease gastrointestinal irritation and bleeding. Acetaminophen is not an appropriate substitute because of the lack of anti-inflammatory properties. Family caregivers must be taught the importance of regular administration of aspirin even when the child is not experiencing pain. The primary purpose of aspirin is not to relieve pain but to decrease inflammation of the joints. When aspirin is no longer effective, nonsteroidal anti-inflammatory drugs (NSAID), indomethacin, gold preparations, antimalarials, steroids, penicillamine, or immunosuppressives may be used. All of these are toxic and must be closely monitored.

Physical therapy for JRA comprises exercise, application of splints, and heat. Implementing this program at home requires the cooperation of the nurse, physical therapist, and physician. Joints must be immobilized dur-

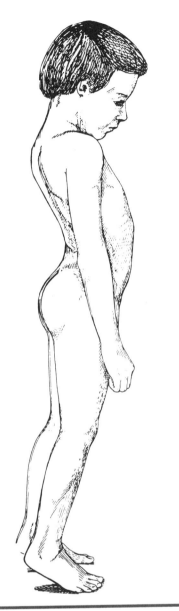

Figure 15-11. Characteristic posture of a child with Duchenne muscular dystrophy. Along with the typical toe gait, the child develops a lordotic posture as Duchenne dystrophy causes further deterioration. (From Brady MH. Lifelong care of the child with Duchenne muscular dystrophy. Am J Matern Child Health 4:227–230, 1979.)

lescence and young adulthood, when the patient usually succumbs to respiratory failure.

The child is encouraged to be as active as possible to delay muscle atrophy and contractures. Physiotherapy, diet to avoid obesity, and parental encouragement help keep the child active.

Once a child becomes bound to a wheelchair, **kyphoscoliosis** (hunchback) develops, causing a decrease in respiratory function and an increase in the incidence of infections. Breathing exercises are a daily necessity for these children.

Table 15-6. Characteristics of Different Types of Juvenile Rheumatoid Arthritis

Characteristic	Polyarthritis	Pauciarticular	Systemic
Frequency of occurrence	40%–50%	40%–50%	10%–20%
Number of joints involved	5 or more	4 or less	Variable
Sex ratio (F:M)	3:1	5:1	1:1
Systemic involvement	Moderate	Not present	Prominent
Uveitis*	5%	20%	Rare
Fever	Rare	Rare	Common
Sensitivity			
Rheumatoid factors	10%	Rare	Rare
Antinuclear bodies	40%–50%	75%–85%	10%
Course	Systemic disease is generally mild; articular involvement may be unremitting	Systemic disease is absent; major cause of morbidity is uveitis	Systemic disease is often self-limited; arthritis is chronic and destructive in 50%
Prognosis	Guarded to moderately good	Excellent except for eyesight	Moderate to poor

* Uveitis—an inflammation of the middle (vascular) tunic of the eye; includes the iris, ciliary body, and choroid.
Adapted from Cassidy JT. Connective tissue diseases and amyloidosis. In FA Oski, et al. (eds). Principle and Practice of Pediatrics. Philadelphia: JB Lippincott, 1990.

ing active disease (accomplished by splinting), but gentle daily exercise is necessary to prevent **ankylosis** (immobility of a joint). The child must be encouraged to perform independent activities of daily living to maintain function and independence. The family caregiver must be patient, allowing the child time to accomplish necessary tasks.

Depending on the degree of disease activity, range-of-motion exercises, isometric exercises, swimming, and riding a tricycle or bicycle may be part of the treatment plan. If exercise triggers increased pain, the amount of exercise should be decreased.

JRA has a long duration, but most (80–90%) of the children who have the disease reach adulthood without serious disability.[4]

Fractures

A fracture is a break in a bone, usually accompanied by vascular and soft-tissue damage, and is characterized by pain, swelling, and tenderness. Children's fractures differ from those of adults in that generally they are less complicated, heal more quickly, and usually occur from different causes. The child has an urge to explore the environment but lacks the experience and judgment to recognize possible hazards. In some instances, caregivers may be negligent in their supervision, but frequently, the child uses immature judgment or is simply too fast for them.

The bones most frequently fractured in childhood are the clavicle, femur, tibia, humerus, wrist, and fingers. Classification of fractures reflects the kind of bone injury sustained. If the fragments of fractured bone are separated, the fracture is said to be complete. If fragments remain partially joined, the fracture is termed incomplete.

Greenstick fractures are one kind of incomplete fracture common in children due to incomplete ossification. When a broken bone penetrates the skin, the fracture is called compound, or open. A simple, or closed, fracture is a single break in the bone without penetration of the skin. Spiral fractures, which twist around the bone, are frequently associated with child abuse and are caused by a wrenching force. The types of fractures are shown in Figure 15-12. Fractures in the area of the epiphyseal plate (growth plate) can cause permanent damage and severely impair growth (Figure 15-13).

Most childhood fractures are treated by realignment and immobilization, using either traction or closed manipulation and casting. A few patients with severe fractures or additional injuries, such as burns and other soft-tissue damage, may require surgical reduction, internal or external fixation, or both. Internal fixation devices include rods, pins, screws, and plates made of inert materials that will not trigger an immune reaction. They make possible early mobilization of the child to wheelchair, crutches, or a walker.

External fixation devices are used primarily in complex fractures often with other injuries or complications. These devices are applied under sterile conditions in the operating room and may be augmented by soft dressings and elevation by means of an overhead traction rope. External fixation devices rarely are used on young children.

Casts

The kind of cast used is determined by the age of the child, the severity of the fracture, the type of bone involved, and the amount of weight bearing. Most casts are

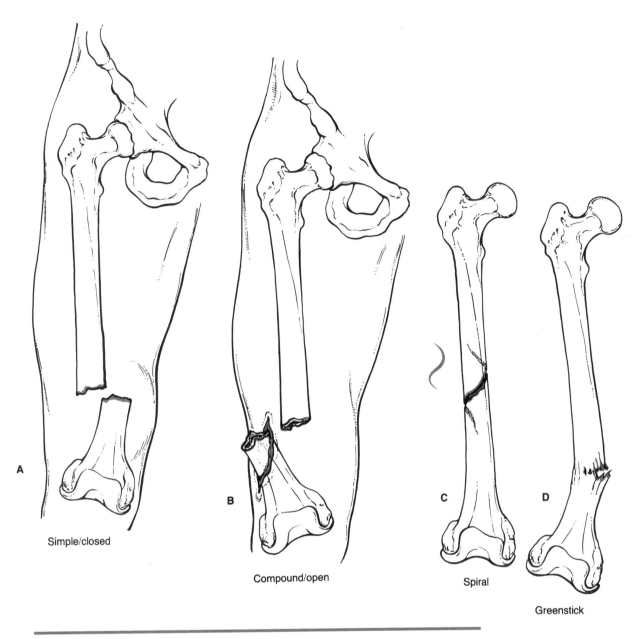

A

Simple/closed

B

Compound/open

C

Spiral

D

Greenstick

Figure 15-12. Types of fractures. All are examples of complete fractures except **D**, which is an incomplete fracture. (Adapted from Jackson DB, Saunders RB. Child Health Nursing. Philadelphia: JB Lippincott, 1993, p. 1728.)

formed from gauze strips impregnated with plaster of Paris or other synthetic material, such as fiberglass or polyurethane resin, that is pliable when wet but hardens when dry. Synthetic materials are lighter in weight and present a cleaner appearance because they can be sponged with water when soiled and even come in colors. Synthetic casts dry more rapidly than plaster of Paris. The lightweight casts tend to be used as arm casts and hip spicas for infants and small children.

The child and the family should be taught what to expect after the cast is applied and how to care for the casted area. A stockinette is applied over the area to be casted, and the bony prominences are padded before the wet plaster rolls are applied. Although the wet plaster of Paris feels cool on the skin when it is applied, evaporation soon causes a temporary sensation of warmth. The cast will feel heavy and cumbersome.

While the cast is wet, it should be handled only with open palms because fingertips can cause indentations and result in pressure points. If the cast has no protective edge, it should be petaled (see Figure 7-22) with adhesive tape strips. If the cast is close to the genital area, plastic should be taped around the edge to prevent wetting and soiling of the cast.

After the fracture has been immobilized, any complaints of pain signal complications and should be re-

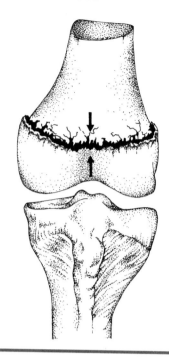

Figure 15-13. One form of epiphyseal injury; a crushing injury (as might occur in a fall from a height) can destroy the layer of germinal cells of the epiphysis, resulting in disturbance of growth. (Redrawn from Specht E. Epiphyseal injuries in childhood. Am Family Physician 10:102, 1974.)

corded and reported immediately. Observing, documenting, and reporting the five P's is essential to good nursing care:

Pain—any sign of pain should be noted and the exact area determined.

Pulse—if an upper extremity is involved, brachial, radial, ulnar, and digital pulses should be checked; if a lower extremity is involved, femoral, popliteal, posterior tibial, and dorsalis pedis pulses should be assessed.

Paresthesia—check for any diminished or absent sensation, or for numbness or tingling.

Paralysis—check hand function by having the child try to hyperextend the thumb or wrist, oppose thumb and little finger, and adduct all fingers; check function of the foot by having the child try to dorsiflex and plantarflex the ankles, and flex and extend the toes.

Pallor—check the color of the extremity and the nail beds distal to the site of the fracture; pallor, discoloration, and coldness indicate circulatory impairment.

In addition to the five P's, any foul odor or drainage on or under the cast, "hot spots" on the cast (warm to touch), looseness or tightness, or any elevation of temperature must be noted, documented, and reported. Family caregivers should be instructed to watch carefully for these same danger signals.

Children and caregivers should be cautioned *not* to put anything down inside the cast, no matter how much the casted area itches. Small toys and sticks or sticklike objects should be kept out of reach until the cast has been removed.

When the fracture has healed, the cast is removed with a cast cutter. This can be a frightening experience for the child unless the person using the cast cutter explains and demonstrates that the device will not cut flesh but only the hard surface of the cast. The child should be told that there will be vibration from the cast cutter, but it will not burn.

After cast removal, the area that was casted should be soaked in warm water to help remove the crusty layer of skin that has accumulated. Application of oil or lotion may prove comforting. Family caregivers and the child must be cautioned against scrubbing or scraping this area because the tender layer of new skin underneath the crust may bleed.

Traction

Traction is a pulling force applied to an extremity or other part of the body. A system of weights, ropes, and pulleys is used to realign and immobilize fractures, reduce or eliminate muscle spasm, and prevent fracture deformity and joint contractures.

There are two basic types of traction: skin traction and skeletal traction. **Skin traction** pulls on tape, rubber, or plastic materials attached to the skin and indirectly exerts pull on the musculoskeletal system. Examples of skin traction are Bryant's traction, Buck extension, Russell traction, and side-arm traction. **Skeletal traction** exerts pull directly on skeletal structures by means of a pin, wire, tongs, or other device surgically inserted through a bone.

Bryant's traction is often used for the treatment of a fractured femur in children younger than 2 years of age. These fractures are frequently transverse or spiral fractures. The use of Bryant's traction entails some risk of compromised circulation and may result in contracture of the foot and lower leg, particularly in an older child.

The child's legs are wrapped with elastic bandages that should be removed at least daily for skin assessment and then rewrapped. Skin temperature and the color of the legs and feet must be checked frequently to detect any circulatory impairment. Severe pain may indicate circulatory difficulty and should be reported immediately. When a child is in Bryant's traction, the hips should not rest on the bed—the nurse should be able to pass a hand between the child's buttocks and the sheet.

Buck extension traction is used for short-term immobilization. The child's body provides the countertraction to the weights. It is used to correct contractures and bone deformities such as Legg-Calvé-Perthes disease.

Russell traction (Figure 15-14) seems to be more effective for older children. A child in either type of trac-

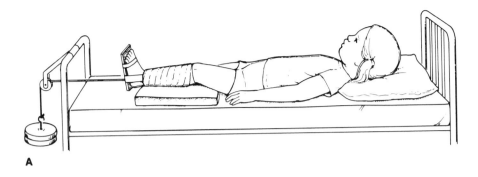

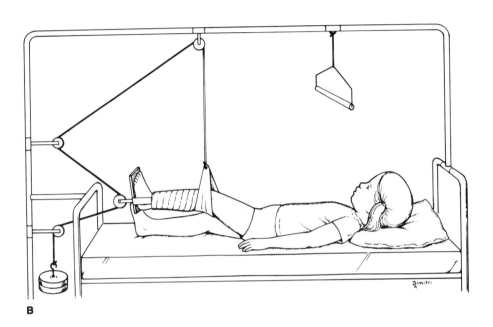

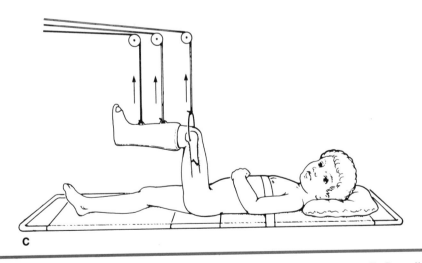

Figure 15-14. Types of traction. **A,** Buck extension, a form of skin traction. **B,** Russell traction, a type of skin traction. Two lines of traction (one horizontal and one vertical) allow for good bone alignment for healing. **C,** 90 degree–90 degree (skeletal) traction. The lower leg is in a boot cast, and a wire pin is inserted into the distal femur. (From Skale N. Manual of Pediatric Nursing Procedures. Philadelphia: JB Lippincott, 1992, pp. 517, 519.)

tion, however, tends to slide down until the weights rest on the bed or the floor. The child should be pulled up to keep the weights free, the ropes must be in alignment with the pulleys, and the alignment should be checked frequently. An older child may coax a roommate to remove the weights or the sandbags used as weights.

Side-arm traction (Figure 15-15) is sometimes used for fractures of the humerus or the elbow. It can be applied as skin traction or, when a pin is inserted into the bone, as skeletal traction.

Children in any kind of traction must be carefully monitored to detect any signs of neurovascular complications. Skin temperature and color, presence or absence of edema, peripheral pulse, sensation, and motion must be assessed every hour for the first 24 hours after traction has been applied and every 4 hours unless ordered otherwise. Skin care must be meticulous. Skin preparation (Skin-Prep) should be used to toughen the skin rather than lotions or oils that soften the skin and contribute to tissue breakdown.

Children in skeletal traction require special attention to pin sites. Pin care should be performed every 8 hours with povidone-iodine or hydrogen peroxide solution. Sterile gloves are worn, and sterile applicators used for the procedure (Figure 15-16). Any sign of infection (odor, local inflammation, or elevated temperature) must be recorded and reported at once.

External Fixation Devices
Children whose fractures are severe enough to require the use of external fixation also need special skin care at pin sites. The sites are left open to the air and should be inspected and cleansed every 8 hours, as described earlier. The appearance of the pins puncturing the skin and the unusual appearance of the device can be upsetting

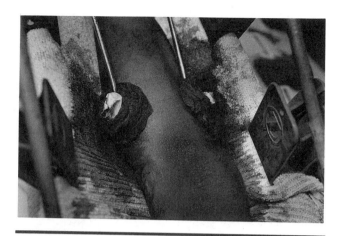

Figure 15-16. Pin sites with povidone-iodine and sterile gauze applied. (From Skale N. Manual of Pediatric Nursing Procedures. Philadelphia: JB Lippincott, 1992, p. 522.)

to the child, and the nurse should be sensitive to any anxiety the child expresses.

As early as possible, the child (if old enough) or family caregivers should be taught to care for the pin sites. External fixation devices are sometimes left in place for as long as 1 year; therefore, it is important that the child accepts this temporary change in body image and learn to care for the affected site. Children with these devices will probably work with a physical therapist during the rehabilitation period and will have specific exercises to perform. Before discharge from the hospital, the child should feel comfortable in moving about and should be able to recognize the signs of pin infection.

Crutches
Children with fractures of the lower extremities and other lower leg injuries often must learn to use crutches to avoid weight-bearing on the injured area. Several types of crutches are available, the most common being axillary crutches, principally used for temporary situations. Forearm, or Canadian, crutches usually are recommended for children who need crutches permanently, such as paraplegic children with braces. Trough, or platform, crutches are more suitable for children with limited strength or function in the arms and hands.

The use of crutches is generally taught by a physical therapist, but it can be the responsibility of nurses. The type of crutch gait to be taught is determined by the amount of weight-bearing permitted, the child's degree of stability, whether or not the knees can be flexed, and the specific goal of treatment for the individual child.

Skin Disorders

The school-age child often has minor bruises, abrasions, or rashes that generally cause few problems. There are, however, common fungal and parasitic disorders that can

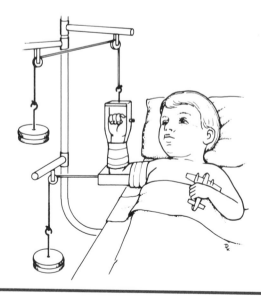

Figure 15-15. Dunlop traction, a variation of sidearm traction. (From Skale N. Manual of Pediatric Nursing Procedures. Philadelphia: JB Lippincott, 1992, p. 518.)

become serious if not controlled and cured. Allergic skin reactions are not uncommon. Because a large part of the school-age child's time is spent away from home, the child is exposed to poisonous plants that cause allergic reactions or to bites from insects, animals, or snakes that need attention.

Fungal Infections

Fungal infections of the skin are superficial infections caused by fungi that live in the outer (dead) layers of the skin, the hair, and nails. **Tinea** (ringworm) is the term commonly applied to these infections, which are further differentiated by the part of the body infected.

Tinea Capitis (Ringworm of the Scalp)

Ringworm of the scalp is called *tinea capitis* or *tinea tonsurans*. The most common cause is *Microsporum audouini*, transmitted from person to person through combs, towels, hats, barber scissors, or direct contact. A less common type, *Microsporum canis*, is transmitted from animal to child.

Tinea capitis begins as a small papule on the scalp and spreads, leaving scaly patches of baldness. The hairs become brittle and break off easily. Griseofulvin, an oral antifungal antibiotic, is the medication of choice. Because treatment may be prolonged (3 months or more), compliance needs to be reinforced. Children who are being properly treated may attend school. Hair loss is not permanent.

Tinea Corporis (Ringworm of the Body)

Tinea corporis is ringworm of the body that affects the epidermal layer of the skin. The lesions appear as a scaly ring with clearing in the center and may occur on any part of the body. They resemble the lesions of scalp ringworm. The child usually contracts *T. corporis* from contact with an infected dog or cat. Topical antifungal agents, such as clotrimazole, econazole nitrate, tolnaftate, and miconazole, are effective. Griseofulvin also is used in this condition.

Tinea Pedis (Ringworm of the Feet; Athlete's Foot)

Tinea pedis (athlete's foot) is the scaling or cracking of the skin between the toes. Examination under a microscope of scrapings from the lesions is necessary for definite diagnosis. Transmission is by direct or indirect contact with skin lesions from infected people. Contaminated sidewalks, floors, and shower stalls spread the condition to those who walk barefoot. Tinea pedis, usually found in adolescents and adults, is becoming more prevalent among school-age children since the popularity of plastic shoes.

Care includes washing the feet with soap and water, then gently removing scabs and crusts and applying a topical agent such as tolnaftate. Griseofulvin by mouth is also useful. During the chronic phase, the use of ointment, scrupulous foot hygiene, frequent changing of white cotton socks, and avoidance of plastic footwear are help-

ful. Continuing application of a topical agent for up to 6 weeks is recommended.

Tinea Cruris (Ringworm of the Inner Thighs and Inguinal Area)

Tinea cruris (jock itch) is caused by the same organisms that cause tinea corporis. It is more commonly seen among athletes and is not common in preadolescent children. Tinea cruris is pruritic and localized to the area. Treatment is the same as tinea corporis. Sitz baths also may be soothing.

Parasitic Infections

Parasites are organisms that live on or within another living organism from which they obtain their food supply. Lice and the scabies mite both live by sucking the blood of the host.

Pediculosis

Pediculosis (lice infestation) may be caused by *Pediculus humanus capitis* (head lice), *Pediculus humanus corporis* (body lice), or *Phthirus pubis* (pubic lice). Head lice are the most common infestation seen in children. Animal lice are not transferred to humans.

Head lice are passed from child to child by direct contact or indirectly by contact with combs, other headgear, or bed linen. Lice, which are rarely seen, lay their eggs, called nits, on the head, attaching them to strands of hair. The nits can be seen as tiny, pearly white flecks attached to the hair shafts. They look much like dandruff, but dandruff flakes can be flicked off easily, whereas the nits are tightly attached and not easily removed. The nits hatch in about 1 week, and the lice become sexually mature in approximately 2 weeks. Severe itching of the scalp is the most obvious symptom. Scratching can cause skin breaks and secondary infections.

Treatment. Use of lindane (Kwell) shampoo, which is prescribed by a physician, gives the most satisfactory results. After wetting the hair with warm water, the Kwell is applied like any ordinary shampoo: about 1 ounce is used. The head should be lathered for 4 minutes, then rinsed thoroughly and dried. After the hair is dry, it should be combed with a fine-toothed comb dipped in warm white vinegar to remove remaining nits and nit shells. Shampooing may be repeated in 2 weeks to remove any lice that may have been missed as nits and since hatched. Care must be taken to avoid getting Kwell into the eyes or on mucous membranes. When treating a child in the hospital for pediculosis, the nurse should wear a disposable gown, gloves, and head cover for protection.

Family caregivers are often embarrassed when the school nurse sends word that the child has head lice. They can be reassured that lice infestation is common and can happen to any child. It is not a reflection on the caregiver's housekeeping. All family members should be inspected and treated as needed. Additional information that the caregiver should follow is provided in the Parent Teaching: Eliminating Pediculi Infestations display.

Scabies

Scabies is a skin infestation caused by the scabies mite *Sarcoptes scabiei*. The female mite burrows in areas between the fingers and toes and in warm folds of the body, such as the axilla and groin, to lay eggs. Burrows are visible as dark lines, and the mite is seen as a black dot at the end of the burrow. Severe itching occurs, causing scratching with resulting secondary infection. The areas are treated with lindane lotion or crotamiton (Eurax). The body is first scrubbed with soap and water, then the lotion is applied on all areas of the body except the face. With lindane, a second coat can be applied, then all washed off in 24 hours. Instructions for crotamiton are to apply a second coat in 24 hours and wait an additional 48 hours to wash off. Caregivers should follow the tips recommended for pediculosis. All who had close contact with the child within a 30- to 60-day period should be treated. The rash and itch may continue for several weeks even though the mites have been successfully eliminated.

Skin Allergies

One of the most common allergic skin reactions is eczema (atopic dermatitis), which is discussed in Chapter 9. Other skin disorders of allergic origin include hives (urticaria) and giant swellings (angioedema) and rashes caused by poison ivy, poison oak, and other plants or drug reactions.

Skin rashes are common in school-age children. Some are caused by infectious diseases and others by allergy. Whatever the cause, rashes are usually treated with topical preparations, such as lotions, ointments, and greases, plus cool soaks. The itching must be relieved as much as possible because scratching can introduce additional pathogens to the affected area.

Hives (Urticaria) and Giant Swellings (Angioedema)

Hives appear in different sizes and on many different parts of the body and are usually caused by foods or drugs. They are bright red and itchy and can occur on the eyelids, tongue, mouth, hands or feet or in the brain or stomach. When affecting the mouth or tongue, hives can cause difficulty in breathing; in the stomach, the swelling can produce pain, nausea, and vomiting. Swelling in brain tissue causes headache and other neurologic symptoms.

Foods such as chocolate, nuts, shellfish, berries or other raw fruit, fish, and highly seasoned foods are likely to cause hives. Possible drug allergens include aspirin and related drugs, laxatives, antiinflammatory drugs, tranquilizers, and antibiotics (penicillin is the most common allergen of this group). Sometimes it is impossible to identify the cause.

Treatment. Treatment is aimed at reducing the swelling and relieving the itching. If the allergen can be identified, it can be removed from the child's environment and desensitization can be performed. Antihistamines (topical or systemic) are used to relieve itching and reduce swelling. Cool soaks also help relieve itching. Fingernails should be kept short and clean. In severe cases, corticosteroids may be necessary. If the allergen is a certain food, that food needs to be eliminated from the child's diet.

Plant Allergies

Poison ivy, oak, and sumac are common causes of contact dermatitis. Of these, poison ivy is the worst offender, particularly during the summer months (Figure 15-17). The cause of the allergy is an oil, urushiol, which is present in all parts of these plants. It is extremely potent. Its effects vary from slight inflammation and itching to severe, extensive swelling that can virtually immobilize the child. This disorder causes intense itching (pruritus) and forms tiny blisters that weep and continue to spread the inflammation. Antihistamines or oral steroids help the child not to scratch; cool soaks, Aveeno baths, Calamine lotion, or topical steroids help minimize the discomfort. The child should be taught to recognize and avoid the poisonous plants. The plants also should be removed from the environment when possible.

Parent Teaching

Eliminating Pediculi Infestations

1. Wash all child's bedding and clothing in hot water, dry in hot dryer.
2. Vacuum carpets, car seats, mattresses, and upholstered furniture very thoroughly. Discard vacuum dust bag.
3. Wash pillows, stuffed animals, and other washable items the same way clothing is washed.
4. Dry clean unwashable items.
5. If items cannot be washed or dry cleaned, seal in plastic bag for 2 weeks to break reproductive cycle of lice.
6. Wash combs, brushes and other hair items (rollers, curlers, barrettes, etc.) in shampoo, soaking for 1 hour.
7. If you discover the infestation yourself, report to child's school or day care.
8. School should disinfect headphones.

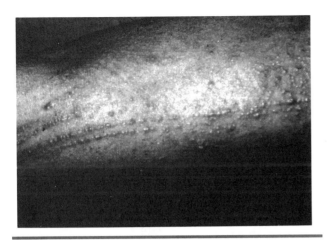

Figure 15-17. The lesions of poison ivy. Note the linear distribution. (Courtesy of the Centers for Disease Control and Prevention, Atlanta, GA.) (Pillitteri A. Maternal and Child Health Nursing. Philadelphia: JB Lippincott, 1992.)

Bites

Because school-age children are active, inquisitive, and not completely inhibited in their actions, they commonly suffer bites, both animal and human, as well as insect stings and bites. Many of these are minor, particularly if the skin is not broken. Some, however, can have life-threatening implications if proper care is not given.

Animal Bites

Children enjoy pets, but often they are not alert to possible dangerous encounters with pets or wild animals. Dog bites are a common occurrence. Fortunately, because of rabies vaccination programs for dogs, few dog bites cause rabies, but cats are the domestic animal most likely to carry rabies. Any pet who bites should be held until it can be determined whether the animal has been vaccinated against rabies. If not, it will be necessary for the child to undergo a series of injections to prevent this potentially fatal disease. The series consists of both active and passive immunizations. Active immunity is established with five injections of human diploid cell vaccine (HDCV) beginning on the day of the bite and on days 3, 7, 14, and 28. Human rabies immune globulin is given on the first day along with the HDCV.

All animal and human bites should be thoroughly washed with soap and water. An antiseptic such as 70% alcohol or povidone-iodine should be applied after the wound has been thoroughly rinsed. The wound must be observed for signs of infection until well healed. Animal bites should be promptly reported to the proper authorities.

Children should be taught at an early age about the danger of animal bites, particularly of strange or wild animals, such as skunks, raccoons, bats, and squirrels.

Spider Bites

Spider bites can cause serious illness if untreated. Bites of black widow and brown recluse spiders and scorpions demand medical attention. Absorption of their poison can be slowed by applying ice to the affected area until medical care is obtained.

Tick Bites

Wood ticks carried by chipmunks, ground squirrels, weasels, and wood rats can cause Rocky Mountain spotted fever. Most cases are found in the South Atlantic, South Central, and Southeastern United States. Dogs are frequently the carriers to humans. People living in areas where ticks are common can be immunized against this disease.

Deer ticks, carried by white-footed mice and white-tailed deer found in the Northeast, Midwest, and West can carry the organism that causes Lyme disease. The first stage of the disease begins with a lesion at the site of the bite. The lesion appears as a macule with a clear center. The second stage occurs several weeks to months later if the patient is not treated. The symptoms of this stage may affect the central nervous system and the heart. The third stage may occur months to years later causing arthritis, neurologic disorders, and bone and joint disease.

Children and adults should wear long pants, long-sleeved shirts, and insect repellent when walking in the woods. Pant legs should be tucked into socks. If a tick is found on the body, alcohol may be applied and the tick carefully removed with tweezers. Care should be taken not to crush the tick to prevent the release of pathogenic organisms. A health care provider must be consulted if there is any suspicion that a child or an adult has been bitten by a deer tick.

Snake Bites

Snake bites demand immediate medical intervention. The wound should be washed, ice should be applied, and the body part involved should be immobilized. Prompt transport to the nearest medical facility is essential.

Insect Stings or Bites

Insect stings or bites can prove fatal to children who are sensitized. Swelling may be localized or include an entire extremity. Circulatory collapse, airway obstruction, and anaphylactic shock can cause death within 30 minutes if the child is untreated. Immediate treatment is necessary and may include injection of epinephrine, antihistamines, or steroids. These children should wear a Medic Alert bracelet and carry an anaphylaxis kit that includes a plastic syringe of epinephrine and an antihistamine. The teacher, school nurse, and alternative caregivers should be alerted to the child's allergy and know where the anaphylaxis kit is and how to use it if needed.

Summary

For most children, the ages from 6 to 10 years are a time of growing and learning. Most illnesses during this period are short term and minor, but for some children this is a time of visits to the hospital and many trips to the health care provider. Children with long-term or chronic diseases such as scoliosis, asthma, rheumatic fever, or diabetes may be self-conscious about being different from their classmates. This is a time when children need to have positive self-esteem. Illness may threaten the child's self-confidence and can contribute to self-doubt.

School-age children are fascinated by their bodies and how they work. Science is a subject that intrigues many of them, and they are eager to learn. School-age children can be involved in their health care, learning how the illness is affecting their bodies, how to help care for themselves, and what the future may hold. They like to feel responsible and usually welcome the chance for new challenges. This age is also a time when children may begin to fear that they could die from their illness. Nurses must be aware of the feelings and fears of these children and plan nursing care with sensitivity and understanding. School-age children can learn good health habits and safety practices and understand why they are important. These children usually wish to please their elders, and this can be an advantage when trying to gain their cooperation in treatment. Throughout the care for this age group, trust must be gained by being truthful and answering questions accurately, acknowledging those aspects of care that may be painful.

Review Questions

1. What is meant by an "elimination" diet?
2. A coworker says to you, "That Jeff in room 204 is bouncing off the walls." You are assigned to him. Using behavior techniques for the ADHD child, tell how you will plan his care.
3. You are in the grocery store and see a child having a grand mal seizure. No other adult is around. What should you do?
4. Six-year-old Alfonse has recovered from a severe asthmatic attack. What teaching would you present to his father, who is a heavy smoker?
5. What response would you make to a 5-year-old child who is having an asthmatic attack and says, "Why is my breathing making music when I want to go to sleep?"
6. What is the danger of giving a laxative or an enema to a child with abdominal pain?
7. Jasmine is a 9-year-old child who had an appendectomy today. Write a postoperative nursing care plan for her.
8. There are five children between 2 and 8 years of age in the household, including cousins. Five-year-old Malcolm has been sent home from kindergarten with a note advising of an outbreak of pinworms. What advice would you give his aunt Eva, who cares for the children?
9. Eight-year-old Raynelle has been diagnosed with rheumatic fever. She has to undergo a brief period of bed rest. Plan some diversional activities for her.
10. Explain the difference between IDDM and NIDDM diabetes.
11. Make a table showing signs and symptoms of hyperglycemia on one side and hypoglycemia on the other.
12. Cody is a 7-year-old diabetic. Approximately 45 minutes before his evening meal, he complains of feeling "funny" and says he has a headache. What would be the best thing to do for him at this time?
13. How might an adolescent's developmental level affect the way she handles being diabetic?
14. Tell how you would teach a 9-year-old diabetic how to self-administer insulin.
15. What teaching would you give 8-year-old Raoul, a diabetic who plans to play Little League Baseball?
16. Ten-year-old Carrie must wear a Milwaukee brace. She has said she thinks it's really ugly. What nursing diagnosis is appropriate for this problem? Indicate planning, implementation, and evaluation for this diagnosis.
17. You are assisting with the cast removal on 6-year-old Felice. What will you do and say to reassure her that her leg won't be cut along with the cast?
18. What signs do you observe for to detect neurovascular complications on a child in traction?
19. Name three drugs commonly used in the treatment of rheumatic fever. What is the purpose of each?
20. What is the best advice you can give someone about avoiding *tinea pedis* (athlete's foot)?
21. Lucy's granddaughter is sent home from school with pediculosis. There are two children and one adult in the home. What would you advise Lucy to do?
22. What is the cause of Lyme disease? How can the disease be prevented?

References

1. Eggleston PA. Asthma. In Oski FA (ed). Principle and Practices of Pediatrics. Philadelphia: JB Lippincott, 1990, pp. 201–207.
2. Kattan M: Managing and preventing asthma emergencies. Contemp Pediatr 5(11):22, 24–26, 28, 30, 32, 1988.
3. Sponseller PD, Toto VT. Bone, joint, and muscle problems. In Oski FA (ed). Principle and Practices of Pediatrics. Philadelphia, JB Lippincott, 1990, pp. 939–969.

4. Cassidy JT. Connective tissue diseases and amyloidosis. In Oski FA (ed). Principle and Practices of Pediatrics. Philadelphia, JB Lippincott, 1990, pp. 226–249.

Bibliography

Amendt LE, Ause-Ellias KL, Eybers JL, et al. Validity and reliability testing of the Scoliometer. Phys Ther 70(2):108–117, 1990.

Austin JK. Childhood epilepsy: Child adaptation and family resources. J Child Adolesc Psychiatr Ment Health Nurs 1(1): 18–24, 1988.

Austin JK. Comparison of child adaptation to epilepsy and asthma. J Child Adolesc Psychiatr Ment Health Nurs 2(4): 139–144, 1989.

Bach JR, Zeelenberg AP, Winter C. Wheelchair-mounted robot manipulators: Long-term use by patients with Duchenne muscular dystrophy. Am J Phys Med Rehabil 69(2):55–59, 1990.

Baciewicz AM, Kyllonen KS. Aerosol inhaler technique in children with asthma. Am J Hosp Pharm 46(12):2510-2511, 1989.

Baydur A, Gilgoff I, Prentice W, et al. Decline in respiratory function and experience with long-term assisted ventilation in advanced Duchenne's muscular dystrophy. Chest 97(4):884-889, 1990.

Bunch D. Baylor Asthma Center offers new concept in asthma education. AARC Times 14(4):62–65, 1990.

Caroselli-Karinja MF. Asthma and adaptation: Exploring the family system. J Psychosoc Nurs Ment Health Serv 28(4):34–41, 1990.

Carpenito LJ. Handbook of Nursing Diagnosis. Philadelphia: JB Lippincott, 1991.

Castiglia PT, Harbin RE. Child Health Care: Process and Practice. Philadelphia: JB Lippincott, 1992.

Chauvin VG. Common skin rashes in children and adolescents. School Nurse 5(1):23–24, 26, 28–33, 1989.

DeWitt S. Nursing assessment of the skin and dermatologic lesions. Nurs Clin North Am 25(1):235–245, 1990.

Drash AL, Arslanian SA. Can insulin-dependent diabetes mellitus be cured or prevented? Pediatr Clin North Am 37(6): 1467–1487, 1990.

Eden-Kilgour S, Gibson DE. Nursing management of children with scoliosis. J Pract Nurs 40(2):34–38, 1990.

Ellett ML. Constipation/encopresis: A nursing perspective. J Pediatr Health Care 4(3):141–146, 1990.

Frost L, Kieckhefer GM, Rubino C. Incorporating research into a community asthma program: Superstuff Program. Pediatr Nurs 14(3):197–200, 1988.

Gibson LY. Bedwetting: A family's recurrent nightmare. MCN 14(8):270–272, 1989.

Gunnoe BA. Adolescent idiopathic scoliosis. Physician Assist 14(9):66-67, 70, 72, 1990.

Hek G. Treating asthma at home: Testing the efficacy of a community asthma nurse. Nurs Times 86(20):64–66, 1990.

Hess V. Diabetes: Stuff and more stuff. Lincoln, NE: HERC, 1989.

Jackson DB, Saunders RB. Child Health Nursing. Philadelphia: JB Lippincott, 1993.

Knox P. School phobia and suicidal depression. Midwife Health Visit Commun Nurse 24(10):431–432, 1988.

Krane EJ. Diabetic ketoacidosis. Pediatr Clin North Am 34(4): 935–960, 1987.

Lord J, Behrman B, Varzos N, et al. Scoliosis associated with Duchenne muscular dystrophy. Arch Phys Med Rehabil 71(1): 13–17, 1990.

Merenda JT. Evaluation and management of idiopathic scoliosis. Physician Assist 13(2):99–100, 102, 105–106, 1989.

Moffitt JE, Moffitt JL. Behavioral and cognitive effects of theophylline. Pediatr Nurs 15(3):277, 1989.

Pillitteri A. Maternal and Child Health Nursing. Philadelphia: JB Lippincott, 1992.

Poussa M, Harkonen H, Mellin G. Spinal mobility in adolescent girls with idiopathic scoliosis and in structurally normal controls. Spine 14(2):217–219, 1989.

Rosen T. Cutaneous fungal infections: I. Dermatophytosis: Practical tips for avoiding common mistakes. Consultant 29(8):29–33, 36, 41, 1989.

Rosen T. Cutaneous fungal infections: II. Tinea versicolor and candidiasis: Practical tips for avoiding common mistakes. Consultant 29(8):46–48, 51, 1989.

Sadler C. Getting dry. Commun Outlook 33, 35, 1990.

Scoloveno MA, Yarcheski A, Mahon NE. Scoliosis treatment effects on selected variables among adolescents. West J Nurs Res 12(5):616–618, 1990.

Scoloveno MA, Yarcheski A, Mahon NE. Scoliosis treatment effects on selected variables among adolescents. West J Nurs Res 12(5):601–615, 1990.

Sharts-Hopko NC. Ritodrine, reexamined. MCN 18(1):56, 1993.

Sperling MA. Outpatient management of diabetes mellitus. Pediatr Clin North Am 34(4):919–934, 1987.

Sprague-McRae JM. Encopresis: Developmental, behavioral and physiological considerations for treatment. Nurse Pract 15(6):8, 11–12, 14–16, 1990.

Strawbridge GW, Gable JF. Strategies for dealing with school phobia. J Am Acad Physician Assist 2(5):368–372, 1989.

Swank SM, Brown JC, Jennings MV, et al. Lateral electrical surface stimulation in idiopathic scoliosis: Experience in two private practices. Spine 14(12):1293–1295, 1989.

Vichyanond P, Sladek WA, Sur S, et al. Efficacy of atropine methylnitrate alone and in combination with albuterol in children with asthma. Chest 98(3):637–642, 1990.

Wallston KA. Scoliosis treatment effects on selected variables among adolescents. West J Nurs Res 12(5):615–616, 1990.

Whaley LF, Wong DL. Nursing Care of Infants and Children, 4th ed. St. Louis: Mosby-Year Book, 1991.

Willis J. Common pests. Commun Outlook 24–25, 27, 29, 1990.

Growth and Development of the Adolescent: 11 to 18 years

Chapter 16

Student Objectives

Upon completion of this chapter, the student will be able to:

1. Define key terms.
2. State the age of the preadolescent; of the adolescent.
3. Describe the psychosocial development of the preadolescent.
4. Name the physical changes that make the child appear uncoordinated in early adolescence.
5. List the secondary sexual characteristics that appear in adolescent boys; in adolescent girls.
6. Name the nutrients that are commonly deficient in the diets of adolescents.
7. State the major cognitive task of the adolescent according to Piaget; the psychosocial task according to Erikson.
8. Discuss the adolescent's need to conform with peers.
9. Explain some of the problems that adolescents face when making career choices today.
10. Discuss the influence of peer pressure on psychosocial development.
11. Discuss the necessity for orderly psychosocial development of identity and trust before adolescents are ready for intimate relationships.
12. Discuss adolescent body image and associated problems.

Marks MG: BROADRIBB'S INTRODUCTORY PEDIATRIC NURSING, 4th ed. © 1994 J.B. Lippincott Company.

Key Terms

early adolescence   menarche

heterosexual   puberty

homosexual

Knowing

by Karen Haynes

There are times
when I have to know
who I am
what I am,
where I am
but really,
who I am.
I have to know
for
a cat just knows she's a cat,
a dog just knows she's a dog;
I must know what I am
for a flower must know it belongs to a plant,
a grain of sand must know it belongs to
a beach.
I must know
where I am
for a leaf must know it is
one in a thousand of others.
Since they all know,
Why can't I?

*A*dolescence comes from the Latin word meaning "to come to maturity," a fitting description of this stage of life. The adolescent is maturing physically and emotionally, growing from childhood toward adulthood and seeking to

know and understand what it means to be "grown up." Adolescents between 13 to 19 years of age are commonly referred to as *teenagers*.

Early adolescence (preadolescence, pubescence) begins at about age 10 in girls and about age 12 in boys with a dramatic growth spurt that signals the advent of **puberty** (reproductive maturity). During this stage, the child's body begins to take on adult-like contours, primary sex organs enlarge, secondary sexual characteristics appear, and hormonal activity increases. This early period ends with the onset of menstruation in the female and production of sperm in the male.

During adolescence, the bone growth that began during intrauterine life continues until, by the end of adolescence, it is usually completed. Other growth during this time includes maturing of reproductive organs and tremendous psychosocial growth.

Adolescents are fascinated, and sometimes fearful and confused, by the changes occurring in their bodies and their thinking processes. They begin to look grown-up, but they do not have the judgment or independence to participate in society as an adult. These young people are strongly influenced by their peer group and often resent parental authority. Roller coaster levels of emotion characterize this age group, as does intense interest in the opposite sex (Figure 16-1).

The adolescent years can be a time of turmoil and uncertainty that creates conflict between family caregivers and children. If these conflicts are successfully resolved, normal development can continue. Unresolved, the conflicts can foster delays in development and prevent the young person from maturing into a fully functioning adult.

Body image is critically important to adolescents. Health problems that threaten body image, such as acne, obesity, dental or vision problems, and traumatic accidents, can seriously interfere with development.

Preadolescence

During the period between 10 and 12 years, there is a great variation in the rate of growth between boys and girls. This variability in growth and maturation can be a concern to the child who develops rapidly or the one who

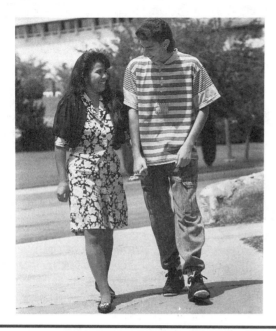

Figure 16-1. Intense interest in the opposite sex characterizes adolescence. (From Castiglia PT, Harbin RE. Child Health Care: Process and Practice. Philadelphia: JB Lippincott, 1992, p. 334.)

develops more slowly than other agemates. Children of this age do not want to be "different" from the rest of their friends. There is much overlapping of developmental characteristics in the preadolescent child between the stages of late school age and early adolescence, but nevertheless there are unique characteristics to set it apart (Table 16-1).

Physical Development

Preadolescence begins in the female between the ages of 9 and 11 years and is marked by a growth spurt that lasts about 18 months. Girls grow approximately 3 inches each year until **menarche** (the beginning of menstruation), after which growth slows considerably. Early in adolescence, girls begin to develop "a figure": the pelvis broadens and axillary and pubic hair begins to appear, along with many changes in hormone levels. The variation between individual girls is great and often is a cause for much concern by the "early bloomer" or the "late bloomer." Young girls who begin to develop physically as early as 9 years of age are often embarrassed by these physical changes. In girls, the onset of menarche marks the end of the preadolescent period.

Boys enter preadolescence a little later, usually between 11 and 13 years of age, and grow generally at a slower, steadier rate than do girls. During this time, the scrotum and testes begin to enlarge, and the skin of the scrotum begins to change in coloring and texture with sparse hair at the base of the penis. Boys who start their

growth spurt later often are concerned about being shorter than any of their peers. In boys, the appearance of nocturnal emissions is often used as the indication that the preadolescent period is ended.

Preparation for Adolescence

Preadolescents need information about their changing bodies and feelings. Sex education that includes information about the hormonal changes that are occurring, or will be occurring, is necessary to help them through this developmental stage. Girls need information that will help them handle their early menstrual periods with minimal apprehension. They need to have answers concerning the regularity of menstrual cycles. Most girls have irregular periods for the first year or so; they need to know that this is not a cause for worry. They have many questions about protection during their menstrual period and the advisability of using sanitary pads or tampons. They may fear that "everybody will know" when they have their first period and need to be able to express this fear and be reassured. Boys also need information about their own bodies. Questions about erections and nocturnal emissions are topics they need to discuss as well as the development of other male secondary sex characteristics. Both boys and girls need information about changes in the opposite sex, including discussions that address their questions. This kind of information helps them increase their understanding of human sexuality.

School programs may provide a good foundation for sex education information, but each preadolescent needs an adult to turn to with particular questions. Even a well-planned program does not address all the needs of the preadolescent. The best school program begins early and builds from year to year as the child's needs progress (see Chapter 14). Preadolescence is an appropriate time for discussions that will help the young teen resist pressures to become sexually active too early. Family caregivers may turn to a nurse acquaintance for guidance in preparing their child. Perhaps the most important aspect of discussions about sexuality is that honest, straightforward answers must be given in an atmosphere of caring concern. Children whose need for information is not met through family, school, or community programs will get their information—often inaccurate—from peers, movies, television, or other media.

Adolescence

Adolescence spans the ages from approximately 13 to 18 years. Some males do not complete adolescence until they are 20 years old. The rate of development during adolescence varies greatly from one teen to another. It is a time during which many physical, emotional, and social changes occur. During this period, the adolescent is en-

Table 16-1. Growth and Development of the Preadolescent: 10–13 Years

Physical	*Motor*	*Personal-Social*	*Language*	*Perceptual*	*Cognitive*
Average height 56¾–59 in (144–150 cm) Average weight 77–88 lb (35–40 kg) Pubescence may begin Girls may surpass boys in height Remaining permanent teeth erupt	Refines gross and fine motor skills May have difficulty with some fine motor coordination owing to growth of large muscles before that of small muscles; hands and feet are first structures to increase in size, thus actions may appear uncoordinated during early preadolescence Can do crafts Uses tools increasingly well	Attends school primarily for peer association Peer relationships of greatest importance Intolerant of violation of group norms Is able to follow rules of group and adapt to another point of view Able to use stored knowledge to make independent judgments	Fluent in spoken language Vocabulary 50,000 words for reading; oral vocabulary of 7200 words Uses slang words and terms, vulgarities, jeers, jokes, and sayings	Can catch or intercept ball thrown from a distance Possible growth spurts may cause myopia	Begins abstract thinking Conservation of volume Understands relationships among time, speed, and distance Ability to sympathize, love, and reason are all evolving Right and wrong become logically clear

gaged in a struggle to master the developmental tasks that lead to successful completion of this stage of development (Table 16-2). The successful completion of these tasks also is based on successful completion of developmental tasks of earlier stages of development.

Physical Development

Rapid growth occurs during adolescence. Girls begin growing during the preadolescent period and achieve 98% of their adult height by the age of 16. Boys start growing around 13 years of age and may continue to grow until 20 years of age. The rapid growth of the skeletal system, which outpaces the muscular system, causes the long, lanky appearance of many teens, contributing to the clumsiness often seen during this age.

When menstruation first begins, ovulation does not occur because it is a result of increasing estrogen levels. However, between 13 and 15 years, menstruation in the female becomes ovulatory, and pregnancy is possible. Breast development takes on the appearance of the adult woman's breasts by age 16, and pubic hair is curly and abundant.

By the age of 16 years, the male's penis, testes, and scrotum are adult in size and shape, and there is production of mature spermatozoa. Male pubic hair also is adult in appearance and amount. After age 13, muscle strength and coordination develop rapidly. The larynx and vocal cords enlarge, and the voice deepens. The "change of voice" makes the teenage male's voice vary unexpectedly, which occasionally causes embarrassment for the teen.

Nutrition

Nutritional requirements are greatly increased during periods of rapid growth in adolescence. Adolescent boys need more calories than do girls throughout the growth period. Appetites increase, and most teens eat frequently. Families with teenage boys often jokingly say that they cannot keep the refrigerator filled. Nutritional needs are related to growth and sexual maturity rather than age.

Even though adolescents understand something about nutrition, they may not relate this understanding to their dietary habits. Their accelerated growth rate and, for some, increased physical activities mean that they need more food to supply their energy requirements. Because adolescents are seeking to establish their independence, their food choices are sometimes not wise ones but tend to be influenced by peer preference rather than parental advice. The era of fast-food meals has given adolescents easy access to high-calorie but nutritionally unbalanced meals. Too many fast-food meals and nutritionally empty snacks can result in nutritional deficiencies.

When good nutritional habits have been established in early childhood, adolescent nutrition is likely to be better balanced than when nutritional teaching has been insufficient. Being part of a family that practices sound nutrition helps ensure that occasional lapses into sweets, fast foods, and other peer group food preferences will not create serious deficiencies. Nutrient needs that frequently are not met by the teen's diet include calcium, iron, zinc, vitamins A, D, B₆, and folic acid. Calcium needs increase in skeletal growth. Girls need additional iron because of

Table 16-2. Developmental Tasks of Adolescence

Basic Task	Associated Tasks
Appreciate own uniqueness*	Identify interests, skills, and talents Identify differences from peers Accept strengths and limitations Challenge own skill levels
Develop independent internal identity*	Value self as a person Separate physical self from psychological self Differentiate personal worth from cultural stereotypes Separate internal value from societal feedback
Determine own value system*	Identify options Establish priorities Commit self to decisions made Translate values into behaviors Resist peer and cultural pressure to conform to their value system Find comfortable balance between own and peer/cultural standards, behaviors, and needs
Develop self-evaluation skills*	Develop basis for self-evaluation and monitoring Evaluate quality of products Assess approach to tasks and responsibilities Develop sensitivity to intrapersonal relationships Evaluate dynamics of interpersonal relationships
Assume increasing responsibility for own behavior*	Quality of work, chores Emotional tone Money management Time management Decision making Personal habits Social behaviors
Finding meaning in life	Accept and integrate meaning of death Develop philosophy of life Begin to identify life or career goals
Acquire skills essential for adult living	Acquire skills essential to independent living Develop social-emotional abilities and temperament Refine sociocultural amenities Identify and experiment with alternatives for facing life Acquire employment skills Seek growth-inducing activities
Seek affiliations outside of family of origin	Seek companionship with compatible peers Affiliate with organizations that support uniqueness Actively seek models or mentors Identify potential emotional support systems Differentiate between acquaintances and friends Identify ways to express one's sexuality
Adapt to adult body functioning	Adapt to somatic (body) changes Refine balance and coordination Develop physical strength Consider sexuality and reproduction issues

*Tasks deemed most crucial to continued maturation.
Adapted from Schuster CS, Ashburn SS. The Process of Human Development: A Holistic Life-Span Approach, 3rd ed.
Philadelphia: JB Lippincott, 1992.

losses that occur during menstruation. Boys also need additional iron during this growth period (Table 16-3).

In their quest for identity and independence, some adolescents experiment with food fads and diets. Adolescent girls, worried about being slim, fall prey to a variety of fad diets. In addition, teens frequently skip meals, particularly breakfast, snack on foods that provide empty calories, and eat a lot of fast foods. Athletes also may follow fad diets that may include supplements in the belief that these diets enhance body building. These diets frequently include increased amounts of protein and amino acids, which cause diuresis and calcium loss. Car-

Table 16-3. Food Sources of Nutrients Commonly Deficient
in Preadolescent and Adolescent Diets

Common Nutrient Deficiencies	Food Sources
Vitamin A	Liver, whole milk, butter, cheese; sources of carotene such as yellow vegetables, green leafy vegetables, tomatoes, yellow fruits
Vitamin D	Fortified milk, fish liver oils
Vitamin B$_6$ (pyridoxine)	Liver, kidney, chicken, fish, pork, eggs, whole-grain cereals, legumes
Folacin (folic acid)	Green leafy vegetables, liver, kidney, meats, fish, nuts, legumes, whole grains
Calcium	Milk, hard cheese, yogurt, ice cream, small fish eaten with bones (e.g., sardines), dark green vegetables, tofu, soybeans, calcium-enriched orange juice
Iron	Lean meats, liver, legumes, dried fruits, green leafy vegetables, whole grain and fortified cereals
Zinc	Oysters, herring, meat, liver, fish, milk, whole grains, nuts, legumes

bohydrate loading, practiced by some during the week before an athletic event, increases muscle glycogen 2 to 3 times normal and may cause injury to heart function. A meal that is low in fat and high in complex carbohydrates eaten 3 to 4 hours before an event is much more appropriate for the teen athlete.

Adolescents need a balanced diet consisting of three servings from the milk–dairy group, 2 or 3 servings (6 to 7 ounces total) from the meat group, 3 or 4 servings from the fruit group, 4 or 5 servings from the vegetable group, and 9 to 11 servings from the grain group (Figure 16-2). Adolescents often resist pressure from family members to eat balanced meals, therefore family caregivers simply must provide adequate nutritious meals and snacks and regular mealtimes. A good example may be the best teacher at this point. A refrigerator stocked with nutritious snacks ready to eat can be a good weapon to prevent snacking on empty calories.

Families with low incomes may have difficulty providing the kind of foods that meet the requirements for a growing teen. These families need help to learn how to make low-cost, nutritious food selections and plan adequate meals and snacks. The nurse can be instrumental in helping these families plan appropriate food purchases. For instance, they might recommend fruit and vegetable stores or farm stands that accept food stamps.

Ethnic and Cultural Influences
Culture also influences adolescent food choices and habits. For example, many Mexican-Americans are accustomed to having their big meal at noon. When school lunches do not provide such a heavy meal, the Mexican-American adolescent may supplement with sweets or fast foods. Within the Asian community, milk is not a popular drink, and this can result in a calcium deficiency. Many Asians have a lactose intolerance; therefore, other products high in calcium, such as tofu (soybean curd), soybeans, and greens should be recommended to increase calcium intake.

Certain religions recommend that their followers observe a vegetarian diet. Other persons follow a vegetarian diet for ecologic or philosophic reasons. With care, vegetarian diets can provide the nutrients that are needed. The most common types of vegetarian diets are the following:

- *Semivegetarian*—includes dairy products, eggs, and fish; excludes red meat and, possibly, poultry
- *Lactoovovegetarian*—includes eggs and dairy products; excludes meat, poultry, and fish
- *Lactovegetarian*—includes dairy products; excludes meat, fish, poultry, and eggs
- *Vegan*—excludes all food of animal origin, including dairy products, eggs, fish, meat, and poultry

Of these, vegan is the diet that may not provide adequate nutrients without careful planning. All vegetarians should include whole-grain products, legumes, nuts, seeds, and fortified soy substitutes if low-fat dairy products are not acceptable.

The nurse must be alert to cultural dietary influences on the adolescent and take these into consideration when helping the adolescent and the family devise an adequate food plan.

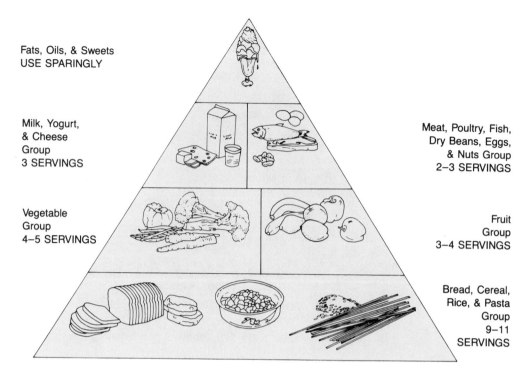

Fats, Oils, & Sweets
USE SPARINGLY

Milk, Yogurt,
& Cheese
Group
3 SERVINGS

Meat, Poultry, Fish,
Dry Beans, Eggs,
& Nuts Group
2–3 SERVINGS

Vegetable
Group
4–5 SERVINGS

Fruit
Group
3–4 SERVINGS

Bread, Cereal,
Rice, & Pasta
Group
9–11
SERVINGS

Smaller number of servings for Teen Girls—Larger number of servings for Teen Boys

What Counts as 1 Serving? ▶

The amount you eat may be more than one serving.
For example, a dinner portion of spaghetti would count as 2 or 3 servings.

Bread, Cereal, Rice & Pasta Group	Vegetable Group	Fruit Group	Milk, Yogurt & Cheese Group	Meat, Poultry, Fish, Dry Beans, Eggs & Nuts Group	Fats & Sweets
1 slice of bread	1/2 cup of chopped raw or cooked vegetables	1 piece of fruit or melon wedge	1 cup of milk or yogurt	2 1/2 to 3 ounces of cooked lean meat, poultry, or fish	LIMIT CALORIES FROM THESE especially if you need to lose weight
1/2 cup of cooked rice or pasta	1 cup of leafy raw vegetables	3/4 cup of juice	1 1/2 ounces of natural cheese	Count 1/2 cup of cooked beans, or 1 egg, or 2 tablespoons of peanut butter as 1 ounce of lean meat	
1/2 cup of cooked cereal		1/2 cup of canned fruit	2 ounces of processed cheese		
1 ounce of ready-to-eat cereal		1/4 cup of dried fruit			

Figure 16-2. Food guide pyramid adapted for adolescent girls and boys. (From United States Department of Agriculture.)

Health Maintenance

Adolescents have much the same need for regular health checkups, protection against infection, and prevention of accidents as do younger children. They also have special needs that can best be met by health professionals with in-depth knowledge and understanding of adolescent concerns (Figure 16-3). The number of adolescent clinics and health centers has increased, along with innovative health services such as school-based clinics, crisis hot lines, homes for runaways, and rehabilitation centers for adolescents who have been involved with alcohol or other drugs or with prostitution. Staffs in these programs work to provide teens with services needed for healthy growth.

Physical Examination, Screening, and Immunization

A routine physical examination is recommended at least twice during the teen years, although annual physical examinations are encouraged. At this time, a complete history of developmental milestones, school problems, behavioral problems, family relationships, and immuniz-

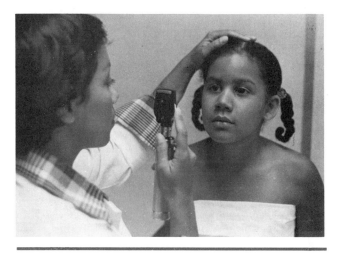

Figure 16-3. Pediatric nurse practitioner examines a young adolescent.

ations should be completed. Immunization for measles, mumps, and rubella (MMR) is given if the second dose of the MMR vaccine was not administered during the late school age; however, a urine pregnancy screening is advisable before the rubella vaccine is administered to a girl of this age. A booster of diphtheria and tetanus toxoid (dT) is given around 14 to 16 years of age (approximately 10 years after the last booster). If the teen has not been immunized with hepatitis B vaccine, immunization also is recommended at this time. Any other immunizations that are incomplete should be updated. Tuberculin testing is included at one visit at least and, depending on the community, may be recommended at both visits if there is an interval of several years between visits.

Height, weight, and blood pressure are measured and recorded. Vision and hearing screening are done if they have not been part of a regular school screening program. Up to the age of 16 years, adolescents need to be screened for scoliosis. Thyroid enlargement should be checked through age 14. Sexually active girls must have a pelvic examination, screening for sexually transmitted diseases (STDs), and a Pap smear. Urinalysis is performed on all female adolescents, and a urine culture is performed if the girl has any symptoms of a urinary tract infection, such as urgency or burning and pain on urination. This is an excellent time for the nurse to counsel the adolescent girl about sexual activity, STDs, and human immunodeficiency viral (HIV) infection.

Adolescents need to be ensured of privacy, individualized attention, confidentiality, and the right to participate in decisions about their health care. They may feel uncomfortable and out of place in a pediatrician's waiting room, where most of the patients are 3 feet tall, or in a waiting room filled with adults. There are adolescent clinics and physicians who specialize in adolescent health care, but many adolescents do not have these facilities available to them.

Continuity of care helps build the adolescent's confidence in the service and the caregivers. Professionals dealing with teens should recognize that the physical symptoms offered as the reason for seeking care are often not the most significant problem about which the adolescent is concerned. An attitude of nonjudgmental acceptance on the part of the health care personnel frequently can encourage the adolescent to share questions, feelings, and concerns about a troubling matter. Adolescents may be accompanied to the health care facility by a family caregiver, but they need to have an opportunity to be interviewed alone. Questions must be asked in a way that is concrete and specific so that the adolescent will give direct answers. The interviewer must be alert to verbal and nonverbal clues.

Health Education and Counseling

Before adolescents can take an active role in their own health care, they need information and guidance on the need for health care and how to most effectively meet that need. Education and counseling about sexuality, STDs, contraception, substance abuse, and mental health are a vital part of adolescent health care. Some of this teaching should, and sometimes does, come from family caregivers, but often the caregivers' lack of information, or their discomfort in discussing these topics, means that the job will have to be done by health professionals.

Sexuality

A good foundation in sex education can help the adolescent take pride in having reached sexual maturity; otherwise, puberty can be a frightening, shameful experience. Girls who have not been taught about menstruation until it occurs are understandably alarmed. Those who have been taught to regard it as "the curse" rather than as an entrance into womanhood will not have positive feelings about this part of their sexuality.

Boys who are unprepared for nocturnal emissions may feel guilty, believing that they have caused these "wet dreams" by sexual fantasies or masturbation. They need to understand that this is a normal occurrence and simply the body's method of getting rid of surplus semen.

Assuming that adolescents are adequately prepared for the events of puberty, sex education during adolescence can deal with the important issues of responsible sexuality, contraception, and venereal disease. More adolescents today are sexually active than ever, resulting in an alarmingly rapid increase in teenage pregnancies and STDs. The incidence of HIV infection, in particular, is increasing among adolescents.

Girls need to learn the importance of regular pelvic examinations and Pap smears and the technique for breast self-examination, a monthly self-care procedure (Figure 16-4). Boys need to learn that testicular cancer is one of the most common cancers in young men between

Breast Self-Examination (BSE)

Here is one way to do BSE:

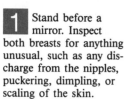

1 Stand before a mirror. Inspect both breasts for anything unusual, such as any discharge from the nipples, puckering, dimpling, or scaling of the skin.

The next two steps are designed to emphasize any change in the shape or contour of your breasts. As you do them you should be able to feel your chest muscles tighten.

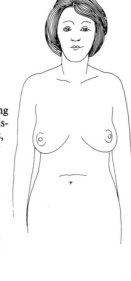

2 Watching closely in the mirror, clasp hands behind your head and press hands forward.

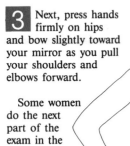

3 Next, press hands firmly on hips and bow slightly toward your mirror as you pull your shoulders and elbows forward.

Some women do the next part of the exam in the shower. Fingers glide over soapy skin, making it easy to concentrate on the texture underneath.

Breast self-examination should be done once a month so you become familiar with the usual appearance and feel of your breasts. Familiarity makes it easier to notice any changes in the breast from one month to another. Early discovery of a change from what is "normal" is the main idea behind BSE.

If you menstruate, the best time to do BSE is 2 or 3 days after your period ends, when your breasts are least likely to be tender or swollen. If you no longer menstruate, pick a day, such as the first day of the month, to remind yourself it is time to do BSE.

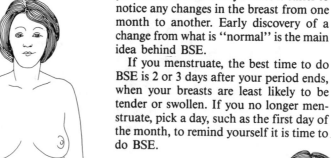

4 Raise your left arm. Use three or four fingers of your right hand to explore your left breast firmly, carefully, and thoroughly. Beginning at the outer edge, press the flat part of your fingers in small circles, moving the circles slowly around the breast. Gradually work toward the nipple. Be sure to cover the entire breast. Pay special attention to the area between the breast and the armpit, including the armpit itself. Feel for any unusual lump or mass under the skin.

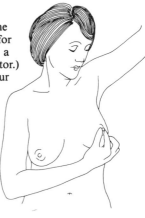

5 Gently squeeze the nipple and look for a discharge. (If there is a discharge, see your doctor.) Repeat the exam on your right breast.

6 Steps 4 and 5 should be repeated lying down. Lie flat on your back, left arm over your head and a pillow or folded towel under your left shoulder. This position flattens the breast and makes it easier to examine. Use the same circular motion described earlier.
     Repeat on your right breast.

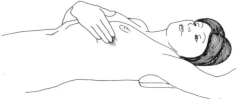

Figure 16-4. Breast self-examination as presented by the National Cancer Institute. (NIH Publication No. 88-1556, 1988.)

the ages of 15 and 34 and must be taught how and when to perform a testicular self-examination (Parent Teaching: Testicular Self-Examination) (Figure 16-5).

Masturbation. Adolescents' growing awareness of their sexuality, sexually provocative material in the media, and lack of acceptable means to gratify sexual desires make masturbation a common practice during adolescence. Unlike young children's genital exploration, adolescent masturbation can produce orgasm in the female and ejaculation in the male. Generally, it is a private, solitary activity, but occasionally it occurs with one or more members of the peer group. Health professionals recognize masturbation as a positive way to release sexual tension and increase one's knowledge of body sensations. The nurse can reassure adolescents that masturbation is common in both males and females and is a normal outlet for sexual urges.

Sexual Responsibility

Not all adolescents are sexually active, but the numbers increase with each year of age. Although abstinence is the only completely successful protection, all adolescents need to have information concerning safe sex practices to be prepared for the occasion when they wish to be sexually intimate with someone. Adolescents do not have a good record of using contraceptives to prevent preg-

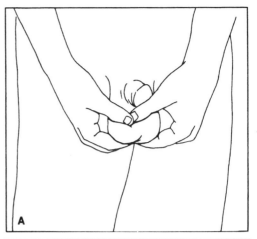

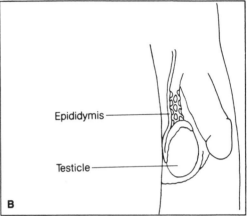

Epididymis

Testicle

Figure 16-5. Drawings from the National Cancer Institute pamphlet, "What You Need to Know About Testicular Cancer," NIH Publication 88-1565, Revised June 1988. **A**, Examine each testicle with index and middle fingers under testicle and thumbs on top; **B**, Cross section of scrotum showing position of the epididymis and the testicle.

Parent Teaching

Testicular Self Examination

1. Perform the examination once a month after a warm bath or shower. The scrotum is relaxed from the warmth. Select a day that is easy to remember, such as the first or last day of the month.

2. Stand in front of a mirror, if possible, and look for any swelling on the skin of the scrotum.

3. Examine each testicle, one at a time, using both hands.

4. Place the index and middle fingers under the testicle and the thumbs on top. Roll each testicle gently between the thumbs and fingers. One testicle is normally larger than the other (see Figure 16-5**A**).

5. The epididymis is the soft, tubelike structure located at the back of the testicle that collects and carries sperm. This must not be mistaken for an abnormal lump (see Figure 16-5**B**).

6. Most lumps are found on the sides of the testicle, although they may appear on the front. Report any lump to your health care provider at once.

7. Testicular cancer is highly curable when treated promptly.

nancy. Many teens give excuses such as "sex shouldn't be planned," because if it is planned, it is wrong or they feel guilty. They need to feel that it just "happened" because of the heat of the moment, not because they really wanted or planned it. Many adolescents are beginning to realize that much more than pregnancy may be at risk, but their attitude of "it won't happen to me," typical of their developmental age, continues to contribute to their increasing sexual activity.

Some adults continue to resist providing contraceptive information to adolescents in school, believing that such information encourages teens to become sexually active. However, as HIV infection becomes a greater threat to every sexually active person, this argument becomes harder to defend. Adolescents need contraceptive information to prevent pregnancy, but, more important, they need straightforward information about using condoms to protect themselves against HIV infection. Both male and female adolescents need this information, and girls must be advised to carry their own condoms if they believe there is any possibility that they may have sexual intercourse.

Condoms have been claimed to have an 85% effectiveness rate. Condoms with spermicidal foam have an effective rate of 95%, but when users are taught how to use them correctly, the rate of effectiveness increases to 99%. The effectiveness of protection from HIV and other STDs should follow the same percentages. The safest choice of condom is one made of latex with a prelubricated tip or reservoir and pretreated with nonoxynol 9 spermicide. Parent Teaching: Safe Condom Use (Figure 16-6) provides guidelines for use.

Parent Teaching

Safe Condom Use

1. Use a new condom each time.
2. The safest type of condom is prelubricated latex with a tip or reservoir that has been pretreated with nonoxynol 9 spermicide.
3. If the condom is not pretreated, you may lubricate with water or water-based lubricant, such as K-Y jelly *and* a spermicidal jelly of foam containing nonoxynol 9.
4. Do not use oil-based products such as mineral oil, cold cream, or petroleum jelly to lubricate; they may weaken the latex.
5. Put condom on as soon as the penis is erect. Retract the foreskin if not circumcised, and unroll the condom over the entire length of the penis.
6. Leave a 1/2-inch space at the end. Press out the tip of the condom to remove air bubbles.
7. The outside of the condom may be lubricated as much as desired with a water-soluble lubricant.
8. If the condom starts to slip during intercourse, hold it on. Do not let it slip off. Condoms come in sizes, so if you have a problem with slipping, look for a smaller size.
9. After ejaculation, hold the rim of the condom at the base of the penis, and withdraw before losing erection.
10. Remove condom and tie a knot in the open end. Dispose of condom so that no one can come in contact with semen.
11. Heat can damage condoms. Store in a cool, dry place.
12. Immediately after intercourse, both partners should wash off any semen or vaginal secretions with soap and water (see Figure 16-6).

Other STDs that sexually active adolescents need to know about are syphilis, gonorrhea, genital herpes, genital warts, and chlamydial and trichomonal infections. Prevention of STDs is the primary aim of education for adolescents. However, if prevention proves ineffective, the most important factor is referral for treatment. Many adolescents are reluctant to seek treatment, fearing that their family caregivers will discover their activity. Crisis hot lines are valuable resources to assure adolescents that treatment is vital for them and their partners, and confidentiality is ensured.

Health care personnel who work with adolescents seeking treatment for an STD must be nonjudgmental, supportive, and understanding. The adolescents need treatment and information about preventing spread of the STD to others as well as how to prevent contracting another STD. (See Chapter 17 for a thorough discussion of STDs and related nursing care.)

Substance Abuse
As adolescents search for identity and independence, they are susceptible to many pressures from society and their peers. Adolescents may indulge in experimentation with a number of substances that may be habit forming or addictive and ultimately will harm them. This may be done just for "kicks," to "go along with the crowd" (peer group), or to rebel against the authority of family caregivers or other adults. Some substances that are abused by adolescents also are abused by many adults, and to some adolescents, using these substances may appear sophisticated. Alcohol and certain other drugs provide an escape, however brief, from the pressures that the adolescent may feel. Alcohol is the mind-altering substance most frequently abused by adolescents.

Substances that adolescents may abuse are tobacco, including smokeless tobacco, alcohol, marijuana, cocaine or "crack," heroin, other "street drugs," and prescription drugs. Programs developed to educate students about substance abuse meet with varying success. Health care personnel must stress to adolescents that abuse of mind-altering drugs frequently is accompanied by irresponsible sexual behavior, further complicating their lives. (Chapter 17 discusses these problems in more detail.)

Accident Prevention
In every part of society, increasing numbers of deaths of adolescents occur as a result of some form of violence. This includes motor vehicle accidents, homicide, suicide, and other causes. The homicide rate is approximately 7 times higher for African-American adolescents than for whites (Figure 16-7), and the overall number of violent deaths is much greater for males than for females in every age group between 10 and 19 years (Figure 16-8). White males between 15 and 19 years are killed in motor vehicle accidents twice as frequently as African-American males in this age group.

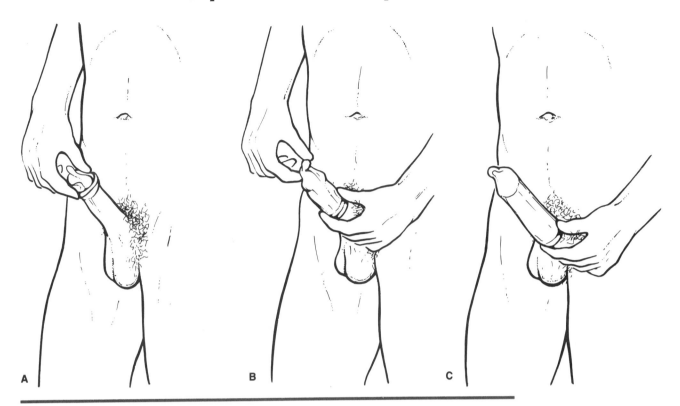

Figure 16-6. Putting on a condom: **A**, Press the air out ½ inch at the tip of the condom; **B**, holding the tip of the condom, carefully roll it down the shaft of the erect penis; **C**, be certain that the condom covers the full length of the penis with the rim of the condom at the base of the penis.

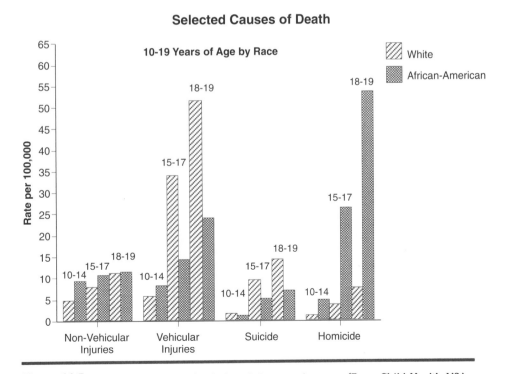

Figure 16-7. Selected causes of death for adolescents by race. (From Child Health USA '90. United States Department of Health and Human Services, HRS-M-CH 90-1, October, 1990.)

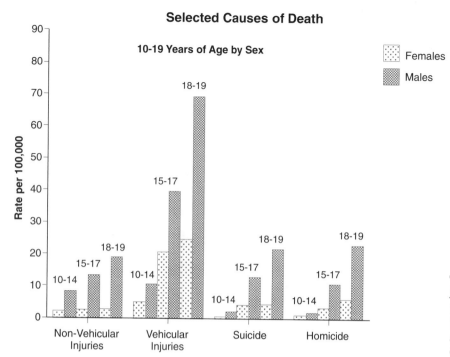

Selected Causes of Death

10-19 Years of Age by Sex

Figure 16-8. Selected causes of death by sex. (From Child Health USA '90. United States Department of Health and Human Services, HRS-M-CH 90-1, October, 1990.)

Alcohol and other drugs are frequently related to the cause of fatal accidents. Deaths are not the only negative outcome of violent acts. Many adolescents are injured and hospitalized or treated in emergency departments. Many also suffer from psychological injury as a result of being the victim of violence.

Violence is on the increase in our nation's schools. This increase is not limited to inner city schools. Weapons are being detected on students in schools all over the country. Guns and knives are the weapons most frequently found. The problem has become so serious that some schools have installed metal detectors to protect students. Adolescents also are victims of violence in their own homes in greater numbers than any other age group of children. Date rape and other violence in a dating relationship has become a concern because such violence has become common.

Students have formed groups such as Students Against Drunk Driving (SADD) to promote safety in driving. Many schools provide support groups that help students work through their grief after schoolmates have met with violent death. Much work needs to be done to understand the reason for this increasing violence. One factor may be that adolescents act recklessly without benefit of mature judgment. Adolescents have access to guns with relative ease and frequently do use them as a means to solve problems. Efforts to control gun sales have met with little success in the United States Congress.

Nurses who have any contact with adolescents must make every effort to help adolescents work through their problems in a nonviolent way. The nurse can become involved at the school or community level, becoming an advocate for adolescents and an educator to promote safe driving as well as helmet wear and safety practices when using a motorcycle, all-terrain vehicle, bicycle, skateboard, or roller blades. Nurses also can support groups that offer counseling to adolescents involved in incidents of date violence. Nurses can provide a positive role model for adolescents as community members and health care workers.

Mental Health

The turmoil that adolescents experience while searching for self-esteem and self-confidence can cause stress that may lead to depression, suicide, and conduct disorders. Academic and social pressures add to that stress. The family also may be under stress due to unemployment or economic difficulties, separation, divorce, or death of one of the caregivers. Health care personnel who work with adolescents must be sensitive to the signs that may indicate that an adolescent is experiencing problems. Adolescents need the opportunity to ventilate their fears, concerns, and frustrations. The rapport between family caregivers and teens may not be such that the adolescent feels able to express these feelings to them. Many schools have mental health personnel on staff who can provide counseling when it is needed. Adolescents need counseling help to work through troublesome situations and avoid chronic mental health problems. Mental health assessment is an important part of the total health assessment of the adolescent.

Psychosocial Development

Adolescence is a time of transition from childhood to adulthood. In the period between the ages of 10 and 18 years, adolescents move from Freud's latency to the genital stage, from Erikson's industry versus inferiority to identity versus role confusion, and from Piaget's concrete operational thinking to formal operational thought. They develop a sense of moral judgment and a system of values and beliefs that will influence their entire life. The foundation provided by their family, school, and community experiences is still a strong influence, but tremendous power is exerted by the peer group. Trends and fads among adolescents dictate clothing choices, hair styles, music, and other recreational choices (Figure 16-9). The adolescent whose family caregivers make it difficult to conform are adding another stress to an already emotion-laden period. Peer pressure to experiment with potentially dangerous practices such as drugs, alcohol, and reckless driving also can be strong, and adolescents may need careful guidance and understanding support to help resist this peer influence.

Personality Development

Erikson considered the central task of adolescence to be the establishment of *identity*. Adolescents spend a lot of time asking themselves, "Who am I as a person? What will I do with my life? Marry? Have children? Will I go to college? If so, where? If not, why not? What kind of career should I choose?"

Adolescents are confronted with a greater variety of choices than ever before. Sex role stereotypes have been shattered in most careers and professions. More women are becoming lawyers, physicians, plumbers, and carpenters; more men are entering nursing or choosing to become house-husbands while their wives earn the primary family income. Transportation has made greater geographic mobility possible, so that many youngsters can spend summers or a full school year in a foreign country, plan to attend college thousands of miles from home, and begin a career in an even more remote location. Making decisions and choices is never simple and, with such a tremendous variety of options, it is understandable that adolescents often are preoccupied with their own concerns.

When identity has been established, generally between the ages of 16 and 18 years, adolescents seek intimate relationships, usually with members of the opposite sex. *Intimacy* means mutual sharing of deepest feelings with another person; intimacy is impossible unless both persons have established a sense of trust and a sense of identity. Intimate relationships are a preparation for long-term relationships, and people who fail to achieve intimacy may develop feelings of isolation and experience chronic difficulty in communicating with others.

Most intimate relationships during adolescence are **heterosexual**, or between members of the opposite sex. Sometimes, however, young people form intimate attachments with members of the same sex, or **homosexual** relationships. Because our culture is predominately heterosexual and is still struggling with trying to understand

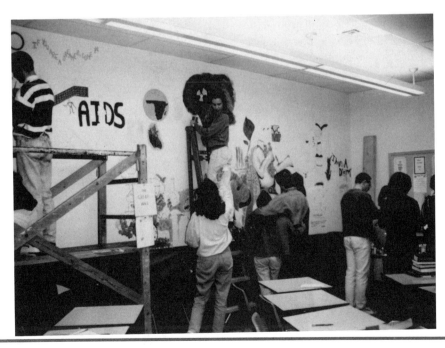

Figure 16-9. Teenagers working together on a wall mural for a high school world cultures class depicting world social concerns. (Photo by Ron Becker.)

homosexual relationships, these relationships can cause great anxiety for family caregivers and children. Although some areas of American society are beginning to accept homosexual relationships as no more than another lifestyle, prejudice still exists. So great a stigma has been attached to homosexuality that many adolescents fear they are homosexual if they are uncomfortable about heterosexual intimacy. However, this is a normal problem that occurs as adolescents move from same-sex peer group activities to dating peers of the opposite sex.

Body Image

A person's concept of body image is closely related to self-esteem. Seeing one's body as attractive and functional contributes to a positive sense of self-esteem. During adolescence, the desire not to be different can extend to feelings about one's body and cause adolescents to feel inadequate about their bodies, even though they are really healthy and attractive.

American culture tends to equate a slender figure with feminine beauty and acceptability and a lean, tall, muscular figure with masculine virility and strength. Adolescents who feel that they are underdeveloped suffer great anxiety, particularly males. Adolescent girls have even undergone plastic surgery to augment their breasts to relieve this anxiety. Girls in this age group often feel that they are too fat and try strange, nutritionally unsound diets to reduce their weight. Some literally starve themselves, and even after their bodies have become emaciated, truly believe that they are still fat and therefore unattractive. This condition is called *anorexia nervosa* and is discussed further in Chapter 17.

It is important that adolescents establish a positive body image by the end of their developmental stage. Because bone growth is completed during adolescence, a person's height will remain basically the same throughout adult life, even though weight can fluctuate greatly. Tall girls who long to be petite and boys who would like to be 6-feet tall may need guidance and support to bring their expectations in line with reality and learn to have positive feelings and acceptance about their bodies the way they are.

norms and an interruption in their search for identity. Adolescents fear loss of control and a loss of privacy. The nurse caring for an adolescent must provide opportunities for the adolescent to make choices whenever possible and protect the adolescent's privacy by providing screening and adequate covering during procedures. Adolescents may react with anger and refuse to cooperate when they feel threatened. The nurse needs to be aware of this possible reaction and avoid labeling such an adolescent as a difficult patient.

The admission interview for an adolescent may be more successful if the family caregiver and the adolescent are interviewed separately. This provides the opportunity to gain information that the adolescent may not want to reveal in the presence of the family caregiver. The nurse who works with hospitalized adolescents needs to thoroughly assess the person's developmental level, listen carefully with empathy to the adolescent's concerns, encourage maximum participation in self-care, and provide sufficient information to make this participation possible. As with all patients, clear, honest explanations about treatments and procedures are essential.

During the admission interview, the adolescent should be advised of the rules and regulations of the nursing unit. Adolescents need to know what limits are set for their behavior while hospitalized. They often will find it helpful to discuss their health problem with a peer who has had the same or a related problem in order to share feelings and gain information.

Adolescents need access to a telephone that they can use to contact peers to keep up social contacts. Recreation areas are important. In settings that are specifically designed for adolescents, recreation rooms can provide an area where teens can gather to do school work, play games, cards, and socialize. In many hospitals with adolescent units, video games as well as television are provided in each patient room for the adolescent's entertainment. Teens are encouraged to wear their own clothes. Girls can be encouraged to shampoo and style their hair and wear their usual makeup. The adolescent's health problem may require a lengthy hospitalization and intense rehabilitation efforts. Adequate preparation and guidance can help make that difficult experience easier and less damaging to normal growth and development.

The Hospitalized Adolescent

When adolescents are hospitalized, it is usually because of a major health problem such as a traumatic injury as a victim of violence or from a motor vehicle accident, substance abuse, attempted suicide, or a chronic health problem intensified by the physiologic changes of adolescence. Adolescents must cope with the stress of hospitalization, possible dramatic alterations in body image, being partially or totally unable to conform with peer group

Summary

The adolescent years are turbulent years during which adolescents often feel confused. Beginning with the preadolescent years, children go through many physical and emotional changes on their way to adulthood. The search for identity and independence brings about many struggles within the adolescent. During these years, they face many pressures and temptations that often make demands on them that are difficult to resist. Adolescents who have a warm, accepting family environment, positive school experiences, and good health have the best chance of reaching adulthood with a positive sense of self, the ability to form close relationships, and the capacity to make sound decisions about their lives.

As a result of the rapid physical growth that occurs during this period, adolescents' nutritional needs are increased. Adolescents may or may not eat nutritionally sound food. Many factors influence an adolescent's nutritional needs and food intake. Caregivers must be alert to adolescents' nutritional deficiencies and make an effort to provide sound nutritional guidance.

Adolescents are trying to identify their career options and determine what they want to do with their lives. Many more career opportunities are available to them than at any previous time. This abundance of choices can place more pressure on them when making decisions.

Although adolescents' health is generally good, they need a program of health maintenance in a setting that meets their needs for privacy, individualized attention, confidentiality, and the right to participate in decisions about their health care.

The issues of substance abuse, sexual decisions, sexual and physical abuse, and accident prevention contribute to additional dilemmas for adolescents. Peer pressure may be extremely influential in affecting the adolescent's attitudes and behaviors related to these issues. The increase in violence in the schools is an additional issue that teens may encounter. Adolescents need a strong support system to help them through this stressful stage of development.

Only after adolescents complete the task of establishing their identity are they ready to establish an intimate relationship, the next task of development according to Erikson. Developing intimate relationships brings an additional set of problems.

In the hospital setting, the adolescent fears loss of control and privacy. The nurse caring for the hospitalized adolescent must be sensitive to the adolescent's needs and provide care that is supportive and provides for as much participation by the adolescent as possible. Health problems that threaten the adolescent's body image may threaten the satisfactory completion of developmental tasks.

Review Questions

1. Mr. K. is the custodial parent of Gina, age 11. He is concerned about providing her with appropriate sex education information. What specific guidelines can you give him?
2. Cathy is the primary family caregiver of Jon, age 11. She asks you what sex education she should be giving Jon. What guidance will you give her?
3. Mattie is the mother of two teenagers. She is concerned about their nutrition. Using Table 16-3, make a list of foods for her that will provide nutrients that are commonly deficient in the adolescent's diet. Include a list of the nutrients that are included.
4. Jamal is an adolescent athlete. He has told you he is planning to use a carbohydrate-loading diet before a big track meet. Using your knowledge about carbohydrate loading, what guidance will you give him?
5. What are the recommended guidelines for routine health care for adolescents?
6. You have the opportunity to talk with a group of 15-year-old girls. What guidance will you give them about breast self-examination and Pap smears?
7. What information would you give an adolescent boy about testicular self-examination?
8. Why is information about condom use considered important for adolescents? Why do many health caregivers believe that all adolescents need this information?
9. Describe the guidelines for condom use.
10. Why are tobacco products and alcohol included in a discussion of substance abuse?
11. How are alcohol and other drugs related to accidents?
12. What are some guidelines to help adolescents adjust to hospitalization?

Bibliography

Castiglia PT, Harbin RE. Child Health Care: Process and Practice. Philadelphia: JB Lippincott, 1992.

Cohall AT, Mayer R, Cohal K, et al. Teen violence: The new morality. Contemp Pediatr 8(9):76–86, 1991.

Cohen MI. Adolescents: Left behind by our health care system. Contemp Pediatr 9(7):33–44, 1992.

Dimond DA. Let's talk about sex. Contemp Pediatr 9(7):19–29, 1992.

Eschleman MM. Introductory Nutrition and Diet Therapy, 2nd ed. Philadelphia: JB Lippincott, 1991.

Jackson DB, Saunders RB. Child Health Nursing. Philadelphia: JB Lippincott, 1993.

Libbus MK. Condoms as primary prevention in sexually active women. MCN 17(5):256–260, 1992.

Pillitteri A. Maternal and Child Health Nursing. Philadelphia: JB Lippincott, 1992.

Schuster CS, Ashburn SS. The Process of Human Development, 3rd ed. Philadelphia: JB Lippincott, 1992.

Starn J, Paperny DM. Computer games to enhance adolescent sex education. MCN 15(4):250–253, 1990.

Whaley LF, Wong DL. Nursing Care of Infants and Children, 4th ed. St. Louis: Mosby-Year Book, 1991.

Health Problems of the Adolescent

Student Objectives

Upon completion of this chapter, the student will be able to:

1. Define key terms.
2. Discuss the goal of caregivers who work with obese adolescents.
3. State two goals of treatment for the hospitalized anorectic patient.
4. Discuss alcohol abuse and its impact on adolescents.
5. List nine types of drugs commonly abused by adolescents, and state at least one negative effect of each.
6. State the third leading cause of death in the 10- to 19-year-old age group.
7. Discuss the factors involved in causing acne vulgaris.
8. List the drugs commonly used for mild acne; for inflammatory acne; and for severe acne.
9. Describe infectious mononucleosis.
10. Identify the only certain way to prevent sexually transmitted diseases.
11. Identify the drug of choice to treat gonorrhea; to treat syphilis.
12. Identify how the human immunodeficiency virus is transmitted.
13. Discuss how the developmental tasks of adolescence conflict with the developmental tasks of pregnancy.

Marks MG: BROADRIBB'S INTRODUCTORY PEDIATRIC NURSING, 4th ed. © 1994 J.B. Lippincott Company.

Key Terms

alcohol abuse	menarche
alcoholism	mittelschmerz
amenorrhea	obesity
anorexia nervosa	overweight
bulimia	polyphagia
chancre	premenstrual syndrome
comedone	sebum
dependence	substance abuse
dysmenorrhea	tolerance
gynecomastia	vaginitis
impunity	withdrawal symptoms

*M*any adolescent health problems result from the rapid physiologic changes that are taking place, the person's reaction to those changes, and the stress, conflict, and confusion that characterize adolescence. As adolescents struggle with questions about identity, independence, career, sexuality, morality, and emotions, alterations in their size and physical appearance make them uncomfortable and unfamiliar even with themselves. Coping with these changes and uncertainties is difficult for every adolescent, but for some it is impossible. Lacking adequate coping mechanisms, many adolescents feel there is no solution but escape and seek that escape through alcohol or drugs, running away, committing suicide, or other self-destructive behavior. Motor vehicle accidents, homicide, and suicide are frequent causes of death in the adolescent age group.

The complex interrelationship between psychological well-being and physical health, although not completely understood, is evident throughout life and particularly during adolescence. Emotions and attitudes affect nutrition and other health behaviors and can result in general or systemic disorders, which in turn can lead to further psychological stress. The high number of adoles-

cent pregnancies also is believed to be a result of inappropriate responses to the stresses of adolescence.

Nurses are assuming an increasingly important role in helping adolescents understand, manage, and prevent health problems. Fulfillment of this role demands an understanding of adolescent growth and development and the ability to listen and observe carefully and project a sensitive, nonjudgmental attitude.

Eating Disorders

Eating disorders are among the most common health problems of adolescents. The most common of these are obesity, anorexia nervosa, and bulimia. Food represents nurturing and security and, as a result, may be consumed inappropriately to try to solve problems, but this misuse can result in health problems that have long-term or permanent effects.

Obesity

Obesity is a national problem in the United States, largely as a result of an overabundance of food and too little exercise. The thin figure, particularly for women, has become so idealized that being fat can handicap a person socially and professionally and severely damage self-esteem. **Obesity** generally is defined as an excessive accumulation of fat that increases body weight by 20% or more over ideal weight (Table 17-1). **Overweight** does not necessarily signify obesity but that a person's weight is more than average for height and body build.

Obesity often begins in childhood and, if not treated successfully, leads to chronic obesity in adult life. The obese adolescent frequently feels isolated from the peer group, normally a source of support during this period. Because of the obesity, the adolescent often is embarrassed to participate in sports activities, thus eliminating one method of burning excess calories. Many use food as a means of satisfying emotional needs, establishing a vicious cycle. Adolescents' eating habits, which include skipping meals, especially breakfast, and indulging in late-night eating, compound the problem because the calories that they consume before going to bed are not used for energy but are stored as fat. Snacking while

Table 17-1. Median Heights and Weights (United States)

Age	Weight		Height	
(years)	(kg)	(lb)	(cm)	(inches)
Infants				
0.0–0.5	6	13	60	24
0.5–1.0	9	20	71	28
Children				
1–3	13	29	90	35
4–6	20	44	112	44
7–10	28	62	132	52
Males				
11–14	45	99	157	62
15–18	66	145	176	69
19–24	72	160	177	70
25–50	79	174	176	70
51 +	77	170	173	68
Females				
11–14	46	101	157	62
15–18	55	120	163	64
19–24	58	128	164	65
25–50	63	138	163	64
51 +	65	143	160	63

food restaurants serving high-fat, high-calorie foods with little nutritional value (Figure 17-1). Diets that emphasize nutritionally sound meals and reduced calorie intake produce results too slowly for impatient teenagers. Thus, the many quick weight-loss programs, diet pills, and diet books find a ready market among adolescents.

Treatment must include a thorough exploration of the obese adolescent's food attitudes. Sometimes, a team approach is necessary, using the skills of a psychiatrist or psychologist, nutritionist, nurse, or other counselor. Summer camps that center on weight reduction with nutritious, calorie-controlled food and that stress exercise and activity are successful for some adolescents but are too costly for many families.

Caregivers who work with obese adolescents should try to make these youngsters feel like worthwhile persons, stressing that obesity does not automatically make them unacceptable. Finding the support of a caring adult who will help the adolescent gain control of this aspect of his or her life can help give the necessary incentive to lose weight (see Parent Teaching: Tips for Caregivers of Obese Teens).

Anorexia Nervosa

Preoccupation with reducing diets and the quest for the "perfect" (ie, thin) figure sometimes leads to **anorexia nervosa**, or self-inflicted starvation. This disorder occurs most frequently in adolescent white females, although

watching prime-time television also contributes to the overindulgence in caloric intake.

Some adolescents suffer from **polyphagia** (compulsive overeating). These persons lack control of their food intake, are unable to postpone their urge to eat, hide food for later secret consumption, eat when not hungry or to escape from worries, and expend a great deal of energy thinking about eating and securing food. Not all compulsive eaters are overweight, and in some ways this disorder resembles anorexia nervosa.

Many factors, including genetic, social, cultural, metabolic, and psychological, contribute to the development of obesity. Children of obese parents are likely to share this problem not only because of some inherited predisposition toward obesity but also because of family eating patterns and the emotional climate surrounding food. Certain cultures equate obesity with being loved and being prosperous. If these values carry over into a modern family, the adolescent is torn between the standards of the peer group and those of the family.

Obesity is difficult to treat in any age group but especially in adolescence. Much of teenage life centers around food, such as after-school snacks, the ice cream shop, the drive-in restaurant, the pizza parlor, and fast-

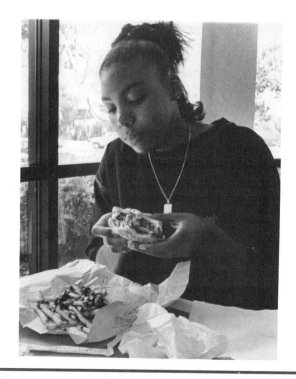

Figure 17-1. Adolescents socializing with food as the "centerpiece."

Parent Teaching

Tips for Caregivers of Obese Teens

1. Have teen keep a food diary for a week. Include food eaten, time eaten, what teen was doing, and how teen felt before and after eating; identify what stimulates urge to eat.

2. Study diary with teen to look for eating triggers.

3. Set a reasonable goal of no more than 1 or 2 pounds a week or perhaps maintaining weight with no gain.

4. Advise teen to eat at only at specific, regular mealtimes.

5. Recommend teen eats only at dining or kitchen table (not in front of TV, or "on the run").

6. Have teen use small plates to make amount of food look like more.

7. Teach to eat slowly—count and chew each bite (25 to 30 is a good goal).

8. Suggest the teen try to leave a little on the plate when done.

9. Have teen survey home and get rid of tempting high-calorie foods.

10. Stock up on low-calorie snacks—carrot sticks, celery sticks, and other raw vegetables.

11. Help teen get involved in an active project that occupies time and also helps to burn calories—any active team sports, or bicycling, walking, hiking, swimming, skating.

12. Promote walking instead of riding whenever possible.

13. Establish group or buddy system.

14. Weigh only once a week, on the same scale, at the same time of day, in the same clothing.

15. Make a chart to keep track of teen's weight.

16. Help teen focus on a positive asset and make the most of it to help build self-concept.

17. Encourage good grooming; group could work on putting on a "mini" fashion show, choosing with guidance clothes that help maximize best features. This could be done simply by using magazine illustrations if actual clothing is not available.

18. Reinforce each small success with positive reinforcement.

19. Enlist cooperation of all family members to support the teen with encouragement and a positive atmosphere.

there are reported cases among males and among African-American, Hispanic, and Asian adolescents. First described more than 100 years ago, anorexia has increased in incidence in recent years, so that anorexia nervosa is currently estimated to affect as many as 1 in 100 adolescent girls and is found in all the developed countries. Two age ranges are identified as the usual age of onset, 11 to 13 years and 19 to 20 years. These adolescents frequently are described as being successful students who tend to be perfectionists, trying always to please parents, teachers, and other adults. Although considered a psychiatric problem, it causes severe physiologic damage and even death.

The adolescent in a controlled family environment, in which the parents do not freely express emotions, appears to try to establish independence and identity by controlling her own appetite and body weight. Depression is common in a large number of these adolescents. The families of anorectic adolescents characteristically show little emotion and display no evidence of conflict within the family. The girl denies her weight loss and actually sees herself as "fat." She frequently adheres to a rigid program of exercise to further her efforts in weight reduction. She also may make demands on herself for cleanliness and order in her environment or engage in rigid schedules for studying and other ritualistic behavior. The adolescent denies hunger but often suffers from fatigue.

These girls are emaciated, almost skeletal, and yet they see themselves as overweight. They appear sexually immature, with dry skin and brittle nails, and often have lanugo (downy hair) over their backs and extremities. Other symptoms include amenorrhea (absence of menstruation), constipation, hypothermia, bradycardia, low blood pressure, and anemia.

The American Psychiatric Association identifies the following criteria for the diagnosis of anorexia nervosa:[1]

- Weight loss 15% below that expected for age and height, or failure to make expected weight gain during a period of growth, leading to body weight 15% below that expected

- Intense fear of gaining weight or becoming fat, even though underweight

- Disturbance in the way the body is experienced (eg, feeling "fat" even when emaciated or perceiving one part of the body to be "too fat," even though underweight)

- Amenorrhea as evidenced by absence of three consecutive menstrual cycles

Treatment

Adolescents diagnosed with anorexia nervosa may be hospitalized to achieve the two goals of treatment: correction of malnutrition and identification and treatment of the psychological cause. An approach involving several disciplines is necessary. Therapy is required to help the adolescent gain insight into her problem. In addition, family therapy, nutritional therapy, and behavior modification are used. The adolescent fears that she will gain an excessive amount of weight, therefore a compromise between what the physician would prefer and what the adolescent desires may be necessary.

Adolescents with anorexia have become experts in manipulating others and their environment. Once hospitalized, they may try to avoid gaining weight by ordering only low-calorie foods; by disposing of their meals in plants, trash, toilets, or dirty linen; or by exercising in the hall or jogging in place in their room. In some instances, nasogastric tube feedings or hyperalimentation is necessary to provide nutritional support.

In treatment based on behavior modification, the patient may be deprived of all privileges, such as visitors, television, and telephone, until she begins to gain weight. Privileges are then gradually restored. These techniques are effective only when the patient and the caregivers understand the program and its purpose and have agreed on individualized goals and rewards. Group therapy may be used, relying on peer support and the opportunity to associate with other patients with the same diagnosis in a nonthreatening setting.

The long-term outlook for the adolescent with anorexia is not clear. Death may occur from suicide, infection, or the effects of starvation. Some adolescents do recover completely, others may have eating problems into adulthood, and still others have problems with social adjustment that are not related to eating. Predicting the outcome is difficult, and more studies are needed before a definitive answer is available.

Bulimia

Bulimia nervosa (usually referred to simply as bulimia) is characterized by binge-eating followed by purging. The bulimic person is usually in late adolescence, is female, and is white. Most often, the bulimic person is of normal weight or overweight. Those who are underweight usually fulfill the criteria for anorexia nervosa. Some anorectic persons periodically practice binging and purging. Bulimia is seen increasingly in young adult women as well.

The binging often occurs late in the day when the adolescent is alone. Secrecy is an important aspect of the process. The adolescent eats large quantities of food within 1 or 2 hours. This binging is followed by guilt, fear, shame, and self-condemnation. To avoid weight gain from the food eaten, the adolescent follows the binging with purging by means of self-induced vomiting, laxatives, diuretics, and excessive exercise.

The clues to bulimia may be few but may include dental caries and erosion from frequent exposure to stomach acid, throat irritation, and endocrine and electrolyte imbalances that may cause cardiac irregularities and menstrual problems. Callouses or abrasions may be noted on the back of the adolescent's hand from frequent contact with the teeth while vomiting is induced. Complications that can occur are esophageal tears and acute gastric dilatation. Hypokalemia also may occur, especially if the adolescent abuses diuretics as part of her effort to keep from gaining weight despite binging.

Other behavior problems seen in many bulimic persons include drug abuse, alcoholism, stealing (especially food), promiscuity, and other impulsive activities.

Treatment of bulimia is varied. Many aspects of the treatment are similar to treatment of the adolescent with anorexia. Food diaries often are used as a tool to assess the adolescent's eating patterns. In some instances, antidepressant drugs may be useful. The nurse can refer the adolescent to a support group that may prove helpful.

Nursing Process for the Adolescent with an Eating Disorder

ASSESSMENT

Assessment of the adolescent with an eating disorder begins with a complete history, including previous illnesses, allergies, a dietary history, and a description of the adolescent's eating habits. The nurse must be aware that the adolescent may not give an accurate dietary history or a description of eating habits. The family caregiver can provide added information, preferably in a separate interview. Physical assessment includes height, weight, blood pressure, temperature, pulse, and respirations. Careful inspection and evaluation of the adolescent's skin condition, mucous membranes, state of nutrition, and state of alertness and cooperation are essential. Complete documentation is important.

NURSING DIAGNOSES

Nursing diagnoses vary with the specific eating disorder, the physical condition of the adolescent, the length of time the adolescent has had the condition, and other accompanying conditions. The following diagnoses may be useful in planning care:

- Altered nutrition: less than body requirements related to self-induced vomiting and use of laxatives or diuretics
- Fluid volume deficit related to self-induced vomiting and use of laxatives and diuretics
- High risk for self-esteem disturbance related to fear of obesity and potential rejection
- High risk for activity intolerance related to fatigue secondary to malnutrition
- Constipation or diarrhea related to decreased food and fluid intake and use of laxatives
- High risk for impaired skin integrity related to loss of

subcutaneous fat and dry skin secondary to malnutrition

- Impaired social interaction related to low self-esteem
- Noncompliance with treatment regimen related to unresolved conflicts over food and eating
- Family health-seeking behaviors related to eating disorders, treatment regimen, and dangers associated with an eating disorder

PLANNING AND IMPLEMENTATION

The major nursing goals for the adolescent with an eating disorder are related to meeting the adolescent's nutritional needs, helping the adolescent and the family understand the condition, and teaching them how to manage the condition and its treatment. The long-term outlook in eating disorders is often poor because of the patient's self-concept and poor self-esteem. After hospitalization for initial treatment, long-term follow-up with counseling for the adolescent and the family is often necessary.

Improving Nutrition. The adolescent with anorexia nervosa has a compulsive desire to be thin and an unrealistic view of her body image. The adolescent with bulimia, on the other hand, may consume large amounts of food followed by purging to avoid the excessive weight gain that could result from such consumption. In either instance, the adolescent's body does not receive the nutrients needed to achieve adequate growth during this period of development. Food intake must be supervised. Daily weights are necessary, but weight fluctuation should not be made an issue with the adolescent. The nurse must be observant when weighing the patient to avoid attempts by the adolescent to add weight by putting heavy objects in pockets, shoes, or other hiding places. Weights should be taken at the same time each day with minimal clothing, preferably a patient gown with no pockets, and bare feet. The adolescent's physician and a dietitian work with the adolescent in devising a food plan to meet the adolescent's nutrition requirements. The food plan is not geared to a sudden weight gain but a slow, steady gain with an established goal that has been agreed on by the health care team and the adolescent. Often, the adolescent keeps a food diary, which is reviewed daily with the health team.

Patients with eating disorders are often manipulative and deceptive. The nurse must observe the patient during and after eating to make certain the teen eats the required food and does not get rid of it after apparently consuming it. Contract agreements frequently are recommended for patients with eating disorders. These agreements, usually part of a behavioral modification plan, specify the adolescent's and the staff's responsibilities for the diet, activity expectations for the teen, and other aspects of the adolescent's behavior. The contract also may spell out specific privileges that can be lost or gained by meeting the contract goals. This places the teen in greater control of the outcome.

In addition to daily weights, testing urine for ketones and regular evaluation of skin turgor and mucous membranes give further indication of the adolescent's nutritional status. Evidence of deteriorating physical condition must be reported and documented immediately. If weight loss continues, nasogastric tube feedings may need to be implemented. This possibility also can be included in the contractual agreement.

Maintaining Fluid Intake. When the adolescent's condition is determined to be at a critical stage, with fluid and electrolyte deficiencies, parenteral fluids are necessary to immediately hydrate the patient before further treatment can be implemented. The adolescent must be observed continuously to prevent any attempt to remove intravenous lines or otherwise disrupt the treatment. Serum electrolytes, cardiac and respiratory status, and renal complications are closely monitored. During administration of parenteral fluids, the adolescent also is encouraged to maintain an oral intake.

Reinforcing Positive Self-Esteem. The nurse must function as an active, nonjudgmental listener to the adolescent. Consistent assignment of the same nursing personnel to care for the adolescent helps establish a climate in which the adolescent can relate to the nurse and begin to build positive feelings about herself. Signs of depression must be reported and documented without delay. Any negative feelings expressed by the adolescent also must be reported and documented. These feelings should never be minimized or ignored. Positive behavior should be positively reinforced. Psychotherapy and counseling groups are necessary to help the adolescent work through negative feelings of self-worth.

Balancing Rest and Activity. Exercise and activity are an important part of the contract agreement that is negotiated with the adolescent. Explain to the adolescent that fatigue is a result of the extreme depletion of energy reserves related to nutritional deficits. Encourage the adolescent to become involved in all activities of daily living. Provide ample rest periods during those times when the adolescent's energy reserves are depleted. The adolescent must be discouraged from pushing beyond endurance and must be closely observed for secretive excessive activity.

Monitoring Bowel Habits. A careful record of bowel movements is necessary. The adolescent may not be reliable as a reporter of bowel habits, therefore methods must be devised to prevent the teen from using the bathroom without supervision. Any occurrence of constipation or diarrhea must be reported and documented at once. The adolescent should be carefully watched so that she has no opportunity to obtain and take a laxative. These patients are devious in their behavior and may go to great lengths to obtain a laxative to purge themselves of food that they have eaten. Any evidence or suspicions of this type of behavior must be reported immediately.

Maintaining Skin Integrity. Good skin care is essential in the care of the adolescent who has severely restricted her nutritional intake. The adolescent's skin may be dry and tend to break down easily because of the lack of a subcutaneous fat cushion. Inspect daily for redness, irritation, or signs of decubitus ulcer formation. Note specifically bony prominences. Adolescents should be encouraged to be out of bed most of the day and, when in bed, should change position regularly so that no pressure areas develop.

Exploring Feelings. The adolescent must be encouraged to express fears, anger, and frustrations and should be helped to recognize that these are feelings that everyone has from time to time. These feelings must never be ridiculed or belittled. Encourage the adolescent to explore ways in which destructive feelings may be changed. These are feelings that can be dealt with in counseling sessions, therefore the nurse must report and document carefully.

Improving Compliance. The long-term outcome for adolescents with eating disorders is precarious. Adolescents with severe eating disorders often have multiple inpatient admissions. During the inpatient treatment, goals should be set and plans made for discharge. Specific consequences must be established for noncompliance. Counseling needs to continue after discharge. A support group referral may be helpful in encouraging compliance. Family involvement is necessary. The adolescent needs to recognize that discharge from the hospital does not mean that the adolescent is "cured."

Teaching the Family and Adolescent. The family of the adolescent needs counseling along with the adolescent. In some instances, the family may deny that the teen has a problem or that the problem is as severe as health care team members perceive it to be. Family therapy meets with varied success. Usually, the earlier the family therapy is initiated, the better the results. Family members must be able to identify behaviors of their own that contribute to the adolescent's problem. Family members also must learn to cooperate with behavior modification programs and, with guidance, carry them out at home when necessary. Ongoing contact between the family, the adolescent, and consistent health team members is essential. (See Nursing Care Plan for the Adolescent with an Eating Disorder.)

EVALUATION

The evaluation of adolescents with an eating disorder is an ongoing process that continues throughout the hospital stay. Goals for implementation include the following:

- The adolescent has a weight gain of a predetermined amount per week, usually not more than 2 lb/wk.

- The adolescent's mucous membranes are moist and skin turgor is good; at least 80% of each meal is eaten by the adolescent.
- The adolescent agrees to, signs, and adheres to a contract agreement.
- The adolescent's electrolyte levels, cardiac and respiratory status, and renal function are within normal limits.
- The adolescent verbally expresses positive attitudes about herself.
- The adolescent is involved in activity as prescribed in a contract; no excessive activity is detected.
- The adolescent paces activity to avoid fatigue.
- The adolescent's bowel elimination is normal.
- The adolescent makes positive statements about her feelings and appearance.
- The adolescent keeps counseling appointments, joins a support group, and continues to gain or maintain weight as per contract agreement.
- The family attends counseling sessions and identifies behaviors that impact negatively on the adolescent's condition.

Skin Disorders

Acne Vulgaris

One of the most common health problems of adolescence, acne, may be only a mild case of oily skin and a few blackheads, or it may be a severe type with ropelike cystic lesions that leave deep scars, both physical and emotional. To adolescents who want to be attractive and popular, however, even a mild case of acne (often called "zits") can cause great anxiety, shyness, and social withdrawal.

Characterized by the appearance of **comedones** (blackheads and whiteheads) and papules and pustules on the face and, to some extent, the back and chest, acne is caused by a variety of factors. Some of these factors are increased hormonal levels, especially androgens; hereditary factors; irritating substances, such as vigorous scrubbing and cosmetics that have a greasy base; and the growth of anaerobic bacteria. Each hair follicle has an associated sebaceous gland that, in adolescents, produces increased **sebum** (oily secretion). The sebum is blocked by epithelial cells and becomes trapped in the follicle. When this collection becomes infected by anaerobic organisms, inflammation occurs, causing papules, pustules, and nodules (Figure 17-2). Several types of acne lesions are frequently present at any time.

(text continued on page 414)

Nursing Diagnosis

Altered nutrition: less than body requirements related to self-induced vomiting or use of laxatives and diuretics

Goal: *Improve nutrition*

Nursing Interventions	Rationale	Evaluation
Supervise intake by observing adolescent during and after meals; monitor weight daily.	The adolescent with an eating disorder may go to any lengths to avoid eating or to fool health care personnel into thinking they are gaining weight.	The adolescent has a weight gain of a predetermined amount per week, usually not more than two pounds per week.
Work with adolescent and other health care providers to establish a mutually agreed upon long-term weight goal and a food plan that provides for a slow, steady, weekly weight gain. A contract agreement that spells out expectations and privileges which can be gained or lost by meeting those expectations may be necessary.	The adolescent is central to the planning process and cannot be made to meet goals set by others. If she participates and agrees to a certain plan, she will feel more in control of the overall outcome and is more likely to make the effort to stick by the program.	

Nursing Diagnosis

High risk for fluid volume deficit related to self-induced vomiting or use of laxatives and diuretics

Goal: *Maintain adequate fluid intake*

Nursing Interventions	Rationale	Evaluation
When parenteral fluids are being administered, observe continuously to prevent any attempts to disrupt the line. Encourage oral fluid intake at the same time.	The anorectic adolescent may deprive herself so much that the fluid and electrolyte deficiencies become life-threatening. A balance must be restored before any further treatment can begin.	The adolescent does not disrupt parenteral fluid administration; the adolescent's mucus membranes are moist; skin turgor is good; electrolytes, cardiac and respiratory status, and renal function are within normal limits.
Test urine for ketones and evaluate skin turgor and mucous membranes regularly.	Provides further indication of adolescent's nutritional status.	

Nursing Diagnosis

High risk for self-esteem disturbance related to fear of obesity and potential rejection

Goal: *Reinforce positive self-esteem*

Nursing Interventions	Rationale	Evaluation
Be an active, nonjudgmental listener; never minimize or ignore feelings expressed by the adolescent.	This is a first step in establishing a climate of trust between the adolescent and the nurse.	The adolescent verbally expresses positive attitudes about herself.

(continued)

Nursing Interventions	Rationale	Evaluation
Report negative feelings or any signs of depression expressed by adolescent without delay.	It is important to know the extent of the adolescent's negative feelings in order to further the therapeutic treatment plan. In addition, it is important that all health care providers be aware if the adolescent is extremely depressed, so that they can take the appropriate precautions.	

Nursing Diagnosis
High risk for activity intolerance related to fatigue secondary to malnutrition

Goal: *Balance rest and activity*

Nursing Interventions	Rationale	Evaluation
Teach the adolescent that a nutritional deficit depletes energy reserves and results in fatigue; encourage the adolescent to engage in activities of daily living, but provide for rest periods when adolescent's energy is low.	The adolescent needs to understand that activity and rest are related to nutritional status and that a healthy balance is crucial to overall health.	The adolescent is involved in activity as prescribed in a contract; no excessive activity is detected; the adolescent paces activity to avoid fatigue.
Discourage the adolescent from pushing herself beyond her physical limits, and observe closely for secretive excessive exercise.	The adolescent with an eating disorder may attempt to burn off excess calories with exercise.	

Nursing Diagnosis
Constipation or diarrhea related to decreased food and fluid intake or use of laxatives.

Goal: *Monitor bowel habits*

Nursing Interventions	Rationale	Evaluation
Keep a careful record of bowel habits; report and document any occurrence of diarrhea or constipation at once.	The adolescent may not be a reliable reporter of bowel habits.	The adolescent's bowel elimination is normal.
Observe adolescent carefully to be sure she has no opportunity for purging or taking a laxative.	These patients can be devious and will go to almost any length to prevent weight gain.	

Nursing Diagnosis
High risk for impaired skin integrity related to loss of subcutaneous fat and dry skin secondary to malnutrition

Goal: *Maintain skin integrity*

(continued)

Nursing Interventions	Rationale	Evaluation
Inspect skin daily for redness, irritation, or signs of decubiti ulcer formation. Provide good skin care and encourage adolescent to remain out of bed as much as possible so as to avoid the formation of pressure ulcers.	The adolescent's skin is likely to break down easily because of the lack of subcutaneous fat tissue cushion.	No pressure ulcers develop.

Nursing Diagnosis

Impaired social interaction related to low self-esteem

Goal: *Improve social interaction*

Nursing Interventions	Rationale	Evaluation
Encourage expression of emotions, and carefully document any destructive or negative feelings.	The adolescent needs the opportunity to express all her feelings, negative or otherwise, in a safe environment. If documented well, these can be explored further in counseling sessions.	The adolescent makes positive statements regarding her feelings and appearance.

Nursing Diagnosis

Noncompliance with treatment regimen related to unresolved conflicts over food and eating

Goal: *Improve compliance*

Nursing Interventions	Rationale	Evaluation
Make plans for discharge and follow-up treatment while the adolescent is still in the hospital. Be sure to establish consequences for noncompliance with program.	Eating disorders cannot be cured with one hospitalization. The treatment plan must include counseling to continue after discharge.	The adolescent keeps counseling appointments; joins support group; continues to gain or maintain weight as per contact agreement.

Nursing Diagnosis

Family health-seeking behaviors related to eating disorders, treatment regimen, dangers associated with eating disorder

Goal: *Improve family's understanding of illness and treatment goals*

Nursing Interventions	Rationale	Evaluation
Provide for family counseling as well as counseling for the adolescent.	It is important for family members to understand the dynamics of the problem and their possible contribution to the disorder.	The family attends counseling sessions; identifies behaviors which impact negatively on adolescent's condition.
Teach family members about the behavior modification program the adolescent is using, providing guidance on how to carry the program out at home.	Eating disorders are not cured simply because the adolescent is discharged. Counseling and a continuation of whatever program or contract agreement the adolescent has signed are essential, thus requiring family involvement.	

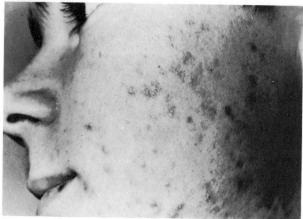

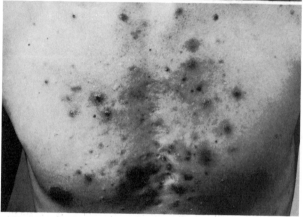

Figure 17-2. Acne of face and chest. (From Sauer GC. Manual of Skin Diseases, 5th ed. Philadelphia: JB Lippincott, 1985.)

Topical medications benzoyl peroxide (Clearasil, Benoxyl) and tretinoin (Retin-A) come in a variety of forms, such as topical cleansers, lotions, creams, sticks, pads, gels, and bars. The usual treatment plan for mild acne is topical application of one of these medications once or twice a day. These medications should not be applied to normal skin or allowed to get into the eyes or nose or on other mucous membranes. Antibiotics, such as erythromycin and tetracycline, may be administered for inflammatory acne. Antibiotic therapy requires an extended treatment course of at least 6 to 12 months followed by tapering of the dosage.

Isotretinoin (Accutane) may be used for severe inflammatory acne. Accutane is a potent, effective oral medication that is used in the treatment of hard-to-treat cystic acne. Side effects are common but frequently diminish when the drug dosage is reduced. Some of the side effects include dry lips and skin, eye irritation, temporary worsening of acne, epistaxis (nose bleed), bleeding and inflammation of the gums, itching, photosensitivity (sensitivity to the sun), and joint and muscle pain. Isotretinoin is a pregnancy category X drug, indicating that it must not be used at all during pregnancy because

of serious risk of fetal abnormalities. Any adolescent girl who is to be treated with isotretinoin must first be given a urine test to rule out pregnancy and must use an effective form of contraception for a month before beginning isotretinoin therapy.

The adolescent's perception of the disfigurement caused by acne may seem out of proportion to the actual severity of the condition, but the nurse must acknowledge and accept the adolescent's feelings. The nurse teaches the adolescent and the family caregiver that the lesions should be washed gently with soap and water and not scrubbed vigorously. Removal of comedones should be performed gently, following the recommendations of the physician and using careful aseptic techniques. Careful removal produces no scarring—a goal for every teen. Understanding and support by the nurse and family caregiver are the most important aspects of caring for the adolescent with acne. The teen can be reassured that consumption of chocolate and fat does not cause acne, but a well-balanced, nutritious diet promotes healing.

Menstrual Disorders

The beginning of menstruation, called **menarche**, normally occurs between the ages of 9 and 16 years, and for many girls this is a joyous affirmation of their womanhood. Other adolescent girls may have negative feelings about this event, depending on how they have been prepared for menarche and for their roles as women. Irregular menstruation is common during the first year until a regular cycle is established.

Some adolescent girls have dull, aching abdominal pain at the time of ovulation (midcycle, hence the name **mittelschmerz**). The cause is not completely understood, but the discomfort usually lasts only a few hours and is relieved by analgesics, a heating pad, or a warm bath.

Premenstrual Syndrome

Women of all ages are subject to the discomfort of **premenstrual syndrome** (PMS), but the symptoms may be alarming to the adolescent. These symptoms include edema (resulting in weight gain), headache, increased anxiety, mild depression, and mood swings. The major cause of PMS is thought to be water retention following progesterone production after ovulation (Figure 17-3).

Generally, the discomforts of PMS are minor and can be relieved by reducing salt intake during the week prior to menstruation and by the administration of mild analgesics and local application of heat. When symptoms are more severe, physicians may prescribe a mild diuretic for the week prior to onset of menstruation to relieve edema or, occasionally, oral contraceptive pills to prevent ovulation.

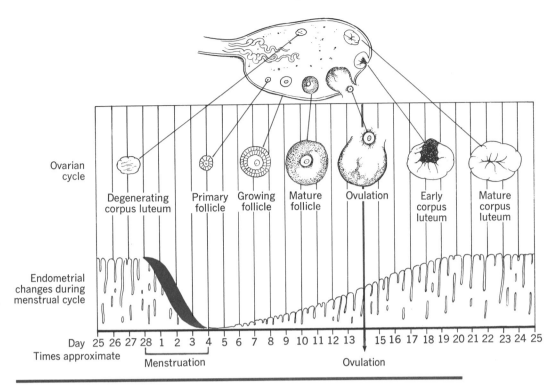

Figure 17-3. Schematic representation of a 28-day ovarian cycle. Menstruation occurs with shedding of the endometrium. The follicular phase is associated with the rapidly growing ovarian follicle and the production of estrogen. Ovulation occurs midcycle, and mittelschmerz may occur. The secretory phase follows in preparation for the fertilized ovum. If fertilization does not occur, the corpus luteum begins to degenerate, estrogen and progesterone levels decline, and menstruation again occurs. (Chaffee EE, Lytle IM. Basic Physiology and Anatomy, 4th ed. Philadelphia: JB Lippincott.)

Dysmenorrhea

Dysmenorrhea (painful menstruation) is classified as primary or secondary. Many adolescent girls experience pain associated with menstruation, including cramping abdominal pain, leg pain, and backache. *Primary dysmenorrhea* occurs as part of the normal menstrual cycle without any associated pelvic disease. The increased secretion of prostaglandins, which occurs in the last few days of the menstrual cycle, is thought to be a contributing factor in primary dysmenorrhea. Nonsteroidal antiinflammatory drugs (NSAIDs), such as ibuprofen (Advil, Motrin), inhibit prostaglandins and are the treatment of choice for primary dysmenorrhea. NSAIDs are most effective when taken before cramps become too severe. Because NSAIDs are irritating to the gastric mucosa, they always should be taken with food and discontinued if epigastric burning occurs.

Secondary dysmenorrhea is the result of pelvic pathologic changes, most often pelvic inflammatory disease or endometriosis. The adolescent girl who has severe menstrual pain should be examined by a physician to determine if any pelvic pathologic changes are present. Treatment of the underlying condition helps relieve severe dysmenorrhea.

Amenorrhea

The absence of menstruation is called **amenorrhea**. It can be primary (no previous menstruation) or secondary (missing three or more periods after menstrual flow has begun). Primary amenorrhea after 16 years of age warrants a diagnostic survey for genetic abnormalities, tumors, or other problems. Secondary amenorrhea can be a sign of pregnancy, the result of discontinuing oral contraceptives and physical or emotional stressors, or a symptom of an underlying medical condition. A complete physical examination, including gynecologic screening, is necessary to help determine the cause.

Infectious Diseases

Infectious Mononucleosis

Sometimes called "kissing disease," infectious mononucleosis ("mono") is caused by the Epstein-Barr virus, one of the herpesvirus group. The organism is transmitted through saliva. There is no immunization available, and treatment is symptomatic. Adolescents and young adults seem to be most susceptible to this disorder, although sometimes it also is seen in younger children.

Clinical Manifestations

Infectious mononucleosis can present a variety of symptoms, ranging from mild to severe and including symptoms that mimic hepatitis. Symptoms include sore throat with enlarged tonsils, fever, palatine petechiae (red spots on the soft palate), swollen lymph nodes, and enlargement of the spleen, accompanied by extreme fatigue and lack of energy. In some instances, headache, abdominal pain, and epistaxis are also present.

Diagnosis

Diagnosis of infectious mononucleosis is based on clinical symptoms, laboratory evidence of lymphocytes in the peripheral blood with 10% or more abnormal lymphocytes present in a peripheral blood smear, and a positive heterophil agglutination test. Monospot is a test that is valuable in diagnosis of this disorder. Rapid, sensitive, inexpensive, and simple to perform, it is capable of detecting significant agglutinins at lower levels, thus making possible earlier diagnosis. Infectious mononucleosis often is confused with streptococcal infections because of the fever and the appearance of the throat and tonsils.

Treatment

No cure exists for infectious mononucleosis; treatment is based on symptoms. An analgesic-antipyretic, such as acetaminophen, usually is recommended for the fever and headaches. Fluids and a soft, bland diet are encouraged to reduce throat irritation. Corticosteroids sometimes are used to relieve the severe sore throat and fever. Bed rest is suggested to relieve fatigue but is not imposed for a specific amount of time. If the spleen is enlarged, the adolescent is cautioned to avoid contact sports that might cause a ruptured spleen. Because the immune system is weakened, the adolescent must take precautions to avoid secondary infections.

The course of mononucleosis is usually uncomplicated. Fever and sore throat last from 1 week to 10 days. Fatigue generally disappears between 2 and 4 weeks after the appearance of acute symptoms but may last as long as 1 year. The limitations that this disorder impose on the teenager's school and social life may cause depression. In most instances, however, the adolescent is able to resume normal activities within 1 month after symptoms present. Nursing care includes encouraging the adolescent to express feelings about the interruptions the illness is causing in school, social, and work plans. Long-term effects rarely are seen.

Pulmonary Tuberculosis

Tuberculosis is present in all parts of the world and is the most important chronic infectious disease in terms of illness, death, and cost.[2] In the United States, the incidence of tuberculosis declined until the late 1980s, when an increasing number of cases were identified. Tuberculosis in patients infected with the human immunodeficiency virus (HIV) has been credited with causing this increase.

Tuberculosis is caused by *Mycobacterium tuberculosis*, a bacillus that is spread through contact with droplets of infected mucus that become airborne when the infected person sneezes, coughs, or laughs. The bacilli, when airborne, are inhaled into the respiratory tract of the unsuspecting person and become implanted in lung tissue. This process is the beginning of a primary lesion.

Primary tuberculosis is the original infection that goes through various stages and ends with calcification. The most common site of a primary lesion is the alveoli of the respiratory tract. In children with poor nutrition or health, the primary infection may invade other tissues of the body, including bones, joints, kidneys, lymph nodes, and meninges. This is called miliary tuberculosis. Most cases, however, arrest with the calcification of the primary infection. Secondary tuberculosis is a reactivation of a healed primary lesion. This frequently occurs in adults and contributes to the exposure of children to the organism.

Diagnosis

The tuberculin skin test is the primary means by which tuberculosis is detected. A skin test can be performed using a multipuncture device that deposits purified protein derivative (PPD) intradermally (Tine test) or by injection of 0.1 mL of PPD intradermally. Either of these tests is administered on the inner aspect of the forearm. The site is marked and read at 48 hours and 72 hours. Redness, swelling, induration, and itching of the site indicate a positive reaction. Persons who have a positive skin test reaction are further examined by radiographic evaluation. Sputum tests of young children are rarely helpful because children do not produce a good specimen. Screening by means of skin testing is recommended for all children at 12 months, before entering school, in adolescence, and annually for those children in high-risk situations or communities, including children in whose family there is an active case, Native Americans, and children who recently immigrated from Central or South America, the Caribbean, Africa, Asia, or the Middle East. Other high-risk children are those who are HIV infected, homeless or live in overcrowded conditions, and immunosuppressed from any cause.

Primary lesions in children generally are unrecognized. In the small number of children with miliary tuberculosis, there may be general symptoms of chronic infection, such as fatigue, loss of weight, and low-grade fever accompanied by night sweats. Secondary lesions occur more frequently in adults but may occur in the adolescent age group. Symptoms resemble those in an adult, including cough with expectoration, fever, loss of weight, malaise, and night sweats.

Treatment

Drug therapy for tuberculosis includes administration of isoniazid (INH), often in combination with rifampin. Although INH has been known to cause peripheral neuritis in children with poor nutrition, few problems occur in children whose diets are well balanced. Rifampin is tolerated well by children, but it causes body fluids such as urine, sweat, tears, and feces to turn orange-red. A possible disadvantage for adolescents is that it may permanently stain contact lenses. Rifamate is an available drug that is a combination of rifampin and INH. Other drugs that may be used are ethambutol, streptomycin, and pyrazinamide.

Drug therapy is continued for 9 to 18 months. After chemotherapy has begun, the child or adolescent may return to school and normal activities unless clinical symptoms are evident. An annual chest radiograph is necessary from that time on.

Prevention

Prevention requires improvements in such undesirable social conditions as overcrowding, poverty, and poor health care. Also needed are health education; availability of medical, laboratory, and radiographic facilities for examination; and control of contacts and suspected persons.

A vaccine called bacille Calmette Guérin (BCG) is used in countries in which the incidence of tuberculosis is high. It is given to tuberculin-negative persons and is said to be effective for 12 years or longer. Mass vaccination is not considered necessary in parts of the world where the incidence of tuberculosis is low. After administration of BCG vaccine, the skin test will result in a positive reaction, so that screening is no longer an effective tool. The use of BCG vaccine remains controversial.

The Sexually Active Adolescent

The age at which adolescents become sexually active has been decreasing in recent years, and with that decrease has come increased complications resulting from sexual activity. Problems that result from sexual activity of adolescents include sexually transmitted diseases (STDs), genital infections, and adolescent pregnancy. These problems are included in this discussion.

Vaginitis

Vaginitis (inflammation of the vagina) can result from a number of causes, such as diaphragms or tampons left in place too long, irritating douches or sprays, estrogen changes caused by birth control pills, and antibiotic therapy. Actually, these causes are precursors, providing opportunity for the organisms to become active. The most common causes of vaginitis are *Candida albicans*, bacterial vaginosis (caused by *Gardnerella vaginalis* and other organisms), or *Trichomonas*. *Trichomonas* is the only one of these organisms transmitted solely by sexual contact (Table 17-2).

Table 17-2. Infectious Causes of Vaginitis

Organism/Incidence	Symptoms	Sexual Transmission	Treatment
Candida albicans First episodes occur in adolescence, especially in sexually active girls	Severe itching, exacerbated just before menstruation Odor not present Milky "cottage cheese"–like discharge may be noted on examination	Normally present in vagina, most often results from glycosuria, antibiotic therapy, birth control pills, steroid therapy, or other factor that alters normal pH of vagina May result from oral-genital sex	Nystatin (Mycotatin), miconazole (Monitstat), or clotrimazole (Gyne-Lotrimin) vaginal suppositories or creams
Bacterial vaginosis (multiple organisms) Common among adolescent girls; sexual partner will probably also be infected	About one half of patients have no symptoms Fishy odor after intercourse Discharge, if present, grayish and thin	Sexually transmitted	Metronidazole (Flagyl) or ampicillin; sexual partners may be treated
Trichomonas Most frequently diagnosed STD	Itching with severe infection, especially after menstruation. Discharge has foul odor and may be frothy, gray or green.	Sexually transmitted	Metronidazole (Flagyl); sexual partners also should be treated

Flagyl is not ordered for the pregnant patient owing to possible danger to fetus
STD, sexually transmitted disease

Sexually Transmitted Diseases

The incidence of STDs is highest in the adolescent population. The diseases range from infections that can be easily treated to life-threatening diseases such as HIV infection (Table 17-3). Infants infected with STDs usually are infected prenatally or during birth. Children infected after the neonatal period must be considered victims of sexual abuse until disproved. Severe or repeated pelvic inflammatory disease (PID) or severe genital warts are warning signs that the girl should be tested for HIV.

Prevention is the most important aspect in the campaign against STDs. The only certain way to avoid contracting an STD is sexual abstinence. However, sexual activity in adolescents indicates that this is frequently not a practical solution. Condoms with spermicide, discussed in Chapter 16, provide protection, although they are not fail-safe. Adolescents must be educated to understand all aspects of consequences of sexual activity.

Gonorrhea

More than 1 million cases of gonorrhea are reported annually, and an equal number of cases are believed to be undiagnosed. It is one of the most commonly reported communicable diseases in the United States. Also called "the clap," "the drips," or "the dose," gonorrhea has mild primary symptoms, particularly in females, and often goes undetected and thus untreated until it progresses to serious pelvic disorders. This disease can cause sterility in males.

There are several drugs that may be used to treat gonorrhea, but the current drug of choice is ceftriaxone (Rocephin) followed by a week of oral doxycycline (Vibramycin) to prevent an accompanying chlamydial infection. Adolescents are asked to name their sexual contacts so that they also may be treated. Penicillin-resistant strains of the organism have developed so that penicillin is no longer an effective method of treatment. Adolescents must learn that their bodies will not develop immunity to the organism and they might become infected again if they continue to expose themselves to the risk.

Chlamydial Infection

Chlamydial infections have replaced gonorrhea as the most common STD in the United States. Symptoms may be mild, causing a delay in diagnosis and treatment until serious complications and transmission to others have occurred.

Adolescents must be made aware of the seriousness of PID, a common result of a chlamydial infection. PID can cause female sterility, primarily by leading to scarring in the fallopian tubes, which prohibits the passage of the fertilized ovum into the uterus. A tubal pregnancy may be the consequence of a chlamydial infection. In the male, sterility may result from epididymitis caused by a chla-

mydial infection. Tetracycline or doxycycline is used to treat chlamydial infection. In the pregnant adolescent, erythromycin can be used to avoid the teratogenic effects of tetracycline and doxycycline. All sexual partners must be treated.

Genital Herpes

Genital herpes has reached epidemic proportions in the United States. Genital herpes begins as a vesicle that ruptures to form a painful ulcer on the genitalia. The initial ulcer lasts 10 to 12 days. Recurrent episodes occur intermittently and last 4 to 5 days. No cure is available, but acyclovir (Zovirax) is useful in relieving or suppressing the symptoms. Genital herpes is associated with a much higher than average risk for cervical cancer; therefore, the female who has genital herpes should have an annual Pap smear. Genital herpes is not transmitted to the fetus in utero, but if there is an active case of genital herpes at the time of delivery, the infant should be delivered by cesarean birth to avoid infection of the newborn during passage through the vagina. In newborns, the infection can become systemic and cause death.

Syphilis

Caused by the spirochete *Treponema pallidum*, syphilis is a destructive disease that can involve every part of the body. Untreated, it can have devastating long-term effects. Infected mothers are highly likely to transmit the infection to their unborn infants.

Syphilis is spread primarily by sexual contact. Symptoms of the primary stage usually appear about 3 weeks after exposure. If allowed to progress without treatment, syphilis has a secondary stage, a latent stage, and a tertiary stage.

The cardinal sign of *primary stage* is the **chancre**, a hard, red, painless lesion at the point of entry of the spirochete. This can appear on the penis in the male or on the vulva or cervix of the female. It also can appear on the mouth, the lips, or the rectal area as a result of oral–genital or anal–genital contact. The *secondary stage* is marked by rash, sore throat, and fever, appearing between 2 and 6 months after the original infection. Signs of both the first and second stages disappear without treatment, but the spirochete remains in the body.

The *latent period* can persist for as long as 20 years without symptoms; however, blood tests are still positive.

In the *tertiary stage*, syphilis causes severe neurologic and cardiovascular damage, mental illness, and gastrointestinal disorders.

Syphilis responds to one intramuscular injection of benzathine penicillin, or if the adolescent is sensitive to penicillin, oral tetracycline can be administered for a 15-day course of treatment. If treatment is not obtained before the tertiary stage, the neurologic and cardiovascular complications can lead to death.

Table 17-3. Major Sexually Transmitted Diseases

Infection and Agent	Transmission	Symptoms	Possible Complications	Prevention
Gonorrhea—gonococcus: *Neisseria gonorrhoeae*	Sexual contact; mother to fetus during vaginal delivery	Yellow mucopurulent discharge of the genital area, painful or frequent urination, pain in the genital area; may be asymptomatic Frequent cause of pelvic inflammatory disease	Sterility, cystitis, arthritis, endocarditis	Public should be educated on safe sex practices; mother should be tested before delivery. Newborn's eyes should be treated with tetracycline ointment, erythromycin ointment, or silver nitrate. All contacts should be treated with antibiotics.
Chlamydia—bacteria: *Chlamydia trachomatis*	Sexual contact; mother to fetus during vaginal delivery	Mucopurulent genital discharge, genital pain, dysuria Frequent cause of pelvic inflammatory disease, often in combination with gonorrhea	Sterility	Public should be educated about safe sex practices Sexual contact should be avoided when lesions are present Infected mothers should have a cesarean delivery
Genital herpes virus: herpes simplex type 2	Sexual contact; mother to fetus during vaginal delivery	Genital soreness, pruritus, and erythema; vesicles appear that usually last for about 10 days, during which time transmission of virus is likely		Public should be educated about safe sex practices Sexual contact should be avoided when lesions are present Infected mothers should have a cesarean delivery.
Syphilis—spirochete: *Treponema pallidum*	Sexual contact; mother to fetus via placenta; blood transfusions if donor is in early stage of disease and undiagnosed	Primary stage: genital lesion, enlarged lymph nodes Secondary stage (6 weeks later): lesions of skin and mucous membrane, with generalized symptoms of headache and fever	Tertiary stage: central nervous system and cardiovascular damage, paralysis, psychosis	Public should be educated about safe sex practices Screen blood donors; do serologic testing before and during pregnancy Avoid contact with body secretions from infected patients
Acquired immunodeficiency syndrome (AIDS)—virus: human immunodeficiency virus	Sexual contact; exposure to blood or blood products; mother to fetus	Active phase: rash, cough, malaise, night sweats, lymphadenopathy Asymptomatic phase: no symptoms, but test is positive for HIV antigens AIDS-related complex: lymphadenopathy, diarrhea, oral candidiasis, weight loss, fatigue, skin rash, recurrent infections, fever AIDS: rare infections such as *Pneumocystis carinii* pneumonia or rare cancers such as Kaposi's sarcoma or B-cell lymphomas	Neurologic impairment	Public should be educated about safe sex practices, especially high-risk groups. Blood or blood products used for transfusion should be carefully screened. Intravenous drug abusers should not share needles. Universal precautions should be used consistently in all health care settings. Institute measures to avoid needlesticks among health care workers

Adapted from Craven RF, Hirnle CJ. Fundamentals of Nursing: Human Health and Function. Philadelphia: JB Lippincott, 1992.

Acquired Immunodeficiency Syndrome

Acquired immunodeficiency syndrome (AIDS) is believed to be caused by HIV, which attacks and destroys the T-helper lymphocytes (CD4 +). The T-helper lymphocytes are the cells that direct the immune response to viral, bacterial, and fungal infections and remove some malignant cells from the body. AIDS has been determined to have four distinct stages: (1) an early stage, during which the patient has symptoms similar to influenza and there is rapid reproduction of the virus; (2) a middle period that may last for years, with few symptoms, during which there is slow reproduction of the virus and loss of T4 cells; (3) a period of transition with symptoms; and (4) a crisis period, which may last months or years. Transmission of HIV is by means of contact with infected blood or sexual contact with an infected person. HIV cannot be transmitted through casual contact. The diagnosis of any STD increases the statistical risk of HIV infection 300%. Because not all persons who test positive for HIV develop AIDS immediately, the Centers for Disease Control and Prevention have established criteria that places patients under AIDS surveillance. The most significant of these criteria for adolescents and adults is a CD4 + T-lymphocyte count of fewer than 200 cells/μL (the normal count is 600 to 1200 cells/μL), or less than 14% of total lymphocytes and, for women, the addition of invasive cervical cancer.[3]

Infants usually are infected through the placenta during prenatal life, in the birth process when contamination of the newborn with the mother's blood is possible, or through breastfeeding after birth. Children and teens also can be infected through sexual abuse. Adolescents are most often infected through intimate heterosexual or homosexual relations and through intravenous drug use. Some hemophiliacs who received blood products before 1985 were infected, but safeguards are now in place, and the blood supply has become much safer.

Although most children with AIDS are between the ages of 1 and 4 years, an alarming increase has occurred among adolescents since 1990, causing great concern in those who work with adolescents. African-American adolescents represent a disproportionately high rate of AIDS among teenagers. In April 1992, the House Select Committee on Children, Youth, and Families completed its study reported in "A Decade of Denial; Teens and AIDS in America." The report stated that "HIV, the virus that causes AIDS, is spreading unchecked among the nation's adolescents, regardless of where they live or their economic status." Exactly how many teens are HIV positive is unknown; however, it is known that the rate of those diagnosed increased more than 6 times between 1989 and 1992. The teenagers' attitude of **impunity** (the belief that nothing can hurt them) and the increasing rate of sexual activity in this age group, often involving multiple partners, contribute to the fear that this group will experience widespread illness from HIV. The incubation period

for HIV can vary from 3 to 8 years; thus, many who contract the disease in adolescence will not have symptoms until they are in their 20s, when they are at their reproductive peak. The proper use of a condom with spermicide (see Parent Teaching: Tips for Safe Condom Use in Chapter 16) during any type of sexual contact is a must to prevent the spread of HIV. Adolescent girls may have sexual experiences with older men who have had many previous sexual partners. This increases the risk for the girl and, in turn, can increase the risk for any adolescent boy with whom she is sexually intimate. Adolescent boys are also at increased risk if they engage in unprotected homosexual relations, use intravenous drugs, have multiple partners, or have sex with a prostitute. Cultural influences may play an important role. The adolescent girl often finds it difficult to insist that her partner use a condom. If the partner refuses and claims to be "safe" (uninfected) or protests that the condom decreases the pleasurable sensations, she might give in for fear that she might otherwise break up the relationship. In addition, in some cultures, the more sexual conquests the boy has, the more manly he is viewed.

Approximately 20% to 30% of the infants born to HIV-infected mothers develop AIDS. Although the infants may test positive in the first year of life, testing is not reliable until 15 months of age because the infant may retain antibodies from the mother for this length of time. However, for those younger than 1 year of age who are affected, the disease can move rapidly to AIDS and serious complications. Failure to thrive, *Pneumocystis carinii* pneumonia, recurrent bacterial infections, progressive encephalopathy, and malignancy are often the illnesses that develop in affected infants. Some of these children progress quickly to terminal illness and death, but with aggressive chemotherapy, some of them are living long enough to become of school age.

Adolescents manifest the symptoms of HIV much the same as do adults. Females rarely have Kaposi's sarcoma, a cancer frequently seen in homosexual men. Many women, including adolescents, present with a chronic infection of vaginitis caused by *C. albicans* that has not responded to local antifungal treatments. These infections may be controlled by oral systemic medications. The female who tests positive for HIV should have a pelvic examination every 6 months to detect early STDs and institute vigorous treatment.

Nursing Process for the Adolescent Girl with AIDS

ASSESSMENT

In assessing the adolescent girl with AIDS, the nurse must gather a complete history, including her chief complaint, the presenting symptoms, her past medical history, immunization status, family history, and social history. A family caregiver may accompany the girl and must be interviewed, but a private admission interview with the adolescent is essential. She may be extremely reluctant to reveal her social and sexual history, especially in the presence of a family member. A careful review of the girl's history of vaginal candidiasis, PID, and sexual activity is critical. Throughout all aspects of the adolescent's care, the nurse must maintain a sensitive, caring, nonjudgmental attitude. The adolescent may be experiencing a variety of emotional feelings, including anger, denial, guilt, and rebelliousness. The nurse must accept all of these emotions as legitimate reactions to the illness.

During the physical assessment, the nurse must maintain strict universal precautions. The physical examination includes vital signs, especially observing for fever, which may indicate infection, and a thorough survey of all body systems, including observations for poor skin turgor, rashes or lesions, alopecia, mucous membrane lesions or thrush, weight loss, mental or neurologic changes, respiratory infections or signs of tuberculosis, diarrhea or abdominal pain, vaginal discharge, perineal lesions, or genital warts. The nurse can assist in preparing the adolescent for diagnostic tests that must be performed.

NURSING DIAGNOSES

Following careful assessment of the adolescent girl, the nurse can develop nursing diagnoses by thoroughly reviewing the assessment data and identifying the actual or potential problems. Nursing diagnoses may include the following:

- High risk for infection related to increased susceptibility secondary to a compromised immune system
- High risk for infection transmission related to the infectious nature of the virus
- High risk for impaired skin integrity related to perineal and anal tissue excoriation secondary to genital candidiasis or genital warts
- Pain related to symptoms of the disease
- Altered nutrition, less than body requirements, related to anorexia, oral or esophageal lesions, or diarrhea
- Social isolation related to rejection by others secondary to the diagnosis of AIDS
- Hopelessness related to the diagnosis and prognosis
- Altered family processes related to the diagnosis of AIDS

PLANNING AND IMPLEMENTATION

Planning the nursing care of the adolescent girl who has AIDS can be challenging. The adolescent needs much support to accept the diagnosis and move in a positive direction to follow the treatment plan to the best of her ability. The nurse can play a critical role in helping the adolescent understand the treatment and prognosis and their impact on her life.

Preventing Infection. In the hospital, strict adherence to appropriate infection control measures is extremely important. Teaching the adolescent to prevent infections is a primary goal. She needs to learn handwashing, with care to wash between fingers and under rings, and to use a pump-type soap. She needs to keep her nails trimmed to avoid harboring microorganisms under her nails. Skin care includes showering (not a tub bath) with a mild soap (no strong perfumed soaps), using an emollient cream, and patting her skin dry, avoiding vigorous rubbing. Foods (fruits and vegetables) that are raw should be washed and peeled or cooked to avoid the danger of bacteria. Unpasteurized dairy products and foods grown in organic fertilizer must be avoided. Meats must be well cooked before eating. Teeth need to be brushed at least 3 times a day with a soft toothbrush and a nonabrasive toothpaste. Routine dental care is vital.

The household in which the adolescent lives must be cleaned carefully and regularly. A household bleach solution of 1 part of bleach to 10 parts of water is a good solution to use. Particular attention should be paid to the refrigerator, the stove, the oven, and the microwave to prevent contamination of foods during preparation or storage. Household items that may be contaminated should be discarded in double plastic bags to prevent spread to others. Laundry bleach should be used when washing any of the adolescent's clothing, especially underwear.[4]

Pets should be cared for by someone other than the adolescent. Cleaning an aquarium, emptying a cat's litter box, and cleaning a bird cage can subject the adolescent to opportunistic organisms that will attack her compromised immune system. The adolescent must learn to avoid persons who have any infectious disease. Prompt attention to an apparently minor infection helps avoid more serious illness. The adolescent with AIDS should not receive any live vaccine immunizations but should continue to receive other immunizations, as indicated.

Preventing Transmission. The good hygienic practices necessary to protect the girl from an acquired or opportunistic infection also help prevent transmission of the virus to others. The adolescent also needs counseling about her sexual practices. One of the most emotionally difficult tasks for the adolescent may be to list her sexual contacts. This is a delicate matter that must be approached in a nonjudgmental, sympathetic manner, but she needs to understand that anyone with whom she has been sexually intimate may be infected and must be identified. In reviewing her sexual contacts, she may find that the sexual partner from whom she contracted the virus already knew that he or she was infected. Infection with HIV does not necessarily mean that the girl was promiscuous. She may have been sexually intimate with only one person, and that person may have assured her that he or she was not infected. The adolescent girl may be extremely angry about her exposure by someone she trusts.

The adolescent must be taught safe sex practices. She needs to understand that is she protecting not only future sexual partners from contracting her disease but also herself from contracting other strains of the virus. The girl needs to have complete instructions on the use of condoms and spermicide (see Parent Teaching: Tips for Safe Condom Use in Chapter 16). She must accept that she must not be sexually intimate with anyone without using a condom, no matter what kind of argument the other person uses to convince her otherwise. Also she needs to learn that HIV is transmitted through vaginal intercourse, oral–genital contact, anal intercourse, or any contact with blood or body fluids, including menstrual discharge. If she practices oral–genital sex, she must use a dental dam, a square of latex worn in the mouth to prevent contact of body fluids with mucous membranes of the mouth.

The adolescent girl needs counseling about pregnancy. The probability of transmitting the virus to her unborn child may be as high as 30%, and there is currently no way to determine if she will pass the virus to her child. She needs to consider that even if her infant is not infected, she will not likely live to see her child reach adulthood. All of these considerations are overwhelming, and the adolescent needs continuous support to successfully understand, accept, and deal with them.

A discussion of the girl's use of illicit, injectable drugs is important. If she is a drug user, she should be counseled about stopping her drug use. A realistic approach must be taken, however, and an explanation of how to sterilize needles using chlorine bleach should be offered. A mixture of 1 part of bleach to 5 parts of water should be drawn through the needle into the syringe, flushing 2 or 3 times and finally rinsing with water. The nurse must recognize that the adolescent girl has the right to decide how she will conduct her life and remain nonjudgmental through all contacts with the girl.

Protecting Skin Integrity. Skin lesions are common symptoms of many STDs. The adolescent needs to report any new skin lesion to her health care provider so that diagnosis and immediate treatment can be undertaken. The best preventive measure the girl can take is to follow careful infection control measures, including careful handwashing, and to protect skin integrity by using skin emollients to guard against dryness, avoiding harsh, perfumed soaps and guarding against injury to her skin. In advanced disease, nursing measures are implemented to protect and pad pressure points and improve peripheral circulation.

Relieving Pain. Pain is present as a result of a number of manifestations of AIDS. Skin and mucous membrane lesions may be very painful. Topical anesthetic solutions, such as viscous lidocaine, and meticulous mouth care can relieve pain caused by oral mucous membrane infections. Smoking, alcohol, and spicy or acidic foods irritate the oral mucous membranes and frequently cause additional pain. PID, a common complication of STDs, is usually accompanied by abdominal pain. The patient with respiratory complications also experiences bouts of chest pain. The nurse can administer analgesics to relieve pain and also should employ all appropriate nursing measures to help the adolescent be more comfortable. As the disease develops, the pain may be greater, and every effort must be made to provide comfort.

Improving Nutrition. Anorexia, or a poor appetite, is a common problem of the patient with AIDS. Dehydration, diarrhea, infection, malabsorption, oral candidiasis, and some drugs also can contribute to the adolescent's poor state of nutrition. Malnutrition can cause additional problems with increased and more serious infections. The adolescent's diet will need to be more nutritious and have a higher caloric content than normal. Several small meals supplemented by high-calorie, high-protein snacks may be desirable. Dietary supplements, such as Ensure and Isocal, also may be useful. The adolescent's food likes and dislikes should be explored and a meal plan developed using this information. If malnutrition becomes severe, the adolescent may need tube feedings or parenteral nutrition.

Easing Social Isolation and Hopelessness. The adolescent girl may fear having others know about her illness because she anticipates a negative reaction from her peers and family. She needs supportive counseling and guidance to help her deal with these fears. She may not feel that she can tell her family for fear of rejection. In fact, many families have rejected their children who have AIDS, but many others have risen to the challenge and, although they may tell the teenager that they do not like his or her behavior, they continue to love and support the teenager. The adolescent girl may need support to help her tell other social acquaintances as well. If there is an adolescent HIV support group available through the hospital or community, she should be referred to that group. Adolescents often find that adult support groups are not as helpful because the adults' needs are different from those of the adolescents. The adolescent is actually facing death before having a chance to experience adulthood.

The fact that the adolescent is facing an early death may give her a special sense of purpose to "spread the word" to others. The adolescent needs support and guidance to decide what the priorities in her life are and help in accomplishing the goals she sets. School officials may need to be told, and the family can be helpful during this time. If the family is not supportive, the adolescent needs even more support from health care providers.

Supporting and Teaching the Family. The adolescent must be involved in telling her family about her diagnosis if they do not already know. The sexual activity of adolescent children is a topic that many family caregivers have a difficult time dealing with, especially if the activity is homosexual or promiscuous in nature. The family caregivers usually need support as much as the adolescent does. They often are devastated by the prospect of their child's illness and early death. If the adolescent is pregnant, or has a child, the family also will have to consider the future of that child. For the family who plays a supportive role in the adolescent's life, a difficult time will follow the initial disclosure of the adolescent's diagnosis. The family must be taught as much about the disease as possible. They must learn how to prevent the spread of the virus among family members and opportunistic infections, the treatments and medication that the adolescent must follow, how to maintain good nutrition in the adolescent, the signs and symptoms to be alert for, the importance of reporting even minor complications to the health care provider, and ways to help support their adolescent child (Table 17-4).

Although teaching the adolescent and the family all of this information is certainly necessary, the nurse must remember that a person can absorb only so much information at one time. To teach them successfully and be ensured that they understand the information, the nurse must not present too much information at one time. The family and the adolescent should be given written materials that review the material for them, and the nurse should review verbally with them, asking questions and clarifying information until they show evidence of clear understanding of the concepts that they need to know. Throughout this time of teaching, the nurse must be sensitive to unspoken feelings and questions and carefully bring them into the discussion to provide the entire family unit with the best possible support and information.

EVALUATION

- The adolescent practices good hygiene measures and identifies ways to prevent infection.
- The adolescent identifies sexual partners and safer sexual practices.
- The adolescent protects her skin and mucous membranes and reports skin lesions or infections.
- The adolescent rests comfortably with minimal pain.
- The adolescent eats nutritionally sound meals and maintains her weight.
- The adolescent voices fears about social isolation and makes plans to maintain relationships.
- The adolescent expresses feelings about her future and begins to make realistic future plans.
- The family voices understanding of the illness and shows support for the adolescent.

Adolescent Pregnancy

The rate of adolescent pregnancy is approximately 1 in 10 girls, resulting in 1 million adolescent pregnancies each year. Approximately half of these result in live births; the remainder are aborted spontaneously or electively. The rate of adolescent pregnancy is higher in the United States than any other country that keeps accurate statistics. In 1989, more than two thirds of the infants born to teenagers were born to single mothers.[5] When this statistic is coupled with the fact that single-parent children are more likely to live in poverty, the magnitude of the problem becomes clear.

There are many factors that may contribute to the high rate of teen sexual activity and pregnancy. Society is mobile, and few people know their neighbors or feel responsible for them, so neighbors do not report a teen's activity as they might in closely knit neighborhoods. Adolescents are continuously bombarded with sex-oriented media. Teenagers have easy access to cars. They have less parental supervision, including after school, when many parents are still at work. Many teenagers take part in sexual activity with no concern about the potential outcome. On the other hand, a girl may want to become pregnant to prove she is "grown up," to prove her femininity, as an act of self-assertion or hostility toward her family, or to fulfill a desire to have a baby to love her and to love. Adolescents from low socioeconomic situations may see motherhood as a form of economic survival with allotments of money, food stamps, and medical and dental care provided. They may see this as a way to escape economic oppression. Unfortunately, they believe this will provide economic and personal independence. More than one of these or other reasons may be involved in any teenage pregnancy.

The pregnant adolescent may have a poor record of success in school, a low self-image, poor family relationships, and inadequate financial means. She frequently is the recipient of inadequate prenatal care. This places her future and the future of her unborn infant in jeopardy.

Pregnancy is associated with its own developmental tasks, and these collide with the normal developmental tasks of adolescence, often with unsatisfactory results. As an adolescent, she is seeking independence; as an expectant mother without adequate resources, she remains dependent. She is seeking identity, but the only identity she gains is that of a young, confused, high-risk mother-to-be. Her acute awareness of body image must accept the silhouette of pregnancy, certainly not in keeping with the slim figure desired by most adolescent girls. Pregnancy brings about many hormonal changes; thus, the adolescent must learn to cope with the hormonal changes of adolescence as well as those brought about by pregnancy. The adolescent's lack of knowledge about pregnancy and parenthood may cause the girl to have increased unrealistic fears about herself and her pregnancy. As an adolescent, she is still trying to clarify her values and develop a positive self-concept, but the pregnancy will have a negative impact on her self-concept, especially if the father of the infant or her parents reject her or her pregnancy.

Once pregnancy has been confirmed, the adolescent must decide whether to terminate the pregnancy by elective abortion or to carry it to term. If she chooses to have

Table 17-4. Counseling Patients at Different Stages of HIV Infection

Stage	Focus
Immediately after learning of positive HIV test (regardless of disease stage)	Assist patient in accepting diagnosis and encourage to verbalize feelings—anger, fear, hopelessness, etc. Explain the difference being HIV positive and having AIDS Explain how HIV is spread (by direct contact with infected body fluids—usually through sex, sharing needles, or blood transfusion) Counsel the patient on how to avoid transmitting the virus to others or contracting yet another strain Teach the patient some safer-sex strategies, such as using condoms, dental dams; use role-playing to demonstrate how to negotiate the use of these barriers Explain the pros and cons of contraceptives, such as intrauterine devices, oral contraceptives, and nonoxynol 9 in women with HIV Discuss why and how to notify sex partners of her infection; explain that partners need counseling, testing, and, if HIV positive, referral for treatment; Offer to help with the notifications process, if necessary Discuss pregnancy and childbearing, as appropriate; explain rates of transmission from mother to newborn; suggest early prenatal care if she is or becomes pregnant If the patient uses illicit, injectable drugs, explain how to sterilize needles with chlorine bleach: use a 5-to-1 ratio of water to bleach, draw the mixture up into the syringe two to three times, then flush with plain water Discuss the importance of primary health care, and provide appropriate referrals Provide educational literature on HIV, and refer patient to local support services and rehabilitation programs
Asymptomatic, CD4 cells > 500 cells/μL blood	Review health maintenance activities: the need for regular gynecologic examinations and Pap smears, adequate diet, regular exercise, 8 to 10 hours sleep/night, cutting back on alcohol, tobacco, and use of recreational drugs (if not ready to stop use) Stress the importance of health care follow-up Assess the patient's support systems: Does she have friends or relatives who can help out when symptoms develop? Does she have physical and economic access to health care? Refer to support groups, financial assistance programs
Asymptomatic, CD4 cells > 500 cells/μL blood, on antiretroviral medicines	Discuss prescribed drugs: indications, scheduled doses, how to recognize and manage side effects Discuss long-term family plans, especially arrangements for child (or children) at the parent's incapacity or death
Visible symptoms: weight loss, thinning hair, darkening nails, skin rashes	Encourage small, frequent meals, or suggest nutritional supplements, such as Ensure, to prevent weight loss Offer strategies for masking signs of illness, such as bright nail polish and attractive scarves or wigs Explore ways for the patient to initiate age-appropriate discussion of her HIV status with family Counsel patient to specify guardianship for any child she has in a legal will Discuss advanced directive alternatives available in your state, such as do-not-resuscitate status and health-care proxy options
After hospitalization for opportunistic infection	Reassess patient's home support—the need to call in a visiting nurse or volunteer buddy Counsel patient to finalize do-not-resuscitate status or health care proxy arrangements per state
End stage	Provide physical comfort through frequent turning on an air mattress, hydration therapy, lubricating skin massages Acknowledge the anticipatory grief of family members and friends

From Kelly PJ, Holman S. The new face of AIDS. AJN 93(3):26–34, 1993.

the baby, she must then decide whether to keep it or relinquish it for adoption. These are difficult choices, particularly for a frightened, often unsupported, immature girl. Health professionals have an obligation to provide the facts and guidance that will enable the girl to make an informed choice. School nurses, social workers, teachers, and counselors may be her only resources. The majority of adolescent mothers choose to keep their babies, whether they marry the father or not. In many instances, the grandmother or grandparents of the newborn help raise the infant.

In most schools, the pregnant adolescent is encouraged to stay in school to continue her education rather than drop out (Fig. 17-4). If this is not the case, the girl should be encouraged to continue her education elsewhere, even if it means relocation. Some urban schools sponsor prenatal classes and child care programs intended to encourage, support, and provide assistance to the girl in continuing her education throughout her pregnancy and parenthood. This often is accomplished through adolescent clinics that are beginning to play a particularly important role in the management of teenage pregnancy. Many of these clinics use a team approach to work with the girl, perhaps the young father, and the girl's parents; the physician, nurse practitioner or nurse midwife, nutritionist, and social worker offer understanding, supportive care, teaching, and counseling during the prenatal period and follow-up care after delivery. If the adolescent has chosen abortion, these clinics also can provide follow-up care and contraceptive counseling.

Adolescent clinics are available in some areas that provide care for adolescents in an environment designed for them and include care for STDs, HIV, substance abuse, and other adolescent health problems. The adolescent clinics help relieve some of the high-risk factors that commonly are seen in a teen pregnancy by providing prenatal care in a setting the teenager finds comfortable and nonthreatening. The adolescent has a higher incidence of pregnancy-induced hypertension (PIH), which may cause fetal and maternal risks; the infant is more likely to be of low birth weight with complications that may even lead to neonatal death; PIH places the infant at risk for inadequate circulation and the mother at risk for convulsions and death. Nutrition of the mother and the fetus may be severely compromised, and there may be social problems that may impact on the mother and the infant for their entire lives.

Nurses who work with pregnant adolescents need to resolve their own feelings to maintain a helpful, nonjudgmental attitude. These teenagers are fragile emotionally and mentally during this crisis. The nurse must develop a trusting relationship with the adolescent. Knowledge and understanding of adolescent psychosocial development are essential. The nurse must never fall into the habit of stereotyping adolescent mothers. As nurses work with the adolescent and develop a trusting relationship, they can help the girl look to the future and guide her in making realistic future plans. The pregnant adolescent has many problems to face and needs strong support, but with good prenatal and postnatal care and planning, the experience can become an opportunity for growth.

Adolescent Fatherhood

Adolescent fathers are often overlooked in discussions about adolescent pregnancy. However, more emphasis recently has been focused on the adolescent father's role. A number of factors enter into the role that the father takes in the pregnancy. The adolescent girl who has had multiple partners may not be sure who the father is, or she may not care enough for the father to want to involve him in her pregnancy and her future. Many boys deny their role in the pregnancy or lose interest in the girl when she announces her pregnancy. All of these factors help determine the degree of responsibility that the teenage father takes. When a cooperative, interested father is involved in education about the pregnancy, parenthood, and future contraception, a better outlook for the couple can be expected. The adolescent couple commonly has serious financial problems, often has unrealistic expectations, and may look forward to years of struggle. Support from the families of both adolescents can help improve the future of the couple. The newborn who has two well-informed parents with a good support system clearly has a brighter future than one who does not.

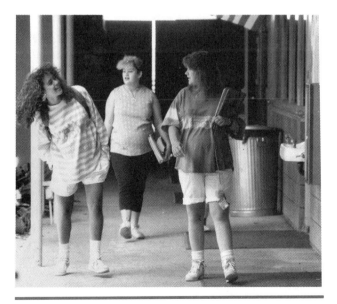

Figure 17-4. Although many adolescent mothers do not complete high school, some are able to continue and complete their education. (From Reeder SJ, Martin LL; Koniak D. Maternity Nursing: Family, Newborn, and Women's Health Care, 17th ed. Philadelphia: JB Lippincott, 1992, p. 903.) (Photo courtesy of St. Anne's Maternity Home.)

Maladaptive Responses to the Stresses of Adolescence

Substance Abuse

Substance abuse is the misuse of an addictive substance that changes the mental state of the user. The addictive substances commonly abused are tobacco, alcohol, and controlled or illicit drugs. Adolescents, influenced by peers and, in some instances, family adults, use drugs and alcohol to avoid facing their problems, trying to escape and forget the pain of life as they see it, or bow to peer pressure. Throughout history, people have used alcohol and other mood-altering drugs as a means of relieving the tensions and pressures of their lives. Many cultures still sanction use of some of these substances but object to their *abuse* (excessive use, or use in a way that is medically, socially, or culturally unacceptable). The unfortunate fact is that frequent use or abuse of these substances can lead to addiction or **dependence** (a compulsive need to use a substance for its satisfying or pleasurable effects). Dependence may be psychological or physical, or both. Psychological dependence means that the substance is desired for the effects or sensations it produces—alertness, euphoria, relaxation, a sense of well-being, and a false sense of control over problems. Physical dependence results from drug-induced changes in body tissue function that require the drug for normal activity. The magnitude of physical dependence determines the severity of **withdrawal symptoms** (physical and psychological symptoms that occur when the drug is no longer being used), including those such as vomiting, chills, tremors, and hallucinations. The symptoms vary with the amount, type, frequency, and duration of drug use. Continued use of an addictive substance can result in **tolerance** (the ability of body tissues to endure and adapt to continued or increased use of a substance), requiring larger doses of the drug to produce the desired effect.

Four stages of use have been identified that help describe the progression of substance abuse (Table 17-5). Using the clues from these stages, the nurse who works in any capacity with adolescents can be more alert to signs of possible substance abuse.

The adolescents at greatest risk of becoming substance abusers are identified as those who:

- Have families in which alcohol or drug abuse is or has been present
- Suffer from abuse, neglect, or loss or have no close relationships as a result of a dysfunctional family
- Have behavior problems, such as aggressiveness, or are excessively rebellious
- Are slow learners, have learning disabilities or attention deficit disorder
- Have problems with depression and low self-esteem[6]

In some instances, early identification of these factors by family, teachers, counselors, or other caregivers and prompt referral for treatment can help avoid the potential tragedy of substance abuse.

The most effective and least expensive treatment for substance abuse is prevention, beginning with education in the early school years. Factual information about drugs and about coping with problems without drugs should be provided. Scare techniques are completely ineffective because they arouse disbelief and often add the tempting thrill of danger. The impact of educational programs may be diluted if children come from a home in which alcohol or other drugs are used by family caregivers.

Alcohol Abuse

In many parts of American culture, drinking alcoholic beverages is considered acceptable and desirable social behavior. Although the purchase of alcohol is legally restricted to adults older than 21 years of age in all states and the District of Columbia, it is available in many homes and, consequently, the first drug most adolescents try. Alcohol is the most commonly abused drug among adolescents. **Alcohol abuse** occurs when a person ingests a quantity sufficient to cause intoxication (drunkenness). **Alcoholism** (chronic alcohol abuse or dependence) has reached epidemic proportions in America—an estimated 4.6 million teenagers have a drinking problem.[5]

Drinking often begins in the late school-age years and increases in frequency throughout adolescence. Some adolescents use alcohol in combination with marijuana and other drugs, potentiating the effects of both substances and increasing the probability of intoxication.

Alcoholism is costly in dollars and in damage to the lives of those who abuse alcohol and their families. During adolescence, alcohol abuse is closely linked to automobile accidents. A car is another symbol of adult status and a means to escape adult supervision. Drinking with friends before or while driving often has tragic results. Most states have a standard of blood alcohol content of 0.1% or higher as the level to determine charges of driving under the influence (DUI). The point that many adolescents miss is that fine motor control and judgment are affected at even lower levels, and driving ability may be decreased. The number of fatal accidents involving adolescents that are related to alcohol has decreased since all states have set 21 years as the legal age for drinking, but it still remains high.

Adolescents who receive treatment and counseling for problem drinking are more likely to recover than adults who have been problem drinkers over a long period. However, adolescents are difficult to treat owing to their feelings of immortality and the rapid progression of the disease in adolescents.

Treatment. Alcoholism is not a weakness of character but a major chronic, progressive, and potentially fatal disease process that affects every organ of the body, mental health

Table 17-5. Progression of Substance Abuse in Adolescents

Stage	Predisposition	Behavior	Family Reaction
Stage 1. Experimentation, Learning the Mood Swing			
Infrequent use of alcohol/ marijuana No consequences Some fear of use Low tolerance	Curiosity Peer pressure Attempt to assume adult role	Learning the mood Feels good Positive reinforcement Can return to normal	Often unaware Denial
Stage 2. Seeking the Mood Swing			
Increasing frequency in use of various drugs Minimal defensiveness Tolerance	Impress others Social function Modeling adult behavior	Using to get high Pride in amount consumed Used to relieve feelings (i.e., anxieties of dating, etc.) Denial of problem	Attempts at elimination Blaming others
Stage 3. Preoccupation with the Mood Swing			
Change in peer group activities revolve around use Steady supply Possible dealing Few or no straight friends Consequences frequent	Using to get loaded, not just high	Begins to violate values and rules Use before and during school Use despite consequences Solitary use Trouble with school Overdoses, "bad trips," blackouts Promises to cut down or attempts to quit Protection of supply, hides use from peers Deterioration in physical condition	Conspiracy of silence Confrontation Reorganization with or without affected person
Stage 4. Using to Feel Normal			
Continue to use despite adverse outcomes Loss of control Inability to stop Compulsion	Use to feel normal	Daily use Failure to meet expectations Loss of control Paranoia Suicide gestures, self-hate Physical deterioration (poor eating and sleep habits)	Frustration Anger May give up

From Hoover A. Adolescent drug abuse. In Oski FA (ed.). Principles and Practice of Pediatrics. Philadelphia: JB Lippincott, 1990.

status, and social competence of afflicted persons. Alcoholism is thought to be inherited, so children with a family history of alcoholism may be prone to alcohol problems. Treatment is lengthy and expensive and has no chance of success until the alcoholic acknowledges the problem and his or her helplessness to deal with it.

Treatment begins with detoxification ("drying out") and management of withdrawal symptoms. After the initial period, nutritional support is essential; a well-balanced diet, high-potency vitamins (especially vitamin B), and plenty of rest help eliminate harmful side effects of the disease.

Counseling to identify the problems that led to compulsive drinking and to help address those problems is an essential part of treatment. Many counselors who work with alcoholic patients are people who are recovering from a drinking problem themselves. This experience gives the counselor additional insight and empathy for the problem and the victim and adds credibility to the counseling offered.

Alcoholics Anonymous (AA) is the best known of all self-help groups; it offers fellowship and understanding to the compulsive drinker. AA has chapters in every sizable community, many of which have special programs for adolescents as well as for families of alcoholics (Alateen and Al-Anon). Anyone who has a desire to stop drinking is welcomed into AA and is helped to stay sober on the basis of taking "one day at a time." Recovery from alcoholism is a lifetime matter. The earlier the problem is diagnosed, the better the person's chances to respond to treatment. Ongoing support from health professionals, peers, family, and community is essential to successful treatment.

Tobacco Abuse

Tobacco is the second most frequently abused drug among adolescents. Any use of tobacco is abuse. More than 70% of young people try tobacco, by either smoking or chewing.[7] Many adolescents smoke because it gives them a feeling of maturity. Threats of long-term physical illnesses are far enough in the future that adolescents tend to ignore them. Many elementary and secondary schools have developed programs that warn children of the dangers of smoking, but the danger seems distant, and children believe that they can quit any time they want to. The use of "smokeless tobacco" (snuff or chewing tobacco) has increased steadily among adolescent males in the last 10 years. These teenagers believe that they are not damaging their lungs, but this type of tobacco use can cause mouth, lip, and throat cancers that are disfiguring and life threatening. The more immediate result of smoking that may stir interest in adolescents is the fact that their hair, breath, and clothes smell bad. Adolescents also have strong feelings of fairness and justice, so they may respond to the fact that children who are around persons who smoke are at increased risk for respiratory illness and cancer.

Adolescents whose family caregivers smoke are especially prone to become smokers, and they have difficulty accepting the fact that they are seriously endangering themselves by smoking. Most hospitals, schools, and public buildings have adopted no-smoking policies. Perhaps the pressure of society will help deter smoking in the future.

Marijuana Abuse

The third most frequently abused drug among adolescents is marijuana. More than 14% of high school seniors claimed they are current users of marijuana and hashish, using it every month. More than 40% have tried the drug at some time.[7] Many adolescents believe that marijuana smoking is not risky.

The effects of marijuana are mostly behavioral. It affects judgment, sense of time, and motivation. These effects make driving hazardous and may even cause hallucinations at higher doses. In addition, marijuana smoke is 3 to 5 times more carcinogenic than is cigarette smoke. Marijuana available today may be 3 to 5 times more potent than that smoked in the 1960s.[7] Adolescents must be informed about the dangers of marijuana to discourage its

use. Because marijuana is illegal, there is no manufacturing control over it, and the user has no idea about where it came from or the additives that may have been used. Although marijuana use has decreased, the rate of smokers is still high, and nurses must make every effort to discourage adolescents from using it.

Cocaine Abuse

Although cocaine does not rank among the first three drugs most commonly used by adolescents, it is an extremely dangerous drug. Fortunately, the use of cocaine and its derivative, "crack," has decreased among adolescents since the late 1980s. Adolescents living in inner city environments are at the greatest risk, but cocaine and crack can be found everywhere.

Cocaine, a fine, white, powdery substance, directly affects the brain cells, causing a physical and psychological effect. It usually is inhaled or smoked and is absorbed through the mucous membranes into the blood stream. The physical results are an increase in pulse, respirations, blood pressure, and temperature. The psychological effect produces a feeling of euphoria and an increased feeling of sociability. The high is reached in about 20 minutes and lasts for 20 to 30 minutes. In contrast, crack enters the blood stream in about 30 seconds, with a fast, powerful, but short "high" that lasts only about 5 minutes. As a result of the rapid, short high from crack, users tend to seek repeated highs over a short period, decreasing the time it takes to become addicted. Because of the rapid absorption of crack, immediate cardiac arrest can occur from its use. After smoking crack, the user may experience a "crash" that causes depression. To relieve this depression, crack users turn to alcohol and marijuana. This multiple use further complicates the effects of the drug. Some cocaine users inject cocaine to obtain a faster high and thus add to their risk of contracting HIV from contaminated needles.

Nurses must stress to adolescents the danger of using cocaine and crack. School education programs should start at the elementary level. Nurses can perform a community service by serving as volunteers to help present programs to local school children. Children and adolescents must be alerted to the dangers of these drugs and taught methods for refusing the offer of drugs. A complete drug program also should include programs and activities that help the child or adolescent increase feelings of self-worth.

Other Abused Drugs

Other mood-altering drugs commonly abused by adolescents include narcotics, psychotomimetic (psychedelic) drugs, hypnotics, amphetamines, and analgesics.

The most commonly abused narcotics are morphine and heroin. These drugs decrease anger, sex drive, and hunger by producing a dreamlike, euphoric state. Highly addictive and extremely expensive, narcotics result in teenage prostitution, pushing (selling) drugs, and robbery as a means to support the drug habit. As mentioned earlier, any of the drugs that are injected subject adolescents to the added risk of contracting HIV from using contaminated needles.

Psychotomimetic (psychedelic) drugs, although not addictive in a physical sense, can create a psychological dependence from the hallucinations that result. This category of drugs includes LSD, PCP ("angel dust"), psilocybin (derived from mushrooms), mescaline, DMT (derived from plants), and airplane glue. Effects can include intoxication, "bad trips," and overdosage.

Hypnotics are equal to narcotics in their addictive potential, and withdrawal from them must be carefully controlled to prevent delirium, seizures, or death. Barbiturates, glutethimide (Doriden), ethchlorvynol (Placidyl), and methaqualone (Quaalude) are the most commonly abused drugs in this group and are sometimes used with alcohol, increasing intoxicating effects such as sleepiness, slurred speech, and impaired cognitive and motor function.

Amphetamines ("uppers") produce several effects on the central nervous system: increased alertness, wakefulness and reduced awareness of fatigue, and increased confidence and energy. Although not physically addicting, they encourage psychological dependence and are abused by millions of Americans, many of whom become trapped in a destructive cycle of uppers and "downers" (barbiturates).

Analgesics, particularly those combining phenacetin, caffeine, and a hypnotic, often are abused by adolescents. Empirin and Fiorinal are two examples; their use often begins for relief of tension headaches, especially in women. Chronic abuse can result in blood and kidney disorders.

Anabolic steroids are not mood-altering drugs, but their abuse among athletes is a cause for great concern. Adolescent athletes take the anabolic steroids to build up muscle mass with the belief that the drug will increase their athletic ability. These athletes take megadoses of the illegally obtained drugs. Other adolescents may take them for the muscle building and "manly" appearance they believe will make them more attractive to girls. The side effects of euphoria and decreased fatigue make these drugs even more inviting to the adolescents. Some use also has been reported in high school female athletes.

The use of excessively large doses of steroids may cause **gynecomastia** (excessive development of mammary glands in the male) or premature fusion of the long bones, stunting growth in the adolescent who has not yet completed growing. Liver damage, predisposition to atherosclerosis, acne, hypertension, aggressiveness, and psychotic and manic symptoms also may result.[8] School

programs about drug abuse should include the topic of anabolic steroid abuse.

Treatment. The best treatment for the abuse of all of these drugs is prevention. When prevention is ineffective, emergency and long-term treatment become necessary. An overdose or a "bad trip" may force the adolescent to seek treatment. Emergency measures may even require artificial ventilation and oxygenation to restore normal respiration.

Long-term treatment involves many health professionals, such as psychiatric nurses, psychologists or psychiatrists, social workers, drug rehabilitation counselors, and community health nurses. The patient is also an important member of the treatment team and must admit the problem and the need for help and be willing to take an active part in treatment. Both outpatient and inpatient treatment programs are available. Many of these programs are geared specifically to adolescents. See the human services section of local telephone directories for specific listings.

Suicide

Suicide is the third leading cause of death in adolescents 10 to 19 years of age, falling just short of the homicide rate (see Figure 16-6). Because some deaths reported as accidents, particularly single car accidents, are thought to be suicides, the rate actually may be higher. Adolescent males commit suicide 4 times more often than do girls, but girls attempt suicide 5 times more often than do boys. Boys use more violent means of committing suicide than do girls and therefore are more often successful. Suicide is twice as common among Native Americans adolescents as among whites and twice as common among white adolescents as among African-Americans.[9]

Adolescents who have attempted suicide once are at greatest risk for attempting again, perhaps more effectively. Attempted suicide rarely occurs without warning and usually is preceded by a long history of emotional problems, difficulty in forming relationships, feelings of rejection, and low self-esteem. Loss of one or both parents through death or divorce, a family history that includes suicide of one or more members, and lack of success in academic or athletic performance are other frequent contributing factors. To this history is added one or more of the normal developmental crises of adolescence: difficulty in establishing independence, identity crisis, lack of intimate relationships, breakdown in family communication, a sense of alienation, and a conflict that interferes with problem solving. The adolescent's situation may be further complicated by an unwanted or unplanned pregnancy, drug addiction, or physical or sexual abuse, leading to depression and a feeling of total hopelessness.

Parent Teaching

Adolescent Suicide Warning Signs for Caregivers

Warning Signs in Teen's Behavior

1. Previous suicide attempt
2. Thoughts of wishing to kill self
3. Plans for self-destructive acts
4. Feeling "down in the dumps"
5. Withdrawal from social activities
6. Loss of pleasure in daily activities
7. Change in activity—increase or decrease
8. Poor concentration
9. Complaints of headaches, upset stomach, joint pains, frequent colds
10. Change in eating or sleeping patterns
11. Strong feelings of guilt, inadequacy, hopelessness
12. Preoccupation with thoughts of people dying, getting sick, or being injured
13. Substance abuse
14. Violence, truancy, stealing, or lying
15. Lack of judgment
16. Poor impulse control
17. Rapid swing in appropriateness of expressed emotions
18. Pessimistic view of self and world

Changes in Teen's Interpersonal Relationships

1. Conflicts with peers
2. Loss of boyfriend or girlfriend
3. School problems—behavioral or academic
4. Feelings of great frustration, being misunderstood, or not being part of the group
5. Lack of positive support from family, peers, or others
6. Family violence
7. Earlier suicide of family member, friend, or classmate
8. Separations, deaths, births, moves, or serious illnesses in the family unit

From Pfeffer CR. Spotting the red flags for adolescent suicide. Contemp Pediatr 6(2):65, 1989.

Health professionals involved with adolescents and family caregivers need to be aware of the factors that place a person at risk for suicide as well as the hints that signal an impending suicide attempt (see Parent Teaching: Adolescent Suicide Warning Signs for Caregivers). Some of these desperate youngsters will verbalize their hopelessness with statements such as, "I won't be around much longer" or "After Monday, it won't matter anyhow." They may begin giving away prized possessions or appear suddenly elated after a long period of acting dejected. These behaviors should *never* be ignored, and an effort should be made to ensure the teen's safety until counseling and treatment resources are in place. The nurse must strive to help the teen understand that although suicide is an option in problem solving, it is a final option, and there are other options available that are not so final. Nurses need to be aware of the resources, such as hot lines and counselors, within the adolescent's community that specialize in working with persons who have attempted suicide.

As part of the initial interview with the adolescent, the nurse should include questions that draw out feelings of alienation, depression, and hopelessness. If any of these indications are present, the nurse must report and document the findings immediately. The nurse also must question the family caregiver about any such signs and follow through with seeking additional help for the adolescent.

Summary

Adolescence, a time during which the teenager usually experiences few health problems, can become a time filled with a multitude of all types of problems for many teens. Minor problems can seem major and major problems insurmountable. Adolescents with a positive sense of self-esteem and a supportive family environment are more likely to weather this turbulence with fewer problems than are youngsters with a poor self-image, fewer successes, and an unfavorable home environment. However, no one is insulated from the stress and temptations that adolescents face.

Today's culture holds many options that have long-term implications for adolescent health and well-being. The choices adolescents make related to nutrition, friends and associates, alcohol and other drugs, sexuality, and school and career plans can affect their entire adult life. Nurses and other health professionals have a critically important part in the care and education of these young people to help guide them toward intelligent, informed choices. Prevention of the health problems that characterize adolescence is the primary objective. Competent, compassionate care of those adolescents who do encounter physiologic and psychological problems is a second objective, and the third is to restore health as quickly and completely as possible.

Review Questions

1. Maria is 14 years old and is obese. She tells you that she hates being "fat." What plans will you make to help her?
2. Tanya is 16 years old. She is 65 inches (165 cm) tall

and weighs 98 pounds (44.5 kg). She moans about how fat her thighs are. You believe she is anorectic. What symptoms in addition to her weight might you expect to find?

3. Tanya's diagnosis of anorexia nervosa is confirmed, and she is hospitalized for treatment. Develop a nursing care plan for Tanya.

4. Leesha, 15 years old, seems to consume an extraordinary amount of food but does not gain weight. In fact, she has lost some weight recently. What clues might you look for if you suspect she may be bulimic?

5. What factors put adolescents at greatest risk of becoming substance abusers?

6. Why is alcohol the most commonly abused drug among adolescents?

7. Mike is 14 years old. He uses snuff and says it is not dangerous because he is not inhaling nicotine like smokers do. What will you say to him?

8. Make a chart listing the substances abused and the effects each has on the user.

9. What are the factors that contribute to placing an adolescent at risk for suicide?

10. Do you think the statement, "The person who threatens suicide won't do it," is true? Defend your answer.

11. Willie is a 15-year-old boy with a mild case of acne. He has been scrubbing his face several times a day with soap, trying to "get rid of the zits." What advice can you give him?

12. Josie, Willie's mother, complains to you that she doesn't understand why he is making such a big fuss about a little acne. What response can you give her?

13. Alan, father of 10-year-old Cathy, asks you when he should start talking to Cathy about menstruation. What help can you give him?

14. When is screening for tuberculosis performed? Why is it important?

15. What is the most common STD?

16. Why is a mother's active case of genital herpes dangerous to the neonate during delivery?

17. Name and describe the stages of syphilis.

18. Name three ways an infant can contract HIV infection from the mother.

19. Why is there great concern about the spread of AIDS among adolescents?

20. What is the most important protection for the nurse against contracting HIV from a patient?

21. Brian is HIV positive and lives with his family. The family is frightened that other members may get the virus. What can you tell his family caregivers to reassure them and to help them protect other family members from spread of the virus in the home?

22. What guidelines will you give Brian's family caregivers to help them protect him from infectious or opportunistic diseases?

23. Brian is admitted to the hospital for evaluation. Develop a nursing care plan for Brian.

24. Explore the options available to a pregnant 10th grade girl in your community. Can she continue school? What sources for maternity care are available if she has no hospitalization insurance? Will child care be available to her after she has the baby so she can return to school?

References

1. American Psychiatric Association. Diagnostic and Statistical Manual of Mental Disorders—Revised, 3rd ed. Washington, DC: American Psychiatric Association, 1987.
2. Starke JR. Tuberculosis. In Oski F: Principles and Practices of Pediatrics. Philadelphia: JB Lippincott, 1990.
3. Centers for Disease Control and Prevention. 1993 revised classification system for HIV infection and expanded surveillance case definition for AIDS among adolescents and adults. MMWR 41(No. RR-17:2), 1992.
4. Kelly PJ, Holman S. The new face of AIDS. Am J Nurs 93(3): 26–34, 1993.
5. Lewit EM. Teenage childbearing. Future of Children 2(2): 186–191, 1992.
6. Adger H. Adolescent drug abuse. In Oski F: Principles and Practices of Pediatrics. Philadelphia: JB Lippincott, 1990.
7. Goldenring JM. 20 questions: A drug talk they'll remember. Contemp Pediatr 9(1):56–79, 1992.
8. Engel NS. Anabolic steroid use among high school athletes. MCN 14(6):417, 1989.
9. Cohall AT, Mayer R, Cohall K, et al. Teen violence: The new morality. Contemp Pediatr 8(9):81, 1991.

Bibliography

Boland MG, Czarniecki L. Starting life with HIV. RN 54(1):54–58, 1991.

Castiglia PT, Harbin RE. Child Health Care: Process and Practice. Philadelphia: JB Lippincott, 1992.

Clarke PF, Byrne MW. A step up from home care: Enhanced care for medically complex HIV infected children. MCN 18(3):94–98, 1993.

Ferraro AR. Bulimia: A look from within. Pediatr Nurs 16(2): 187–191, 1990.

Fleming BW, Munton MT, Clarke BA, et al. Assessing and promoting positive parenting in adolescent mothers. MCN 18(1): 32–37, 1993.

Jackson DB, Saunders RB. Child Health Nursing. Philadelphia: JB Lippincott, 1993.

Jaffe ES. Working with troubled teens. RN 54(2):58–62, 1991.

Novotny J. Adolescents, acne, and the side effects of accutane. Pediatr Nurs 15(3):247–248, 1989.

Pfeffer CR. Spotting the red flags for adolescent suicide. Contemp Pediatr 6(2):59–60, 65–66, 68–70, 1989.

Pillitteri A. Maternal and Child Health Nursing. Philadelphia: JB Lippincott, 1992.

Roller CG. Drawing out young mothers. MCN 17(5):254–255, 1992.

Ungvarski PJ, Schmidt J. AIDS patients under attack. RN 55(11): 37–45, 1992.

Washburn P. Identification, assessment, and referral of adolescent drug abusers. Pediatr Nurs 17(2):137–140, 1991.

Whaley LF, Wong DL. Nursing Care of Infants and Children, 4th ed. St. Louis: Mosby-Year Book, 1991.

Whatley JH. Effects of health locus of control and social network on adolescent risk taking. Pediatr Nurs 17(2):145–148, 1991.

Williams AD. Nursing management of the child with AIDS. Pediatr Nurs 15(3):259–261, 1989.

The Child in a Troubled Society

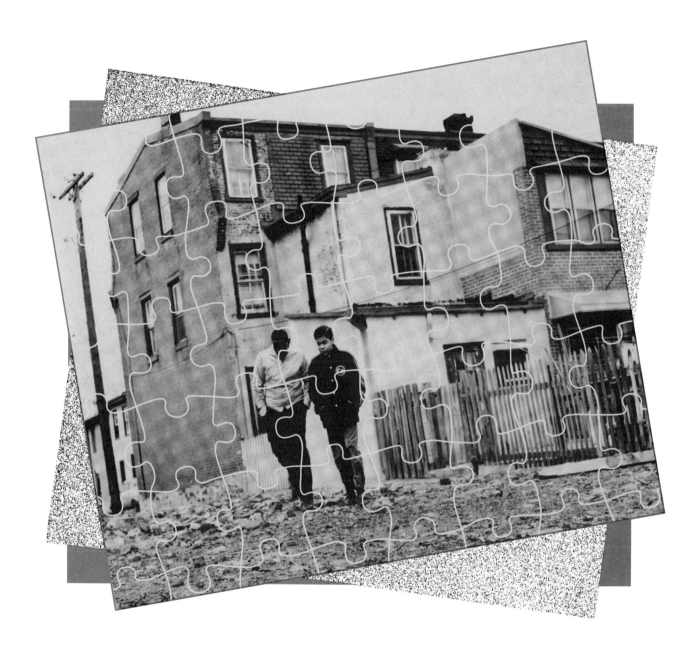

Unit IV

The Child
and Substance Abuse

Chapter 18

Student Objectives

Upon completion of this chapter, the student will be able to:

1. Define the key terms.
2. Identify the behaviors of the pregnant drug abuser that put her fetus in danger.
3. Describe the effects that cocaine abuse during pregnancy may have on the fetus.
4. Identify nursing care that may be helpful when caring for crack cocaine infants.
5. Describe characteristics of the infant with fetal alcohol syndrome.
6. Describe the unpredictable behavior of an addicted parent and its effect on the child.
7. List six behaviors that offer the nurse a clue that there may be a problem of addiction in the child's family.
8. Identify common inhalant products that children may use as deliriants.
9. Discuss principles that a family caregiver can use to teach children about substance abuse.

Marks MG: BROADRIBB'S INTRODUCTORY PEDIATRIC NURSING, 4th ed. © 1994 J.B. Lippincott Company.

Key Terms

co-dependent parent

deliriants

fetal alcohol syndrome

inhalants

microcephaly

micrognathia

neonatal abstinence syndrome

palpebral fissures

philtrum

*S*ubstance abuse is a family problem. If one member of the family abuses alcohol or drugs, every member of that family is affected. The problem has grown to alarming proportions since the early 1980s. The number of infants born to substance-abusing mothers has grown consistently during this time, resulting in a large number of babies who face great physical and emotional challenges with few or limited family resources. In addition, children who have at least one parent who is a substance abuser are at risk for a variety of problems that researchers relate to substance abuse in the family. Behavior problems, school failures, and child abuse are just a few of the negative results that can occur.

The Infant of a Substance-Abusing Mother

Maternal substance abuse takes an enormous toll on the unborn child. Most illicit drugs cross the placenta easily, and it is estimated that the concentration of these drugs in the fetus can be as high as 50% of that in the mother. The substances that affect the neonate most severely are cocaine and alcohol, although cigarette smoking and other drugs are also detrimental to fetal health. The pregnant substance abuser frequently has no prenatal care or may receive irregular care. The pregnant woman who is dependent on drugs may be more interested in getting her next supply of drugs than in keeping an appointment. If the woman's financial status does not provide enough money for food, health care, and drugs, she is likely to use her limited her resources to get more drugs. As a result the unborn child suffers not only from the effects of the drugs but from nutritional deprivation and inadequate care. In addition, the drug abuser is often sexually promiscuous, perhaps practicing prostitution to obtain money to support her habit. Thus, she puts herself in jeopardy for sexually transmitted diseases. If she injects drugs, she also may be at great risk for human immunodeficiency viral infection or hepatitis. Many women with a substance abuse problem deny or try to hide their drug dependence, avoiding contact with health care workers in fear of detection.

The Effect of Cocaine on the Neonate

During pregnancy, cocaine (often used in the form of "crack" because it is cheaper) causes vasoconstriction of the placental blood vessels, resulting in a variety of problems. Spontaneous abortion, premature birth, and premature separation of the placenta are common. The decrease in circulation to the fetus can cause intrauterine growth retardation. Congenital anomalies such as missing fingers or toes, seizures, necrotizing enterocolitis, apnea, atresia of the ileum, occlusion of heart valves, cerebral infarction (a type of stroke), **microcephaly** (small head), and permanent neurologic damage can occur. Many cocaine users also use other drugs, specifically alcohol, marijuana, and cigarettes, further endangering the health of the fetus.

At birth, newborns who have been exposed to cocaine ("crack cocaine infants") often are irritable, quivery, easily startled, and cry at any sound or even the softest touch. Most newborns of drug-dependent women show signs of **neonatal abstinence syndrome** (NAS), characterized by signs and symptoms of central nervous system hyperirritability; gastrointestinal dysfunction; respiratory distress; and vague autonomic symptoms, including yawning, sneezing, sweating, stuffy nose, mottling, increased tearing, and fever.[1] At birth, these infants frequently have a low birth weight and poor Apgar scores. The infant may not be able to take nutrition normally and may need to be fed by means of gavage feeding. Breast feeding is not attempted because cocaine can stay in breast milk for 60 hours after drug use. Crack cocaine infants have a high rate of sudden infant death syndrome.

Many of these newborns are admitted to the neonatal

intensive care unit for care because of prematurity, very low birth weight, and other birth problems. The mother often leaves the infant in the hospital, and the infant is sent to a foster home when ready for discharge.

Nursing Care of the Crack Cocaine Infant
Caring for crack cocaine infants is challenging. These infants frequently suffer from poor sleep patterns, diarrhea, and dehydration. They often do not respond to usual means of quieting infants, such as swaddling, offering pacifiers, and rocking. Wrapping the infant securely with arms brought to the midline and holding the infant snugly against the body in an upright position may be helpful. When the infant is rocked, the movement should be in a vertical (up and down) motion rather than the usual back-and-forth method. Reducing stimuli, such as noise, bright lights, and sudden movements, helps quiet the infant. Soft music also may be helpful. These infants seem to take nourishment better when held in an upright position and fed slowly. They may need to have smaller, more frequent feedings because they tire so quickly.

In the event that the mother plans to take the baby home, intensive teaching is required. The mother must be drug free and enrolled in a program to support her resolve to quit using drugs. The mother needs to learn basic parenting skills. In addition, the caregiver must be helped to understand that the infant may show many signs that can be interpreted as rejection of the caregiver but that these behaviors are general reactions and not specifically directed at the caregiver. Caregivers must be provided with complete instructions, including written materials. The nurse must be certain that the teaching materials are presented at a level and in language the caregiver can understand. Close home contact should be planned to follow up on the infant after discharge. The caregiver can be encouraged to telephone for help when facing a problem with the infant. Ongoing support for these families is essential.

The Effect of Heroin and Other Opiates on the Neonate

Crack cocaine has clearly become the most frequently abused narcotic since its appearance in the 1980s. However, heroin and other opiates continue to be used, and in some parts of the country, heroin use is increasing. The death rate for neonates of heroin-addicted mothers is 4 times greater than that of nonaddicted mothers. The effects of maternal abuse of these drugs is similar to those of crack cocaine infants. Hypoxia during labor may cause meconium staining and aspiration pneumonia in the newborn, contributing to increased illness and possible death. These infants often have jaundice, aspiration pneumonia, transient tachypnea, respiratory distress syndrome, and congenital malformations. Prenatal care frequently is poor. The infants may have a high-pitched cry

and increased muscle tone and may be irritable. They have a marked rooting reflex, sucking on fists or thumbs, but are poor feeders with frequent regurgitation, resulting from ineffective sucking and swallowing reflexes.[2] Infants of mothers who have been taking methadone have much the same withdrawal symptoms. However, these infants may have a higher birth weight because the mother had more consistent prenatal care.

Withdrawal symptoms apparently are related to the drug habit of the mother. Those newborns whose mothers have taken large doses over a long period have the most severe withdrawal. Timing of withdrawal symptoms also is related to how close to delivery the mother took heroin. The closer to delivery the last dose occurred, the later the withdrawal symptoms appear. These symptoms may continue for 2 months or more.

Nursing care of the infant of a heroin or opiate abuser is similar to the care of the crack cocaine infant. Paregoric is used to treat infants with opiate-induced NAS to manage the symptoms. Phenobarbital is used in infants who have nonopiate NAS. Some physicians may prescribe the two drugs in combination.

The Neonate with Fetal Alcohol Syndrome

Alcohol is the substance most commonly abused by pregnant women. Any ingestion of alcohol during pregnancy is considered unwise. Moderate maternal drinking has been demonstrated to produce poor infants with intrauterine growth and congenital anomalies, and heavy maternal drinking produces greater abnormalities than does moderate drinking. The collection of abnormalities that are characteristically seen in the infant whose mother consumed alcohol during pregnancy is commonly referred to as **fetal alcohol syndrome** (FAS). These infants are shorter and lower in birth weight and may have microcephaly (small head), facial deformities, hearing disorders, poor coordination, minor joint and limb abnormalities, heart defects, delayed development, and mental retardation. The facial deformities are characteristic and include short **palpebral fissures** (opening between the eyes); flat **philtrum** (a vertical groove in the middle of the upper lip); thin upper lip; short, upturned nose; and **micrognathia** (a small lower jaw) (Figure 18-1). Infants may have a few or many of these abnormalities. Neonates are jittery and may evidence failure to thrive.

The fetus may be affected by a number of factors related to the mother's drinking: the alcoholic mother may be malnourished; the mother may have an alcohol-induced illness, such as gastric hemorrhage and cirrhosis of the liver; and alcohol crosses the placental "barrier" easily, directly affecting the fetus as well as being present in the amniotic fluid that the fetus ingests. In addition, many mothers who consume alcohol also smoke and use other drugs, adding the effects of these drugs to the fetus's state of well-being. At birth, the infant may be hypo-

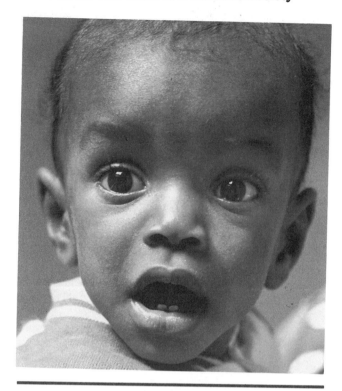

Figure 18-1. A 15-month-old child with fetal alcohol syndrome (From Castiglia PT, Harbin R. Child Health Care. Philadelphia: JB Lippincott, 1992.)

glycemic from the effect of the alcohol. All infants at risk should be screened with a reagent strip in the nursery within the first few hours after birth. Symptoms of neonatal hypoglycemia for which the nurse should be alert include tremors, lethargy, seizures, irregular respirations, and apnea. These neonates also may have respiratory distress syndrome.

Newborns with fetal alcohol syndrome need a quiet, nonstimulating environment. Intravenous fluids are administered as needed to avoid dehydration, and anticonvulsant drugs are administered if the infant is having seizures.

As infants and toddlers, children with FAS often have difficulty with feedings. They also may be hyperactive or have attention deficit disorders, intellectual slowness, poor fine-motor control, and developmental delay of gross motor skills. These children need a supportive educational environment throughout their school years.

Parents Addicted to Drugs or Alcohol

More than 10% of children come from a home that is affected by the alcoholism of one or both parents. Alcoholism exacts a terrible toll on the functioning of the family. Children of alcoholics are 4 times more likely to become alcoholics themselves. When other substances are included in the statistics, the number of affected homes increases substantially.

The Effect of Parental Substance Abuse on the Family

Developmental delays occur in young children of substance abusers. Infants of cocaine abusers avoid the caregiver's gaze, contributing further to bonding delays. The parent who is addicted may be so involved in procuring the drug that any pretense of good parenting is forgotten. The parent, caught up in the ups and downs of addiction, is not dependable and is unable to provide any stability for the child. The parent may waver between overindulgence—giving the child more than is appropriate, "smothering" the child in attention, leniency, and gifts—and the opposite behavior of irritability, unreasonable accusations, threats, and anger. This unpredictable behavior of the parent has a severe impact on the relationships in the family. Children of substance-abusing parents often become "loners," avoiding the development of relationships with others in fear that the substance-abusing parent might do or say something to embarrass them in front of their peers. As the parent's substance abuse increases, there is an increase in the dysfunction and social isolation of the family. The **co-dependent parent** supports, directly or indirectly, the addictive behavior of the other parent. This behavior usually involves making excuses for the addicted person's actions, expecting others (ie, the children) to overlook their moodiness, erratic behavior, and consumption of alcohol or drugs. Co-dependency of the other parent may add to the dilemma of children living with an addicted parent.

Children Coping with Parental Addiction

Children rarely talk about the parent's problem, even to the other parent. These children often suffer from guilt, anxiety, confusion, anger, depression, and addictive behavior. Children react in a variety of ways. An older child, frequently a girl, may take on the responsibility of running the household, taking care of the younger children, making meals, and performing the tasks that the parent normally should do. These children may become "overachievers" in school but remain isolated emotionally from their peers and teachers. Another child in the family may try to deflect the embarrassment and anger of the other siblings, trying to make everyone feel good. As these children become adolescents or young adults, they may have problems such as substance abuse or eating disorders. The child in the family who acts out and engages in delinquent behavior is the child most likely to come to the attention of social services and be identified as a child who needs help.

Behaviors of children that may alert nurses and other

health care personnel that there may a problem of addiction in the family are the following:

- The "loner" child who avoids interaction with classmates
- The child who is failing in school or has numerous episodes of unexcused absences or truancy
- The child with frequent minor physical complaints, such as headaches or stomach aches
- The child who demonstrates behavior such as stealing and committing acts of violence
- The child who is aggressive to others
- The child who is abusing drugs or alcohol

Nurses and others who work with children must be alert to these signals for help. Children can benefit from programs that support them and help them understand what is happening in the home. Such a program can be a type of group therapy program based in a school setting in which the child learns that others have the same problems. The child's feelings of isolation are reduced when others are seen to have the same kind of problems. Other programs may work with the whole family, perhaps as part of the program for the addicted parent who is trying to break the addiction. Professional help is necessary to prevent the child from developing more serious problems. The earlier the child can be identified and treatment begun the better the prognosis.

Substance Abuse by Children

Despite the stereotype that children who engage in abusing substances are children of the ghetto, age, race, and socioeconomic status are not limiting factors in this problem. The use of alcohol and other substances to provide mind-altering excitement occurs in children as young as 8 or 9 years of age. Many children, even as young as elementary school age, from every level of society engage in smoking cigarettes. The risk for starting to smoke is greatest in the sixth and seventh grades, according to research findings. Forty percent of children try cigarettes before reaching high school, with the total reaching 70% before completing high school. Twelve percent of boys

Box 18-1

Common Products Inhaled as Deliriants

Model glue
Rubber cement
Cleaning fluids
Kerosene vapors
Gasoline vapors
Butane lighter fluid
Paint sprays
Paint thinner
Varnish
Shellac
Nail polish remover
Liquid typing correction fluid
Propellant in whipped cream spray cans
Aerosol paint cans
Upholstery fabric protection spray cans
Solvents

Box 18-2

Guidelines to Prevent Substance Abuse

1. Openly communicate values by talking about the importance of honesty, responsibility, and self-reliance. Encourage decision making. Help child see how each decision builds on previous decisions.

2. Provide a good role model for the child to copy. Children tend to copy parents' habits of smoking and drinking alcohol and accept attitudes about drug use, whether they are over-the-counter, prescription, or illicit drugs.

3. Avoid conflicts between what you say and what you do. For example, don't ask the child to lie that you are not home when you are or encourage the child to lie about age when trying to get lower admission price at amusement centers.

4. Talk about values during family times. Give the child "what if" examples, and discuss the best responses when faced with a difficult situation. For example, "What would you do if you found money that someone dropped?"

5. Set strong rules about using alcohol and other drugs. Make specific rules with specific punishments. Discuss these rules and the reason for them.

6. Be consistent in applying the rules that you set.

7. Be reasonable; don't make wild threats. Respond calmly, carrying out the expected punishment.

8. Get the facts about alcohol and other drugs, and provide children with current, correct information. This helps you in discussions with children and also helps you recognize symptoms if a child has been using them.

(From Growing Up Drug Free: A Parent's Guide to Prevention. Washington, DC: U.S. Department of Education, 1990.)

Box 18-3

Resources for Information and Help with Drug and Alcohol Problems

Abraxas Foundation, Inc. (adolescents only)—Telephone (800) 227-2927

Alcoholics Anonymous—listed in telephone white pages

Al-Anon for family and friends of alcoholics—listed in telephone white pages

American Council for Drug Education provides information, books, newsletter; develops media campaigns; reviews scientific data; offers films and curriculum materials for preteens, 204 Monroe Street, Rockville, MD 20850. Telephone (301) 294-0600

Families Anonymous, Inc.—a 12-step program for family and friends of people with problems of drug abuse. P.O. Box 528, Van Nuys, CA 91408. Telephone (818) 989-7841

Hazeldon Foundation distributes educational material and self-help literature for 12-step recovery participants and professionals. Pleasant Valley Road, P.O. Box 176, Center City, MN 55012-0176. Telephone (800) 328-9000

Institute on Black Chemical Abuse provides training and technical assistance for programs serving African Americans and others of color. 2614 Nicollett Avenue, Minneapolis, MN 55408. Telephone (612) 871-7878

"Just Say No" clubs, through workshops, newsletters, and other activities, provide support and positive reinforcement for children. 1777 North California Boulevard, Suite 200, Walnut Creek, CA 94596. Telephone (800) 258-2766/(415) 939-6666

Nar-Anon Family Group Headquarters supports friends and families of drug abusers; similar to Al-Anon. World Service Office, P.O. Box 2563, Palos Verdes Peninsula, CA 90274. Telephone (213) 547-5800

Narcotics Anonymous is similar to Alcoholics Anonymous. World Service Office, P.O. Box 9999, Van Nuys, CA 91409. Telephone (818) 780-3951

National Clearinghouse for Alcohol and Drug Information (NCAD) is a resource for alcohol and other drug information. P.O. Box 2345, Rockville, MD 20852. Telephone (301) 468-2600

National Council on Alcoholism, Inc., through local affiliates, provides information on alcohol and alcoholism. 12 West 21st Street, New York, NY 10010. Telephone (212) 206-6770

National Crime Prevention Council develops materials such as audiovisuals and reproducible brochures for parents and children. 1700 K Street, N.W., Washington, DC 20006. Telephone (202) 466-NCPC

National Federation of Parents for Drug-Free Youth, Inc., sponsors the National Red Ribbon Campaign to reduce demand for drugs and the Responsible Educated Adolescents Can Help (REACH) program to educate junior and senior high school students about drug abuse. Communications Center, 1423 North Jefferson, Springfield, MO 65802. Telephone (417) 836-3709

National PTA Drug and Alcohol Abuse Prevention Project provides kits, brochures, posters, and publications on alcohol and drugs for parents, teachers, and PTA organizations. 700 North Rush Street, Chicago, IL 60611. Telephone (312) 577-4500

Safe Homes encourages parents to sign a contract stipulating that strict no-alcohol/no-drug-use rule will prevail at home parties. P.O. Box 702, Livingston, NJ 07039

Toughlove is a self-help group for parents, children, and communities emphasizing cooperation, personal initiative, and action. Provides newsletter, brochures, books, and workshops. P.O. Box 1069, Doylestown, PA 18901. Telephone (800) 333-1069/(215) 348-7090

(From Growing Up Drug Free: A Parent's Guide to Prevention. Washington, DC: U.S. Department of Education, 1990.)

have chewed tobacco or snuff, which is just as addictive and harmful as smoking.

Children may experiment with **inhalants** (substances whose volatile vapors can be abused) because they are readily available and may seem no more threatening than an innocent prank. Inhalants classified as **deliriants** contain chemicals that give off fumes that can produce symptoms of confusion, disorientation, excitement, and hallucinations. Many inhalants are products commonly found in most homes (Box 18-1). The fumes are mind altering when inhaled. The child initially may experience a temporary "high," giddiness, nausea, coughing, nosebleed, fatigue, lack of coordination, or loss of appetite. Overdose can cause loss of consciousness and possible death from suffocation by replacing oxygen in the lungs or depressing the central nervous system, causing respiratory arrest. Permanent damage to the lungs, the nervous system, or the liver can result. Children who experiment with inhalants may proceed to abuse other drugs in an attempt to get similar effects. Addiction occurs in younger children more rapidly than in adults.

Family caregivers must work to develop a strong, loving relationship with the children in the family, teach the children values of the family and the difference between right and wrong, set and enforce rules for acceptable behavior of family members, learn facts about drugs and alcohol, and actively listen to the children in the family (Box 18-2). An excellent reference for family caregivers is "Growing up Free: A Parent's Guide to Prevention," which is published by the United States Department of Education and can be ordered free by calling the Department of Education's toll-free number: 1-800-624-0100. Other resources for alcohol and drug abuse help may be found in Box 18-3.

Summary

Substance abuse is a widespread social problem that affects every aspect of family life and takes a terrible toll on our nation's children. From the fetus carried by the substance-abusing woman to the children who grow up in homes deeply affected by parental addiction, children suffer physical, emotional, and social consequences that affect them throughout their lives.

Children may begin to abuse alcohol or drugs as early as their elementary school years. Inhalation of fumes from products that are commonly found in many homes may be the way they first experiment with drugs. Because of the danger of this type of substance abuse, children may suffer permanent injury or death. Smoking and other tobacco use may start at the elementary school level. Alcohol use sometimes begins in this age group.

Review Questions

1. What are some of the factors occurring in substance abuse that may affect the unborn fetus?
2. You are talking with Tasha, a high school student. Explain to her the problems of pregnancy that result from vasoconstriction resulting from crack cocaine use.
3. Continue your discussion with Tasha to include the congenital anomalies that crack cocaine use during pregnancy may cause.
4. What are the characteristics that may be seen in neonatal abstinence syndrome?
5. Maria is a pregnant teen who has been bragging about the "partying" she has been doing. What can you tell her about the use of alcohol during pregnancy and the symptoms of fetal alcohol syndrome?
6. What are some typical behaviors of the co-dependent parent?
7. Children react differently to living with a family caregiver who is addicted. What are the behaviors that may be seen in a child that may indicate a family problem?
8. Survey your home and make a list of all the products available that a child could use as a inhalant for a deliriant effect.

References

1. Kaltenbach K, Finnegan LP. Neonatal abstinence syndrome: Pharmacotherapy and developmental outcome. Neurobehav Toxicol Teratol 8(4):353–355, 1986.
2. Finnegan LP. Effects of maternal opiate abuse on the newborn. Fed Proc 44:2314–2317, 1985.

Bibliography

Bresnahan K, Brooks C, Zuckerman B. Prenatal cocaine use: Impact on infants and mothers. Pediatr Nurs 17(2):123–129, 1991.

Chasnoff IJ. Cocaine, pregnancy, and the neonate. Women Health 15(3):23–35, 1989.

Culverwell M. Perinatal effects of cocaine. Childbirth Instr 1(1):10–13, 16–17, 1991.

Free T, Russell F, Mills B, et al. A descriptive study of infants and toddlers exposed prenatally to substance abuse. MCN 15(4): 245–249, 1990.

Kaltenbach KA, Finnegan LP. Prenatal narcotic exposure: Perinatal and developmental effects. Neurotoxicology 10:597–604, 1989.

Kelley SJ, Walsh JH, Thompson K. Birth outcomes, health problems, and neglect with prenatal exposure to cocaine. Pediatr Nurs 17(2):130–136, 1991.

Lewis KD, Bennett B, Schmeder ND. The care of infants menaced by cocaine abuse. MCN 14(5):324–329, 1989.

Mutch PB. Infant addicts: A preventable rage. Vibrant Life 16: 26–27, 1990.

The Child in a Stressed Family

Chapter 19

Student Objectives

Upon completion of this chapter, the student will be able to:

1. Define the key terms.
2. Identify how poor parenting skills may lead to child abuse.
3. State the amount of time that a health care facility can hold a child while investigating for possible child abuse.
4. Identify under what circumstances physical punishment can be classified as abusive.
5. Describe the differences between bruises that occur accidentally to a young child and those that have been inflicted in an abusive manner.
6. Define Munchausen syndrome by proxy.
7. Identify ways that a child may be emotionally abused.
8. List the services offered by the National Runaway Hot Line.
9. Describe emotional reactions a child may have to divorce.
10. Describe the effects of homelessness on the health care of children.

Marks MG: BROADRIBB'S INTRODUCTORY PEDIATRIC NURSING, 4th ed. © 1994 J.B. Lippincott Company.

Key Terms

child neglect   latchkey child

dysfunctional family   sexual abuse

incest   sexual assault

*E*very family faces many types of stress at one time or another. Events that create stress for a family include illness, job loss, economic crisis, relocation, birth, death, and trauma. How the family handles these stresses impacts greatly on the emotional, social, and physical health of the family and its children. A **dysfunctional family** is one that is not able to resolve these stresses and work through them in a positive, socially acceptable manner. The atmosphere in such a family creates additional stress for all family members. Because of the lack of support within the family for individual members, these members respond negatively to real or perceived problems. This may set the stage for child abuse, runaway children, substance abuse, and other unhealthy coping behaviors. The single-parent family often faces multiple pressures occurring at the same time, creating additional stress and adding to the risk of dysfunctional coping.

Child Abuse

Although child abuse has occurred throughout the ages, the evolution of cultural practices in the United States during the last few decades of the 20th century has emphasized the rights of children; thus, any sort of mistreatment and abuse of children is regarded as totally unacceptable. The term *child abuse* has come to mean any intentional act of physical, emotional, or sexual abuse, including acts of negligence, committed by a person responsible for the care of the child.

Each year increasing numbers of child abuse cases are brought to the attention of authorities. Estimates of the number of children treated in emergency departments of hospitals range from 500,000 to 1 million annually. How-

ever, this may be only the "tip of the iceberg" because the abuse of many more children may go without detection. Child abuse is not limited to just one age group but can be detected at any age. The courts have even viewed the exposure of the fetus in utero to the effects of drugs and alcohol as child abuse. Surprisingly, adolescents have the greatest incidence of abuse. In children younger than 2 years of age, the rate is estimated at 6 in 1000 and the rate in children between 15 and 17 years of age escalates to more than than 14 in 1000.[1]

The effects of child abuse are long term. The child who has been abused may be hyperactive; may exhibit angry, antisocial behavior; or may be especially withdrawn. Abusing parents often have been abused themselves as children; thus, the problem of child abuse continues in a cyclical fashion from generation to generation. Abusive parents can be found at all socioeconomic levels; however, those families with greater financial means may be able to evade detection more easily. Families with low income show greater evidence of violence, neglect, and sexual abuse according to some studies. Frequently, abusive parents do not have adequate parenting skills; therefore, they have unrealistic expectations of the child and do not respond to the child's behavior appropriately.

State laws require health care personnel to report suspected child abuse cases. Loss of nursing license is the usual penalty for the nurse who does not report suspected child abuse. This requirement overrides the concern for confidentiality. In most instances, the health care facility can hold the child for 72 hours after suspected abuse has been reported so that a caseworker will have time to investigate the charge. After this 72-hour period, a hearing is held to determine if the charges are true and placement of the child is decided.

Physical Abuse

Frequently, physical abuse occurs when the caregiver is unfamiliar with normal child behavior. Young caregivers do not know what is normal behavior for a child and become frustrated when the child does not respond to them in the way that they expect. Some young girls become pregnant to have a child to love, expecting that love to be returned in full measure. When the child resists the mother's control or seems to do the opposite of what she expects, she feels that it is a personal affront to her and becomes angry, responding with physical punishment, sometimes in an uncontrolled manner. Some cultural patterns support physical punishment for children, citing the old principle, "spare the rod, spoil the child." The practice of physical punishment has been debated over many years, but despite the evidence that physical punishment frequently results in negative behavior whereas other forms of punishment are more effective, corporal punishment continues to be approved, even in some schools. However, physical punishment that leaves marks, causes injury, or threatens the child's physical or emotional well-being is considered abusive.

When a child is brought to a physician or hospital because of physical injuries, family caregivers may attribute the injury to some action of the child that is not in keeping with the child's age or level of development. The caregiver may also attribute the injury to some action of a sibling. Any time health care personnel observe injuries that do not correspond to the injury the caregiver says has occurred, health care personnel must be on the alert for possible abuse. The nurse should be careful not to accuse the caregiver, however, before a complete investigation takes place.

Young, active children often have a number of bruises that occur from their usual activities. Most of these bruises occur over bony areas such as knees, elbows, shins, and the forehead. Bruises that occur in areas of soft tissue, such as the abdomen, the buttocks, the genitalia, the thighs, and the mouth, may be suspect. Bruises in the inner aspect of the upper arms may indicate that the child raised his or her arms to protect the face and head from blows. Bruises may be distinctive in outline, clearly indicating the instrument that was used. Hangers, belt buckles, electrical cords, hand prints, teeth (from biting), and sticks are all instruments that leave marks that can be identified. Bruises may be in varying stages of healing, indicating that all of the injuries did not occur during one episode (Figures 19-1 and 19-2). On radiograph, bone fractures in various stages of healing may be noted. Spiral fractures of the long bones of a young child are considered a cardinal sign of abusive injury. Infants who have been harshly shaken may not demonstrate a clear picture of abuse, but through use of computed tomography scanning, cerebral edema or cerebral hemorrhage may be detected.

Burns are another common type of injury seen in the abused child. Although young children may be burned because of accidental circumstances, certain types of burns are highly suspect as deliberate burns. Cigarette burns are common abuse injuries. Also, burns from immersion of a hand in hot liquid; a hot register, as evidenced by the grid pattern; a steam iron; or a curling iron are not uncommon. Caregivers have immersed the buttocks of a child into hot water when the child was judged to be uncooperative in toilet training. Caregivers are often unaware of how quickly a child can be seriously burned.

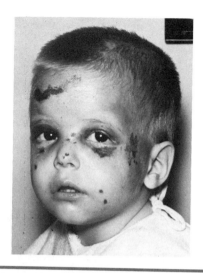

Figure 19-1. The child who has been physically abused usually has old and fresh bruises about the head, face, and body and may either look sad and forlorn or be actively seeking to please, sometimes even particularly involved with and attentive to the abusing parent. (From Jackson DB, Saunders RB. Child Health Nursing. Philadelphia: JB Lippincott, 1993.)

A burn that is neglected or not reported immediately must be considered suspicious until all of the facts can be gathered and examined.

Munchausen Syndrome

Munchausen syndrome is a syndrome in which one person either fabricates or induces illness in another to get attention. The mother is most often the person who has the syndrome when injury to a child is involved. Often, the mother injures the child to get the attention of medical personnel. She may slowly poison the child with prescription drugs, alcohol, or other drugs, or she may suffocate the child to cause apnea. These types of circumstances are most frustrating for the health care personnel. Close observation of caregiver interactions with the child are necessary to adequately assess this possibility. For instance, if episodes of apnea occur only in the presence of the mother, health care personnel should be on the alert for this syndrome. The caregiver who suffers from this syndrome must receive psychiatric help.

Emotional Abuse and Neglect

Injury from emotional abuse can be just as serious and long term as physical abuse, but it is much more difficult to identify. Several types of emotional abuse can occur, including verbal abuse, such as humiliation, scapegoating, unrealistic expectations with belittling, and erratic discipline; emotional unavailability when caregivers are absorbed in their own problems; insufficient or poor nurturing or threatening to leave the child or otherwise end

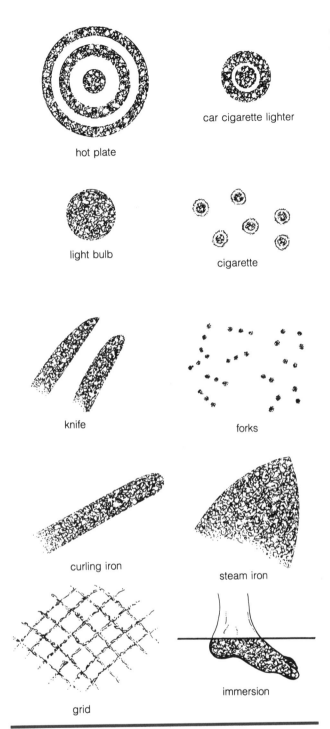

Figure 19-2. Burn patterns from objects used for inflicting burns in child abuse.

the relationship; and role reversal, in which the child must take on the role of parenting the parent and is blamed for the problems of the parent.

Children may show evidence of emotional abuse by appearing worried or fearful or having vague complaints of illness or nightmares. Caregivers may display signs of inappropriate expectations of the child when in the health care facility, sometimes mocking or belittling them for age-appropriate behavior. In young children, failure to thrive may be a sign of emotional abuse. In the older child, poor school performance and attendance, poor self-esteem, and poor peer relationships may be clues. **Child neglect** is failing to provide adequate hygiene, health care, nutrition, love, nurturing, and supervision that is needed for growth and development. If a child is not provided with adequate care for a serious medical condition, the caregivers are considered neglectful. For example, if a child is seriously burned (even though it is accidental) and the caregivers do not take the child for evaluation and treatment of the burn until several days later, the caregiver may be judged to be neglectful. Often, the child with failure to thrive as a result of being under-fed, deprived of love, or constantly "picked at" and criticized can be classified as neglected; however, the nurse must be careful not to make an unsubstantiated accusation of neglect.

Sexual Abuse

Sexual abuse of children has existed in all ages and cultures, but seldom has it been admitted when it is perpetrated by parents or other relatives in the home. Estimates indicate that **incest** (sexually arousing physical contact between family members not married to each other) occurs in 240,000 to 1 million American families annually, and that number is growing each year. As with other types of child abuse, sexual abuse knows no socio-economic, racial, religious, or ethnic boundaries. However, substance abuse, job loss, and poverty are contributing factors. Like other forms of child abuse, sexual abuse is being recognized and reported more often. The National Center for Child Abuse and Neglect defines **sexual abuse** as contacts or interactions between a child and an adult when the child is being used for sexual stimulation of the perpetrator or other person. Sexual abuse also may be committed by someone younger than 18 years of age if that person is in a position of power or control over the other.[2]

Several terms are frequently used when sexual abuse is discussed. From a legal viewpoint, sexual contacts between a child and another person in a caretaking position, such as a parent, babysitter, or teacher, is classified as sexual abuse. Sexual contacts made by someone who is not functioning in a caretaker role with the child is classified as **sexual assault**. Incest includes fondling of breasts, genitalia, intercourse (vaginal or anal), oral–genital contact, exhibitionism, and voyeurism. Regardless of the relationship of the perpetrator to the child, the outcome of the abuse is devastating. Episodes of sexual abuse that involve a person the child trusts seem to be the most damaging. Incest often goes unreported because the person committing the act uses intimidation by means of threats, appealing to the child's desire to be loved and to please, convincing the child of the importance of keeping the act secret.

When a child is sexually assaulted by a stranger, the child's caregivers usually become aware of the incident, promptly report it, and take the child for a physical examination. However, in the case of incest, the child rarely tells another person what is happening. The child may exhibit physical complaints, such as various aches and pains; gastrointestinal upsets; changes in bowel and bladder habits, including enuresis; nightmares; and acts of aggression or hostility. Some of these complaints or behaviors may be the presenting problem when the child is seen in a health care facility.

Nursing Process in the Care of an Abused Child

ASSESSMENT

When assessing the child who may have been abused or neglected, the nurse must be thorough and complete in observation and documentation. The child should have a complete physical assessment, and all bruises, blemishes, lacerations, areas of redness and irritation, and marks of any kind on the child's body must be carefully described and accurately documented. The nurse may need to request that photographs be taken, if appropriate. The nurse must be observant of the interaction between the child and the caregiver and carefully document what is observed in nonjudgmental terms. The child's body language may be revealing, and the nurse must be alert to record significant information. For example, if the child shrinks away from contact by the caregiver or the nurse or if, on the other hand, the child is especially clinging to the caregiver, the nurse should be alert for other signs of inappropriate behavior. These assessments vary with the age of the child. Perhaps the most difficult part for the nurse may be to maintain a nonjudgmental attitude throughout the assessment and examination (Table 19-1). The nurse should be calm and reassuring with the child, letting the child lead the way, when possible.

Table 19-1. Nursing Assessments: Signs of Abuse in Children

Physical Signs	*Behavioral Signs*
Physical Abuse	
Bruises and welts: may be on multiple body surfaces or soft tissue; may form regular pattern (e.g., belt buckle)	Less compliant than average
	Signs of negativism, unhappiness
Burns: cigar or cigarette, immersion (stocking/glovelike on extremities or doughnut-shaped on buttocks or genitals), or patterned as an electrical appliance (e.g., iron)	Anger, isolation
	Destructive
	Abusive toward others
	Difficulty developing relationships
Fractures: single or multiple; may be in various stages of healing	Either excessive or absent separation anxiety
Lacerations or abrasions: rope burns; tears in and around the mouth, eyes, ears, or genitalia	Inappropriate caretaking concern for parent
	Constantly in search of attention, favors, food, etc.
Abdominal injuries: ruptured or injured internal organs	Various developmental delays (cognitive, language, motor)
Central nervous system injuries: subdural hematoma, retinal or subarachnoid hemorrhage	
Physical Neglect	
Malnutrition	
Repeated episodes of pica	Lack of appropriate adult supervision
Constant fatigue or listlessness	Repeated ingestions of harmful substances
Poor hygiene	Poor school attendance
Inadequate clothing for circumstances	Exploitation (forced to beg or steal; excessive household work)
Inadequate medical or dental care	Role reversal with parent
	Drug or alcohol use

(continued)

Table 19-1. Nursing Assessments: Signs of Abuse in Children (*Continued*)

Physical Signs	Behavioral Signs
Sexual Abuse	
Difficulty walking or sitting	Direct or indirect disclosure to relative, friend, or teacher
Thickening and/or hyperpigmentation of labial skin	Withdrawal with excessive dependency
Vaginal opening measures >4 mm horizontally in preadolescence	Poor peer relationships
Torn, stained, or bloody underclothing	Poor self-esteem
Bruises or bleeding of genitalia or perianal area	Frightened or phobic of adults
Lax rectal tone	Sudden decline in academic performance
Vaginal discharge	Pseudomature personality development
Recurrent urinary tract infections	Suicide attempts
Nonspecific vaginitis	Regressive behavior
Venereal disease	Enuresis or encopresis
Sperm or acid phosphatase on body or clothes	Excessive masturbation
Pregnancy	Highly sexualized play
	Sexual promiscuity
Emotional Abuse	
Delays in physical development	Distinct emotional symptoms and/or functional limitations
Failure to thrive	Deteriorating conduct
	Increased anxiety
	Apathy or depression
	Developmental lags

(From Jackson DB, Saunders RB. Child Health Nursing. Philadelphia: JB Lippincott, 1993.)
Data from Council on Scientific Affairs. AMA diagnostic and treatment guidelines concerning child abuse and neglect. JAMA 254(6):796–800, 1985.

NURSING DIAGNOSES

The nursing diagnoses vary with the type of abuse or neglect that the child may have experienced. Appropriate nursing diagnoses for a child with fractures, for example, include care of the child before and after the fracture has been set and casted. A child with burns has a variety of nursing diagnoses that correspond to the care for the burns; a child who is nutritionally deprived needs diagnoses that address nutritional needs. Several nursing diagnoses that may be of use include the following:

- Anxiety of child related to history of abuse and fear of abuse from others
- Ineffective individual coping by nonabusive parent related to fear of violence from abusing partner or feelings of powerlessness
- Ineffective family coping: disabling related to unknown cause
- Ineffective family coping: disabling related to unrealistic expectations of child by parent

PLANNING AND IMPLEMENTATION

When planning the care of the abused child, the nurse includes diagnoses that are suitable to the injuries that the child has experienced. In addition, the following nursing care is appropriate.

Relieving the Child's Anxiety. Observe the child for behavior that indicates anxiety, such as withdrawal, ducking or shying away from the nurse or caregivers, guarding, and avoidance of eye contact. One nurse should be assigned to take care of the child so that the child has a consistent person to relate to. Physical contact of hugging, rocking, and caressing should be given only if the child accepts it. Nursing actions that seem to comfort the child should be identified and used consistently. The nurse must be calm, reassuring, and kind, and he or she should provide a safe atmosphere in which the child has an opportunity to express feelings and fears. Play can be used to help the child express some of these emotions. The nurse should be careful not to do anything that might alarm or upset the child. Psychological support is provided through social services or an abuse team.

Supporting the Nonabusive Caregiver. One caregiver in the family may be the abuser, and the other is not. The nonabusive caregiver is a victim as well as the child. The nurse can provide the nonabusive caregiver an opportunity to express fears and anxieties. The nonabusive caregiver may feel powerless in the situation. The nurse can help the passive caregiver to seek help in solving the dilemma of whether to continue the relationship or to leave it. These are not easy decisions to make, and the nurse must use complex problem-solving skills to successfully guide the caregiver and conserve that person's self-esteem. The nurse must remember that confidentiality is absolutely essential when discussing such problems.

Observing Interaction Between the Caregiver and Child. While caring for the abused child, the nurse has an opportunity to observe how the caregiver relates to the child when the caregiver is present and how the child reacts to the caregiver. The nurse must be careful to give the caregiver every courtesy that is extended to all caregivers. The nurse should comment positively when the caregiver does something well in caring for the child. The caregiver may need an opportunity to talk with the nurse privately, during which time the nurse may be able to gain the caregiver's confidence.

Promoting Parenting Skills. Often, abuse occurs when a child's caregiver is not familiar with normal growth and development and the behaviors that are common to a particular stage of development. The nurse can design a teaching plan to help the caregiver develop realistic expectations. Including the caregiver in caring for the child is a positive way to help accomplish this goal. The nurse can teach the caregiver expected responses from the child and increase the caregiver's understanding of normal development. The caregiver should be encouraged and praised for positive behaviors. Pointing out specific behaviors of the child and explaining them to the caregiver also can be helpful. The nurse can explore the reasons for the caregiver's absence when the caregiver is not visiting regularly. Discuss with the caregiver specific behaviors of the child that are upsetting to the caregiver and help the caregiver understand that these are common behaviors of the child's age group.

The caregiver may be facing temporary or permanent placement of the child in another home. The caregiver and the child both need to be assisted in accepting this change. The assistance of social services and a child life specialist is beneficial in these situations. The nurse can function as a member of the team to aid in the transition. The foster parents may need support from the nursing

staff to help ease the transition of the child to the new home. Emotions and feelings that a caregiver has had over a long period cannot be easily "switched off." Abused children need to be followed carefully after discharge from the health care facility to ensure that the children's well-being is protected.

EVALUATION

- The child's play is relaxed; the child's facial expressions and posture are relaxed; the child displays no withdrawal or guarding during contacts with the nursing staff
- The nonabusive caregiver expresses fears and concerns and makes plans to resolve problems
- An abusive caregiver is cooperative when present
- Caregivers are involved in child's care, are able to verbalize recognition of age-appropriate behavior, can discuss ways to handle the child's irritating behavior, and are involved in counseling or other discharge plans

The Runaway Child

In the United States, as many as 750,000 to 2 million adolescents run away from home each year. A child can be considered a runaway after being absent from home overnight or longer without permission from a family caregiver. Most children who run away from home are between 10 and 17 years of age, although runaways are commonly thought of as teenagers.

A child may run away from home in response to circumstances that he or she views as too difficult to tolerate. Circumstances of physical abuse, incest, alcohol or drug abuse, divorce, stepfamilies, pregnancy, school failure, and truancy may contribute to the child's desire to escape. However, some adolescents are not runaways but rather "throwaways" who have been forced to leave home and are not wanted back by the adults in the home. Frequently, the throwaways have been forced out of the home because their behavior is unacceptable to family caregivers or because of other family stresses such as divorce, remarriage, and job loss.

Runaway (or throwaway) adolescents frequently turn to stealing, drug dealing, and prostitution to provide money for alcohol, drugs, food, and possibly, shelter. Many of these adolescents may live on the streets because they are not able to pay for shelter and avoid going to public shelter for fear of being found by police. They may become victims of pimps or drug dealers who use and manipulate the adolescents for their own gain. There are numerous programs to help runaways, especially in urban areas. A 24-hour National Runaway Hot Line (1-800-231-6946) is available to give runaways information and referral to help the runaway find a safe place to stay as well as resources available to the runaway, counseling, shelter, medical clinics for health care, legal aid when needed, message relay to the family if the runaway chooses, and transportation home, if desired. They are not forced to go home but may be encouraged to let their family know that they are all right. Other free hot line numbers are also available.

Symptoms of a sexually transmitted disease, pregnancy, acquired immunodeficiency syndrome, or drug overdose are the usual reasons that runaway children may be seen at a health care facility. When caring for such a child, the nurse should be careful to be nonjudgmental. Any indication of being disturbed or disgusted by the adolescent's lifestyle may end any possible cooperation and cause the adolescent to avoid giving any additional information. The nurse must try to build a trusting relationship with the child. The nurse must remember that the runaway viewed his or her problems so great that they could not be resolved in any other way than by trying to escape them. Counseling will be necessary to attempt to begin to resolve the problems.

Health teaching for the runaway must be geared to a level that the child can understand and that is practical for the way that the runaway lives. Without prying excessively, the nurse can try to find out the runaway's living circumstances and adjust the teaching plans to these circumstances. The nurse must remember that the child's problems did not come about in a short time, and they will not be resolved quickly. Caring for a runaway can be frustrating, challenging, and sometimes rewarding for the health care staff.

The Latchkey Child

As a result of the increased number of families with both caregivers working and the increase in single-parent families in which the parent must work, many children need after-school care and supervision, but adequate or appropriate child care is not readily available. A **latchkey child** is one who has to come home to an empty house after school each day because the family caregivers are at work. The term latchkey child was coined because these children frequently wear the house key around their neck. These children usually have to spend several hours alone before an adult comes home from work (Figure 19-3). The number of latchkey children may be as high as 10 million in the United States.

Latchkey children often have fears about being at home alone. When there is more than one child and the older child has to be responsible for the younger one, conflicts can arise. The older child may have to assume responsibility that is beyond the normal expectations for the child's age. This can be a difficult situation for the

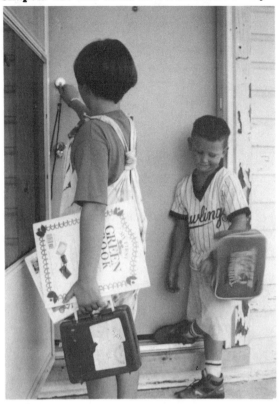

Figure 19-3. A 10-year-old girl and her 6-year-old brother come home to an empty house to await the arrival of their mother.

caregivers and the children. Extra attention must be given to outline with the children activities permitted and rules for safety. The caregiver should have a plan in place to help the older child solve any problem that may arise that involves both children. The older child should not have to feel that the complete responsibility is his or hers alone, but rather it is a shared responsibility with the caregiver. Some schools have after-school latchkey programs that provide safe activities for children. In addition, some communities have programs in which an adult telephones the child regularly every day after school or there is a telephone hot line that the child can call (see Parent Teaching: Tips for Latchkey Children).

Despite concerns that latchkey children are more likely to become involved with smoking, stealing, or taking drugs, researchers have not found sufficient data to support this fear. Children who are given responsibility of this kind and who are recognized for their dependability usually live up to the expectations of the adults in their social environment.

Nurses must recognize the need for after-school services for these children and take an active role in the community to plan and support such services. Nurses should maintain a list of the facilities available to support families with latchkey children. The nurse can give care-

Parent Teaching

Tips for Latchkey Children

1. Teach child to keep key hidden and not show it to anyone.
2. Plan with the child the routine to follow when arriving home; plan something special each day.
3. Plan a telephone contact on child's arrival at home—either have the child call you or you call the child.
4. Always let the child know if you are going to be delayed.
5. Review safety rules with the child. Post them on the refrigerator for reminder.
6. Use a refrigerator chart to spell out daily responsibilities, and have child check them off as they are completed.
7. Let the child know how much you appreciate his or her responsible behavior.
8. Have a trusted neighbor for backup if the child needs help; be sure the child knows the telephone number and that it is also posted by the phone.
9. Post telephone emergency numbers the child can use; practice with the child when to use them.
10. Teach the child to tell any telephone caller that caregiver is busy but never to say that caregiver is not home.
11. Teach the child to not open door to anyone.
12. Be specific about activities that are allowed and those that are not allowed.
13. Carefully survey your home for any hazards or other dangerous temptations (ie, guns, motorcycle, all-terrain vehicle, swimming pool). Eliminate them, if possible, or discuss with the child so that rules about them are clear.
14. Investigate to see if your community has a telephone friend program available for latchkey children.
15. A pet can relieve loneliness, but be certain that you give the child clear guidelines about care of the pet during your absence.

givers guidance in planning for children's after-school activities and offer support to the caregivers in their attempts to provide for their children.

Divorce and the Child

Divorce has increased to the point where one in two marriages ends in divorce. Approximately 50% of the children experience the separation or divorce of their parents before they complete high school. Some children may experience more than one divorce because 40% of those who remarry divorce for the second time.[3] Divorce can be traumatic for children but may be better than the constant tension and turmoil that they have lived through in their home.

Children often feel responsible for the breakup and believe that it would not have occurred if they had just done the right thing or been "good." On the other hand, children may blame one of the parents for deciding to end the marriage and thus cause the children grief and unhappiness. Children frequently feel unloved and, in a sense, feel that they too are being divorced. Through counseling, children can be helped to acknowledge and understand the anger they feel and the need they have to place blame on one or the other of the parents. This is a process that may take a considerable amount of time to resolve. Both parents should make every effort to eliminate the child's feeling of guilt and avoid using the child as a spy or go-between with the estranged spouse. Parents must avoid trying to buy the affection of the children. This is especially true for the noncustodial parent who must not shower the children with special gifts, trips, and privileges when the children are visiting.

Children should be encouraged to ask questions about the separation and divorce. A child who does not ask questions may be afraid to ask for fear of retaliation by one of the parents. Children should be discouraged from thinking that they might be able to do something that would get the parents back together again. They must be helped to recognize the finality of the divorce. Plans for the children should be made (eg, whom will the children live with, where will they live, and where will the children go to school) and shared with the children as soon as possible. This can give the children a sense of security in their chaotic personal world. Each child's confidence and self-esteem must be strengthened through careful handling of the transition.

When a child of a divorce is hospitalized, the nurse must be certain to have clear documentation concerning who is the custodial parent as well as who may visit or otherwise contact the child. The custodial parent's instructions and wishes should be honored.

The nurse may encourage the child to express feelings of fear and guilt. The nurse also can help the child understand that other children have divorced parents. The school nurse may function as an advocate for a counseling program in the school setting that brings together children of divorces so that they can voice their fears and concerns and begin to work through them with the help of an objective counselor in a protected environment. One of the most important aspects of such groups is the reassurance the children get that they are not alone in this crisis in their lives.

When the custodial parent begins to date and plans to remarry, the child may again have strong emotions that must be worked through. If the remarriage brings together a blended family of children from the previous marriages of both adults, the children may need extra support in accepting the new stepparent and stepsiblings. The adults who seek preventive counseling when planning to form a stepfamily have greater success than those who seek help only after problems are overwhelming. Children react in a variety of ways to the impending new marriage for a

parent, depending in part on each child's age. The new marriage may introduce additional problems of a new home, new neighborhood, and new school that can cause anxiety for any child. Although children should not be permitted to veto the parent's choice of a new partner, every effort should be made to help them adjust to this new family member and view the change in a nonthreatening way.

The Homeless Family

A growing number of families are among the homeless population in the United States. The causes of this homelessness are attributed to job loss, loss of housing, drug addiction of adult caregivers, insufficient income, domestic turmoil, and separation or divorce. Single mothers with children make up an increasing number of these families. Many of these homeless single mothers and their families have multiple problems. In one study, homeless mothers in Los Angeles reported more than twice as many instances of abuse, drug use, and mental health problems as did those who were classified as housed poor.[4] In urban areas, most homeless families are from minority groups, but in nonurban areas, the homeless families are primarily white.[5] Many of these family units may have lived with relatives for a time before actually being reduced to living in a car, an empty building, a welfare hotel, or perhaps, a cardboard box. These families sometimes seek temporary housing in a shelter for the homeless. Frequently, they move from one living situation to another, living in a shelter for the time allowed, moving elsewhere, only to return after a while to repeat the cycle (Figure 19-4).

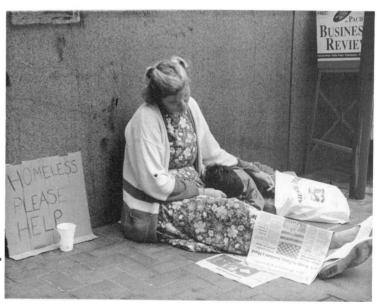

Figure 19-4. The homeless family has become a growing concern across the United States. (Photo by Kathy Sloane.)

Homelessness creates additional stresses for the family. Many of the homeless families have young children but have problems gaining entry into health care even though these children are at high risk for developing an acute or chronic condition. Health care for these families commonly occurs as crisis intervention instead of the more effective preventive intervention. Pregnant homeless women receive little, if any, prenatal care, suffer from poor nutrition, and give birth to low-birth-weight infants with their attendant problems. Most of the children of homeless families do not have adequate immunizations. Homeless children suffer from chronic illnesses at twice the rate of the general population.[5] These chronic conditions include anemia, heart disease, peripheral vascular disease, and neurologic disorders. Many homeless children have developmental delays, perform poorly when they attend school, and suffer from anxiety and depression in addition to having behavioral problems.

Many shelters available to the homeless are overcrowded, lack privacy (including bathroom facilities that are used by many people), and have no personal bedding, no cribs for infants, or no facilities for cooking or refrigerating food. Because of limits to the length of stay, many families must move from one shelter to another. This adds to the problems these families face, contributing to a lack of consistency in services and programs available to them.

Nurses can set the tone of the interaction between the homeless family and the health care facility. It is important to establish an environment in which the caregiver feels respected and comfortable. Focusing initially on the positive factors in the caregiver's relationship with the children alleviates some of the caregiver's guilt and fear of being criticized. The nurse must make every effort to offer down-to-earth suggestions and help the family in the most practical manner.

On admission of the child to the health care facility, the nurse needs to perform a complete admission assessment. During this time the nurse also can ask the caregiver questions about living arrangements that will help in the care and planning for the child. During this interview, the nurse may become aware of problems of other family members that need attention. When giving assistance and guidance, the nurse must be careful to supplement the family's functioning, not to take it over. For instance, the nurse should tell the family how to go about getting a particular benefit and should be certain that they have complete and accurate information but must not do it for them. These families need to feel self-reliant and in control and need realistic solutions to their problems.

Outreach programs have been established in many major cities. These programs conduct screening, treat acute illnesses, and help families contact local health care services when they are needed. The nurse should provide information to the family about any assistance that is available.

Summary

Job loss, financial crisis, illness, injury, loss of a home, and death are among the stresses that cause a family to respond in a dysfunctional way. Many families handle this type of stress and manage to function adequately, perhaps because of a strong support system, but a growing number of families are unable to do so. As a result, physical, emotional, and sexual child abuse may occur, often complicated by the use of drugs and alcohol. Children become victims of the adult's frustration and anger. The nurse must serve as an advocate for children in abusing homes and is required to report any suspected maltreatment of a child. Older children try to escape home situations that they view as unacceptable by running away. Unfortunately, runaways find that life in the "outside world" can be even more traumatic than life with their families.

Latchkey children are on their own every afternoon after school until an adult comes home to supervise them. Many latchkey children are able to handle this responsibility, but the family caregivers need to plan for them to provide appropriate activities and security.

Children become torn in the process of their parents' divorce and often are used as pawns in the parents' power struggles. Children actually may have an improved home life after the divorce, but the emotional toll can still be enormous for involved children.

The number of homeless families is increasing each year. These families move from place to place and suffer from poor nutrition, inadequate shelter, and minimal health care. As a result, children in these families are developmentally and physically deprived. Many infants born to homeless women begin their lives as low-birth-weight infants and have multiple problems as a result. Shelter programs do not fulfill the needs of these families. When caring for children from dysfunctional families, the nurse needs to be sensitive to the underlying needs of the children and assist in providing guidance for the whole family.

Review Questions

1. Your neighbor, 17-year-old Kari, has an active 18-month-old toddler named Jason. You overhear Kari screaming at him and saying, "I'm going to beat you if you don't listen to me." What is your reaction? How can you diplomatically help Kari?
2. You are on duty in the emergency department when an infant is admitted with injuries that cause you to suspect that the infant was abused. The mother says her boyfriend was babysitting for her. How do you feel about this? What observations will you make when assessing the infant? How will you approach the mother?

3. What observations will you be certain to make about the infant's bruises?

4. What type of burns indicate a child may have been abused?

5. You have an opportunity to talk to a youth group about the hazards of becoming a runaway. What are some of the points you will make?

6. You have an 8-year-old child who must stay alone every day until you get home from work. How will you prepare her? What plans will you make?

7. Seven-year-old Mike's parents are divorcing. What guidance can you give Mike's mother to help him make the adjustment?

8. How can a school counseling program help children of divorce?

9. How does homelessness affect the health of children?

References

1. Wissow LS. Child maltreatment. In Oski FA (ed): Principle and Practices of Pediatrics. Philadelphia: JB Lippincott, 1990.
2. Paradise JE. The medical evaluation of the sexually abused child. Pediatr Clin North Am 37(4):839–862, 1990.
3. Green M. Reaching out to the children of divorce. Contemp Pediatr 5(2):22–42, 1988.
4. Wood D, Valdez RB, Hayashi T, et al. Homeless and housed families in Los Angeles: A study comparing demographic, economic, and family function characteristics. Am J Public Health 80(9):104, 1990.

5. Weinreb LF, Bassuk EL. Health care of homeless families: A growing challenge for family medicine. J Fam Pract 31(1): 74–80, 1990.

Bibliography

Bassuk E, Rosenberg L. Psychosocial characteristics of homeless children and children with homes. Pediatrics 85(3): 257–261, 1990.

Castiglia PT, Harbin RE. Child Health Care: Process and Practice. Philadelphia: JB Lippincott, 1992.

D'Avanzo CE. Incest: Break the silence, break the cycle. RN 53(10):34–36, 1990.

Davidhizar R, Frank B. Understanding the physical and psychosocial stressors of the child who is homeless. Pediatr Nurs 18(6):559–562, 1992.

Jackson DB, Saunders RB. Child Health Nursing. Philadelphia: JB Lippincott, 1993.

Jurgrau A. How to spot child abuse. RN 53(10):26–33, 1990.

Malloy C. Children and poverty: America's future at risk. Pediatr Nurs 18(6):553–557, 1992.

Melnyk BM. Changes in parent–child relationships following divorce. Pediatr Nurs 17(4):337–341, 1991.

Pillitteri A. Maternal and Child Health Nursing. Philadelphia: JB Lippincott, 1992.

Weitzman M, Adair R. Divorce and children. Pediatr Clin North Am 35(6):1313–1323, 1988.

Whaley LF, Wong DL. Nursing Care of Infants and Children, 4th ed. St. Louis: Mosby-Year Book, 1991.

A Child Faces Chronic or Terminal Illness

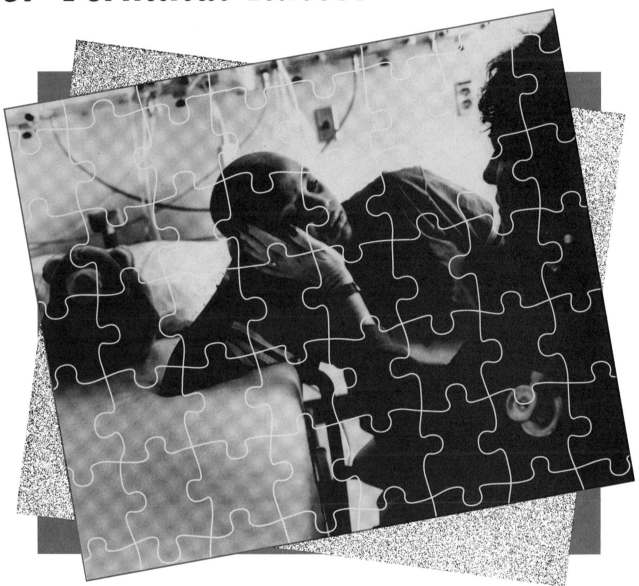

Unit V

The Child with a Chronic Health Problem

Chapter 20

Student Objectives

Upon completion of this chapter, the student will be able to:

1. Define the key terms.
2. Identify 10 conditions that cause chronic illness.
3. Identify 10 concerns that are common to many families of a child with a chronic illness.
4. Describe economic pressures that can overwhelm families of chronically ill children.
5. Discuss the importance of respite care.
6. Discuss the effect a developmental stage may have on the child's needs.
7. Identify positive and negative responses that well siblings may manifest in response to an ill sibling.
8. Describe how the nurse can assist the family to adjust to the child's condition.
9. Identify several ways the nurse may encourage self-care by the child.
10. Discuss general guidelines for preparing the family for home care of the child.

Marks MG: BROADRIBB'S INTRODUCTORY PEDIATRIC NURSING, 4th ed. © 1994 J.B. Lippincott Company.

Key Terms

chronic illness   rejection denial

gradual acceptance   respite care

overprotection   stigma

*C*hronic illness is a leading health problem in the United States. The numbers are growing as more infants and children survive prematurity, difficult births, congenital anomalies that once were fatal, previously fatal illnesses, and accidents. Most children experience only brief, acute episodes of illness; however, a significant number are affected with chronic health problems. Diseases that cause chronic illness include congenital heart disease, cystic fibrosis, juvenile arthritis, asthma, hemophilia, muscular dystrophy, leukemia and other malignancies, spina bifida, and immunodeficiency syndromes. When a family member has a chronic illness, the entire family is affected in many ways. The chronic illness of a child may affect the child's physical, psychosocial, and cognitive development. Because nurses are usually involved from the early stages of diagnosis, and because the child and family have ongoing, long-term needs, the nurse can play a vital role in helping the family adjust and adapt to the condition.

Common Problems in Chronic Illness

Chronic illness is defined as a condition that interferes with daily functioning for more than 3 months in a year, causes hospitalization of more than 1 month in a year, or (at time of diagnosis) is likely to do either of these.[1]

Specific chronic health problems of children have been discussed in earlier chapters. Each requires individualized management based on the disease process and the ability of the patient and family to understand and comply with the treatment regimen. All chronic health problems, however, create some common difficulties for patients and families, and these are the focus of this chapter. Some of these concerns are the following:

- Financial concerns—paying for treatment; living expenses at a distant hospital; caregiver's loss of job because of lost time
- Administration of prescribed treatments and medications at home
- Disruption of family life—vacations, family goals, two-parent careers
- Concerns about educational opportunities for child
- Possible social isolation due to child's condition
- Changing course of disease causes need for family adjustments
- Reaction of well siblings
- Stress among family caregivers
- Guilt and acceptance of chronic condition
- Care of the child when family caregivers are no longer able to provide care

Effects of Chronic Illness on the Family

The diagnosis of a chronic health problem causes a crisis in the family, whether it happens during the first few hours or days of the child's life or much later. How a family copes with the illness varies greatly from one family to another. Although the diagnoses of the children vary from family to family, the families have many of the same problems.

Parents and Chronic Illness

When family caregivers first learn of the child's diagnosis, their first reaction may be shock, disbelief, and denial. These reactions may last for a varied amount of time, from days to months. The initial response may be one of mourning for the "perfect" child that they lost, combined with guilt, blame, and rationalization. The caregivers may react by seeking advice from other professionals and actually may go "shopping" for another physician. They may refuse to accept the diagnosis or refuse to talk about it, or they may delay in seeking or agreeing to treatment. Gradually, they adjust to the diagnosis. However, they frequently enter a period of chronic sorrow, in which they adapt to the child's state of chronic illness but do not necessarily accept it. They often waver between the stages and experience highs and lows of emotions as they work through caring for the child and meeting the challenges of daily life. Families who have a strong support system usually are better able to meet these challenges.

Economic pressures can become overwhelming to the families of chronically ill children. If the family does not have adequate health insurance, the costs of treatment may be enormous. Away-from-home living costs may become a problem if the child has to be taken to a distant hospital for further diagnosis or treatment. To keep health care benefits, a family caregiver may feel tied to a job, which creates additional stress. The time required to take a child for health care appointments can be excessive and may cause an additional threat to job security because of the time lost from the job.

Families need to make many adjustments to cope with the care of the chronically ill child. The family caregivers may have to learn to perform treatments and give medications to their child. Family life is often disrupted. Vacations may be nonexistent, and the family may be limited in how they can spend their leisure time. Families may have difficulty finding adequate babysitters and have little opportunity for a break in their routine. In some situations, the family may be isolated from their customary social activities because of the responsibilities of caring for their child. **Respite care** (care of the ill child so that the family caregivers can have a period of rest and refreshment) is often desperately needed but is not readily available in many communities. Two-career families often have to forgo the second income so that one caregiver can stay home with the child.

As the child grows, concerns about education may become foremost among the family caregivers' worries. These concerns include the availability of appropriate education, early learning opportunities, physical accessibility of the facilities, acceptance of the child by school personnel and classmates, mainstreaming versus segregated classes, availability and quality of homebound teaching, and general flexibility of the school's teaching and administrative personnel. Few schools are prepared to easily accommodate treatments at school that may otherwise require that the child leave school during the school day. Family caregivers frequently have to become the child's advocate to preserve as much normalcy as possible in the child's educational experience.

As the child's condition changes, the family must make additional changes. All of these stresses may create strain on the marriage. Although the marriage may suffer much stress, the divorce rate does not seem to be affected by the presence of a chronically ill child in the family.[2] However, single caregivers have significant needs to which health care personnel must be especially sensitive.

The Child and Chronic Illness

The child with a chronic illness may face many problems that interfere with normal growth and development. These problems vary with the child's diagnosis and condition. The child's attitude toward the condition is a critical element in the long-term management and in the family's adjustment. For instance, the child who must be immobilized during school age while in the stage of industry versus inferiority is unable to complete tasks of industry, such as helping with household chores or working on special projects with siblings or peers.

The child's response to the chronic condition is influenced by the response of family caregivers (Figure 20-1). Several typical responses have been identified: **overprotection**, **rejection**, **denial**, and **gradual acceptance**. Overprotective caregivers try to protect the child at all costs, preventing the child from achieving new skills by hovering, avoiding the use of discipline, and using every means to prevent the child from experiencing any frustration. Rejecting caregivers distance themselves emotionally from the child and, although they provide physical care, they tend to continuously scold and correct the child. Caregivers in denial behave as though the condition does not exist, encouraging the child to overcompensate for any disabilities. The caregivers who respond with gradual acceptance take a common-sense approach to the child's condition, helping the child to set realistic goals for self-care and independence, and encouraging the child to achieve social and physical skills that are within the child's capability.

Children often perceive any illness as punishment for a bad thought or action. The child's perception of chronic illness is subject to the same "magical thinking," depending on the child's developmental stage at the time of diagnosis. This perception is also influenced by attitudes of parents and peers and by whether or not the dysfunctional body part is visible or invisible. Problems such as asthma, allergies, and epilepsy are difficult for children to understand because "what's wrong" is inside, not outside. The child's family, peers, and school personnel make up the support system than can have an impact on the child's adaptation. Sometimes the efforts necessary to meet the child's physical needs are so great that finding time and energy to meet the child's emotional needs can be difficult for members of the support team. The older child with a chronic illness also has developing sexual needs that should not be ignored but must be acknowledged and provided for. Additional stresses continue to occur as the disease progresses. For instance, Hodgkin's disease can be successfully treated for a time with chemotherapy and radiotherapy, but that means adding the side effects of treatment (steroid-induced acne, edema, and alopecia) to the disease manifestations of night sweats, chronic fatigue, pruritus, and gastrointestinal bleeding. Also, consider the boy with Duchenne's muscu-

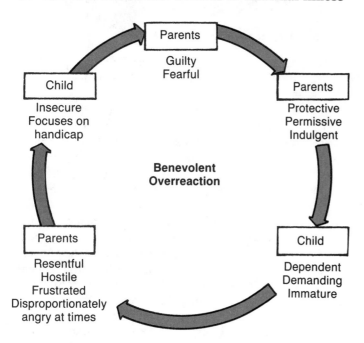

Figure 20-1. Common cyclical response between parents and handicapped child. (Boone DR, Hartman BH. The benevolent over-reaction. Clin Pediatr 11, 5: 268–271, 1972.)

lar dystrophy who gradually weakens so that in adolescence he is wheelchair bound when his peers are actively involved in sports and exploring sexual relationships. These stresses can add up to more than one young person can cope with for long.

Siblings and Chronic Illness

Some degree of sibling rivalry can be found in most families with healthy children, so it is not surprising that a child with a chronic health problem can seriously disrupt the lives of brothers and sisters. By necessity, much of the family caregivers' time, attention, and money is directed toward management of the ill child's problem. This can cause anger, resentment, and jealousy in the well siblings. The caregivers' failure to set limits for the ill child's behavior while maintaining discipline for the healthy siblings can cause further resentment. Some family caregivers unknowingly create feelings of guilt in the healthy children by overemphasizing the ill child's needs.

Siblings may feel **stigma** (embarrassment or shame) because of a brother or sister with a chronic illness, especially if the ill child has a physical disfigurement or apparent cognitive deficit. Siblings may choose not to tell others about the ill child or they may be selective in who they tell, choosing only those persons who they believe they can trust. The older siblings are more likely to tell others than younger ones, perhaps because the older child tends to understand more about the illness and its effect. Both positive and negative influences can be found in the behaviors of well siblings. Some siblings react with anger, hostility, jealousy, increased competition for attention, social withdrawal, and poor school performance. On the other hand, many siblings demonstrate positive be-

haviors, such as caring and concern for the ill sibling, cooperating with family caregivers in helping with the care of the ill child, protecting the ill child from negative reaction of others, and including the ill child in activities with peers. How well siblings react to a chronically ill sibling may ultimately depend on how the family copes with stress and how its members feel about one another. Families that seem to adapt most successfully to the presence of a child with chronic illness are those in which the caregivers find time for special activities with the healthy children, explain the ill child's condition as simply as possible, involve the healthy siblings in the care of the ill child according to their developmental ability, and set behavioral limits for all children in the family. This is a delicate balance that is challenging and takes great effort and caring for a family to sustain but well worth the end results.

Nursing Process in Caring for a Child with a Chronic Illness

ASSESSMENT

The assessment of the family and the child with a disability or chronic illness is an ongoing process that is reviewed and updated with each visit the child makes to the health care facility. The child should be included in the assessment interview if old enough and able to participate. The child may have had many visits and treatments in the past that have left a negative memory, so the nurse must approach the child in a low-key, kind, gentle manner to gain cooperation. Unless the child is newly diagnosed, the family caregivers may have a good understanding of the condition. The nurse needs to assess this knowledge so that plans can be included to supplement it.

During the assessment interview, the nurse must determine how the family is coping with the child's condition and assess the family's strengths, weaknesses, and their acceptance of the diagnosis. Needs may change as the child's condition changes, and the nurse must identify these changing needs to include them in planning care. Needs that change with the child's growth and development also must be considered.

The type of illness determines the physical assessment that is appropriate. Throughout the physical assessment, the nurse must make every effort to gain the child's cooperation and should explain what is being done in terms that the child can understand. Praising the child for cooperating throughout the assessment is an important method to gain the child's (and the family caregivers') good will.

NURSING DIAGNOSES

The nursing diagnoses vary depending on the illness or disability that the child has, but certain developmental diagnoses are appropriate regardless of the medical diagnosis. Some of those diagnoses are included here.

- Altered family processes related to adjustment requirements for the child with chronic illness or disability
- Altered growth and development related to impaired ability to achieve developmental tasks or family caregivers' reactions to the child's condition
- Anxiety related to procedures, tests, or hospitalization
- Self-care deficit related to limitations of illness or disability
- Grieving of family caregiver related to anticipated losses secondary to condition
- High risk for social isolation of the child or family related to the child's condition
- Family caregivers health-seeking behaviors related to home care of a child with chronic illness

PLANNING AND IMPLEMENTATION

Assisting Family in Adjusting to Child's Condition. The family's adjustment to the child's condition is assessed during the assessment interview. The adjustment may depend on how recently the child has been diagnosed. After determining the family's needs, the nurse can provide opportunity for the family members to express feelings and anxieties. The nurse can help family caregivers explore feelings of guilt or blame about the child's condition. The caregivers may express doubts about their ability to cope with the child's future, and the nurse may explore these concerns with them, helping them to take a realistic look at their resources and giving them positive suggestions for ways to cope. The nurse

serves as a role model when caring for the child, expressing a positive attitude toward the child and the child's illness or disability. The nurse can explore with the family to determine the resources and support systems available to them. These support systems include immediate family members, extended family, friends, community services, and health care providers. Needs of the siblings of the ill child are important to discuss at this time. The family caregivers can be encouraged to discuss needs of the well siblings and their adjustment to the ill child's condition. The nurse can give the family guidance in fulfilling the needs of the well siblings and in helping them feel comfortable with the ill child's problems and needs. The nurse can help the family set reasonable expectations for all of their children.

Encouraging Optimal Growth and Development. The family caregivers may respond to the child's condition with overprotectiveness, preventing the child from exhibiting growth and development appropriate for his or her age and disability. The nurse can help the caregivers recognize the child's potential and assist in setting realistic growth and development goals for the child. Consistent care by the same staff helps provide a sense of routine in which the child can be encouraged to have some control and perform age-appropriate tasks within the limitations of the disability. Age-appropriate limits can be set and appropriate discipline established. This must be accomplished gradually, with a kind and caring attitude. The child can be permitted choices within the limits of treatments and other aspects of required care. Encouraging the child to dress when appropriate can help reduce some of the feeling of being an "invalid." The child can learn about the condition and meet other children with the same or a similar condition to help dispel feelings of being the only person with such a condition. An older child or adolescent benefits from social interaction with peers with or without disabilities (Figure 20-2). Family caregivers can be encouraged to assist the adolescent in joining in age-appropriate activities. The adolescent also may need some help in dressing or using makeup to maximize appearance and minimize a physical disability.

Reducing Anxiety About Procedures and Treatments. Periodically, perhaps over a long period, the child may need to be hospitalized and have procedures, tests, and treatments performed. Many of the procedures may be painful, or at least uncomfortable. The child needs to have tests, treatments, and procedures explained ahead of time and be encouraged to ask questions. The nurse can acknowledge that a particular procedure is painful and can help the child plan ways to handle the pain. Family caregivers should also prepare the child for hospitalization ahead of time whenever possible.

Promoting Self-Care. To encourage the child to assist in self-care, the nurse can devise aids to ease tasks. When appropriate, play and toys can be integrated into

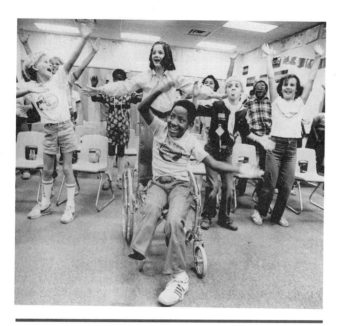

Figure 20-2. Children with disabilities engaged in an adapted sports activity. (From Castiglia PT, Harbin RE. Child Health Care. Philadelphia: JB Lippincott, 1992; Photo courtesy of Stock, Boston.)

the care to help encourage cooperation. Praise for tasks that are attempted, even if not totally completed, must be genuine and generous. The nurse must take care to avoid expecting the child to perform tasks beyond the child's capabilities. The child should be well rested before any energy-taxing tasks are attempted. A chart or other visual aid with tasks listed is a useful tool to help a child reach a desired goal. Stickers can record the child's progress. School-age children often respond well to contracts, for instance, when a set number of stickers are earned, a special privilege or other incentive is awarded. The nurse must remember that these tasks often are hard work for the child.

Preventing Social Isolation. A child who requires constant or frequent attention often is wearing on the family caregivers. The family with no close extended family and few close friends may find getting away for rest and relaxation, even for an evening, almost impossible. Family caregivers need help finding resources available to them for respite care. Any caregiver, no matter how devoted, needs to have a break from everyday cares and concerns. The nurse can refer the family to social services, where they can get help. Sometimes a caregiver may feel that another person cannot take care of the child adequately. The nurse can encourage the caregiver to express fears and anxieties about leaving the child. In this way, the nurse can help the caregiver work through some of these anxieties and feel more confident about getting away for a period of rest.

The child also may feel isolated from peers. When the child is hospitalized, the nurse can make arrangements

for contact with peers by phone, in writing, or through visits. Regular school attendance should be encouraged for the child after discharge. If the child is mainstreamed in a regular classroom the caregiver can make arrangements with the school for rest periods as needed. The nurse can ask the child about interests that may give some clues about suitable after-school activities that increase the child's interactions with peers. The nurse can make suggestions and confer with family caregivers to ensure that proposed plans are carried out. The nurse needs to listen carefully to the child during discussions about social activities to gain insight into the child's feelings about socialization.

Aiding Caregivers' Acceptance of the Condition. When anyone suffers a serious loss, a grief reaction occurs. This is true of family caregivers when they first learn that their child has a chronic or disabling illness. They must mourn the loss of their desired or "perfect" child. The family caregivers must be encouraged to express these feelings and helped to understand that this reaction is common and acceptable. Denial is usually the first reaction that family caregivers have to the information they receive about their child's condition. This is a time when they say, "How could this be?" or "Why my child?" During this time, the nurse can let them express their emotions and respond in a nonjudgmental way. Remaining with them and offering quiet, accepting support may be helpful. Statements by the nurse such as "It will seem better in time" are definitely not appropriate. The nurse must acknowledge the caregivers' feelings as acceptable and reasonable. During the following stage of guilt, the nurse can listen to the caregivers express feelings of guilt and remorse. Again, acknowledging the feelings of the caregivers is useful. The nurse must accept expressions of anger by family caregivers without viewing them as a personal attack. Using listening techniques reflecting the caregivers feelings, such as "You sound very angry," is a helpful method of handling these emotions.

Grief reactions also may occur when the family caregivers are informed that their child is deteriorating or has had a setback. Although caregivers usually cycle through these reactions much more quickly at this time, the same methods are useful.

Preparing for Home Care. Home care planning begins when the child is admitted to the health care facility and continues until discharge. Plans for care at home focus on the continuing care, medications, and treatments the child will need. During the child's hospitalization, family caregivers need to be included in caring for the child so that they become comfortable with the care. Children are frequently sent home with sophisticated equipment and treatments; therefore, the use of the equipment and treatments must be demonstrated, and family caregivers need the opportunity to perform the treatments under the guidance of a nurse. A discussion of

(text continued on page 466)

Nursing Care Plan
for the Chronically Ill Child and Family

Nursing Diagnosis

Altered family processes related to adjustment requirements for the child with chronic illness or disability

Goal: Assist family in adjustment to child's condition

Nursing Interventions	*Rationale*	*Evaluation*
Provide opportunities for family members to express feelings, including doubts about their ability to adequately care for their child in the future.	The family may need encouragement in order to talk about some of their fears.	Family caregivers express fears and anxieties about the child's condition.
Maintain a positive but realistic attitude about the child and the child's illness or disability both when providing care and when discussing the impact of the child's illness on the family.	The nurse serves as a role model for the family; modeling a positive attitude will help family caregivers take the same approach at home.	Family speaks in positive way about the child.
Explore with the family various resources or support systems that may be available to help them. Encourage discussion of needs of other siblings in the family when planning.	The family needs to make plans for meeting the long-term needs of their entire family.	Family caregivers identify community resources or support groups they will contact for help in adjusting to child's illness. Family caregivers set reasonable goals for all the children in the family.

Nursing Diagnosis

High risk for altered growth and development related to impaired ability to achieve developmental tasks or family's reactions to child's condition

Goal: Encourage optimal growth and development

Nursing Interventions	*Rationale*	*Evaluation*
Help caregivers recognize the child's potential and assist in setting realistic growth and development goals.	Family caregivers may not know what to expect in terms of their child's development, and may automatically assume that the child's illness will prevent the child from achieving certain milestones. It is as important to dispel these ideas early on as it is to discuss realistic limitations.	Family caregivers acknowledge the child's capabilities, encourage the child, and set realistic goals for the child.
Discuss the effects of overprotectiveness of family caregivers on the child's development.	Many families react to a child's illness by shielding the child from challenges that the child could cope with if allowed to do so.	

(continued)

Nursing Care Plan
for the Chronically Ill Child and Family (Continued)

Nursing Interventions	Rationale	Evaluation
Encourage the child to carry out self-care as appropriate for age and limitations of illness; permit the child to make choices as possible; establish age-appropriate limits for activities, with appropriate discipline.	Promotes feelings of control and self-worth in the child; shows the child that the illness or disability should not stop developmental growth or activity.	

Nursing Diagnosis
Anxiety related to procedures, tests, or hospitalization

Goal: Reduce anxiety

Nursing Interventions	Rationale	Evaluation
Explain procedures to child ahead of time (but not too far ahead); encourage the child to ask questions.	Understanding exactly what a procedure entails prevents the child from imagining more traumatic possibilities.	Child's anxiety is minimized as evidenced by cooperation with care and treatments.
Acknowledge when a procedure could be painful.	The child needs to trust the nurse and family caregivers; if you promise a particular procedure will be painless and it turns out to cause the child pain, the child will lose trust quickly.	

Nursing Diagnosis
Self-care deficit related to limitations of illness or disability

Goal: Promote self-care

Nursing Interventions	Rationale	Evaluation
Encourage and reinforce any self-care performed with generous praise; take care not to expect the child to perform tasks beyond capabilities.	Positive reinforcement gives the child self confidence and pride in accomplishments.	Child participates in self-care as appropriate for age and capabilities
When a child is having trouble accomplishing some task, devise aids to make the task easier whenever possible, instead of doing the task for the child.	Reinforces importance of self-care and independence; demonstrates creative problem-solving, which the child can use in the future.	

(continued)

Nursing Care Plan
for the Chronically Ill Child and Family (Continued)

Nursing Diagnosis

High risk for social isolation of the child or family related to the child's condition

Goal: Prevent social isolation

Nursing Interventions	Rationale	Evaluation
Encourage the family to establish or maintain the child's contacts with friends and schoolmates. Discuss that this may require some advance planning and contact with other parents in order to establish conditions of playtime necessitated by child's illness.	The child needs to feel that he or she is a part of the outside world, with friends and activities to look forward to.	Family and child use opportunities to socialize with others; the family seeks and finds adequate respite care for the child.
Help family caregivers find resources for respite care, making referrals to social services or other resources as necessary.	The caregiver who periodically gets away from the responsibilities of caring for the child will be able to re-energize and return with a refreshed spirit.	
Encourage the family caregiver to express anxieties about leaving the child.	Talking about such fears helps the caregiver work through anxieties, dismiss those fears that may not be realistic, and make specific plans for those that are. This will allow for a much better period of rest when the caregiver does get away.	

Nursing Diagnosis

Grieving of family caregivers related to anticipated losses secondary to child's illness

Goal: Promote caregivers' acceptance of the child's condition

Nursing Interventions	Rationale	Evaluation
Encourage family members to express their feelings of grief, guilt, or anger and listen, acknowledge, and respond in a nonjudgmental way.	Families need a chance to simply vent their emotions before they are able to come to terms with their child's condition.	Family caregivers receive support while expressing feelings of denial, guilt, and anger during the time they are working through acceptance of the child's condition.

(continued)

Nursing Care Plan
for the Chronically Ill Child and Family (Continued)

Nursing Diagnosis

Family caregivers health-seeking behaviors related to home care of a child with a chronic illness

Goal: Provide adequate family teaching

Nursing Interventions	Rationale	Evaluation
Explain thoroughly and demonstrate the use of any equipment or treatments the family will need to perform at home; provide opportunities for all family members participating in the child's care to practice under the guidance of a nurse.	Watching someone who knows how to perform a technique well and performing that technique yourself are very different matters. Practice is essential!	Family caregivers demonstrate ability to perform care and treatments; family caregivers ask pertinent questions; family caregivers make contact with support groups and community agencies for help.
Provide family with a list of community services and organizations to which they can turn for help and support; include the name and telephone number of a contact person from the discharging health facility whom the family can call with questions or concerns.	Knowing who to contact and how to reach that person will give families reassurance that help is close by and add to self-confidence about being able to handle their child's care.	

home facilities may be appropriate to help the family plan how to accommodate any special needs that the child may have. Family caregivers need a list of community services and organizations to which they can turn for help and support. Many organizations are disease or disability specific, and these should be included in the referrals the caregivers receive. The nurse also should include growth and development guidelines for the caregivers so that they have a realistic concept of what to expect as the child develops. Throughout the child's stay, family caregivers must be encouraged to express their fears, anxieties, and concerns so that the nurse can help solve whatever problems the family anticipates while caring for the child at home. Providing the family with the name and telephone number of a contact person who they can call is reassuring. Families face many hurdles while caring for the child, but with the reassurance that help is just a telephone call away, they are more likely to feel that they can competently face the future. Caring for a chronically ill child can be an overwhelming task that requires cooperation of all who are involved with the child and the family. Family caregivers deserve all the help they can get. (See Nursing Care Plan for the Chronically Ill Child and Family.)

EVALUATION

- Family caregivers express fears and anxieties about the child's condition; family caregivers set reasonable goals for all children in the family
- Family caregivers acknowledge the child's capabilities, encourage the child, and set realistic goals for the child
- Child's anxiety is minimized as evidenced by cooperation with care and treatments
- Child participates in self-care as appropriate for age and capabilities
- Family and child use opportunities to socialize with others; the family seeks and finds adequate respite care for the child
- Family caregivers receive support while expressing feelings of denial, guilt, and anger during the time they are working through acceptance of the child's condition
- Family caregivers demonstrate ability to perform care and treatments; family caregivers ask pertinent questions; family caregivers make contact with support groups and community agencies for help

Summary

Advances in medical technology have brought about an increase in the number of families who have to cope with caring for a child with a chronic illness or disability because many have a longer, and often more productive, life than they once would have had. Caring for such a child over a long period can create much stress in the family, however. When family caregivers first realize they have a child with serious, long-term problems, they often react with denial, guilt, and anger. Nurses can help them through this difficult period with kind, positive support. All members of the family are affected—the child, family caregivers, siblings, and others of the extended family. Although family members sometimes tend to focus on the ill child and that child's problems and care, they must not forget the needs of the well siblings. Often, well siblings respond positively to an ill sibling, especially when the well child's needs are met and the child has a clear understanding of the ill child's condition. Volunteer and community agencies provide support and guidance for families, often specific to the condition of the child. Nurses need to help families set realistic goals for all family members and encourage the family to use all of the support systems available to them.

Review Questions

1. You are caring for 5-year-old Angel, who is a bright young girl with cystic fibrosis. Her mother, Mattie, has been overprotective and has always done everything for her. How will you plan her care to involve her in self-care? What can you say or do to help Mattie encourage Angel to do more of her own care?

2. Nine-year-old Tyson is angry. He tells you that he hates his 6-year-old brother, Josh, who has Down syndrome. What are you going to say to him? If you have the opportunity to talk to his family caregiver, what would you say?

3. Examine Figure 20-1 and discuss how benevolent overreaction affects the chronically ill child and family.

4. Teena and José are the young parents of Nina, a 12-month-old with meningomyelocele (spina bifida). Nina must be catheterized at least 4 times a day and also has mobility problems. What are some of the economic and other stresses that this young couple faces?

5. Cassie is a 16-year-old girl with cerebral palsy. She wants to go to the school prom, but her family caregivers are very resistant to the idea. Cassie pleads with you to talk to them. How will you approach this problem? What will you say to the caregivers?

6. Eight-year-old Jason is a patient in your pediatric unit undergoing a series of chemotherapy. He seems very lonely and sad although his family visits him regularly. You decide he may need contact with children his own age. What plans can you make to provide contact with peers?

7. Using your local phone book, make a list of agencies to which you could refer families for assistance and support in the care of a chronically ill child.

References

1. Hobbs N, Perrin JM (eds). Issues in the Care of Children with Chronic Illness. San Francisco: Jossey-Bass, 1985.
2. Longo OC, Bond L. Families of the handicapped child: Research and practice. Family Relat 33:57–65, 1984.

Bibliography

Austin JK. Assessment of coping mechanisms used by parents and children with chronic illness. MCN 15(2):98–102, 1990.

Clements DB, Copeland LG, Loftus M. Critical times for families with a chronically ill child. Pediatr Nurs 16(2):157–161, 1990.

Clubb RL. Chronic sorrow: Adaptation patterns of parents with chronically ill children. Pediatr Nurs 17(5):461–466, 1991.

Davis BD, Steele S. Case management for young children with special health care needs. Pediatr Nurs 17(1):15–19, 1991.

Gallo AM, Breitmayer BJ, Knafl KA, et al. Stigma in childhood chronic illness: A well sibling perspective. Pediatr Nurs 17(1):21–25, 1991.

Selekman J. Pediatric rehabilitation: From concepts to practice. Pediatr Nurs 17(1):11–14, 1991.

The Dying Child

Chapter 21

Student Objectives

Upon completion of this chapter, the student will be able to:

1. Describe the role of anticipatory grief in the grieving process.
2. Identify reasons why nurses may have difficulty working effectively with dying children.
3. Identify how a nurse can personally prepare to care for a dying child.
4. List the factors that affect the child's understanding of death.
5. Describe how a child's understanding of death changes at each developmental level.
6. State the importance of encouraging families to complete unfinished business.
7. Describe why a family may suffer excessive grief and guilt when a child dies suddenly.
8. Describe possible reactions in a sibling when a child dies.
9. Identify settings for caring for the dying child and the advantages and disadvantages of each.

Marks MG: BROADRIBB'S INTRODUCTORY PEDIATRIC NURSING, 4th ed. © 1994 J.B. Lippincott Company.

Key Terms

anticipatory grief   thanatologist

hospice   unfinished business

I sat in silence

rocking the baby,

    reflecting upon life and death.

And as I felt the small bundle of warmth

    stir within my arms,

I realized that

    while life's essence had died within one,

    it had been born anew within another—

    continuing and completing the cycle.

And that there is never really death—

only a passing from this world into another,

    that the spiritual flame is never

    extinguished—

    only shared and passed on.

And as I held the baby closer still

I felt how young and innocent she was

    —how very much she had to experience and

    learn.

and I felt her vulnerability

    as my own,

    realizing that the child in my arms

    was me,

    just as she was a symbol of all of humanity—

    and the child within each one of us.

by Karen Wapner, written at age 17 while working through her grief after the death of a very close friend.

*T*he most difficult death to accept is the death of a child. We can accept that elderly patients have lived a full life and that life must end, but the life of a child still holds the hopes, dreams, and promises of the future. When a child's life ends early, whether abruptly as the result of an accident or after a prolonged illness, we ask ourselves "Why?" "What's the justice of this?" Caring for a dying child and the family is stressful, but it can be extremely rewarding.

Caring for a family facing the death of their child calls on every personal and professional skill of the nurse. It means offering sensitive, gentle physical care and comfort measures for the child and continuing emotional support for the child, the family caregivers, and the siblings. This kind of caring demands an understanding of the nurse's own feelings about death and dying, knowledge of the grieving process that terminally ill patients and families experience, and a willingness to become involved.

Like chronic illness, terminal illness creates a family crisis with the potential for destroying or strengthening the family as a unit and as individuals. Nurses and other health professionals who can offer knowledgeable, sensitive care to these families help make the remainder of the child's life more meaningful and the family's mourning experience more healing. Helping a family struggle through this crisis and emerge stronger and closer can yield deep satisfaction.

Diagnosis of a fatal illness initiates the grieving process in the child and the family: denial and isolation, anger, bargaining, depression and acute grief, and finally, acceptance. Not every child or family will complete the process because each family, as well as each death, is personal and unique.

When death is expected, the family begins to mourn, a phenomenon called **anticipatory grief**. For some people, this shortens the period of acute grief and loss after the child's death. Unexpected death offers no chance for preparation, and grief may last longer and be more difficult to resolve.

Death is a tragic reality for thousands of children each year. Accidents are the leading cause of death in children between the ages of 1 and 14 years; cancer is the number one fatal disease in this age group. Nearly every one of these childhood deaths means at least one grieving family caregiver and perhaps brothers, sisters, and grandparents. Nurses who care for children and families need to be prepared for encounters with the dying and the bereaved.

The Nurse's Reaction To Dying And Death

I am a student nurse. I am dying. I write this to you who are, and will become, nurses in the hope that by my sharing my feelings with you, you may someday be better able to help those who share my experience. . . . You slip in and out of my room, give me medications and check my blood pressure. Is it because I am a student nurse, myself, or just a human being, that I sense your fright? And your fears enhance mine. Why are you afraid? I am the one who is dying!

I know you feel insecure, don't know what to say, don't know what to do. But please believe me, if you care, you can't go wrong. Just admit that you care. . . . Don't run away—wait—all I want to know is that there will be someone to hold my hand when I need it. . . . If only we could be honest, both admit our fears, touch one another. If you really care, would you lose so much of your valuable professionalism if you even cried with me? Just person to person? Then it might not be so hard to die—in a hospital—with friends close by.[1]

The feelings expressed by this young student nurse are not uncommon. Health care workers often are uncomfortable with dying patients, so they avoid them, afraid the patients will ask questions they cannot or should not answer. These caregivers signal by their behavior that the patient should avoid the fact of his or her impending death and should keep up a show of bravery. In effect, they are asking the patient to meet their needs instead of trying to meet the patient's needs.

Death reminds us of our own mortality, a thought with which many of us are uncomfortable. The thought that someone even younger than we are is about to die makes us feel more vulnerable. Every nurse needs to examine his or her own feelings about death and the reason for these feelings. How has the nurse reacted to the death of a friend or a family member? When growing up, was talking and thinking about death avoided because of family caregivers' attitudes? Admitting that death is a part of life, and that patients should be helped to live each day to the fullest until death, is a step toward understanding and being able to communicate with those who are dying. A workshop, conference, or seminar in which the nurse goes through self-examination of feelings about life and death is useful in preparing the nurse to care for the dying child and family (Box 21-1).

Learning to care for the dying means talking with other professionals, sharing concerns, and comforting each other in stressful times. It means reading the studies that have been done on death to discover how dying patients feel about their care, their illness, their families, and how they want to spend the rest of their lives. It also means being a sensitive, empathic, nonjudgmental listener to patients and families who need to express their feelings, even if they may not be able to express feelings to each other. Caring for the dying is usually a team effort that may involve a nurse, a physician, a chaplain, a social worker, a psychiatrist, a hospice nurse, or a **thanatologist** (a person trained especially to work with the dying and their families, sometimes a nurse), but often the nurse is the person who coordinates the care.

The Child's Understanding of Death

Stage of development, cognitive ability, and experiences influence children's understanding of death. The death of a pet or a family member may be a child's first experience with death. How the family deals with the death has a great impact on the child's understanding of death, but children usually do not have a realistic comprehension of the finality of death until they are nearing preadolescence. Although the dying child may be unable to understand death, the emotions of family caregivers and others alert the child that something is threatening his or her secure world. Dealing with the child's anxieties with openness and honesty restores the child's trust and comfort.

Developmental Stage

Infants and toddlers have little if any understanding of death. The toddler may fear separation from beloved caregivers but have no recognition of the fact that death is nearing and irreversible. A toddler may be able to verbalize that "Nana's gone bye-bye to be with God" or "Grampy went to heaven" but in a few moments ask to go visit the deceased person. This is an opportunity to explain to the child that Nana or Grampy is in a special place and cannot be visited, but the family has many memories of him or her that they will always treasure. The child should not be scolded for not understanding. Questions are best answered simply and honestly.

If the infant or toddler's own death is approaching, family caregivers can be encouraged to stay with the child to provide comfort, love, and security. Maintaining routines as much as possible helps give the toddler a greater sense of security. The egocentric thinking of preschool children contributes to a belief that they may have caused a person or pet to die by thinking angry thoughts. Magical

Box 21-1

Questions to Cover in a Self-Examination About Death

Some Considerations in the Resolution of Death and Dying

1. What was your first conscious memory of death—what were your feelings and reactions?

2. What is your most recent memory of death—how was it the same or different from your first memory?

3. What experience of death had the most effect on you—why?

Get Comfortable and Imagine Now—

You have just been told you have 6 months to live—What is your *first* reaction to that news?

3 months later—What relationships might require you to tie up loose ends? What unfinished business do you have to deal with? You and your significant other are trying to cope with the news. What changes occur in your relationship?

1 month remaining—What do you need to have happen in the remaining time? What hopes, dreams, and plans can or need to be fulfilled?

1 week remains—You are very weak and barely have enough energy to talk. You don't want to even look at yourself. Nausea and vomiting are constant companions. Write a letter to the one person you feel would be the most affected by your dying.

24 hours remain—You are dying. Your breathing is difficult, you feel very hot inside; overwhelming fatigue is ever present. How would you like to spend this last day?

These questions can be used in a group with a hospice or other facilitator. They can be used to help you increase or heighten your awareness of yourself—who you are; how you have gotten to the place in life where you are today; what you are doing with your life and why; how you would change the way you live; your feelings about death—in general, in relationship to your own circle of friends and family, in regard to your own death.

With permission from Ruth Anne Sieber, Hospice: The Bridge, Lewistown, PA.

thinking also plays an important part in the preschooler's beliefs about death. It is not unusual for a preschool child to insist on burying a dead pet or bird and then in a few hours, or a day or two, dig it up to see if it is still there (Figure 21-1). This may be especially true if the child has been told that it will "go to heaven." Frequently, preschoolers think of death as a kind of sleep, not understanding that the dead person will not "wake up"; they may fear going to sleep after the death of a close family member because they fear *they* may not wake up. Family caregivers must be watchful for this kind of reaction so that the child can be encouraged to talk about these fears and be reassured that he or she need not fear dying while sleeping. The child's feelings must be acknowledged as real, and the child must be assisted to resolve them. The feelings must never be ridiculed.

A preschool child may view personal illness as punishment for thoughts or actions. Because preschoolers do not have an accurate concept of death, they fear separation from family caregivers. Caregivers can provide security and comfort by staying with the child as much as possible.

The child who is 6 or 7 years of age is still in the magical thinking stage and continues to think of death in the same way as the preschool child. At about 8 or 9 years of age, school-age children gain the concept that death is universal and irreversible. Around this age, death is personified, that is, it is given characteristics of a person and may be called the devil, God, a monster, or the bogeyman. Children of this age often believe they can protect themselves from death by avoiding stepping on cracks, running past a cemetery while holding their breath, keeping doors locked, staying out of dark rooms, and staying away from funeral homes and dead people.

When faced with the prospect of their own death, school-age children usually are sad that they will be leaving their family and the people they love. They may be apprehensive about how they will manage when they no

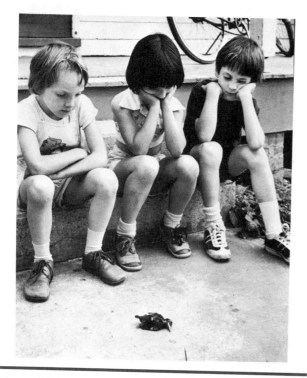

Figure 21-1. A funeral and burial for an animal facilitate respect for life as well as an emerging concept of death. (From Schuster CS, Ashburn SS. *The Process of Human Development*, 3rd ed. Philadelphia: JB Lippincott, 1992.)

terminal illness, but they generally choose to concentrate on living as fully as possible for the time that they have.[2]

Adolescents may be upset by the results of treatments that make them feel weak and alter their appearance, such as alopecia, edema resulting from steroid therapy, and pallor. They may need assistance in presenting themselves as attractively as possible to their peers. Adolescents need opportunities to acknowledge their impending death and can be encouraged to express fears, anxieties, and questions about death. Permitting and encouraging usual activities help the adolescent feel in control.

Experience with Death and Loss

Every death that touches the life of a child makes an impression that affects the way the child thinks about every other death, including his or her own. Attitudes of family caregivers and other family members are powerful influences. Family caregivers must be able to discuss death with children when a grandparent or other family member dies, even though the discussion may be painful. Otherwise, the child thinks that death is another one of those forbidden topics, which undiscussed, leaves im-

longer have their parents around to help them. Often, they view death as another new experience, like going to school, leaving for camp, or flying in an airplane for the first time. They may fear the loss of control that death represents to them, expressing this fear through vocal aggression. Family caregivers and nurses must recognize this as an expression of their fear and avoid scolding or disciplining them for this behavior. This is a time when those people close to the child can help the child voice anxieties about his or her future and provide an outlet for these aggressive feelings. The presence of family members and maintenance of relatively normal routines help give the child a sense of security.

Adolescents have an adult understanding of death but feel that they are immortal; that is, death will happen to others but not to themselves. This belief contributes to adolescents' behaviors that are acknowledged as dangerous and life threatening. This denial of the possibility of serious personal danger may contribute to an adolescent's delay in reporting symptoms or seeking help. Diagnosis of a life-threatening or terminal illness creates a crisis for the adolescent. The adolescent must draw on his or her level of cognitive functioning, past experiences, family support, and ability to problem solve. Depression, feelings of helplessness, anger, fear of pain, and hopelessness often may be expressed by adolescents with a

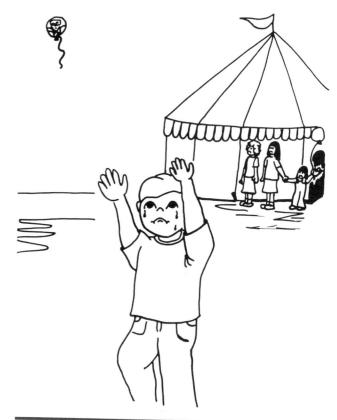

Figure 21-2. Nathan cried and kept jumping and reaching after everyone else had given up. (Courtesy of Ruth Anne Sieber.)

measurable room for fantasy and distortion in the child's imagination.

Many books are available to help a child deal with loss and death. *A Balloon Story*, for example, a simply produced, 13-page coloring storybook by Ruth Anne Sieber, a hospice nurse, is an introduction to a discussion of loss appropriate for the young child. This story of two children who go to a fair with their mothers is illustrated with large line drawings to color. The children in the story each select and purchase a helium balloon, of which they are quite proud. Unfortunately, Nathan's balloon slips from his hand and floats away, forever. Nathan displays typical grief reactions of protest, anger, and finally, acceptance. As the story is read to a child and the pictures are colored, the opportunity to discuss loss provides the adult with the perfect opening. A small booklet for parents, caregivers, and other adults accompanies *A Balloon Story*; it contains excellent guidelines for discussing death and loss with a child (Figure 21-2).* Another small booklet that is excellent to use with any age group is *Water Bugs and Dragonflies*. It is the story that approaches life and death as stages of existence by illustrating that after a water bug turns into a dragonfly, he can no longer go back and tell the other curious water bugs what life is like in this beautiful new world to which he has gone. This story can serve as the foundation for further discussion about death (Figure 21-3).

A number of the books that are available focus on the death of an animal or pet. Many of the stories deal with death as a result of old age. Several books have an accident as the cause of death. Most of the books are fiction, but several nonfiction sources are available for older children (Box 21-2). There is no discussion of one's own death in these resources, which is consistent with Western philosophy to see death as something that happens to others but not to oneself.[3]

Awareness of Impending Death

Children know when they are dying. They sense and fear what is going to happen even if they are unable to specifically identify it by name. Their play activities, their artwork, their dreams, and their symbolic language demonstrate this knowledge. Family caregivers who insist that a child not learn the truth about his or her illness place health care professionals at a disadvantage because they are not free to help the child deal with fears and concerns.

Family caregivers who permit openness and honesty in communication with a dying child offer the health care staff an opportunity to meet the child's individual needs most effectively, to dispel misunderstandings that may need to be confronted, and to see that the child and the

* *A Balloon Story* can be obtained from Hospice: The Bridge, Lewistown Hospital, Lewistown, PA 17044.

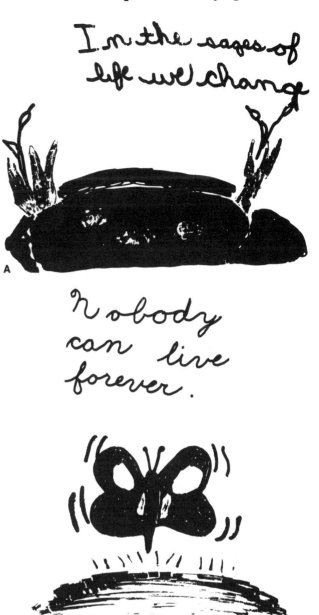

Figure 21-3. Drawings done by fourth grade students after a presentation about death that included a reading of *Water Bugs and Butterflies*. **A**, In the s[t]ages of life we change. At the center of the drawing is a pond with three lily pads. The stems at the end represent plants that waterbugs crawl up on before turning into dragonflies. **B**, Nobody lives forever. (Courtesy of Ruth Anne Sieber.)

family are able to resolve any problems or "unfinished business."

Openness does not mean that caregivers offer information not asked for by the child but simply that the child be given the information desired, using words that the child can understand, in a gentle and straightforward

Box 21-2

Books about Death for Children

Book	Who Died	Cause of Death	Age Appropriate
Anderson L. *It's OK to Cry.* Chicago: Chicago Press, 1979	Uncle	Accident	5–11
Anderson L. *Death.* New York: First Book, 1980 (nonfiction)	Various	Various	11–15
Bradley B. *Endings: A Book About Death.* Reading, MA: Addison-Wesley, 1979 (nonfiction)	Various	Various	11–14
Brandenberg A. *The Two of Them.* New York: Greenwillow, 1979	Grandpa	Old age	5–12
Brown M. *The Dead Bird.* Reading, MA: Addison-Wesley, 1965	Bird	Unknown	3–12
Bunting E. *The Happy Funeral.* New York: Harper & Row, 1982	Grandpa	Old age	3–8
Buscaglia L. *The Fall of Freddie the Leaf.* Thorofare, NJ: Charles B. Slack, 1982	Leaf	Old age	All
Carrick C. *The Accident.* New York: Seabury, 1976	Dog	Accident	4–9
Clifton L. *Everett Anderson's Good-bye.* New York: Holt, Rinehart, & Winston, 1983	Parent	Unknown	3–9
Cohen M. *Jim's Dog Muffin.* New York: Greenwillow, 1984	Dog	Accident	3–7
Herriot J. *The Christmas Day Kitten.* New York: St. Martin's Press, 1976	Cat	Illness	All
Hurd E. *The Black Dog Who Went into the Woods.* New York: Harper & Row, 1980	Dog	Unknown	5–8
Kantrowitz M. *When Violet Died.* New York: Parents' Magazine Press, 1975	Bird	Old age	5–11
Keller H. *Good-bye Max.* New York: Greenwillow, 1987	Dog	Old age	3–7
Leshan E. *Learning to Say Good-bye.* New York: Macmillan, 1976	Parent	Various	10–13
Patterson K. *Bridge to Terabithia.* Santa Barbara, CA: Cornerstone, 1977	Friend	Accident	10–15
Pringle L. *Death is Natural.* New York: Four Winds, 1977 (nonfiction)	—	Old age	8–12
Rofes E. *The Kids' Book About Death and Dying.* Boston: Little Brown, 1985 (nonfiction)	Various	Various	11–15
Sanford D. *It Must Hurt a Lot.* Portland, OR: Multnomah, 1985	Dog	Accident	5–11
Simon N. *The Saddest Time.* Niles, IL: Albert Whitmont, 1986	Uncle	Illness	9–15
Smith D. *A Taste of Blackberries.* New York: Thomas Y. Crowall, 1973	Friend	Accident	9–14
Stein S. *About Dying.* New York: Walker & Company, 1974	Bird and grandpa	Old age	3–8
Stevens M. *When Grandpa Died.* Chicago: Chicago Press, 1979	Grandpa	Old age	5–9
Tobias T. *Petey.* New York: G.P. Putnam's Sons, 1978	Gerbil	Old age	4–8
Viorst J. *The Tenth Good Thing About Barney.* Atheneum, NY: Connecticut Printers, 1971	Cat	Unknown	5–14

Adapted from Bowden VR. Children's literature: The death experience. Pediatr Nurs 19(1):17–21, 1993.

manner. The truth can be kind as well as cruel. Honest, specific answers leave less room for misinterpretation and distortion.

Adolescents are usually sensitive to what is happening to them and may need the nurse to be an advocate for them if they have wishes that they want to fulfill before dying. An adolescent may sense the nurse's willingness and ability to discuss feelings that the adolescent is uncomfortable discussing with family caregivers. The nurse can talk with the adolescent and work with the family caregivers to help them understand the adolescent's desires and needs. The nurse can call on the hospice, social or psychiatric services, or a chaplain or rabbi to help the family express and resolve their concerns and recognize the adolescent's needs.

The Family's Reaction to Dying and Death

Diagnosis of a potentially fatal disease, such as acquired immunodeficiency syndrome, cystic fibrosis, or cancer sends feelings of shock, disbelief, and guilt through every family member. Anticipatory grief begins then and continues until remission or death occurs. When the disease is a rapidly advancing illness, anticipatory grief may be short lived as the death of the child nears.

Family Caregivers

The family caregivers of children in the final stages of a terminal illness may have had to cope with many hospital admissions between periods at home. During this time, the family may be faced with decisions about the physical care of the child as well as learning to live with a dying child. As the child's condition deteriorates, the family can be encouraged to talk to their child about dying. This is a task that they may find difficult. Support from a religious counselor, hospice nurse, or social service or psychiatric worker can help them through this difficult task. Family caregivers can be encouraged to provide as much normalcy as possible in the child's schedule. School attendance and special trips can be encouraged, within the capabilities and desires of the child.

During this time, family caregivers may find themselves going through a grief process of anger, depression, ambivalence, and bargaining over and over again. The caregivers may direct anger at the hospital staff, themselves (because of guilt), at each other, or at the child. The nurse can reassure the caregivers that this is a normal reaction but must avoid taking sides.

If the child improves enough to go home again, parents may find that they tend to be overprotective of the child. As in chronic illness, this overprotective attitude reinforces the child's sick behavior and dependency and is usually accompanied by a lack of discipline. Failure to set limits accentuates the child's feelings of being different and creates problems with siblings. The child learns to manipulate family members, only to find that this kind of behavior does not bring positive results when attempted with peers or health care personnel.

When the child has to return to the hospital because of increasing symptoms, family caregivers may experience all the stages of the grieving process again. The family caregivers fear the child's approaching death, the possibility that the child will be in great pain, and the possibility that the child may die when they are not pres-

ent. Nurses can help relieve these fears by keeping them informed about their child's condition, by making the child as comfortable as possible, and by reassuring the family that they will be summoned if they are not with the child when death appears to be near. When death comes, it is perfectly appropriate to share the family's grief, to cry with the family, and then provide them with privacy to express their sorrow. The nurse can stay with the family for a while, remaining quietly supportive, with an attitude of a comforting listener. The nurse can say "I am so sorry" or "This is a very sad time" but must keep the focus on the family's grief and should never share personal experiences of loss.[4] The family may want to hold the child to say a final good-bye, and the nurse can encourage and assist them in this. Intravenous lines and other equipment can be removed to make holding the child easier. The family may be left alone during this time if they desire. The nurse must be sensitive to the family's needs and desires in order to provide them with comfort.

During anticipatory grief, the family of a child with a terminal illness has an opportunity to complete any **unfinished business**, such as spending more time with the child, helping siblings understand the child's illness and impending death, and providing family members a chance to share their love with the child. This can help them prepare for the child's death. However, when a child dies suddenly and unexpectedly, the family has not had the opportunity to go through anticipatory grief. Such a family may have excessive guilt and remorse for something they felt they left unsaid or undone. Even if a child has had a traumatic death with disfigurement, the family needs to be given the opportunity to be with, see, and hold the child to help with closure of the child's life. The nurse can prepare the family for seeing the child, explaining why parts of the body may be covered. Viewing the child, even if severely mutilated, helps the family have a realistic view of the child and aids in the grief process.

The family may face a number of decisions that must be made rather quickly, especially when the death of the child was unexpected. Families of terminally ill children usually have made some plans for the child's death and may know exactly what they want done. However, when the child dies unexpectedly, decisions may be necessary concerning organ donation, funeral arrangements, and autopsy. If the death has been the result of violence or is unexplained, an autopsy is required by law, but there may be other reasons that an autopsy is desired. Organ donation can be discussed with the family by the hospital's organ donor coordinator or other designated person. The family needs to be well informed and must be supported throughout these difficult decisions.

Grief for the death of a child is not limited in time but may continue for years. Sometimes, professional counseling is necessary to help family caregivers work through grief. The support of others who have experienced the same sort of loss can be helpful to some people. Two national organizations founded for the purpose of offering support are the following:

Candlelighters Childhood Cancer Foundation
1901 Pennsylvania Avenue, NW
Washington, DC 20006
(202) 659-5136

Compassionate Friends
PO Box 3696
Oak Brook, IL 60522-3696
(708) 990-0010

These organizations have many local chapters.

The Child

The dying child may exhibit a lessened level of consciousness, but the child's level of hearing remains intact. Family members at the bedside and health care personnel may need to be reminded of this. Care must be taken to avoid saying anything in the child's presence that would not be said if the child was fully conscious. Gentle touch and caressing may provide comfort to the child. Excellent nursing care is required. Medications for pain are given intravenously because they are poorly absorbed from muscle owing to poor circulation. Mucous membranes are kept clean, and petroleum jelly (Vaseline) can be applied to the lips to prevent drying and cracking. The conjunctiva of the eyes can be moistened with normal saline eye drops, such as Artificial Tears, if drying occurs. The child's skin is kept clean and dry, and the child is turned and positioned regularly to provide comfort and prevent skin breakdown. While caring for the child, the nurse should talk to the child and explain everything that is being done.

As death approaches, internal body temperature increases; thus, dying patients seem to be unaware of cold, even though their skin feels cool. Family caregivers need to have this explained to them so they do not think the child needs additional covering.

In the period immediately before death, children who have remained conscious may experience restlessness followed by a time of peace and calm. The nurse and family caregivers should be aware of these reactions and know that death is near.

Siblings

Just as in chronic illness, siblings resent the attention given the ill child and are angry about the disruption in the family. Reaction varies according to the developmental age of the sibling and parental attitudes and actions. Younger children find it almost impossible to understand what is happening; it is difficult even for older children to grasp. Reaction to the illness and its accompanying stresses can cause classroom problems for school-age siblings, which may be incorrectly labeled as learning disabilities or behavioral disorders unless school personnel are aware of the family situation.

When the child dies, young siblings who are still prone to magical thinking may feel much guilt, particularly if a strong degree of rivalry existed before the illness. These children need continued reassurance that they did not cause or help cause their sibling's death.

The decision of whether a sibling should or should not attend funeral services for the child may be difficult. Although there has been little research regarding this, the current thinking among many health professionals supports the presence of the sibling. The sibling may be encouraged to leave a token of love and good-bye with the child. This can be a drawing, a note, a toy, or other special memento. Siblings can visit the dead child in privacy when there are not a lot of other mourners present. As with family caregivers, siblings most likely benefit from being able to deal with the realities of the child's death rather than anything that they may imagine (Box 21-3).

Settings for Care of the Dying Child

The family and the child's responses to and acceptance of a child's death can be greatly influenced by where the child dies. While dying in a hospital, a child may receive the most professional care and the most technologically advanced treatment, but this also can contribute to family separation, a feeling of loss of control, and a sense of isolation. An increasing number of families and children are choosing to keep the child at home to die.

Hospice Care

In medieval times, the **hospice** was a refuge for travelers, not only those who traveled through the countryside but those who were leaving this life for another, the terminally ill. Hospices often were operated by religious orders and became havens for the dying.

The current hospice movement in health care began in England, when Dr. Cicely Saunders founded St. Christopher's Hospice in London in 1967. This institution has become the model for others in the United States and Canada, with emphasis on sensitive, humane care for the dying. Hospice principles of care include relief of pain, attention to the needs of the total person, and absence of heroic life-saving measures.

The first hospice in the United States was the New Haven Hospice in New Haven, Connecticut. Many communities now have hospice programs that may or may not be affiliated with a hospital. Some of the programs offer a hospice setting to which patients go when in terminal stages of their illness, whereas many others provide support and guidance for the patient and family while the patient remains in the hospital or is cared for at home.

Box 21-3

Guidelines for Helping Children Cope with Death

DO	DON'T
1. Know your own beliefs.	1. Praise stoicism (detached, unemotional behavior).
2. Begin where the child is.	2. Use euphemisms (mild expressions substituted for ones that might be offensive).
3. Be there.	
4. Confront reality.	
5. Allow and encourage expression of feelings.	3. Be nonchalant.
6. Be truthful.	4. Glamorize death.
7. Include the child in family rituals.	5. Tell fairy tales or half truths.
8. Encourage remembrance.	6. Close the door to questions.
9. Admit when you don't know the answer.	7. Be judgmental of feelings and behaviors.
10. Use touch to communicate.	8. Protect the child from exposure to experiences with death.
11. Start death education early, simply, using naturally occurring events.	9. Encourage forgetting the deceased.
12. Recognize symptoms of grief, and deal with the grief.	10. Encourage the child to be like the deceased.
13. Accept differing reactions to death.	

(Courtesy of Alice Demi, President, Grief Education Institute, PO Box 623, Englewood, CO 80151.)

Most of these hospice programs are established primarily for adult patients, and only about 200 of the estimated 1700 accept children as patients.[5]

Children's Hospice International (CHI), founded in 1983, is an organization dedicated to hospice support of children. Through an individualized plan of care, CHI addresses the physical, developmental, psychological, social, and spiritual needs and issues of children and families in a comprehensive and consistent way. It serves as a resource and advocacy center, providing education for parents and professionals. CHI conducts training seminars and conferences, publishes training manuals, and supports a clearinghouse of information available through a national hot line (1-800-24-CHILD). CHI is planning to open a pediatric center in the Washington, DC area for critically ill children to be named Melinda House, in memory of Melinda Lawrence, who had muscular dystrophy and lived her life to the fullest until her death in March, 1993.

Home Care

Caring for the dying patient, young or old, at home has become increasingly more common in recent years. More families are choosing to keep their child at home during their terminal stage of illness. Factors that contribute to the decision to care for a child at home include the following:

- Concerns about cost, both for the hospitalization and for the nonmedical expenses of travel, housing, and food for families to be near the dying child
- Stress from repeated family separations
- Loss of control over the care of the child and family life

Families feel that the more loving, caring environment that the home provides for the child draws the family closer together and helps reduce the guilt that often is part of bereavement. All members of the family can be involved to some extent in the child's care and in this way gain a feeling of usefulness. Family caregivers feel that they remain in control. Not all of the factors are positive ones, however. Costs that would have been covered by health care insurance if the child was hospitalized may not be covered when the child is cared for at home. Caring for a dying child can be extremely difficult, both emotionally and physically. Not every family has the resource of someone who is able to carry out procedures that may need to be performed regularly. In some instances, home nursing assistance may be available, but this varies from community to community. Usually, the home care nurse visits the home several days a week for a period and may be on call for the remainder of the time. In some communities, hospice nurses may provide the teaching and support that families need. Deciding to care for a dying child at home is an extremely difficult decision for a family to make, and the family needs support and guidance from the health care personnel involved in caring for the child when it is trying to make the decision, as well as after the decision is made, until after the death of the child.

Hospital Care

Dying in the hospital has limitations and advantages. Both the child and family may find support from others in the same situation. Family members may not have the physical or emotional strength to cope with total care of the child at home, but they can participate in care that is supported by the hospital staff. Hospital care is much more expensive, as mentioned earlier, but this fact may not be important to some families, especially if they have health insurance coverage. The hospital is still the culturally accepted place, in which to die, and this is also important to some persons. Those who do choose hospital care need to know that they have rights and can exert some control over what happens to them and their families.

◣ Nursing Process for the Dying Child

ASSESSMENT

The assessment of the terminally ill child and family is an ongoing process that is developed over a period of working with the child and family. The assessment covers the developmental level of the child, the influence of cultural and spiritual concerns, the family's support system, present indications of grieving (ie, anticipatory grief), members of the family and their interactions, and unfinished business. To understand the child's view of death, the nurse must consider the child's previous experiences as well as developmental level and cognitive ability.

NURSING DIAGNOSES

Nursing diagnoses for the dying child include those that are appropriate for the child's illness as well as those that are specific to the dying process. The following diagnoses are specific to the dying process:

- Pain related to illness and weakened condition
- High risk for social isolation related to the child's terminal illness
- Anxiety related to condition and prognosis
- High risk for ineffective family coping related to the child's approaching death

- Powerlessness of family caregivers related to inability to control child's condition

PLANNING AND IMPLEMENTATION

Providing Relief from Pain and Discomfort. The child may be experiencing pain for many reasons. Pain can result from chemotherapy; nausea, vomiting, and gastrointestinal cramping; pressure caused by positioning; constipation; and any of a number of other causes. Until the child is comfortable and relatively pain free, all other nursing interventions are fruitless. Pain becomes the primary focus of the child until relief is provided. Nursing measures to relieve pain may include positioning, using pillows as needed; changing linens; providing conscientious skin and mouth care; protecting skin surfaces from rubbing together; back rubs and massages; and administering antiemetics, analgesics, and stool softeners as appropriate to provide comfort.

Providing Appropriate Diversional Activities for the Child. Encourage the child's peers (siblings and school or social friends) to maintain contact. Provide opportunities for peers to visit, write, or telephone as the child is able. Read to the child, and engage in other activities that the child is interested in and physically can tolerate. Encourage the child to make decisions, when possible, to foster the child's feeling of control. Explain all procedures and how they will affect the child. Provide the child with privacy, but be cautious not to neglect the child. Provide ample periods of rest. Continue to talk to and tell the child what you are doing, even though the child may not seem to be responsive.

Easing the Child's Anxiety. Ask family caregiver about the child's understanding of death and previous experiences with death. Observe how the child exhibits fear, and ask family caregivers for any additional information. Encourage the child to use a doll, a pillow, or another special "warm fuzzy" for comforting fears. Do use words such as "dead" or "dying" if appropriate in conversation, because this may give the child an opening to talk about his or her own death. Nighttime is an especially frightening time for children because they often think they will die at night. Provide company and comfort, and be alert for periods of wakefulness during which the child may need someone to talk to. Be honest, straightforward, and avoid injecting your beliefs into the conversation. If appropriate, a book about death may be read to the child to initiate conversation, although this method should have been used much earlier in the child's care.

Assisting the Family to Cope. Family caregivers may need encouragement to discuss their feelings about the child. Emotions and fears must be acknowledged and caregivers reassured that their reactions are normal. The support of a spiritual counselor may be helpful during this time. Assist the family in contacting their own spiritual

(text continued on page 481)

Nursing Care Plan
for the Dying Child and Family

Nursing Diagnosis
Pain related to illness and weakened condition

Goal: Relieve pain

Nursing Interventions	*Rationale*	*Evaluation*
Make pain relief the primary focus of all nursing care until the child is comfortable.	Pain is the child's primary focus, and until it is relieved, all other nursing interventions are fruitless.	The child rests quietly; denies pain when asked.
Administer pain-relief medications, but also include such nursing measures as positioning, providing back rubs and massages, changing linens, providing conscientious skin and mouth care, and protecting skin surfaces from rubbing together to make child as comfortable as possible.	Each child experiences pain uniquely. Some measures may work to relieve pain in one child but not in another; the nurse needs to find out which measures are the most effective for this child.	

Nursing Diagnosis
High risk for social isolation related to child's terminal illness

Goal: Promote social interactions

Nursing Interventions	*Rationale*	*Evaluation*
Encourage the child's siblings and peers (including school friends) to maintain contact; provide opportunities for such contact by arranging for convenient visiting hours, providing paper and pens for writing, and making telephone available.	The child needs to feel that he or she is not cut off from everyone and everything.	The child engages in social interactions and activities within his or her physical capabilities.
Spend time with, and talk to the child, even when you are not sure the child is responsive.	Hearing is often the last sense to shut down; the child will feel reassured by your voice and presence.	

Nursing Diagnosis
Anxiety related to condition and prognosis

Goal: Ease the child's and family's anxiety

Nursing Interventions	*Rationale*	*Evaluation*
Discuss with the family caregivers their perception of their child's understanding of death and note how the child exhibits fear.	The child may or may not have discussed death with the family, and it is important for the nurse to respond to the child appropriately. Also, the nurse is able,	The child keeps a "warm fuzzy" close by for comfort; the child talks about death to the nurse and/or family.

(continued)

Nursing Care Plan
for the Dying Child and Family (Continued)

Nursing Interventions	Rationale	Evaluation
	at the same time, to get a sense of how the family views the child's death and what sort of help they may need in discussing the topic with their child and each other.	
Encourage the child to keep a favorite object or "warm fuzzy" for comforting fears. Provide company and comfort, particularly during the night.	Many children think they will die at night; periods of wakefulness are common, and if they are left alone, fears may compound.	

Nursing Diagnosis

High risk for ineffective family coping related to child's approaching death

Goal: *Assist the family to cope*

Nursing Interventions	Rationale	Evaluation
Encourage family caregivers to discuss their feelings about the child and to acknowledge their fears and emotions; reassure them that their reactions are normal.	It may be very difficult to family members to talk about their child's death; they may feel they need to "keep up a brave front" for the child or siblings; however, it is important for them to acknowledge the death and begin to let out some of their emotions.	Family caregivers express their feelings and identify signs in the child that indicate approaching death.
Assist the family in contacting their own spiritual advisor or help them make contact with a hospital chaplain if they desire.	The support of a spiritual counselor, particularly one already known to the family, may be helpful to family members.	
Make sure family caregivers are resting and eating adequately.	It would not help the child if parents collapsed or became ill from exhaustion; lack of sleep and inadequate nutrition will only make it harder for family members to cope.	

(continued)

Nursing Care Plan
for the Dying Child and Family (Continued)

Nursing Diagnosis
Powerlessness of family caregivers related to inability to control child's condition

Goal: Assist the family to participate in child's care

Nursing Interventions	Rationale	Evaluation
Suggest specific care measures individual family members might perform to provide comfort for the child.	Caregivers' need to feel they are doing something to help their child.	Family caregivers provide comfort measures for the child, talk to the child, and complete unfinished business with the child.
Encourage family members to talk to the child, even when the child seems non-responsive.	The child may well be able to hear their loved ones voices, even when the child is unable to respond; family caregivers will feel better when they can still communicate love and support.	
Explain the meaning of "unfinished business" to the family and encourage them to complete any unfinished business on their agenda.	Caregivers need the nurse's support and guidance through an experience they may have never before encountered; discussion of unfinished business provides another opportunity for family members to engage in meaningful activity with their child before the child's death.	

counselor, or offer to contact the hospital chaplain if the family desires. Family caregivers need to be encouraged to eat and rest properly so that they will not become ill or exhausted themselves. The nurse can explain the child's condition to the family and answer any questions. The family can be reassured that everything is being done to keep the child as comfortable and pain free as possible. The nurse can ask the family about siblings of the ill child—what they know, how much they understand, and whether or not the family has spoken to them about their sibling's approaching death. The nurse can offer help to the caregivers in talking with siblings. Signs of approaching death can be interpreted for the family.

Assisting the Family to Feel Involved in the Child's Care. Respond to the family caregivers' needs to feel some control over the situation by suggesting specific measures they can perform to provide comfort for the child, such as positioning, moistening lips, and reading or telling a favorite story. Encourage the caregivers to talk to the child, even if the child does not respond. Discour-

age whispered conversations in the room. Encourage and help the family carry out cultural customs if they wish. Explain unfinished business to the family caregivers, and assist them in completing any unfinished business on their agenda. This may include the need for the child to go home to die. Contact support persons, such as hospice or social services, to help complete unfinished business, if necessary. (See Nursing Care Plan for the Dying Child and Family.)

EVALUATION

- The child rests quietly; denies pain when asked
- The child engages in activities within his or her physical capabilities
- The child keeps a "warm fuzzy" close by for comfort; the child talks about death to the nurse or family; the child is comforted when awake at night by the presence of someone to talk to

- Family caregivers express their feelings and identify signs in the child that indicate approaching death
- Siblings visit and verbally demonstrate an understanding of the child's approaching death
- Family caregivers provide comfort measures for the child, talk to the child, and complete unfinished business with the child

Summary

When a child dies, the family and the health care personnel are all greatly affected. Because nurses and other health care personnel have not worked through their own feelings about death, they are often uncomfortable working with dying patients.

The child's stage of development, cognitive ability, and life experiences contribute to the child's understanding of death. Before the age of 8 or 9 years, the concept of death is greatly influenced by magical thinking. The adolescent has an attitude of self-immortality, which may contribute to the adolescent's denial of the possibility of his or her own death. There are a number of books available that can facilitate a discussion about death with a child of any age.

The grief process is a multistep process that does not follow a predictable schedule from one person to another. When a child has been diagnosed with a terminal illness and has been ill for some time, the family experiences anticipatory grief, which gives them an opportunity to complete unfinished business and helps them resolve their grief when death occurs. However, when a child dies suddenly or unexpectedly, the family has not had that opportunity and may experience grief more profoundly.

Hospital, home, and hospice care are all options that the child and family may exercise in the terminal stage of the child's illness. Each type of care has advantages and disadvantages that must be considered when making the choice.

Review Questions

1. What are some advantages of caring for the terminally ill child at home?
2. Why do some families feel unable to care for a dying child at home?
3. Why are nurses often upset by the death of a child they have been caring for?
4. What is your feeling about the story *Nurse's Reaction to Dying and Death* in this chapter?
5. How does a preschooler typically respond to the death of a family caregiver? of a pet?
6. In what kinds of settings can a children's hospice take place?
7. Is there a hospice in your area? How does it function? Does it take children as patients?
8. How does a 9-year-old child view death?
9. What developmental characteristics of adolescents affect their view of death?

References

1. American Journal of Nursing, 70(2), 1070.
2. Peronne J. Adolescents with cancer: Are they at risk for suicide? Pediatr Nurs 19(1):22–25, 1993.
3. Bowden VR. Children's literature: The death experience. Pediatr Nurs 19(1):17–21, 1993.
4. Miles A. Caring for families when a child dies. Pediatr Nurs 16(4):346–347, 1990.
5. Armstrong-Dailey A. About our children. Am J Hospice Care 4(5):11–12, 1987.

Bibliography

Castiglia PT, Harbin RE. Child Health Care: Process and Practice. Philadelphia: JB Lippincott, 1992.

Consolvo CA. Jeff's last wish . . . A dying child wanted to go home to his rocking chair. Nursing 20(9):152, 1990.

Coody D. High expectations: Nurses who work with children who might die. Nurs Clin North Am 20(1):131–142, 1985.

Davies B, Eng B. Factors influencing nursing care of children who are terminally ill. Pediatr Nurs 19(1):9–14, 1993.

Grogan LB. Grief of an adolescent when a sibling dies. MCN 15(1):21–24, 1990.

Jackson DB, Saunders RB. Child Health Nursing. Philadelphia: JB Lippincott, 1993.

Pazola KJ, Gerber AK. Privileged communication: Talking with a dying adolescent. MCN 15(1):16–21, 1990.

Pillitteri A. Maternal and Child Health Nursing. Philadelphia: JB Lippincott, 1992.

Rushton CH, Hogue EE, Billet CA, et al: End of life care for infants with AIDS: Ethical and legal issues. Pediatr Nurs 19(1):79–83, 1993.

Rushton CH, Hogue EE. When parents demand "everything." Pediatr Nurs 19(2):180–183, 1993.

Schuster CS, Ashburn SS. The Process of Human Development, 3rd ed. Philadelphia: JB Lippincott, 1992.

Stickney D. Water Bugs and Dragonflies. New York: Pilgrim Press, 1982.

Whaley LF, Wong DL. Nursing Care of Infants and Children, 4th ed. St. Louis: Mosby-Year Book, 1991.

Glossary

abdominal paracentesis surgical puncture into the abdomen to drain fluid.

abuse misuse, excessive use, rough or bad treatment; is used to refer to misuse of alcohol or drugs (substance abuse) and mistreatment of children or family members (child abuse, domestic abuse).

achylia absence of pancreatic enzymes in gastric secretions.

acid–base balance a state of equilibrium between the acidity and the alkalinity of body fluids.

acrocyanosis cyanosis of the hands and feet seen periodically in the newborn.

actual nursing diagnoses diagnoses that identify existing health problems.

adenoids a mass of lymphoid tissue in the nasal pharynx, extending from the roof of the nasal pharynx to the free edge of the soft palate.

adenopathy enlarged lymph glands.

alcohol abuse drinking sufficient alcoholic beverages to induce intoxication.

alcoholism chronic alcohol abuse.

allergen antigen that causes an allergic reaction.

allograft skin graft taken from a genetically different person for temporary coverage during burn healing; skin from a cadaver sometimes is used.

alopecia loss of hair.

amblyopia dimness of vision from disuse of the eye, sometimes called "lazy eye."

amenorrhea absence of menstruation.

amniocentesis analysis of amniotic fluid that reveals much about the fetus including sex, state of fetal health, and fetal maturity. A sample of amniotic fluid is withdrawn for early diagnosis of possible disorders, such as chromosomal abnormalities and blood disorders. The procedure is done by inserting a needle through the abdominal and uterine walls into the amniotic sac and withdrawing a small amount of fluid (10 to 20 mL) through a syringe.

amniotic sac the strong translucent membrane that encloses the fetus suspended in amniotic fluid, the environment that provides protection for the developing child. This membrane is large and elastic enough to permit the fetus to move about and turn at will during most of its intrauterine life.

ankylosis immovability of a joint.

anorexia nervosa an eating disorder characterized by loss of appetite due to emotional causes, usually excessive fear of becoming (or being) fat.

anthelmintic medication that expels intestinal worms; vermifuge.

anticipatory grief preparatory grieving that often helps the caregivers mourn the loss of their child when death actually comes.

antigen a protein substance found on the surface of red blood cells capable of inducing a specific immune response and reacting with the products of that response.

antigen–antibody response the response of the body to an antigen causing the formation of antibodies that protect the body from an invading antigen.

anuria absence of urine.

apnea temporary interruption of the breathing impulse.

archetype predetermined patterns of human development, which according to Carl Jung, replace instinctive behavior of other animals; prototype.

areola the darkened area around the nipple.

arthralgia painful joints.

ascites edema in the peritoneal cavity.

associative play being engaged in a common activity without any sense of belonging or fixed rules.

astigmatism error in refraction of light on the retina caused by unequal curvature in the cornea of the eye bending light rays in different directions, producing a blurred image.

ataxia a lack of coordination caused by disturbances in the kinesthetic and balance senses.

atresia the absence of a normal body opening or the abnormal closure of a body passage.

aura a sensation that signals an impending epileptic attack; may be visual, aromatic, or other sensation.

autistic totally self-centered and unable to relate to others, often exhibiting bizarre behaviors; autistic children can sometimes be destructive to themselves and others.

autograft skin taken from an individual's own body; it is the only kind of skin accepted permanently by recipient tissues, except for the skin of an identical twin.

autonomy the ability to function in an independent manner.

autosomal recessive trait a trait or condition that is not expressed unless both parents are carrying the gene for that trait.

autosomal dominant trait a trait or condition appearing in a heterozygous person resulting from a dominant gene within a pair.

autosomes twenty-two pairs of chromosomes that are alike in the male and female; the sex chromosomes are not autosomes.

azotemia nitrogen containing compounds in the blood.

Babinski reflex the flaring open of the infant's toes when the lateral plantar surface is stroked. Also called the plantar reflex, this reaction usually disappears by the end of the first year.

bilateral pertaining to both sides; eg, bilateral cleft lip involves both sides of the lip.

binocular vision normal vision that is maintained through the muscular coordination of eye movements of both eyes, so that a single vision results.

blended family both partners in a marriage bring children from a previous marriage into the household; his, hers, and theirs.

body surface area (BSA) most reliable formula to calculate dosages. Using a West nomogram, the child's weight is marked down on the right scale and the height is marked on the left scale. A straight edge is used to draw a line between the two marks. The point at which it crosses the column labelled SA (surface area) is the BSA expressed in square meters (m^2).

bonding the development of a close emotional tie between the newborn and the parent or parents.

bottle mouth (nursing bottle) caries condition caused by the erosion of the enamel on deciduous teeth of the infant caused by sugar from the formula or sweetened juice, which coats the teeth for long periods. This condition also can occur in infants who sleep with their mother and nurse intermittently throughout the night.

brachycephaly shortness of the head.

bulimia nervosa an eating disorder characterized by episodes of binge eating followed by purging by self-induced vomiting or with use of laxatives.

caput succedaneum an edematous swelling of the soft tissues of the scalp caused by prolonged pressure of the occiput against the cervix during labor and delivery. The edema disappears within a few days.

carditis inflammation of the heart.

cataract a development of opacity in the crystalline lens that prevents light rays from entering the eye.

cavernous hemangioma congenital malformations that are subcutaneous collections of blood vessels with bluish overlying skin. Although these lesions are benign tumors, they may become so large and extensive as to interfere with the functions of the body part on which they appear.

celiac syndrome term used to designate the complex of malabsorptive disorders.

centromere the portion of the chromosome by which the chromosome is attached to the spindle during cell division.

cephalhematoma a collection of blood between the periosteum and the skull caused by excessive pressure on the head during birth.

chancre a hard, red, painless primary lesion of syphilis at the point of entry of the spirochete.

chelating agent an agent that binds with metal.

child neglect failing to provide adequate hygiene, health care, nutrition, love, nurturing, and supervision that is needed for growth and development.

child-life programs program to make hospitalization less threatening for children and their parents. These programs are usually under the direction of a child-life specialist whose background is in psychology and early childhood development.

chordee a chordlike anomaly that extends from the scrotum to the penis, pulling the penis downward in an arc.

chorea rapid, jerky involuntary movements that are continuous.

chromosomes threadlike structures that occur in pairs and carry genetic information.

chronic illness condition that interferes with daily functioning for more than 3 months in a year, causes hospitalization of more than 1 month in a year, or (at time of diagnosis) is likely to do either of these.

circumcision surgical removal of all or part of the foreskin (prepuce) of the penis.

classification ability to group objects by order of rank, grade, or class.

clonus rapid involuntary muscle contraction and relaxation.

clove hitch restraints restraints used to secure an arm or leg, most often when a child is receiving an intravenous infusion. The restraint is made of soft cloth formed in a figure eight.

co-dependent parent the parent who supports, directly or indirectly, the other parent's addictive behavior.

cognitive development progressive change in the intellectual process, including perception, memory, and judgment.

colic recurrent paroxysmal bouts of abdominal pain that are fairly common among young infants and that usually disappear around the age of 3 months.

colostrum thin, yellowish, milky fluid secreted by the mother's breasts during pregnancy or just after delivery (before the secretion of milk).

comedones a collection of keratin and sebum in the hair follicle; blackhead; whitehead.

communal family alternative family in which members share responsibility for homemaking and child-rearing; all children are the collective responsibility of adult members.

conception occurs when a sperm cell reaches and penetrates an ovum.

conduction heat loss that occurs when the neonate's skin is in direct contact with a cooler solid object.

congenital hip dysplasia abnormal fetal development of the acetabulum that may or may not cause dislocation of the hip. If the malformed acetabulum permits dislocation, the head of the femur displaces upward and backward. May be difficult to recognize in early infancy.

congestive heart failure (CHF) the result of impaired pumping capability of the heart. It may appear the first year of life in infants with conditions such as large ventricular septal defects, coarctation of the aorta, and other defects that place an increased workload on the ventricles.

conjunctivitis an acute inflammation of the conjunctiva that may be caused by a virus, bacteria, allergy, or foreign body.

conservation ability to recognize that change in shape does not necessarily mean change in amount or mass.

contractures fibrous scarring that forms over a movable body part that had been burned; this part of the healing process can cause serious deformities and limit movement.

convection heat loss similar to conduction but increased by moving air currents.

cooperative play children play with each other, as in team sports.

coryza runny nose.

cradle cap an accumulation of oil and dirt that often forms on an infant's scalp; seborrheic dermatitis.

craniotabes softening of the occipital bones caused by a reduction of mineralization of the skull.

croup a general term that typically exhibits symptoms of a barking cough, hoarseness, and inspiratory stridor.

currant jelly stools stools that consist of blood and mucus.

cyanotic heart disease a congenital heart disease that causes right-to-left shunting of blood in the heart resulting in a depletion of oxygen to such an extent that the oxygen saturation of the peripheral arterial blood is 85% or less. Defects that permit right-to-left shunting may occur at the atrial, ventricular, or aortic level.

dawdling wasting time; whiling away time; being idle.

débridement removal of necrotic tissue.

decentration ability to see several aspects of a problem at the same time and understand the relationship of various parts to the whole situation.

deciduous teeth primary teeth that usually erupt between 6 and 8 months of age.

deliriants inhalants that contain chemicals that give off fumes that can produce symptoms of confusion, disorientation, excitement, and hallucinations.

denial a defense mechanism in which the existence of unpleasant actions or ideas is unconsciously repressed; in the grieving process, one of the stages many people go through; also, a type of response of caregivers when caring for chronically ill children exhibited by the caregivers' denial of the existence of the condition and caregivers' encouragement of the child to overcompensate for any disabilities.

dependence a compulsive need to use a substance for its satisfying or pleasurable effects.

dependent nursing actions nursing actions that the nurse performs as a result of a physician's orders, such as administering analgesics for pain.

desensitization immunization therapy by injection; immunotherapy.

development the progressive change in the child's maturation.

developmental tasks basic achievements associated with each stage of development; these tasks must be mastered to successfully move on to the next developmental stage. Developmental tasks must be completed successfully at each stage for a person to achieve maturity.

diabetic acidosis characterized by drowsiness, dry skin, flushed cheeks, cherry red lips, acetone breath with a fruity smell as a result of excessive ketones in the blood in uncontrolled diabetes.

differentiation changes in the dividing cells, creating specialized tissues necessary to form an organized, coordinated, unique individual.

diplopia double vision.

discipline to train or instruct to produce a particular behavior pattern, especially moral or mental improvement, and self-control.

dominant gene gene that is expressed in only one of a chromosomal pair.

ductus arteriosus the prenatal blood vessel between the pulmonary artery and the aorta that closes functionally within the first 3 or 4 days of life.

ductus venosus the prenatal blood vessel between the umbilical vein and the inferior vena cava; does not achieve complete closure until the end of the second month of life.

dysarthria poor speech articulation.

dysfunctional family family that is not able to resolve routine stresses in a positive, socially acceptable manner.

dysmenorrhea painful menstruation.

dysphagia difficulty in swallowing.

early adolescence begins at about age 10 in girls and about age 12 in boys with a dramatic growth spurt that signals the advent of puberty; preadolescence; pubescence.

echolalia "parrot speech" typical of autistic children; they echo words they hear, such as a television commercial, but do not appear to understand the words.

ego in psychoanalytic theory, the conscious self that controls the pleasure principle of the id by delaying the instincts until an appropriate time.

egocentric concerned only with one's own activities or needs; unable to put oneself in another's place or to see another's point of view.

elbow restraints restraints made of muslin with two layers. Pockets wide enough to fit tongue depressors are placed vertically along the width of the fabric. The restraints are wrapped around the arm to prevent the infant from bending the arm.

elderly primigravida woman becoming pregnant for the first time after the age of 35 years.

electrolytes chemical compounds (minerals) that break down into ions when placed in water.

embryo the products of conception from the second to the eighth week of pregnancy.

emetic an agent that causes vomiting.

en face position establishment of eye contact in the same vertical plane between the caregiver and infant; extremely important to parent–infant bonding. This is also called mutual gazing.

encephalopathy degenerative disease of the brain.

encopresis chronic involuntary fecal soiling with no medical cause.

enteric precautions procedures issued by the Centers for Disease Control required in the care of children with gastroenteritis to prevent the spread of possibly infectious organisms to other pediatric patients.

enuresis involuntary urination, especially at night; bedwetting beyond the usual age of control.

epiphyses growth centers at the end of long bones and at the wrists.

epistaxis nose bleed.

erythema toxicum fine rash of the newborn that may appear over the trunk, back, abdomen, and buttocks. It appears about 24 hours after birth and disappears in several days.

erythroblastosis fetalis hemolytic disease of the newborn in which maternal antiRh antibodies in the infant's system destroy the infant's Rh containing red blood cells producing severe anemia and hyperbilirubinemia.

eschar hard crust or scab.

esotropia eye deviation toward the other eye.

evaporation heat loss through conversion of a liquid to a vapor.

exotropia an eye turning away from the other eye.

extended family consists of one or more nuclear families plus other relatives, often crossing generations to include grandparents, aunts, uncles, and cousins. The needs of individual members are subordinate to the needs of the group, and the children are considered an economic asset.

external hordeolum a purulent infection of the follicle of an eyelash, generally caused by *Staphylococcus aureus*. Localized swelling, tenderness, and pain are present with a reddened lid edge; a sty.

extracellular fluid fluid situated outside a cell or cells.

extravasation escape of fluid into surrounding tissue.

extrusion reflex infant's way of taking food by thrusting his or her tongue forward as if to suck, which has the effect of pushing the solid food right out of the mouth.

febrile seizure seizure occurring in infants and young children commonly associated with high fever of 102°F to 106°F (38.9°C to 41.1°C).

fertilization the process by which the male's sperm unites with the female's ovum.

fetal alcohol syndrome (FAS) symptoms seen in an infant born to a woman who abused alcohol during pregnancy, including shorter stature, lower birth weight, possible microcephaly, facial deformities, hearing disorders, poor coordination, minor joint and limb abnormalities, heart defects, delayed development, and mental retardation.

fetus the term for the organism after it has reached the eighth week of life and acquires a human likeness.

fiberoptic blanket a specialized pad with illuminating plastic fibers used to break down bilirubin in an infant's blood: The blanket is covered with a disposable protective cover that disperses therapeutic light when wrapped around the infant; an alternative type of phototherapy.

fontanelle a "soft spot" covered by a tough membrane at the junctures of the six bones of a newborn's skull. At birth the two fontanelles can be detected—the anterior fontanelle at the juncture of the frontal and parietal bones and the posterior fontanelle at the junction of the parietal and occipital bones. They are ossified (filled in by bone) during the normal growth process.

foramen ovale an opening between the left and right atria of the fetal heart that closes with the first breath.

forceps marks noticeable marks on the infant's face if delivery was assisted with the use of forceps. These marks usually disappear within a day or two.

gag reflex the reaction to any stimulation of the posterior pharynx by food, suction, or the passage of a tube that causes elevation of the soft palate and a strong involuntary effort to vomit. The gag reflex continues throughout life.

galactosemia a recessive hereditary metabolic disorder in which the enzyme necessary for converting galactose into glucose is missing. The infants generally appear normal at birth, but experience difficulties after the ingestion of milk.

gastroenteritis infectious diarrhea caused by infectious organisms, including salmonella, *Escherichia coli*, dysentery bacilli, and various viruses, most notable rotaviruses.

gastrostomy tube surgically inserted through the abdominal wall into the stomach, this procedure is performed under general anesthesia. It is used in children who have obstructions or surgical repairs in the mouth, pharynx, esophagus, or cardiac sphincter of the stomach or who are respiratory dependent.

gavage feeding nourishment provided directly through a tube passed into the stomach.

genes units threaded along chromosomes that carry genetic instructions from one generation to another. Like chromosomes, genes also occur in pairs. There are thousands of genes in the chromosomes of each cell nucleus.

genetic counseling study of the family history and tissue analysis of both partners to determine chromosome patterns for couples concerned about transmitting a specific disease to their unborn children.

genetic code blueprint for the development of the individual organism.

genotype each person's unique set of genes.

gestation the period of development from fertilization to birth; the length in time of a pregnancy.

goniotomy surgical opening into Schlemm's canal that provides drainage of aqueous humor; performed to relieve intraocular pressure in glaucoma.

gradual acceptance a type of response of caregivers when caring for chronically ill children exhibited by the caregivers' adoption of a common sense approach to the child's condition, encouraging the child to function within the child's capabilities.

granulocytes a type of white blood cell; divided into eosinophils, basophils, and neutrophils.

growth result of cell division and marked by an increase in size and weight; the physical increase in size and appearance of the body caused by increasing numbers of new cells.

gynecomastia excessive growth of the mammary glands in the male.

halo traction a metal ring attached to the skull is added to a body cast using stainless steel pins inserted into the skull and into the femurs or iliac wings.

health maintenance organizations (HMOs) professional groups of physicians, laboratory service personnel, nurse practitioners, nurses, and consultants who care for the health of a family on a continuing basis and are geared to health care and disease prevention. The family pays a set fee for total care; any necessary hospitalization is covered by that fee. The emphasis is on health and prevention.

hemarthrosis bleeding into the joints.

hemolysis destruction of red blood cells with the release of hemoglobin into the plasma.

hernia the abnormal protrusion of a part of an organ through a weak spot or other abnormal opening in a body wall.

heterograft a graft of tissue obtained from an animal; for burn patients, pig skin (porcine) is often used.

heterosexual relationship intimate relationship of two people of opposite sex.

heterozygous term used to describe a particular trait of an individual when each member of a pair of genes carries different instructions for that trait.

hierarchical arrangement grouping by some common system, such as rank, grade, or class.

high risk nursing diagnoses a category of diagnoses that identify those health problems to which the patient is especially vulnerable.

hirsutism abnormal body and facial hair growth.

homeostasis a uniform state; signifies biologically the dynamic equilibrium of the healthy organism.

homosexual relationship intimate relationship of two people of the same sex.

homozygous term used to describe a particular trait of

an individual when any two members of a pair of genes carry the same genetic instructions for that trait.

hospice provides comforting and supportive care to terminally ill patients and their families. There are few hospice programs for children in the United States.

hyaline membrane disease also known as respiratory distress syndrome (RDS); occurs due to immature lungs, which lack sufficient surfactant to decrease the surface tension of the alveoli; affects about half of all preterm newborns.

hydrops fetalis excessive edema, marked anemia, jaundice, and enlargement of the liver and spleen resulting from erythroblastosis fetalis.

hydrotherapy use of water in a treatment.

hyperalimentation also called total parenteral nutrition (TPN). The administration of dextrose, lipids, amino acids, electrolytes, vitamins, minerals, and trace elements into the circulatory system to meet the nutritional needs of the child whose needs cannot be met through the gastrointestinal tract.

hyperlipidemia an increase in the level of cholesterol in the blood.

hyperopia a refractive condition in which the person can see objects better at a distance; farsightedness.

hyperpnea increase in depth of breathing.

hyperthermia excessive overheating of an infant.

hypocholia diminished flow of pancreatic enzymes.

hypothermia low body temperature; may be a symptom of a disease or dysfunction of the temperature-regulating mechanism of the body, or it may be deliberately induced, such as during open heart surgery, to reduce the child's oxygen needs and provide a longer window of time for the surgeon to complete the operation without brain damage. When caring for the newborn, it is important to remember that heat loss can lead to hypothermia because of the infant's immature temperature-regulating system.

hypovolemia decreased volume of circulating plasma.

id in psychoanalytic theory, part of the personality that controls physical needs and instincts of the body; dominated by the pleasure principle.

imperforate anus congenital disorder in which the rectal pouch ends blindly above the anus, and there is no anal orifice.

impunity belief, common among adolescents, that nothing can hurt them.

incest sexually arousing physical contact between family members not married to each other.

independent nursing actions nursing actions that may be performed based on the nurse's own clinical judgment.

induration hardness.

inhalants substance that may be taken into the body through inhaling; substances whose volatile vapors can be abused.

insulin reaction excessively low blood sugar caused by insulin overload, resulting in too rapid metabolism of the body's glucose; insulin shock; hypoglycemia.

intercurrent infection infections that occur during the course of an already existing disease.

interdependent nursing actions nursing actions that the nurse must work with other health team members to accomplish, such as meal planning with a dietary therapist and teaching breathing exercises with a respiratory therapist.

interstitial fluid also called intracellular or tissue fluid, has a composition similar to plasma except that it contains almost no protein. This reservoir of fluid outside the body cells decreases or increases easily in response to disease.

interstitial keratitis inflammation of the cornea, often caused by congenital syphilis and usually accompanied by lacrimation, photophobia, and opacity of the lens; may lead to blindness.

intracellular fluid fluid contained within the cell membranes; constitutes about two-thirds of the total body fluids.

intrathecal administration injection into the cerebrospinal fluid by lumbar puncture.

intravascular fluid fluid situated within the blood vessels or blood plasma.

invagination telescoping; the infolding of one part of a structure into another.

karyotype the chromosomal constitution of the cell nucleus; the photomicrograph of chromosomes used to locate malformations and translocations.

kernicterus severe brain damage as a result of excessive bilirubin levels.

Kussmaul breathing abnormal increase in the depth and rate of the respiratory movements.

kwashiorkor syndrome occurring in infants and young children soon after weaning, resulting from severe deficiency of protein. Symptoms include a swollen abdomen, retarded growth with muscle wasting, edema, gastrointestinal changes, thin dry hair with patchy alopecia, apathy, and irritability.

kyphoscoliosis backward and lateral curvature of the spine; hunchback.

lacrimation secretion of tears.

lactose a sugar found in milk that, when hydrolyzed, yields glucose and galactose.

lactose intolerance inability to digest lactose because of an inborn deficiency of the enzyme lactase.

lanugo fine, downy hair that covers the skin of the fetus.

latchkey child child who comes home to an empty house after school each day because the family caregivers are at work.

lecithin major component of surfactant.

leukemia the uncontrolled reproduction of deformed white blood cells.

leukopenia leukocyte count less than 5000 mm^3.

libido the sexual drive.

lordosis forward curvature of lumbar spine; swayback.

lymphoblasts a lymphocyte that has been changed by antigenic stimulation to a structurally immature lymphocyte.

lymphocytes single nucleus, nonphagocytic leukocytes that are instrumental in the body's immune response.

magical thinking child's belief that thoughts are powerful and can cause something to happen (eg, illness or death of a loved one occurs because the child wished it in a moment of anger).

marasmus deficiency in calories as well as protein. The child suffers from growth retardation and wasting of subcutaneous fat and muscle.

meconium the first stools of the newborn; a sticky, greenish black substance composed of bile, mucus, cellular waste, intestinal secretions, fat, hair, and other materials swallowed during fetal life, together with amniotic fluid.

menarche beginning of menstruation.

metered dose inhaler hand-held plastic device that delivers a premeasured dose of medicine.

microcephaly small head.

micrognathia abnormal smallness of the lower jaw.

milia pearly white cysts usually seen over the bridge of the nose, chin, and cheeks of a newborn. They are usually retention cysts of sebaceous glands or hair follicles and disappear within a few weeks without treatment.

mittelschmerz pain experienced midcycle of the menstrual cycle, at the time of ovulation.

mongolian spots areas of bluish-black pigmentation resembling bruises. Most often seen over the sacral or gluteal regions of infants of African, Mediterranean, Native American, or Asian descent, and they usually fade within 1 or 2 years.

monocytes 5% to 10% of white blood cells that defend the body against infection.

Moro reflex abduction of the arms and legs and flexion of the elbows in response to a sudden loud noise, jarring, or abrupt change in equilibrium: fingers flare except the forefinger and thumb, which are clenched to form a C-shape. Occurs in the normal newborn up to the end of the 4th or 5th month.

mother-baby nursing the cross-education of postpartum and nursery nurses, so that one nurse takes care of both mother and infant. The infant's bassinet is kept beside the mother who participates in caring for her newborn while being carefully guided and taught by the nurse.

mummy restraint used to restrain an infant or small child during procedures that involve only the head or neck.

mutation fundamental change that takes place in the structure of a gene, resulting in the transmission of a trait different from that normally carried by that particular gene.

mutual gazing see *en face position*.

myopia the ability to see objects clearly at close range but not at a distance; nearsightedness.

myringotomy incision of the eardrum performed to establish drainage and to insert tiny tubes into the tympanic membrane to facilitate drainage of serous or purulent fluid in the middle ear.

nebulizer tube attached to a wall unit or cylinder that delivers moist air via a face mask.

necrotizing enterocolitis (NEC) an acute inflammatory disease of the intestine that occurs most often in small preterm infants; necrotic patches develop interfering with digestion and can result in perforation and peritonitis.

negativism opposition to suggestion or advice; associated with the toddler age group because the toddler in search of autonomy, frequently responds "no" to almost everything.

neonatal abstinence syndrome (NAS) symptoms seen in the newborn of the woman who has abused substances during pregnancy; withdrawal symptoms.

neonate term used to describe a newborn in the first 28 days of life.

noncommunicative language egocentric speech exhibited by children who talk to themselves, toys, or pets without any purpose other than the pleasure of using words.

nuchal rigidity stiff neck.

nuclear family family structure that consists of only the father, the mother, and the children living in one household.

nursing process a proven form of problem solving based on the scientific method. The nursing process consists of five components: assessment, nursing diagnosis, planning, implementation, and evaluation.

obesity   an excessive accumulation of fat that increases body weight by 20% or more over ideal weight.

objective data   in the nursing assessment, the data gained by direct observation by the nurse.

oliguria   decrease production of urine, especially in relation to fluid intake.

onlooker play   an interest in the observation of an activity without participation.

opisthotonos   arching of the back so that the head and the heels are bent backward and the body is forward.

orchiopexy   surgical procedure used to bring an undescended testis down into the scrotum and anchor it there.

organogenesis   process by which cells differentiate into major organ systems; commences shortly after conception and is almost completed by the end of the eighth week.

orthoptics   therapeutic exercises to improve the quality of vision.

overprotection   a type of response of caregivers when caring for chronically ill children exhibited by the caregivers' protecting the child at all costs, preventing the child from achieving new skills by hovering, avoiding the use of discipline, and using every means to prevent the child from suffering any frustration.

overriding aorta   in Tetralogy of Fallot the aorta shifts to the right over the opening in the ventricular septum so that blood from both the right and left ventricles are pumped into the aorta.

overweight   generally considered to be characteristic of people more than 10% over their ideal weight.

palmar grasp reflex   phenomenon that results as pressure on the palms of the hands or soles of the feet near the base of the digits causes flexion of hands or toes.

palpebral fissures   the opening between the eyes.

papoose board   a commercial restraint board for use with toddlers or preschool age children that uses canvas strips to secure the child's body and canvas strips to secure the extremities. One extremity can be released to allow treatment to be performed on that extremity.

parallel play   child play alongside another child or children involved in the same type of activity, but not interacting with each other.

patient controlled analgesia (PCA)   a programmed intravenous infusion of narcotic analgesia that an individual may control within set limits.

pediatric nurse practitioner (PNP)   a professional nurse prepared at the postbaccalaureate level to give primary health care to children and families; use pediatricians or family physicians as consultants, but offer day-to-day assessment and care.

pedodontist   dentist who specializes in the care and treatment of children's teeth.

petechiae   small bluish purple spots caused by tiny broken capillaries; pinpoint hemorrhages beneath the skin.

phenylketonuria (PKU)   a recessive hereditary defect of metabolism that results in a congenital disease due to a defect in the enzyme that normally changes the essential amino acid, phenylalanine, into tyrosine. If untreated, PKU results in severe mental retardation.

philtrum   the vertical groove in the middle of the upper lip.

phimosis   adherence of the foreskin to the glans penis.

photophobia   intolerance to light.

photosensitivity   sensitivity to sunlight.

phototherapy   exposure of newborns to fluorescent lights to prevent bilirubin concentration from reaching dangerous levels.

physiologic jaundice   (icterus neonatorum) jaundice that occurs in a large number of newborns that has no medical significance; the result of the breakdown of fetal red blood cells.

pica   compulsive eating of nonfood substances.

placenta   organ linking the fetus to the mother; performs four functions for the developing fetus: respiration, nutrition, excretion, and protection; also called afterbirth.

play therapy   a technique of psychoanalysis that psychiatrists or psychiatric nurse clinicians use to uncover a disturbed child's underlying thoughts, feelings, and motivations to help understand them better.

polyarthritis   inflammation of several joints.

polydipsia   abnormal thirst.

polyphagia   increased food consumption.

polyuria   dramatic increase in urinary output; often with enuresis.

postterm (postmature) infant   one born after completion of the 42nd week of gestation, regardless of birth weight.

premenstrual syndrome (PMS)   symptoms in the period before menstruation, including edema (resulting in weight gain), headache, increased anxiety, mild depression, or mood swings; premenstrual tension.

preterm (premature) infant   any infant of less than 37 weeks' gestation.

priapism   a perpetual abnormal erection of the penis.

primary nursing   a system whereby one nurse plans the total care for a child and directs the efforts of nurses on the other shifts.

pruritus itching.

pseudomenses (false menstruation) a slight red-tinged vaginal discharge in female infants resulting from a decline in the hormonal level after birth compared with the higher concentration in the maternal hormone environment before birth.

pseudostrabismus the cross-eyed look found in infants due to incomplete development of the nerves and muscles that control focusing and coordination; begins to disappear in the sixth month.

puberty the period during which secondary sexual characteristics begin to develop and reproductive maturity is attained.

pulmonary stenosis a narrowing of the opening between the right ventricle and the pulmonary artery, decreasing the flow of blood to the lungs.

pulse oximeter a photoelectric device used to measure oxygen saturation in an artery. Can be attached to a finger, toe, or the heel of an infant.

punishment penalty given for wrongdoing.

purpura hemorrhages into the skin or the mucous membranes.

purpuric rash a rash consisting of ecchymoses (bruises) and petechiae caused by bleeding under the skin.

radiation in heat loss it is the transfer of body heat to cooler solid objects that are not in direct contact with the infant.

recessive gene a gene carrying different information for a trait within a pair that is not expressed (eg, blue eyes versus brown eyes). A recessive gene is only detectable when present on both chromosomes.

refraction the way light rays bend as they pass through the lens of the eye to the retina.

regurgitation spitting up of small quantities of milk, which occurs rather easily in the young infant.

rejection a type of response of caregivers when caring for chronically ill children exhibited by the caregivers' distancing themselves emotionally from the child and, although they provide physical care, a tendency to continuously scold and correct the child.

respiratory distress syndrome (RDS) see *hyaline membrane disease*.

respite care care of the child by someone other than the usual caregiver so that the caregiver can have an opportunity to get temporary relief and rest.

retinopathy of prematurity (ROP) an overgrowth of blood vessels of the eye caused by constriction of the capillaries of the retina due to high blood concentration of oxygen.

retrolental fibroplasia (RLF) the final stage of ROP in which scarring occurs resulting in retinal detachment and blindness.

reversibility ability to think in either direction.

RhoGAM a commercial preparation of Rh_o (D antigen) immune globulin given to nonsensitized Rh negative mothers.

right ventricular hypertrophy increase in thickness of the myocardium of the right ventricle.

ritualism practice employed by the young child to help develop security; consists of following a certain routine, making rituals of simple tasks.

rooming-in an arrangement in which the health care facility permits a family caregiver to stay with a child and that provides a cot or sleeping chair for the caregiver to rest.

rooting reflex the infant's response of turning the head when the cheek is stroked toward the stroked side.

rumination voluntary regurgitation.

runaway child a child who is absent from home for overnight or longer without the permission of the caregiver.

school phobia fear of child resulting in dread of a school situation or fear of leaving home; can be a combination of both.

scoliosis lateral curvature of the spine.

sebum oily secretion of the sebaceous glands.

seizure a series of involuntary contractions of voluntary muscles; convulsion.

sex chromosomes one pair of chromosomes that differ in the male and the female.

sexual assault sexual contact made by someone who is not functioning in a role of caretaker of the child.

sexual abuse sexual contact between a child and another peron in a caretaking position, such as a parent, a babysitter, or a teacher.

single-parent family household headed by one adult of either sex; there may be one or more children in the family.

skeletal traction pulls exerted directly on skeletal structures by means of pins, wire, tongs, or another device surgically inserted through the bone.

skin traction pulls on tape, rubber, or plastic materials attached to the skin and indirectly exerting pull on the musculoskeletal system.

small for gestational age (SGA) expression used to signify term infants of low birth weight.

smegma the cheese-like secretion of the sebaceous glands found under the foreskin.

socialization the process by which a child learns the rules of the society and culture in which the family lives: its language, values, ethics, and acceptable behaviors.

soft neurological signs signs of clumsiness or poor coordination that may be appropriate for a younger child.

solitary independent play playing apart from others without making an effort to be part of the group or their activity.

spina bifida the failure of the posterior laminate of the vertebrae to close, leaving an opening through which the spinal meninges and spinal cord may protrude.

startle reflex follows any loud noise; similar to the Moro reflex, but the hands remain clenched, and this reflex is never lost.

steatorrhea fatty stools.

step reflex also called the dance reflex, the tendency of infants to make stepping movements when held upright.

stepfamily consists of custodial parent, children, and a new spouse.

stigma negative perception of a person because that person is believed to be different from the general population; may cause a feeling of embarrassment or shame by the person being stigmatized.

strabismus the failure of the two eyes to direct their gaze at the same object simultaneously; squint; crossed eyes.

striae stretch marks.

stridor shrill, harsh respiratory sound, usually on inspiration.

subjective data in the nursing assessment, the data spoken by the child or family.

sublimation process of directing a desire or impulse into more acceptable behaviors.

sucking reflex the infant's response of strong, vigorous sucking when a nipple, finger, or tongue blade is put in the infant's mouth.

superego in psychoanalytic theory the conscience or parental value system; acts primarily as a monitor over the ego.

supernumerary excessive in number (eg, more than the usual number of teeth).

surfactant a surface-active agent produced in the alveoli of the lungs that reduces surface tension inside the alveoli and bronchioles, preventing collapse and allowing free air exchange.

suture a narrow band of connective tissue that divides the six ununited bones of a newborn's skull.

swaddling wrapping securely in a small blanket.

sympathetic ophthalmia an inflammatory reaction of the uninjured eye; symptoms can include photophobia, lacrimation, and some dimness of vision.

synovitis inflammation of a joint, most commonly the hip in children.

talipes equinovarus clubfoot with plantar flexion.

temper tantrum behavior in children that springs from frustrations caused by their urge for independence. A violent display of temper. The child reacts with enthusiastic rebellion against the wishes of the caregiver.

teratogens (from the Greek *terato*, meaning monster, and *genesis*, meaning birth), an agent or influence that causes a defect or disruption in the prenatal growth process. The effect of a teratogen depends on when it enters the fetal system and in the stages of differentiation of the various organs or organ systems at that time. Generally, the fetus is most vulnerable to teratogens during the first trimester.

term infant infant born between the beginning of the 38th week and the end of the 42nd week of gestation, regardless of birth weight.

thanatologist a person trained especially to work with the dying and their families, sometimes a nurse.

therapeutic play play technique that may be used by play therapists, nurses, child-life specialists, or trained volunteers.

thermoregulation regulation of the infant's temperature.

throwaway child child (frequently a teenager) who has been forced to leave home and is not wanted back by the adults in the home.

tinea ringworm.

tissue perfusion circulation of blood through the capillaries carrying nutrients and oxygen to the cells.

tolerance in substance abuse, the ability of body tissues to endure and adapt to continued or increased use of a substance.

tonic neck reflex also called the fencing reflex; seen when the infant lies on the back, with the head turned to one side and the arm and leg on that side extended, the opposite arm flexed as if in a fencing position.

tonsils two oval masses attached to the side walls of the back of the mouth between the anterior and posterior pillars (folds of mucous membranes at the side of the passage from the mouth to the pharynx).

total parenteral nutrition (TPN) often called hyperalimentation; the administration of dextrose, lipids, amino acids, electrolytes, vitamins, minerals, and trace elements into the circulatory system to meet the nutritional needs of the child whose needs cannot be met through the gastrointestinal tract.

traction force applied to an extremity or other part of the body to maintain proper alignment and facilitate healing for a fractured bone or dislocated joint.

trimester period of 3 months; pregnancy is divided into 3 trimesters.

tympanic membrane sensor device used to determine the temperature of the tympanic membrane by rapidly sensing infrared radiation from the membrane. The tympanic thermometer offers the advantage of recording the temperature rapidly with little disturbance to the child.

umbilical cord connects the fetus to the placenta; contains one vein and two arteries that carry the blood supply between the developing fetus and the placenta.

unfinished business completing those matters that will help to ease the death of a loved one; saying the unsaid and doing the undone acts of love and caring that may seem difficult to express. Recognizing time is limited and filling that time with the important issues that need to be taken care of.

unilateral one side, such as in cleft lip only one side of the lip is cleft.

unoccupied behavior daydreaming, fingering clothing or a toy without any apparent purpose.

urticaria hives.

vaginitis inflammation of the vagina.

vascular nevus commonly known as a strawberry mark, a slightly raised, bright-red collection of hypertrophied skin capillaries that does not blanch completely on pressure.

ventricular septal defect an abnormal opening in the septum of the heart between the ventricles, allowing blood to pass directly from the left to the right side of the heart. The most common intracardiac defect.

ventriculoatrial shunting implanting of a plastic tubing into the cerebral ventricle passing under the skin to the cardiac atrium, providing drainage for excessive cerebrospinal fluid.

ventriculoperitoneal shunting implanting of a plastic tubing into the cerebral ventricle passing under the skin to the peritoneal cavity, providing drainage for excessive cerebrospinal fluid. Excessive tubing can be inserted to accommodate the child's growth.

vernix caseosa a greasy cheese-like substance that protects the skin during fetal life consisting of a sebum and desquamated epithelial cells.

viability able to maintain life after birth; the age of viability is the earliest gestation age at which a fetus can survive outside the uterine environment.

wellness nursing diagnoses diagnoses that identify the potential of an individual, family, or community to move from one level of wellness to a higher level.

West nomogram a graph with several scales arranged so that when two values are known, the third can be plotted by drawing a line with a straight edge; commonly used to calculate BSA.

wheezing sound of expired air being pushed through obstructed bronchioles.

withdrawal symptoms in substance abuse, physical and psychological symptoms that occur when the drug is no longer being used.

zygote a fertilized ovum.

Resources for Families and Caretakers of Children

Appendix A

American Anorexia/Bulimia Association, Inc.
418 E. 76th St.
New York, NY 10021
212-734-1114

American Cleft Palate Association
1218 Grandview Ave.
Pittsburgh, PA 15211
800-24-CLEFT (800-242-5338)

Association for the Care of Children's Health
7910 Woodmont Ave., Ste. 300
Bethesda, MD 20814
301-654-6549

Association of Retarded Citizens of the United States
PO Box 6109
Arlington, TX 76005
817-640-0204

Autism Society of America
8601 Georgia Ave., Ste. 503
Silver Springs, MD 20910
301-565-0433

Children's Hospice International
901 Washington St., Ste. 700
Alexandria, VA 22314
800-24-CHILD (800-242-4453)

Clearinghouse for Disability Information
Room 3132, Switzer Building, C St. S.W.
Washington, DC 20202
202-732-1250

John T. Tracey Clinic
806 West Adams Blvd.
Los Angeles, CA 90007
213-748-5481

Leukemia Society of America
733 Third Ave.
New York, NY 10017
212-573-8484

March of Dimes Birth Defect Foundation
1275 Mamaroneck Ave.
White Plains, NY 10605
914-428-7100

National Association of Anorexia Nervosa and Associated Disorders, Inc. (ANAD)
PO Box 7
Highland Park, IL 60035
312-831-3438

National Childhood Grief Institute
6200 Colonial Way
Minneapolis, MN 55436
616-920-0737

National Clearinghouse for Alcohol and Drug Abuse Information
PO Box 2345
Rockville, MD 20852
800-729-6686

National Down Syndrome Society
666 Broadway, Ste. 810
New York, NY 10012
800-221-4602

National Easter Seal Society
2023 West Ogden Ave.
Chicago, IL 60612
312-243-8400

National Hydrocephalus Foundation
Route One, River Road, Box 210 A
Joliet, IL 60436
815-467-6548

National Self-Help Clearinghouse (families of chronically ill)
CUNY Graduate Center
33 W. 42nd St., Room 620 N
New York, NY 10036
212-642-2944

National Sudden Infant Death Syndrome Foundation
10500 Little Patuxen Parkway, Ste. 420
Columbia, MD 21044
800-221-5105

Parents Anonymous
7120 Franklin Ave.
Los Angeles, CA 90046
800-421-0353

Parents of Down Syndrome Children
11600 Nebel St.
Rockville, MD 20852
301-984-5792

Special Olympics
1350 New York Ave. N.W., Ste. 500
Washington, DC 2005-47009
202-628-3630

Spina Bifida Association of America
1700 Rockville Pike, Ste. 540
Rockville, MD 20852
800-621-5141

Sudden Infant Death Syndrome Clearinghouse
8201 Greensboro Drive, Ste. 600
McLean, VA 22102
703-821-8955

Youth Suicide National Center
1825 I St., N.W.
Washington, DC 20006
202-429-0190

Growth Charts

Appendix B

BOYS: BIRTH TO 36 MONTHS
PHYSICAL GROWTH
NCHS PERCENTILES*

NAME_____ RECORD #_____

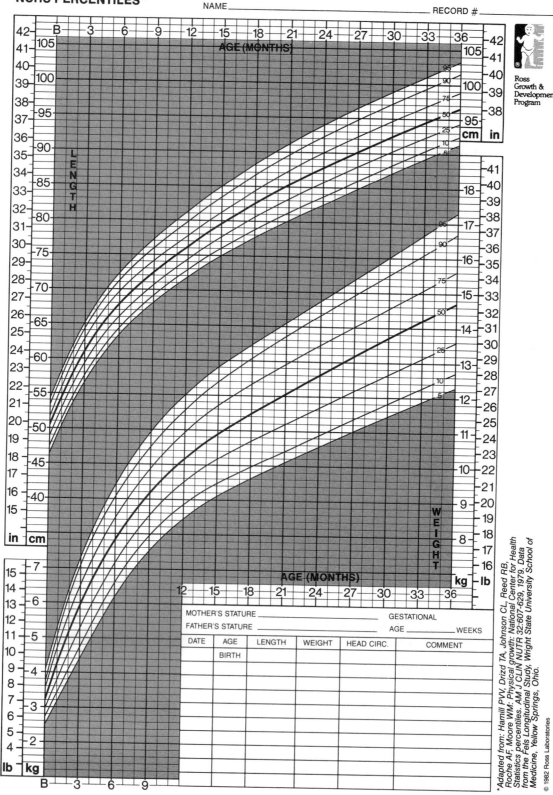

MOTHER'S STATURE _____ GESTATIONAL

FATHER'S STATURE _____ AGE _____ WEEKS

DATE	AGE	LENGTH	WEIGHT	HEAD CIRC.	COMMENT
	BIRTH				

Ross
Growth &
Development
Program

*Adapted from: Hamill PVV, Drizd TA, Johnson CL, Reed RB, Roche AF, Moore WM: Physical growth: National Center for Health Statistics percentiles. AM J CLIN NUTR 32:607-629, 1979. Data from the Fels Longitudinal Study, Wright State University School of Medicine, Yellow Springs, Ohio.

© 1982 Ross Laboratories

BOYS: BIRTH TO 36 MONTHS
PHYSICAL GROWTH
NCHS PERCENTILES*

NAME _____

RECORD # _____

AGE (MONTHS)

B 3 6 9 12 15 18 21 24 27 30 33 36

95
90
75
50
25
10
5

HEAD CIRCUMFERENCE

WEIGHT

LENGTH

cm 50 55 60 65 70 75 80 85 90 95 100
in 19 20 21 22 23 24 25 26 27 28 29 30 31 32 33 34 35 36 37 38 39 40

*Adapted from: Hamill PVV, Drizd TA, Johnson CL, Reed RB, Roche AF, Moore WM: Physical growth: National Center for Health Statistics percentiles. AM J CLIN NUTR 32:607-629, 1979. Data from the Fels Longitudinal Study, Wright State University School of Medicine, Yellow Springs, Ohio.

© 1982 Ross Laboratories

DATE	AGE	LENGTH	WEIGHT	HEAD CIRC.	COMMENT

COLUMBUS, OHIO 43216
DIVISION OF ABBOTT LABORATORIES, USA

ROSS

G105(0.05)/JANUARY 1986

LITHO IN USA

GIRLS: BIRTH TO 36 MONTHS
PHYSICAL GROWTH
NCHS PERCENTILES*

NAME _____ RECORD # _____

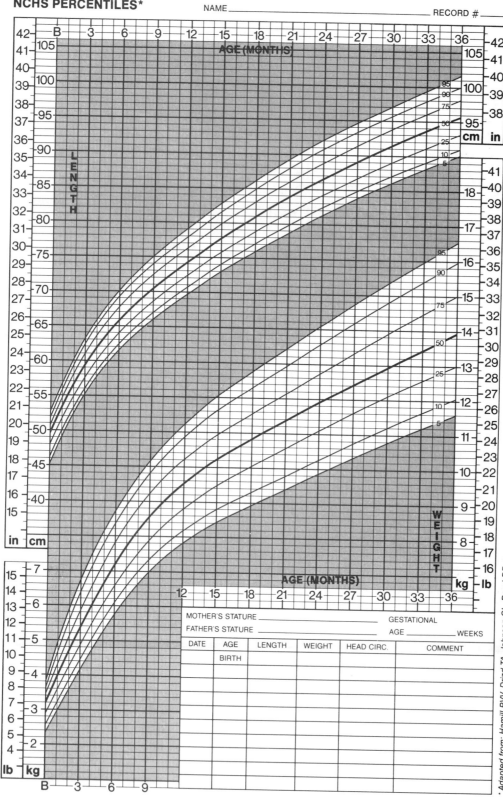

MOTHER'S STATURE _____ GESTATIONAL
FATHER'S STATURE _____ AGE _____ WEEKS

DATE	AGE	LENGTH	WEIGHT	HEAD CIRC.	COMMENT
	BIRTH				

* Adapted from: Hamill PVV, Drizd TA, Johnson CL, Reed RB, Roche AF, Moore WM: Physical growth: National Center for Health Statistics percentiles. AM J CLIN NUTR 32:607-629, 1979. Data from the Fels Longitudinal Study, Wright State University School of Medicine, Yellow Springs, Ohio.

© 1982 Ross Laboratories

Ross
Growth &
Development
Program

GIRLS: BIRTH TO 36 MONTHS
PHYSICAL GROWTH
NCHS PERCENTILES*

NAME_____ RECORD #_____

*Adapted from: Hamill PVV, Drizd TA, Johnson CL, Reed RB, Roche AF, Moore WM: Physical growth: National Center for Health Statistics percentiles. AM J CLIN NUTR 32:607-629, 1979. Data from the Fels Longitudinal Study, Wright State University School of Medicine, Yellow Springs, Ohio.

© 1982 Ross Laboratories

DATE	AGE	LENGTH	WEIGHT	HEAD CIRC.	COMMENT

ROSS LABORATORIES
COLUMBUS, OHIO 43216
DIVISION OF ABBOTT LABORATORIES, USA

G106(0.05)/APRIL 1989   LITHO IN USA

BOYS: 2 TO 18 YEARS
PHYSICAL GROWTH
National Center for Health Statistics Percentiles   NAME_____   RECORD #_____

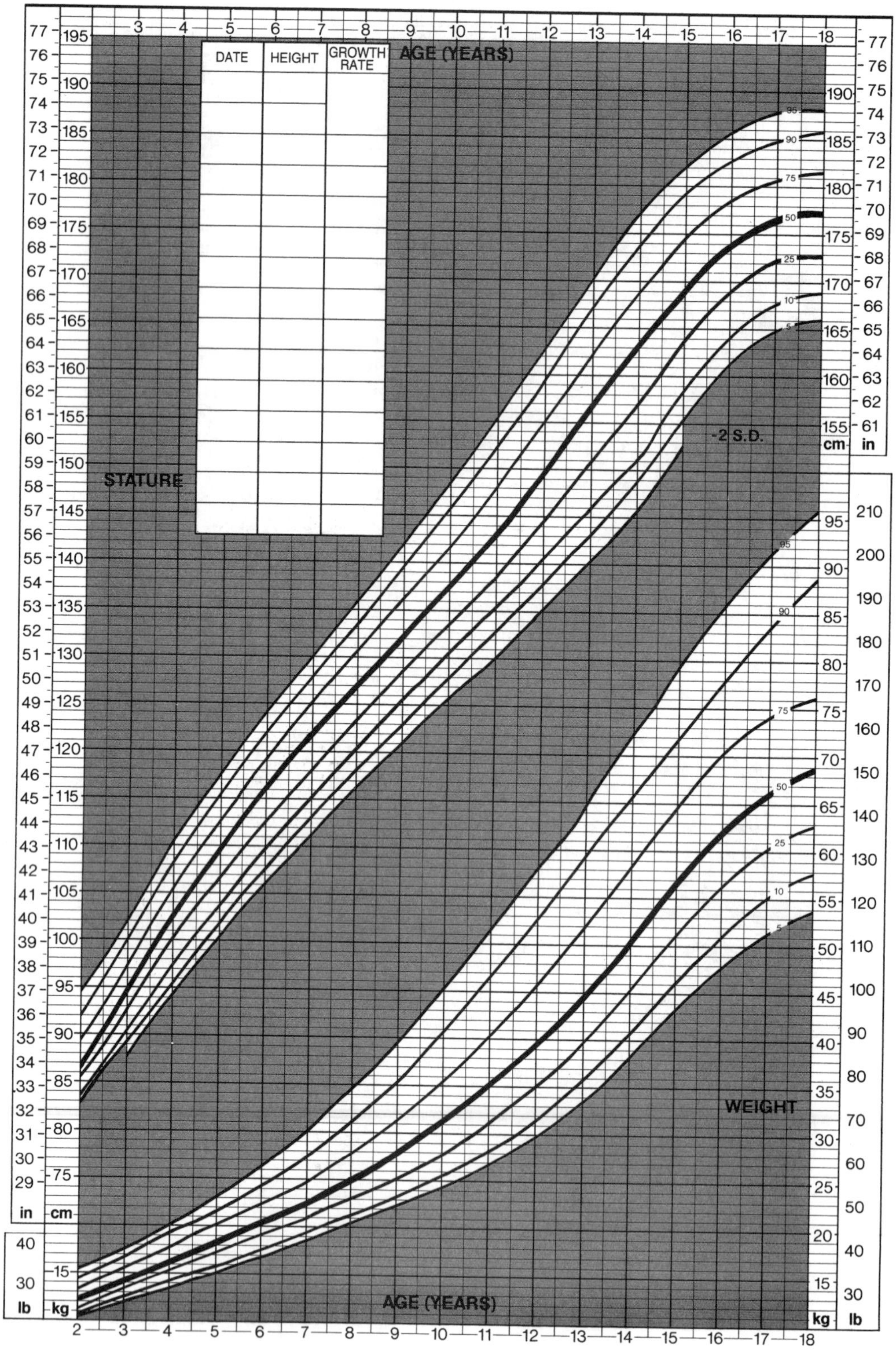

DATE	HEIGHT	GROWTH RATE

AGE (YEARS)

STATURE

WEIGHT

-2 S.D.

Provided as
a service of
Genentech, Inc

G70048-RO

GIRLS: 2 TO 18 YEARS
PHYSICAL GROWTH
National Center for Health Statistics Percentiles   NAME _____ RECORD # _____

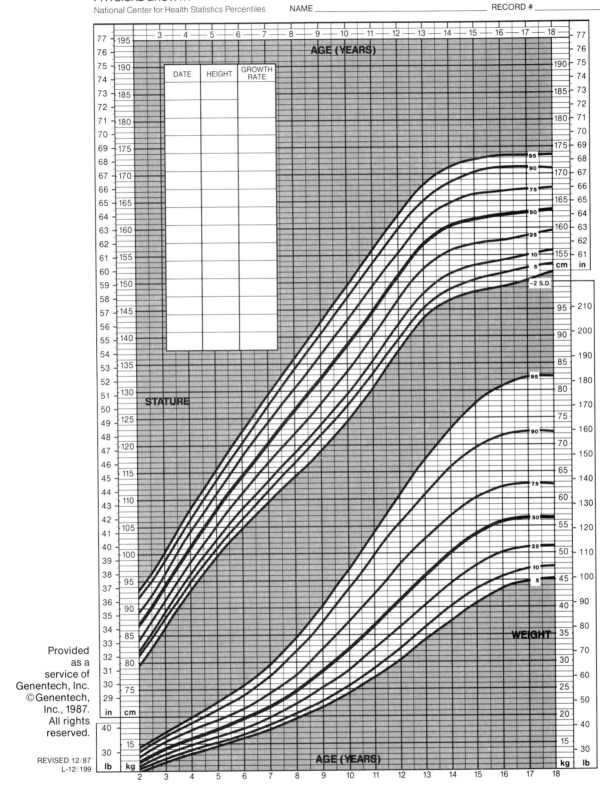

Provided
as a
service of
Genentech, Inc.
© Genentech,
Inc., 1987.
All rights
reserved.

REVISED 12/87
L-12/199

Pulse, Respiration, and Blood Pressure Values for Children

Appendix C

Normal Pulse Ranges in Children

Age	Normal Range	Average
0–24 hours	70–170 bpm	120 bpm
1–7 days	100–180 bpm	140 bpm
1 month	110–188 bpm	160 bpm
1 month–1 year	80–180 bpm	120–130 bpm
2 years	80–140 bpm	110 bpm
4 years	80–120 bpm	100 bpm
6 years	70–115 bpm	100 bpm
10 years	70–110 bpm	90 bpm
12–14 years	60–110 bpm	85–90 bpm
14–18 years	50–95 bpm	70–75 bpm

bpm, beats per minute.
From Skale N. Manual of Pediatric Nursing Procedures. Philadelphia: JB Lippincott, 1992, p. 35.

Variations in Respirations with Age

Age	Rate per Minute
Newborn	40–90
1 year	20–40
2 years	20–30
3 years	20–30
5 years	20–25
10 years	17–22
15 years	15–20
20 years	15–20

Lowrey GH. Growth and Development of Children, 6th ed. Copyright © 1973 by Year Book Medical Publishers, Inc., Chicago. Used by permission.

Normal Blood Pressure Ranges

Age	Systolic (mm Hg)	Diastolic (mm Hg)
Newborn—12 hr (less than 1000 g)	39–59	16–36
Newborn—12 hr (3000 g)	50–70	24–45
Newborn—96 hr (3000 g)	60–90	20–60
Infant	74–100	50–70
Toddler	80–112	50–80
Preschooler	82–110	50–78
School-age	84–120	54–80
Adolescent	94–140	62–88

From Skale N. Manual of Pediatric Nursing Procedures. Philadelphia: JB Lippincott, 1992, p. 46.

Conversion Charts

Conversion of Pounds to Kilograms

Pounds	0	1	2	3	4	5	6	7	8	9
0	—	0.45	0.90	1.36	1.81	2.26	2.72	3.17	3.62	4.08
10	4.53	4.98	5.44	5.89	6.35	6.80	7.25	7.71	8.16	8.61
20	9.07	9.52	9.97	10.43	10.88	11.34	11.79	12.24	12.70	13.15
30	13.60	14.06	14.51	14.96	15.42	15.87	16.32	16.78	17.23	17.69
40	18.14	18.59	19.05	19.50	19.95	20.41	20.86	21.31	21.77	22.22
50	22.68	23.13	23.58	24.04	24.49	24.94	25.40	25.85	26.30	26.76
60	27.21	27.66	28.12	28.57	29.03	29.48	29.93	30.39	30.84	31.29
70	31.75	32.20	32.65	33.11	33.56	34.02	34.47	34.92	35.38	35.83
80	36.28	36.74	37.19	37.64	38.10	38.55	39.00	39.46	39.91	40.37
90	40.82	41.27	41.73	42.18	42.63	43.09	43.54	43.99	44.45	44.90
100	45.36	45.81	46.26	46.72	47.17	47.62	48.08	48.53	48.98	49.44
110	49.89	50.34	50.80	51.25	51.71	52.16	52.61	53.07	53.52	53.97
120	54.43	54.88	55.33	55.79	56.24	56.70	57.15	57.60	58.06	58.51
130	58.96	59.42	59.87	60.32	60.78	61.23	61.68	62.14	62.59	63.05
140	63.50	63.95	64.41	64.86	65.31	65.77	66.22	66.67	67.13	67.58
150	68.04	68.49	68.94	69.40	69.85	70.30	70.76	71.21	71.66	72.12
160	72.57	73.02	73.48	73.93	74.39	74.84	75.29	75.75	76.20	76.65
170	77.11	77.56	78.01	78.47	78.92	79.38	79.83	80.28	80.74	81.19
180	81.64	82.10	82.55	83.00	83.46	83.91	84.36	84.82	85.27	85.73
190	86.18	86.68	87.09	87.54	87.99	88.45	88.90	89.35	89.81	90.26
200	90.72	91.17	91.62	92.08	92.53	92.98	93.44	93.89	94.34	94.80

Conversion of Fahrenheit to Celsius

Celsius	Fahrenheit	Celsius	Fahrenheit	Celsius	Fahrenheit
34.0	93.2	37.0	98.6	40.0	104.0
34.2	93.6	37.2	99.0	40.2	104.4
34.4	93.9	37.4	99.3	40.4	104.7
34.6	94.3	37.6	99.7	40.6	105.2
34.8	94.6	37.8	100.0	40.8	105.4
35.0	95.0	38.0	100.4	41.0	105.9
35.2	95.4	38.2	100.8	41.2	106.1
35.4	95.7	38.4	101.1	41.4	106.5
35.6	96.1	38.6	101.5	41.6	106.8
35.8	96.4	38.8	101.8	41.8	107.2
36.0	96.8	39.0	102.2	42.0	107.6
36.2	97.2	39.2	102.6	42.2	108.0
36.4	97.5	39.4	102.9	42.4	108.3
36.6	97.9	39.6	103.3	42.6	108.7
36.8	98.2	39.8	103.6	42.8	109.0
				43.0	109.4

$(°C) \times (9/5) + 32 = °F.$

$(°F - 32) \times (5/9) = °C.$

Index

Note: Page numbers in *italics* indicate illustrations; page numbers followed by t indicate tables; page numbers followed by b indicate boxed material

Universal Precautions

Human immunodeficiency virus (HIV), the virus that causes acquired immunodeficiency syndrome (AIDS), is transmitted during sexual contact, through the sharing of intravenous drug needles and syringes while "shooting" drugs, through exposure to infected blood or blood components, and perinatally from mother to neonate. Currently there is neither a cure for nor an immunization to prevent AIDS. The increasing prevalence of HIV increases the risk that health care workers will be exposed to blood from patients infected with HIV.

The Centers for Disease Control in Atlanta has developed "Universal Precautions" (formerly called "Universal Blood and Body Fluid Precautions") as recommendations to all health care workers. Under universal precautions, blood and certain body fluids of **all** patients are considered potentially infectious for HIV, hepatitis B virus (HBV), and other bloodborne pathogens. Universal precautions are intended to prevent parenteral, mucous membrane, and nonintact skin exposures of health care workers to bloodborne pathogens. In addition, immunization with HBV vaccine is recommended as an important adjunct to universal precautions for health care workers who have been exposed to blood. (The implementation of control measures for HIV and HBV does not obviate the need for continued adherence to general infection-control principles and general hygiene measures.) The following is a summary of the CDC's recommendations.

Body Fluids to Which Universal Precautions Apply

Universal precautions apply to blood and other body fluids containing visible blood. **Blood is the single most important source of HIV, HBV, and other bloodborne pathogens in the health care facility.** Infection control efforts for HIV, HBV, and other bloodborne pathogens must focus on both preventing exposures to blood and delivering HBV immunization. Universal precautions also apply to semen and vaginal secretions, tissues, and the following fluids: cerebrospinal, synovial, pleural, peritoneal, pericardial, and amniotic.

Body Fluids to Which Universal Precautions Do Not Apply

Universal precautions *do not* apply to feces, nasal secretions, sputum, sweat, tears, urine, and vomitus unless they contain visible blood. The risk of transmission of HIV or HBV from these fluids is extremely low or nonexistent.

General Precautions

- Use universal precautions for **all** patients.
- Use appropriate barrier precautions routinely when contact with blood or other body fluids of any patient is anticipated.
  Wear gloves when touching blood and body fluids, mucous membranes, or nonintact skin; when handling items or surfaces soiled with blood or body fluids; and when performing venipuncture and other vascular access procedures.
  Change gloves after each contact with patients.
  Wear masks and protective eyewear or face shields during procedures that are likely to generate drops of blood or other body fluids to prevent exposure of mucous membranes of mouth, nose, and eyes.
  Wear gowns or aprons during procedures that are likely to generate splashes of blood or other body fluids.
- Wash hands and other skin surfaces immediately and thoroughly if contaminated with blood or other body fluids.
- Wash hands immediately after gloves are removed.
- Take precautions to prevent injuries caused by needles, scalpels, and other sharp instruments or devices during procedures; when cleaning used instruments; during disposal of used needles; and when handling sharp instruments after procedures.

Discard needle units uncapped and unbroken after use.
Place disposable syringes and needles, scalpel blades, and other sharp items in puncture-resistant containers.
Place puncture-resistant containers as near as practical to the area of use.
- Although saliva has not been implicated, to minimize the need for emergency mouth-to-mouth resuscitation, make mouthpieces, resuscitation bags, or other ventilation devices available for use in areas where the need for resuscitation is predictable.
- If you have exudative lesions or weeping dermatitis refrain from all direct patient care and from handling patient care equipment until the condition resolves.

Precautions for Invasive Procedures

- If you participate in invasive procedures, use appropriate barrier methods: gloves, surgical masks, protective eyewear, face shields, gowns, and aprons.
- If you perform or assist in vaginal or cesarean deliveries, wear gloves and gowns when handling the placenta or the infant until blood and amniotic fluid have been removed from the infant's skin and during postdelivery care of the umbilical cord.
- If a glove is torn or a needlestick or other injury occurs, remove the gloves and use a new glove as promptly as patient safety permits; remove the needle or instrument used in the incident from the sterile field.

Environmental Considerations

- Standard sterilization and disinfection procedures currently recommended for use in health care settings are adequate.
- Sterile instruments or devices that enter sterile tissue or the vascular system before reuse.
- Clean and remove soiled surfaces on walls, floors, and other surfaces routinely; extraordinary attempts to disinfect or sterilize are not necessary.
- Use chemical germicides approved as hospital disinfectants (and tuberculocidals) to decontaminate spills of blood and other body fluids.

Precautions with Soiled Linen

- Observe hygienic and common-sense storage and processing of clean and soiled linens.
- Handle soiled linen as little as possible and with minimum agitation.
- Bag all soiled linen at the location where it is used.
- Place and transport linen soiled with blood or body fluids in bags that prevent leakage.

Infective Waste

- It is practical to identify those wastes with the potential for causing infection during handling and disposal and for which some special precautions seem prudent (e.g., microbiology laboratory waste, pathology waste, and blood specimens or blood products).
- Incinerate or autoclave infective waste before disposal in a sanitary landfill.
- Carefully pour bulk blood, suctioned fluids, excretions, and secretions down a drain connected to a sanitary sewer.

From Guidelines for Prevention of Transmission of Human Immunodeficiency Virus and Hepatitis B Virus to Health-Care and Public-Safety Workers. U.S. Department of Health and Human Services, Centers for Disease Control, Atlanta, GA, February 1989; Update: Universal Precautions for Prevention of Transmission of Human Immunodeficiency Virus, Hepatitis B Virus, and Other Bloodborne Pathogens in Health-Care Settings. Morbidity and Mortality Weekly Report, 1988; Recommendations for Prevention of HIV Transmission in Health-Care Settings. Morbidity and Mortality Weekly Report, 1987.